Current Approaches in Gene Therapy

Current Approaches in Gene Therapy

Edited by **Harvey Summers**

FOSTER ACADEMICS

New Jersey

Published by Foster Academics,
61 Van Reypen Street,
Jersey City, NJ 07306, USA
www.fosteracademics.com

Current Approaches in Gene Therapy
Edited by Harvey Summers

International Standard Book Number: 978-1-63242-099-2 (Hardback)

Printed in the United States of America.

Contents

Preface

This book intends to present updated reviews of the swiftly rising field of gene therapy. Gene therapy has the capability to be a suitable therapeutic with enhanced specificity and reduced side effects that can offer a cure for several disorders. The book encompasses a broad spectrum of topics including methodologies of gene delivery and recognition of targets in cancer gene therapy. The ultimate aim is to achieve the complete benefit of such an innovative approach for the treatment of several diseases, including cancer, by educating the readers regarding the true nature and potential of gene therapy.

This book is the end result of constructive efforts and intensive research done by experts in this field. The aim of this book is to enlighten the readers with recent information in this area of research. The information provided in this profound book would serve as a valuable reference to students and researchers in this field.

At the end, I would like to thank all the authors for devoting their precious time and providing their valuable contribution to this book. I would also like to express my gratitude to my fellow colleagues who encouraged me throughout the process.

Editor

Section 1

Approaches to Gene Therapy

Chapter 1

Targeted Gene Delivery: Importance of Administration Routes

Shintaro Fumoto, Shigeru Kawakami,
Mitsuru Hashida and Koyo Nishida

Additional information is available at the end of the chapter

1. Introduction

Gene therapy is a promising approach to treat intractable and refractory diseases at the genetic level. Basically, in gene therapy, target gene expression is induced by delivering foreign genes. Downregulation of target gene expression or gene silencing can also be performed using miRNA, siRNA or shRNA expression vectors [1]. Gene therapy is useful for both genetic and acquired diseases. For genetic diseases, the first clinical trial was performed for adenosine deaminase deficiency in 1990 [2]. Subsequently, numerous clinical trials were carried out for other congenital genetic defects such as familial hypercholesterolemia and cystic fibrosis [3]. Gene therapy clinical trials were also performed for acquired diseases such as cancers, cardiovascular diseases and infectious diseases [3].

There are two strategies to perform gene therapy, that is, *ex vivo* methods and *in vivo* methods. In *ex vivo* gene transfer, once cells are taken from a patient, *in vitro* gene transfer is performed, and then transfected cells are introduced into the patient. Since *ex vivo* gene transfer requires a cell culture facility, the procedure is cumbersome. On the other hand, *in vivo* gene transfer is performed by directly administering genetic medicine into the patient. When foreign genes are administered into systemic circulation as a naked form, they are rapidly taken up by the reticuloendothelial system and degraded by nuclease in the blood [4]; thus, foreign genes themselves are generally inactive in gene transfer. As such, to achieve *in vivo* gene transfer, both viral and non-viral vectors have been utilized. In both cases, the selectivity of transgene expression in target organs/sites/cells would determine the therapeutic outcome. Uncontrolled transgene expression in non-target organs/sites/cells is problematic due to high biological activities of transgene products. Furthermore, undesirable biodistribution of vectors leads to their loss and vector-dependent side effects. Thus, gene delivery systems that are targeted to specific organs/sites/cells are important for not only efficacy but also safety.

2. Overview of targeted gene delivery

There are several strategies to achieve targeted gene delivery. Among them, modification with a ligand for specific receptors on target cells is a rational approach. Viral vectors natively utilize specific receptors. For example, adenoviral vector serotype 5 utilizes coxsackievirus and adenovirus receptor (CAR) and integrin, which are abundant on mouse hepatocytes [5, 6]. On the other hand, the receptor for adenoviral vector serotype 35 is CD34, which is expressed on human hematopoietic stem cells [7]. As another good example, sugar modification of vectors is useful. Galactosylation of vectors is useful for targeting to hepatocytes via asialoglycoprotein receptors [8], whereas mannosylation is useful for targeting to macrophages [9]. Furthermore, antibodies against cell surface proteins are also a useful tool for targeting. Antibody against transferrin receptors is utilized for targeting to the brain [10, 11].

Activation of vectors by target cell-specific enzymes is also a rational strategy. In most tumor cells, protein kinase Cα (PKCα) is hyper-activated. A cationic polymer having a peptide substrate of PKCα is specifically phosphorylated in tumor cells; subsequently, the polymer is detached from DNA and transgene expression is turned on [12]. As a similar strategy, a polymer having HIV proteinase-cleavable cationic residues has been developed [13].

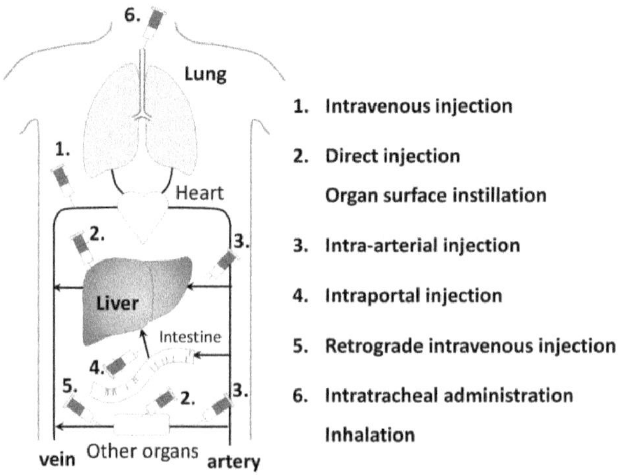

Figure 1. Scheme of administration routes for targeted gene delivery.

To regulate transgene expression in target cells, a tissue-selective promoter can be utilized. For example, albumin promoter and human α1-antitrypsin promoter selectively work in liver hepatocytes [14]. Tumor-selective promoters such as AFP promoter [15] and CAE promoter [16] are useful to improve tumor-selective transgene expression.

Selection of administration routes is a simple and useful way to control the *in vivo* fate of both viral and non-viral vectors. Selection of administration routes can be combined with other strategies. Depending on the administration routes, accessibilities of vectors to target organs/sites/cells vary significantly. Thus, selection of administration routes is important.

3. Administration routes

Figure 1 shows a schematic representation of administration routes for targeted gene delivery. When target cells are distributed throughout the body, various administration routes can be chosen. Antigen-presenting cells such as macrophages and dendritic cells are good examples. Factors affecting transgene expression, such as interaction with blood components and retention time, are different in each administration route. In addition, transfected cell types are dependent on administration routes. When target cells have polarity, secretion polarity of transgene products is subject to the route of transfection, that is, apical or basal route. Thus, we should cautiously select administration routes in accordance with the purpose. We explain the characteristics of each administration route below.

3.1. Oral route

The oral route is one of the most attractive and challenging routes. Non-invasive administration could be theoretically achieved by the oral route. The potential for daily intake of genetic medicine is also one of the merits of oral administration. Cells in the gastrointestinal tract are transfected via oral routes. Using foreign genes encoding secretion proteins, the transgene products can be secreted into systemic circulation. However, the epithelial barrier, acidic pH in the stomach and digestive fluids are major obstacles for gene transfer via the oral route.

The *in vivo* stability of a recombinant adeno-associated virus (rAAV) type 2 vector could be improved by gastric acid neutralization with sodium bicarbonate and protease inhibition with aprotinin [17]. Despite these changes, the transduction efficiency after oral administration of this vector remained low. We also failed to detect transgene expression after intragastric injection of plasmid DNA in mice [18]. To overcome these obstacles, microparticles and nanoparticles are a promising approach. Chitosan-DNA microparticles could protect the encapsulated plasmid DNA from nuclease degradation [19]. In *in vivo* animal studies, a blue color was observed upon X-gal staining of histological stomach and small intestine sections after oral administration of chitosan-DNA microparticles. Furthermore, chitosan nanoparticles using quaternized chitosan (60% trimethylated chitosan) that were given via a gastric feeding tube exhibited green fluorescent protein expression in the mucosa of the stomach, duodenum, jejunum, ileum and large intestine [20]. Bhavsar and Amiji developed a hybrid system dubbed the nanoparticles-in-microsphere oral system (NiMOS), which consists of gelatin nanoparticles containing plasmid DNA and a poly(epsilon-caprolactone) outer shell [21]. NiMOS resided in the stomach and small intestine for longer than gelatin nanoparticles alone.

In the case of DNA vaccines, transfection into only a subset of antigen-presenting cells may be sufficient for the vaccination to exhibit its required effect. The feasibility of DNA vaccination via the oral route may be high since one or a few administrations is theoretically enough to maintain immunity. In fact, oral DNA vaccines against Mycobacterium tuberculosis using liposome [22] and attenuated Salmonella vector [23] were developed and elicited immune responses.

3.2. Intravenous route

Various targeted gene delivery systems via the intravenous route have been developed worldwide. By intravenous administration, various organs and cells can be targeted. However, undesirable and broad biodistribution of vectors can easily lead to side effects.

Adenoviral vectors have liver tropism after intravenous injection [24]. If the target is not the liver, it is necessary to reduce hepatic transgene expression. Fiber-shaft exchange from adenovirus serotype 5 to serotype 35 in combination with both CAR- and αv integrin-binding ablation by mutation reduced liver tropism [25]. Such mutation may be suitable for retargeting from the liver to other organs/tissues. Capsid engineering of adenoviral fibers from serotype 19p based on phage display technology is useful for targeting to the kidney [26]. On the other hand, when cationic liposome/plasmid DNA complex (lipoplex) was injected intravenously, transgene expression mainly occurred in the lung [27]. Galactosylation of the lipoplex reduced transgene expression in the lung after intravenous injection, while it maintained transgene expression in the liver; however, it remained unselective to the liver [28]. In contrast, we successfully delivered foreign genes to the liver Kupffer cells via the intravenous route by mannosylation of the lipoplex [9].

Innate and adaptive immune responses caused by vector administration are problematic. Recombinant adenoviral vectors induce the production of neutralizing antibodies by single administration [29]. Moreover, neutralizing antibodies to human adenovirus serotype 5 have a prevalence of 60% in Europe [30, 31], 35–70% in North America [32, 33] and 75–100% in Asia [34]; thus, many patients already have neutralizing antibodies before administration of recombinant adenoviral vectors. Neutralizing antibodies also induce complement activation upon administration of recombinant adenoviruses [35]. In addition, an alternative pathway is also activated by recombinant adenoviruses [36]. Neutrophils recognize opsonized adenoviral vectors [37]. These immune responses can cause adverse side effects. In fact, administration of recombinant adenoviral vectors causes liver damage and elevates c-reactive protein in cynomolgus monkey [38]. Moreover, human mortality upon the administration of recombinant adenoviral vectors was reported [39]. On the other hand, non-viral vectors also induce immune responses. Plasmid DNA generally contains an immunostimulatory CpG motif, which is recognized by Toll-like receptor 9 [40, 41]. Lipoplex containing plasmid DNA causes the production of inflammatory cytokines and subsequent liver damage [42, 43]. Immunostimulatory CpG motifs in plasmid DNA also inhibit transgene expression by lipoplex [44]. In addition, dexamethasone treatment was found to improve transgene expression by lipoplex [44]. Here, immunostimulatory CpG motifs can be depleted from plasmid DNA. As expected, depletion of immunostimulatory CpG motifs from plasmid DNA improves the safety and transgene expression over a long period [45].

When using the intravenous route, it should be considered that interaction with blood components can affect transfection using viral and non-viral vectors. A low level of neutralizing antibodies against adenovirus inhibits CAR-dependent transfection, whereas neutralized adenoviral vector can transfect Fcγ receptor-positive cells [46]. However, this Fcγ receptor-mediated delivery of adenoviral vectors can induce liver inflammation [37, 47]. Binding of coagulation factor X to adenoviral vector serotype 5 determines liver and spleen tropism via heparan sulfate proteoglycan [48-50]. On the other hand, the lipoplex interacts with various blood components due to its cationic nature. Interaction of the lipoplex with serum inhibits *in vitro* transfection, but the inhibitory effect of serum can be overcome by increasing the charge ratio, which is the molar ratio of cationic residues of lipids to anionic residues of DNA [51]. The inhibitory effect of serum on transfection can also be overcome by increasing the lipoplex particle size [52-54]. The lipoplex interacts with complement proteins after intravenous administration in mice; however, the lipofection efficiency and biodistribution of the lipoplex did not change when complement proteins were depleted from mice [55]. Interaction of the lipoplex with plasma lipoproteins decreased transfection efficiency [56, 57]. In contrast, interaction of the lipoplex with erythrocytes greatly inhibited *in vivo* transfection, whereas interaction with serum did not [58, 59]. The lipoplex also induced hemagglutination upon an increase in the charge ratio [60]. Thus, it is necessary to control interaction with blood components for successful and safe *in vivo* transfection using lipoplex. To prevent hemagglutination, coating of cationic carriers with anionic polymers such as γ-polyglutamic acid [61, 62] and chondroitin sulfate [63, 64] is a useful strategy.

Physicochemical properties such as surface charge and particle size of vectors affect *in vivo* transfection, as mentioned above. The size of lipoplex is dependent on the charge ratio and can determine pulmonary transfection efficiency after intravenous injection [65]. In addition, neutral lipids, so-called 'helper lipids', are also important for *in vivo* transfection using lipoplex. While incorporation of DOPE to liposomes is effective in cell culture, incorporation of cholesterol to liposomes enhances pulmonary transfection efficiency [66]. The combination of mannosylated cationic cholesterol derivative with DOPE exhibited superior *in vivo* disposition and transgene expression in the liver than that with DOPC [67]. Incorporation of N-lauroylsarcosine into cationic liposomes in addition to cholesterol inhibited hemagglutination observed in the case of incorporation of DOPE, and increased the pulmonary transfection efficiency [68].

3.3. Local administration

For transfection into a specific organ/tissue/site, local administration is a useful strategy. Local administration can be categorized into the following two routes: vasculature route and non-vasculature route.

Administration routes	Target organs/tissues	Vectors	References
ia	Liver	Naked plasmid DNA	[69]
ia	Pancreas	Adenoviral vector	[70]
ia	Hind limb	Naked plasmid DNA	[71]
ia	Cecum	AAV	[72]
ia	Brain tumor	Adenoviral vector and lipoplex	[73]
ip	Liver	Lipoplex	[28]
riv	Kidney	Naked plasmid DNA	[74]

Abbreviations: ia, intra-arterial; ip, intraportal; riv, retrograde intravenous

Table 1. Administration routes for targeted gene delivery to specific organs/tissues

3.3.1. Vasculature route

Intra-arterial, intraportal and retrograde intravenous routes have been investigated for transfection into a specific target organ. Table 1 summarizes the administration routes and tested target organs.

We developed galactosylated cationic lipoplex targeted to the liver parenchymal cells [8, 28]. Liver-selective transgene expression was observed after intraportal injection of the galactosylated lipoplex, whereas transgene expression was ineffective and non-selective to the liver after intravenous injection [9]. We also developed galactosylated polyethylenimine (PEI)/plasmid DNA complex (polyplex) and analyzed the molecular weight dependence of PEI [75]. For targeted delivery to the liver parenchymal cells, penetration through fenestrated endothelium is one of the major obstacles. We analyzed the intrahepatic disposition characteristics of galactosylated lipoplex [76] and galactosylated PEI polyplex [77]. While galactosylation of carriers was useful to deliver plasmid DNA to the liver, it was proposed that reduction of the particle size of lipoplex would further improve parenchymal cell selectivity by enhancing the penetration through fenestrated endothelium. Here, larger lipoplex exhibited superior transfection efficiency; however, liver parenchymal cell selectivity was low in large lipoplex [78]. In terms of the particle size of lipoplex and polyplex, the composition of the solution is important. Particle sizes of lipoplex and polyplex in non-ionic solution are smaller than those in ionic solution [79, 80]. In the case of siRNA, the particle size of lipoplex is relatively small; using such lipoplexes, several reported studies succeeded in delivering siRNA to hepatocytes *in vivo* [81, 82].

In terms of interaction of the lipoplex with serum, we reported that transgene expression in the liver after intraportal injection of galactosylated lipoplex was increased by pre-incubation of the lipoplex with serum [83]. This enhancement of transgene expression in the liver was also observed in conventional lipoplex [84]. Multiple components in serum including calcium ion, aggregation-inhibiting components, fibronectin and complement component C3 were responsible for increased transgene expression in the liver [84].

Target organs/tissues	Vectors	References
Skeletal muscle	Naked plasmid DNA	[85]
Heart	Naked plasmid DNA	[86]
Heart	AAV	[87]
Liver	Naked plasmid DNA	[88]
Kidney	Lentiviral vector	[89]
Spleen	Naked plasmid DNA	[90]
Stomach	Naked plasmid DNA	[91]
Thymus	Adenoviral vector and others	[92]
Tumor	Naked plasmid DNA	[93]
Tumor	Naked plasmid DNA and lipoplex	[94, 95]

Table 2. Direct injection for targeted gene delivery to specific organs/tissues

3.3.2. Non-vasculature route

Direct injection to the target organ such as the liver or spleen has been investigated (Table 2). By direct injection to the target organ, the use of naked plasmid DNA without carrier systems is sufficient to detect transgene expression. However, in general, transgene expression is limited to the injection site. To overcome a limited transfection area, electroporation after intramuscular injection of plasmid DNA increased the number of transfected myofibers [96].

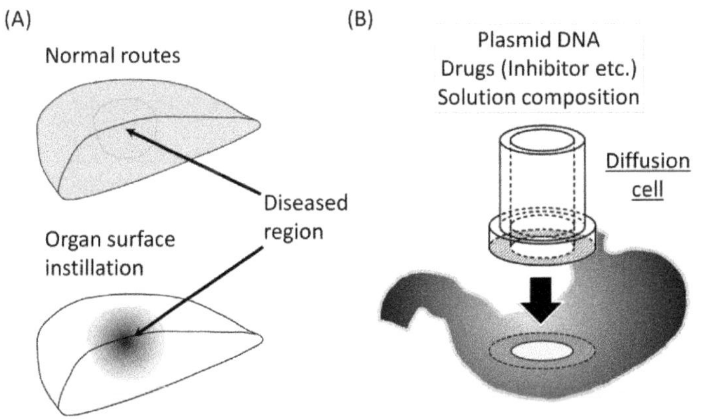

Figure 2. Scheme of organ surface instillation. Panel (A) represents the proposed drug distribution after systemic administration and organ surface instillation of drugs. Panel (B) represents attachment of a glass-made cylindrical diffusion cell onto the organ surface.

For other routes of gene transfer, retrograde intrabiliary injection of naked plasmid DNA, polyethylenimine-plasmid DNA complex and chitosan-plasmid DNA complex resulted in transgene expression in the liver [97]. Intranasal administrations of adenoviral vector [98], lipoplex and polyplex [99] were also tested. In addition, inhalation of chitosan/plasmid DNA nanoparticles resulted in pulmonary transgene expression [100]. Intracerebroventricular administration of lentiviral vector was utilized to deliver foreign genes to the brain [101]. Gene gun bombardment of plasmid DNA with gold particles resulted in efficient gene transfer to the skin [102]. After intraperitoneal injection of adenoviral vector, not only mesothelium but also parenchymal cells of the liver were transduced [103]. This non-specific biodistribution was overcome by ablation of native CAR and integrin receptor binding [103].

3.4. Organ surface route

We developed a novel route for targeted gene delivery to intra-abdominal and intra-thoracic organs, namely, the organ surface route (Fig. 2A). When diseases are limited to a certain region, the organ surface route enables us to target the diseased region, while drugs are distributed to the whole organ via the normal route. Naked plasmid DNA was utilized to transfect target organs/sites. As a first report of this approach, the liver was targeted and successfully transfected in mice [104]. Selectivity of transgene expression in the applied liver lobe was high. Laparotomy was performed in the first reported study, but it is not essential since catheter-based administration through the abdominal wall is available [105]. This catheter-based administration is essential to the safety of liver surface instillation of plasmid DNA [106].

We developed an experimental system using a glass-made cylindrical diffusion cell attached to the organ surface (Fig. 2B) [107]. Using this experimental system, we can precisely limit the area of drug application. Specific transgene expression in the applied area of the liver was achieved [108]. The effect of solution composition on naked plasmid DNA transfer was also examined [109]. Use of hypotonic solution enhanced the transfection efficiency in the applied site of the liver. As for the mechanism of transfection, we analyzed endocytic routes for naked plasmid DNA transfer *in vivo*. While the lipoplex and polyplex are taken up via clathrin- and caveolae-mediated endocytosis [110-113], macropinocytosis is essential for naked plasmid DNA uptake in mesothelial cells in mice [114].

As for other organs, unilateral kidney [115], unilateral lung [116], spleen [117] and stomach surface [118, 119] were transfected with naked plasmid DNA in mice. To improve organ selectivity, microinstillation of naked plasmid DNA onto the stomach was performed [18]. Since specific transgene expression in the stomach was observed in rats [120], organ size would be an important factor for target selectivity of gene transfer. Moreover, specific transgene expression in the applied liver lobe was also achieved in mice by controlling instillation speed using an infusion pump [121].

3.5. Comparison of administration routes

We summarize the advantages and disadvantages of each administration route for targeted gene delivery in Table 3.

Administration routes	Advantages	Disadvantages
Oral	Ease of administration, Frequent dosing (daily intake)	Barriers (epithelium, digestive fluids), Low selectivity
Intravenous	Frequent dosing, Vast distribution	Non-specificity
Intra-arterial, Intraportal, Retrograde intravenous	Selective delivery	Necessity of cannulation
Direct injection	Effective gene transfer, High selectivity	Physical force against the organ, Limited region, Limited frequency of dosing
Intraperitoneal	Effective gene transfer	Low selectivity
Organ surface	Effective gene transfer, High selectivity	Necessity of laparoscopy

Table 3. Advantages and disadvantages of vector transfer routes.

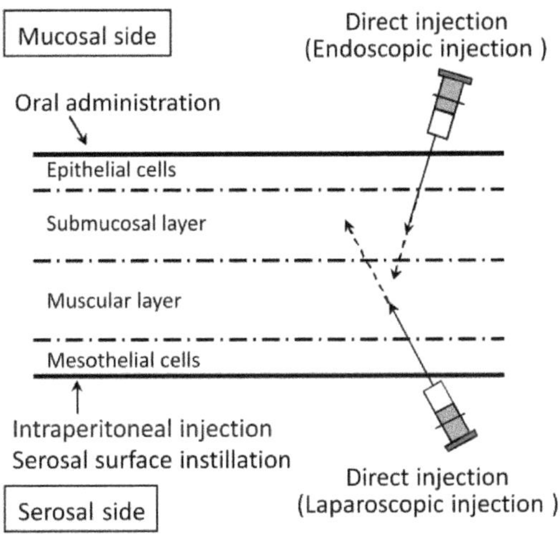

Figure 3. Scheme of administration routes for targeted delivery of foreign genes to the stomach

Direct injection of rAAV vector to the liver exhibited faster and stronger transgene expression than intravenous and intraportal injections of rAAV vector [122]. Similar results were obtained for direct injection of the lipoplex into localized intrahepatic tumors [123]. Moreover, direct intrahepatic injection of adenoviral vector reduced inflammation and increased transgene expression in comparison with intravenous injection [124]. On the other hand, retrograde infusion of lentiviral vector into the ureter, injection into the renal vein or artery, and direct injection into the renal parenchyma were compared [89]. Parenchymal or ureteral administration appeared to be more efficient than other routes of administration.

Figure 3 depicts the administration routes for targeted gene delivery to the stomach. Via the oral route, there are many barriers such as digestive fluids and acidic pH that hamper effective gene transfer. Although effective gene transfer can be achieved by direct injection, it is necessary to consider tissue damage. In contrast, safe and effective gene transfer is possible by serosal surface instillation of naked plasmid DNA. Although transgene expression is limited to the surface layer in the case of serosal surface instillation, limited vertical distribution of transgene products can be overcome by the use of the secretory form of proteins [121].

4. Improving methods for targeted gene delivery

Various strategies have been tested to improve targeted gene delivery. Methods for improved targeted gene delivery can be categorized as physical approaches and chemical approaches.

Physical forces such as electroporation, sonoporation and mechanical massage have been employed to improve targeted gene delivery. Naked plasmid DNA can be delivered to the liver by intravenous injection with electroporation [125, 126]. Intravenous injection of naked plasmid DNA with tissue electroporation resulted in significant transgene expression in the liver, spleen and kidney, but not in the skin or muscle [127].

Utilization of microbubbles with ultrasound exposure can deliver naked plasmid DNA to the muscle [128, 129], liver [130] and lung [131]. Use of PEGylated liposomal bubbles containing perfluoropropane with ultrasound exposure was also effective to deliver naked plasmid DNA via the femoral artery [132]. Mannosylated lipoplex and liposomal bubbles with ultrasound exposure can transfect the liver and spleen [133]. In addition, mannosylated PEGylated bubble lipoplexes selectively transfected antigen-presenting cells *in vivo* [134]. DNA vaccination by this type of lipoplex with ultrasound exposure resulted in suppression of melanoma growth and metastasis [135]. The timing of ultrasound exposure was important [136]. As a mechanism of high transgene expression, a transcriptional process activated by ultrasound exposure was involved [137].

Hydrodynamics-based transfection, with rapid large volume injection of naked plasmid DNA via the intravascular route, is an efficient method to transfect the liver [138, 139]. It was also reported that pig liver can be transfected by retrograde hydrodynamic injection of plasmid DNA via an isolated segment of the inferior vena cava [140]. In terms of the mechanism of high efficiency of gene transfer in hydrodynamics-based transfection, both the generation of transient pores [141, 142] and a transcriptional process activated by hydrodynamic injection [143, 144] are important.

Naked plasmid DNA was also intravenously delivered to the liver by mechanical massage of the liver [145]. Pressure-mediated deliveries of naked plasmid DNA to the kidney [146], liver and spleen [147] were also achieved. As the mechanism of high transgene expression, a transcriptional process activated by pressure to the tissue was involved [148].

Chemical modification of gene carriers has also been investigated. PEGylation of carriers improves blood circulation of the carrier and tumor accumulation by the enhanced permeability and retention effects [149]. However, transfection efficiencies of PEGylated vectors are generally low. Although PEGylation of lipoplex reduced retention in the lung and heart, PEGylated lipoplex failed to deliver foreign gene into tumors [150]. PEGylation of adenoviral vectors generally prevents CAR recognition. Hexon-specific PEGylation of adenoviral vector improved *in vitro* transfection efficiency in the presence of neutralizing antibodies, *in vivo* blood retention and tumor accumulation after intravenous administration; however, transfection efficiency in tumor remained low [151]. To overcome this dilemma of PEGylation, that is, high retention and low uptake, cleavable PEG-lipids have been developed. PEG-lipids, which were designed to exhibit cleavage of the PEG moiety by tumor-specific matrix metalloproteinase, were incorporated into a multifunctional envelope-type nano-device [152]. As a result, transgene expression in the tumor was stimulated after intravenous injection of this carrier in comparison with that with normal PEGylated gene carrier.

It was reported that incorporation of human serum albumin to lipoplex enhanced the transfection efficiency *in vitro* and *in vivo* [153]. Moreover, utilization of serum components such as asialofetuin [154], transferrin [155] and fibronectin [156] was tested for the development of vectors.

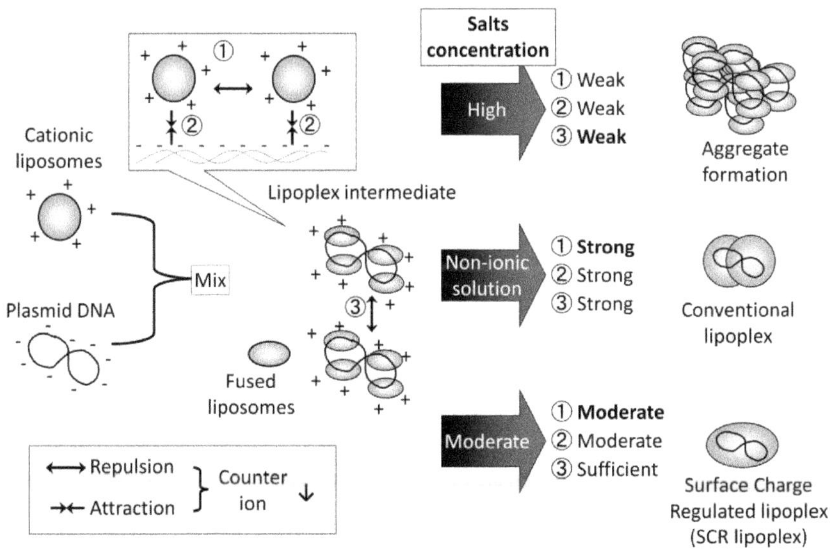

Figure 4. Schematic representation of surface charge-regulated lipoplex.

Intravenous sequential injection of cationic liposome and plasmid DNA resulted in significant pulmonary transgene expression with reduced inflammatory cytokine production compared with those with the lipoplex [157]. Sequential injection resulted in lower DNA uptake by the liver and higher DNA levels in the lung than with the lipoplex administration [158]. Interaction with several serum proteins including albumin reduced inflammatory cytokine production by sequential complex (liposome mixed with serum proteins before mixing with plasmid DNA), whereas interaction of the lipoplex with serum proteins did not reduce inflammatory cytokine production by lipoplex [159].

We successfully developed surface charge-regulated (SCR) lipoplex, which improved targeted gene delivery by stabilizing the lipoplex. Figure 4 shows a scheme of the salt-dependent formation of lipoplex. For *in vivo* preparation of the lipoplex, the concentrations of plasmid DNA and liposomes are high; consequently, a physiological concentration of salts induces aggregation of the lipoplex. This problem can be overcome using a non-ionic solution such as 5% glucose solution. Here, we hypothesized that repulsion between cationic liposomes was too strong to induce sufficient fusion of lipid membranes for stable lipoplex formation. Moderate concentration of salts in the solution of the lipoplex would reduce repulsion among cationic liposomes and enhance fusion of lipid membranes, while maintaining sufficient repulsion among lipoplex particles. This hypothesis was proved by a series of physicochemical experiments including fluorescent resonance energy transfer assessments and measurements of particle size changes in the presence of physiological concentration of salts [160]. This stable galactosylated SCR lipoplex exhibited superior hepatocyte-selective gene transfer than conventional lipoplex after intraportal injection [160]. Furthermore, the stabilization effect of SCR lipoplex was also evident in pulmonary gene transfer after intravenous injection [161].

As for the organ surface instillation method, we succeeded in enhancing the transfection efficiency of naked plasmid DNA by several strategies. Pretreatment with epidermal growth factor (EGF) enhanced transgene expression and increased transgene-positive cells on the stomach after instillation of naked plasmid DNA onto it [162]. Rubbing the gastric serosal surface with a medical spoon after instillation of naked plasmid DNA onto the stomach was more effective than EGF pretreatment [163]. However, rubbing the organ surface with a medical spoon may be impractical for future clinical application. Thus, we searched for various materials to reproduce the effect of rubbing an organ's surface. Among them, concomitant use of calcium carbonate suspension with naked plasmid DNA was similarly effective as rubbing the gastric serosal surface [164]. Unfortunately, sedimentation of calcium carbonate suspension occurs rapidly and is problematic. To obtain slowly settling particles of calcium carbonate, we tested various conditions for calcium carbonate synthesis. We succeeded in synthesizing a novel form of calcium carbonate with a flower-like shape, named calcium carbonate microflowers [164]. Sedimentation of calcium carbonate microflowers was sufficiently slow to perform *in vivo* experiments. Fortunately, the suspension of calcium carbonate microflowers containing naked plasmid DNA was a more effective transfection reagent than commercially available calcium carbonate, especially at a low concentration of calcium carbonate. Intraperitoneal injection of the suspension of calcium carbonate microflowers containing naked plasmid DNA resulted in effective and peritoneal cavity-selective gene transfer. However, the mechanism of effective *in vivo* transfection remains to be elucidated.

5. Disease-dependent strategies in targeted gene delivery

Among the above-mentioned methods, intramuscular injection of naked plasmid is one of the simplest methods since it can be applied without surgery and carriers. Not only muscular diseases, such as dystrophy, but also systemic diseases may be cured using the secretory form of proteins. Intramuscular injection of plasmid DNA encoding hepatocyte growth factor rescued critical limb ischemia with high safety in a phase I/IIa clinical trial [165]. Muscular delivery of naked plasmid DNA encoding erythropoietin resulted in an increase of hematocrits [166]. In general, however, targeted gene delivery to specific organs/sites/cells is required since high biological activities of proteins may lead to side effects. For example, in suicide gene therapy to treat tumors, thymidine kinase gene expression should be restricted to tumor cells [167]. Since hepatocyte growth factor is mitogenic, liver-directed gene transfer is a rational approach to treat liver cirrhosis [168]. To treat inherited gene deficiency diseases such as familial hypercholesterolemia (LDL receptor deficiency in hepatocytes) [169] and Crigler-Najjar syndrome (uridine diphospho-glucuronosyl transferase 1A1 deficiency in hepatocytes) [170], targeted gene delivery is also reasonable due to its efficacy.

As for DNA vaccination, Kasinrerk et al. compared intramuscular, intraperitoneal, intravenous and intrasplenic immunizations with a single dose of naked plasmid DNA and observed that only the intrasplenic route induced specific antibody production [171]. In contrast, to develop DNA vaccine to induce cellular immunity, intradermal injection of naked plasmid DNA with electroporation was better than intrasplenic injection, even though there was high transfection efficiency in the spleen [172]. Gene gun bombardments of naked plasmid DNA to the skin were not effective to induce cellular immunity in comparison with intracutaneous injections of antigen-transduced dendritic cells [102]. Gene gun bombardments of naked plasmid DNA to the skin induced Th2 response and anaphylactic shock upon antigen recall [173]. On the other hand, transgene expression of fusion proteins of the immunodominant domain of human type XVII collagen and dendritic cell-specific antibody targeted to dendritic cells in the skin induced tolerance to human type XVII collagen in a skin transplantation model [174]. Intraperitoneal injection of mannosylated lipoplex resulted in efficient transgene expression in antigen-presenting cells and induced cellular immunity [175, 176]. As for the intravenous route, mannosylated lipoplex initiated a Th1 response [177]. As mentioned above, mannosylated PEGylated bubble lipoplexes with ultrasound exposure more effectively and selectively transfected antigen-presenting cells than an approach without ultrasound exposure after intravenous injection, and induced strong cellular immunity [134, 135]. Thus, the success or failure of DNA vaccination is dependent on transfection methods including transfection routes.

6. Conclusions

Selection of administration routes is important in targeted gene delivery for not only efficacy but also safety of the vector. Administration routes can be categorized as systemic routes and local routes. Via the systemic routes, administration is simple and does not require a complicated operation. However, very wide distribution of the vectors after their systemic administration may lead to systemic side effects. This problem can be overcome by changing the administration route from a systemic route to a local route. In addition, target selectivity can be improved by modification of the vectors with a ligand, combination with targeted application of physical forces and utilization of tissue-specific promoters. Importantly, selection of administration routes can be combined with these strategies to improve targeted gene delivery. The importance of selection of administration routes is dependent on the kind of target disease. Taking safety including germline conservativeness into consideration, further improvement of targeted gene delivery systems should be pursued.

Acknowledgements

This work was supported in part by a Grant-in-Aid for Scientific Research from the Ministry of Education, Culture, Sports, Science and Technology, Japan.

Author details

Shintaro Fumoto[1], Shigeru Kawakami[2], Mitsuru Hashida[2,3] and Koyo Nishida[1]

1 Graduate School of Biomedical Sciences, Nagasaki University, Japan

2 Graduate School of Pharmaceutical Sciences, Kyoto University, Japan

3 Institute for Integrated Cell-Material Sciences (iCeMS), Kyoto University, Japan

References

[1] Boudreau RL, Davidson BL. Generation of hairpin-based RNAi vectors for biological and therapeutic application. *Methods in Enzymology* 2012;507 275-296.

[2] Blaese RM, Culver KW, Miller AD, Carter CS, Fleisher T, Clerici M, Shearer G, Chang L, Chiang Y, Tolstoshev P, Greenblatt JJ, Rosenberg SA, Klein H, Berger M, Mullen CA, Ramsey WJ, Muul L, Morgan RA, Anderson WF. T lymphocyte-directed gene therapy for ADA- SCID: initial trial results after 4 years. *Science* 1995;270(5235) 475-480.

[3] Edelstein ML, Abedi MR, Wixon J. Gene therapy clinical trials worldwide to 2007--an update. *Journal of Gene Medicine* 2007;9(10) 833-842.

[4] Kawabata K, Takakura Y, Hashida M. The fate of plasmid DNA after intravenous injection in mice: involvement of scavenger receptors in its hepatic uptake. *Pharmaceutical Research* 1995;12(6) 825-830.

[5] Wickham TJ, Mathias P, Cheresh DA, Nemerow GR. Integrins αv β3 and αvβ5 promote adenovirus internalization but not virus attachment. *Cell* 1993;73(2) 309-319.

[6] Tomko RP, Xu R, Philipson L. HCAR and MCAR: the human and mouse cellular receptors for subgroup C adenoviruses and group B coxsackieviruses. *Proceedings of the National Academy of Science of the United States of America* 1997;94(7) 3352-3356.

[7] Sakurai F, Mizuguchi H, Hayakawa T. Efficient gene transfer into human CD34+ cells by an adenovirus type 35 vector. *Gene Therapy* 2003;10(12) 1041-1048.

[8] Kawakami S, Yamashita F, Nishikawa M, Takakura Y, Hashida M. Asialoglycoprotein receptor-mediated gene transfer using novel galactosylated cationic liposomes. *Biochemical and Biophysical Research Communications* 1998;252(1) 78-83.

[9] Kawakami S, Sato A, Nishikawa M, Yamashita F, Hashida M. Mannose receptor-mediated gene transfer into macrophages using novel mannosylated cationic liposomes. *Gene Therapy* 2000;7(4) 292-299.

[10] Shi N, Pardridge WM. Noninvasive gene targeting to the brain. *Proceedings of the National Academy of Science of the United States of America* 2000;97(13) 7567-7572.

[11] Shi N, Zhang Y, Zhu C, Boado RJ, Pardridge WM. Brain-specific expression of an exogenous gene after i.v. administration. *Proceedings of the National Academy of Science of the United States of America* 2001;98(22) 12754-12759.

[12] Toita R, Kang JH, Kim JH, Tomiyama T, Mori T, Niidome T, Jun B, Katayama Y. Protein kinase Cα-specific peptide substrate graft-type copolymer for cancer cell-specific gene regulation systems. *Journal of Controlled Release* 2009;139(2) 133-139.

[13] Asai D, Kuramoto M, Shoji Y, Kang JH, Kodama KB, Kawamura K, Mori T, Miyoshi H, Niidome T, Nakashima H, Katayama Y. Specific transgene expression in HIV-infected cells using protease-cleavable transcription regulator. *Journal of Controlled Release* 2010;141(1) 52-61.

[14] Jacobs F, Snoeys J, Feng Y, Van Craeyveld E, Lievens J, Armentano D, Cheng SH, De Geest B. Direct comparison of hepatocyte-specific expression cassettes following adenoviral and nonviral hydrodynamic gene transfer. *Gene Therapy* 2008;15(8) 594-603.

[15] Dai M, Liu J, Chen DE, Rao Y, Tang ZJ, Ho WZ, Dong CY. Tumor-targeted gene therapy using Adv-AFP-HRPC/IAA prodrug system suppresses growth of hepatoma xenografted in mice. *Cancer Gene Therapy* 2012;19(2) 77-83.

[16] Liu T, Zhang G, Chen YH, Chen Y, Liu X, Peng J, Xu MH, Yuan JW. Tissue specific expression of suicide genes delivered by nanoparticles inhibits gastric carcinoma growth. *Cancer Biology and Therapy* 2006;5(12) 1683-1690.

[17] Shao G, Greathouse K, Huang Q, Wang CM, Sferra TJ. Gene transfer to the gastrointestinal tract after peroral administration of recombinant adeno-associated virus type 2 vectors. *Journal of Pediatric Gastroenterology and Nutrition* 2006;43(2) 168-179.

[18] Nishi J, Fumoto S, Ishii H, Kodama Y, Nakashima M, Sasaki H, Nakamura J, Nishida K. Improved stomach selectivity of gene expression following microinstillation of plasmid DNA onto the gastric serosal surface in mice. *European Journal of Pharmaceutics and Biopharmaceutics* 2008;69(2) 633-639.

[19] Guliyeva Ü, Öner F, Özsoy Ş, Haziroğlu R. Chitosan microparticles containing plasmid DNA as potential oral gene delivery system. *European Journal of Pharmaceutics and Biopharmaceutics* 2006;62(1) 17-25.

[20] Zheng F, Shi XW, Yang GF, Gong LL, Yuan HY, Cui YJ, Wang Y, Du YM, Li Y. Chitosan nanoparticle as gene therapy vector via gastrointestinal mucosa administration: results of an in vitro and in vivo study. *Life Sciences* 2007;80(4) 388-396.

[21] Bhavsar MD, Amiji MM. Gastrointestinal distribution and in vivo gene transfection studies with nanoparticles-in-microsphere oral system (NiMOS). *Journal of Controlled Release* 2007;119(3) 339-348.

[22] Wang D, Xu J, Feng Y, Liu Y, Mchenga SS, Shan F, Sasaki J, Lu C. Liposomal oral DNA vaccine (mycobacterium DNA) elicits immune response. *Vaccine* 2010;28(18) 3134-3142.

[23] Wang QL, Pan Q, Ma Y, Wang K, Sun P, Liu S, Zhang XL. An attenuated Salmonella-vectored vaccine elicits protective immunity against Mycobacterium tuberculosis. *Vaccine* 2009;27(48) 6712-6722.

[24] Honigman A, Zeira E, Ohana P, Abramovitz R, Tavor E, Bar I, Zilberman Y, Rabinovsky R, Gazit D, Joseph A, Panet A, Shai E, Palmon A, Laster M, Galun E. Imaging transgene expression in live animals. *Molecular Therapy* 2001;4(3) 239-249.

[25] Koizumi N, Mizuguchi H, Sakurai F, Yamaguchi T, Watanabe Y, Hayakawa T. Reduction of natural adenovirus tropism to mouse liver by fiber-shaft exchange in combination with both CAR- and αv integrin-binding ablation. *Journal of Virology* 2003;77(24) 13062-13072.

[26] Denby L, Work LM, Seggern DJ, Wu E, McVey JH, Nicklin SA, Baker AH. Development of renal-targeted vectors through combined in vivo phage display and capsid engineering of adenoviral fibers from serotype 19p. *Molecular Therapy* 2007;15(9) 1647-1654.

[27] Liu F, Qi H, Huang L, Liu D. Factors controlling the efficiency of cationic lipid-mediated transfection in vivo via intravenous administration. *Gene Therapy* 1997;4(6) 517-523.

[28] Kawakami S, Fumoto S, Nishikawa M, Yamashita F, Hashida M. In vivo gene delivery to the liver using novel galactosylated cationic liposomes. *Pharmaceutical Research* 2000;17(3) 306-313.

[29] Gahéry-Ségard H, Juillard V, Gaston J, Lengagne R, Pavirani A, Boulanger P, Guillet JG. Humoral immune response to the capsid components of recombinant adenoviruses: routes of immunization modulate virus-induced Ig subclass shifts. *European Journal of Immunology* 1997;27(3) 653-659.

[30] Kostense S, Koudstaal W, Sprangers M, Weverling GJ, Penders G, Helmus N, Vogels R, Bakker M, Berkhout B, Havenga M, Goudsmit J. Adenovirus types 5 and 35 seroprevalence in AIDS risk groups supports type 35 as a vaccine vector. *AIDS* 2004;18(8) 1213–1216.

[31] Mast TC, Kierstead L, Gupta SB, Nikas AA, Kallas EG, Novitsky V, Mbewe B, Pitisuttithum P, Schechter M, Vardas E, Wolfe ND, Aste-Amezaga M, Casimiro DR, Coplan P, Straus WL, Shiver JW. International epidemiology of human pre-existing adenovirus (Ad) type-5, type-6, type-26 and type-36 neutralizing antibodies: correlates of high Ad5 titers and implications for potential HIV vaccine trials. *Vaccine* 2010;28(4). pp. 950–957.

[32] Nwanegbo E, Vardas E, Gao W, Whittle H, Sun H, Rowe D, Robbins PD, Gambotto A. Prevalence of neutralizing antibodies to adenoviral serotypes 5 and 35 in the adult populations of The Gambia, South Africa, and the United States. *Clinical and Diagnostic Laboratory Immunology* 2004;11(2) 351–357.

[33] Sumida SM, Truitt DM, Lemckert AA, Vogels R, Custers JH, Addo MM, Lockman S, Peter T, Peyerl FW, Kishko MG, Jackson SS, Gorgone DA, Lifton MA, Essex M, Walker BD, Goudsmit J, Havenga MJ, Barouch DH. Neutralizing antibodies to adenovirus serotype 5 vaccine vectors are directed primarily against the adenovirus hexon protein. *Journal of Immunology* 2005;174(11) 7179–7185.

[34] Pilankatta R, Chawla T, Khanna N, Swaminathan S. The prevalence of antibodies to adenovirus serotype 5 in an adult Indian population and implications for adenovirus vector vaccines. *Journal of Medical Virology* 2010;82(3) 407–414.

[35] Cichon G, Boeckh-Herwig S, Schmidt HH, Wehnes E, Müller T, Pring-Akerblom P, Burger R. Complement activation by recombinant adenoviruses. *Gene Therapy* 2001;8(23) 1794-800.

[36] Jiang H, Wang Z, Serra D, Frank MM, Amalfitano A. Recombinant adenovirus vectors activate the alternative complement pathway, leading to the binding of human complement protein C3 independent of anti-ad antibodies. *Molecular Therapy* 2004;10(6) 1140-1142.

[37] Cotter MJ, Zaiss AK, Muruve DA. Neutrophils interact with adenovirus vectors via Fc receptors and complement receptor 1. *Journal of Virology* 2005;79(23) 14622-14631.

[38] Sakurai F, Nakamura S, Akitomo K, Shibata H, Terao K, Kawabata K, Hayakawa T, Mizuguchi H. Transduction properties of adenovirus serotype 35 vectors after intravenous administration into nonhuman primates. *Molecular Therapy* 2008;16(4) 726-733.

[39] Marshall E. Gene therapy death prompts review of adenovirus vector. *Science* 1999;286(5448) 2244-2245.

[40] Hemmi H, Takeuchi O, Kawai T, Kaisho T, Sato S, Sanjo H, Matsumoto M, Hoshino K, Wagner H, Takeda K, Akira S. A Toll-like receptor recognizes bacterial DNA. *Nature* 2000;408(6813) 740-745.

[41] Cornélie S, Hoebeke J, Schacht AM, Bertin B, Vicogne J, Capron M, Riveau G. Direct evidence that toll-like receptor 9 (TLR9) functionally binds plasmid DNA by specific cytosine-phosphate-guanine motif recognition. *Journal of Biological Chemistry* 2004;279(15) 15124-15129.

[42] Loisel S, Le Gall C, Doucet L, Ferec C, Floch V. Contribution of plasmid DNA to hepatotoxicity after systemic administration of lipoplexes. *Human Gene Therapy* 2001;12(6) 685-696.

[43] Ito Y., Kawakami S, Charoensit P, Higuchi Y, Hashida M. Evaluation of proinflammatory cytokine production and liver injury induced by plasmid DNA/cationic liposome complexes with various mixing ratios in mice. *European Journal of Pharmaceutics and Biopharmaceutics* 2009;71(2) 303-309.

[44] Tan Y, Li S, Pitt BR, Huang L. The inhibitory role of CpG immunostimulatory motifs in cationic lipid vector-mediated transgene expression in vivo. *Human Gene Therapy* 1999;10(13) 2153-2161.

[45] Yew NS, Zhao H, Przybylska M, Wu IH, Tousignant JD, Scheule RK, Cheng SH. CpG-depleted plasmid DNA vectors with enhanced safety and long-term gene expression in vivo. *Molecular Therapy* 2002;5(6) 731-738.

[46] Leopold PL, Wendland RL, Vincent T, Crystal RG. Neutralized adenovirus-immune complexes can mediate effective gene transfer via an Fc receptor-dependent infection pathway. *Journal of Virology* 2006;80(20) 10237-10247.

[47] Muruve DA, Barnes MJ, Stillman IE, Libermann TA. Adenoviral gene therapy leads to rapid induction of multiple chemokines and acute neutrophil-dependent hepatic injury in vivo. *Human Gene Therapy* 1999;10(6) 965-976.

[48] Bradshaw AC, Parker AL, Duffy MR, Coughlan L, van Rooijen N, Kähäri VM, Nicklin SA, Baker AH. Requirements for receptor engagement during infection by adenovirus complexed with blood coagulation factor X. *PLoS Pathogens* 2010;6(10), e1001142.

[49] Zaiss AK, Lawrence R, Elashoff D, Esko JD, Herschman HR. Differential effects of murine and human factor X on adenovirus transduction via cell-surface heparan sulfate. *Journal of Biological Chemistry* 2011;286(28) 24535-24543.

[50] Corjon S, Gonzalez G, Henning P, Grichine A, Lindholm L, Boulanger P, Fender P, Hong SS. Cell entry and trafficking of human adenovirus bound to blood factor X is

determined by the fiber serotype and not hexon:heparan sulfate interaction. *PLoS One* 2011;6(5), e18205.

[51] Yang JP, Huang L. Overcoming the inhibitory effect of serum on lipofection by increasing the charge ratio of cationic liposome to DNA. *Gene Therapy* 1997;4(9) 950-960.

[52] Ross PC, Hui SW. Lipoplex size is a major determinant of in vitro lipofection efficiency. *Gene Therapy* 1999;6(4) 651-659.

[53] Turek J, Dubertret C, Jaslin G, Antonakis K, Scherman D, Pitard B. Formulations which increase the size of lipoplexes prevent serum-associated inhibition of transfection. *Journal of Gene Medicine* 2000;2(1) 32-40.

[54] Almofti MR, Harashima H, Shinohara Y, Almofti A, Li W, Kiwada H. Lipoplex size determines lipofection efficiency with or without serum. *Molecular Membrane Biology* 2003;20(1) 35-43.

[55] Barron LG, Meyer KB, Szoka FC Jr. Effects of complement depletion on the pharmacokinetics and gene delivery mediated by cationic lipid-DNA complexes. *Human Gene Therapy* 1998;9(3) 315-323.

[56] Tandia BM, Vandenbranden M, Wattiez R, Lakhdar Z, Ruysschaert JM, Elouahabi A. Identification of human plasma proteins that bind to cationic lipid/DNA complex and analysis of their effects on transfection efficiency: implications for intravenous gene transfer. *Molecular Therapy* 2003;8(2) 264-273.

[57] Tandia BM, Lonez C, Vandenbranden M, Ruysschaert JM, Elouahabi A. Lipid mixing between lipoplexes and plasma lipoproteins is a major barrier for intravenous transfection mediated by cationic lipids. *Journal of Biological Chemistry* 2005;280(13) 12255-12261.

[58] Sakurai F, Nishioka T, Saito H, Baba T, Okuda A, Matsumoto O, Taga T, Yamashita F, Takakura Y, Hashida M. Interaction between DNA-cationic liposome complexes and erythrocytes is an important factor in systemic gene transfer via the intravenous route in mice: the role of the neutral helper lipid. *Gene Therapy* 2001;8(9) 677-686.

[59] Sakurai F, Nishioka T, Yamashita F, Takakura Y, Hashida M. Effects of erythrocytes and serum proteins on lung accumulation of lipoplexes containing cholesterol or DOPE as a helper lipid in the single-pass rat lung perfusion system. *European Journal of Pharmaceutics and Biopharmaceutics* 2001;52(2) 165-172.

[60] Eliyahu H, Servel N, Domb AJ, Barenholz Y. Lipoplex-induced hemagglutination: potential involvement in intravenous gene delivery. *Gene Therapy* 2002;9(13) 850-858.

[61] Kurosaki T, Kitahara T, Fumoto S, Nishida K, Nakamura J, Niidome T, Kodama Y, Nakagawa H, To H, Sasaki H. Ternary complexes of pDNA, polyethylenimine, and γ-polyglutamic acid for gene delivery systems. *Biomaterials* 2009;30(14) 2846-2853.

[62] Kurosaki T, Kitahara T, Kawakami S, Higuchi Y, Yamaguchi A, Nakagawa H, Kodama Y, Hamamoto T, Hashida M, Sasaki H. γ-polyglutamic acid-coated vectors for effective and safe gene therapy. *Journal of Controlled Release* 2010;142(3) 404-410

[63] Kurosaki T, Kitahara T, Kawakami S, Nishida K, Nakamura J, Teshima M, Nakagawa H, Kodama Y, To H, Sasaki H. The development of a gene vector electrostatically assembled with a polysaccharide capsule. *Biomaterials* 2009;30(26) 4427-4434.

[64] Kurosaki T, Kitahara T, Fumoto S, Nishida K, Yamamoto K, Nakagawa H, Kodama Y, Higuchi N, Nakamura T, Sasaki H. Chondroitin sulfate capsule system for efficient and secure gene delivery. *Journal of Pharmacy & Pharmaceutical Sciences* 2010;13(3) 351-361.

[65] Templeton NS, Lasic DD, Frederik PM, Strey HH, Roberts DD, Pavlakis GN. Improved DNA: liposome complexes for increased systemic delivery and gene expression. *Nature Biotechnology* 1997;15(7) 647-652.

[66] Liu Y, Mounkes LC, Liggitt HD, Brown CS, Solodin I, Heath TD, Debs RJ. Factors influencing the efficiency of cationic liposome-mediated intravenous gene delivery. *Nature Biotechnology* 1997;15(2) 167-173.

[67] Hattori Y, Suzuki S, Kawakami S, Yamashita F, Hashida M. The role of dioleoylphosphatidylethanolamine (DOPE) in targeted gene delivery with mannosylated cationic liposomes via intravenous route. *Journal of Controlled Release* 2005;108(2-3) 484-495.

[68] Kurosaki T, Kitahara T, Teshima M, Nishida K, Nakamura J, Nakashima M, To H, Hukuchi H, Hamamoto T, Sasaki H. Exploitation of De Novo helper-lipids for effective gene delivery. *Journal of Pharmacy & Pharmaceutical Sciences* 2008;11(4) 56-67.

[69] Kanemura H, Iimuro Y, Takeuchi M, Ueki T, Hirano T, Horiguchi K, Asano Y, Fujimoto J. Hepatocyte growth factor gene transfer with naked plasmid DNA ameliorates dimethylnitrosamine-induced liver fibrosis in rats. *Hepatology Research* 2008;38(9) 930-939.

[70] Tang MM, Zhu QE, Fan WZ, Zhang SL, Li DZ, Liu LZ, Chen M, Zhang M, Zhou J, Wei CJ. Intra-arterial targeted islet-specific expression of Sirt1 protects β cells from streptozotocin-induced apoptosis in mice. *Molecular Therapy* 2011;19(1) 60-66.

[71] Zhang G, Ludtke JJ, Thioudellet C, Kleinpeter P, Antoniou M, Herweijer H, Braun S, Wolff JA. Intraarterial delivery of naked plasmid DNA expressing full-length mouse dystrophin in the mdx mouse model of duchenne muscular dystrophy. *Human Gene Therapy* 2004;15(8) 770-782.

[72] Porvasnik SL, Mah C, Polyak S. Targeting murine small bowel and colon through selective superior mesenteric artery injection. *Microsurgery* 2010;30(6) 487-493

[73] Rainov NG, Ikeda K, Qureshi NH, Grover S, Herrlinger U, Pechan P, Chiocca EA, Breakefield XO, Barnett FH. Intraarterial delivery of adenovirus vectors and liposome-DNA complexes to experimental brain neoplasms. *Human Gene Therapy* 1999;10(2) 311-318.

[74] Maruyama H, Higuchi N, Nishikawa Y, Hirahara H, Iino N, Kameda S, Kawachi H, Yaoita E, Gejyo F, Miyazaki J. Kidney-targeted naked DNA transfer by retrograde renal vein injection in rats. *Human Gene Therapy* 2002;13(3) 455-468.

[75] Morimoto K, Nishikawa M, Kawakami S, Nakano T, Hattori Y, Fumoto S, Yamashita F, Hashida M. Molecular weight-dependent gene transfection activity of unmodified and galactosylated polyethyleneimine on hepatoma cells and mouse liver. *Molecular Therapy* 2003;7(2) 254-261.

[76] Fumoto S, Nakadori F, Kawakami S, Nishikawa M, Yamashita F, Hashida M. Analysis of hepatic disposition of galactosylated cationic liposome/plasmid DNA complexes in perfused rat liver. *Pharmaceutical Research* 2003;20(9) 1452-1459.

[77] Fumoto S, Kawakami S, Ishizuka M, Nishikawa M, Yamashita F, Hashida M. Analysis of hepatic disposition of native and galactosylated polyethylenimine complexed with plasmid DNA in perfused rat liver. *Drug Metabolism and Pharmacokinetics* 2003;18(4) 230-237.

[78] Higuchi Y, Kawakami S, Fumoto S, Yamashita F, Hashida M. Effect of the particle size of galactosylated lipoplex on hepatocyte-selective gene transfection after intraportal administration. *Biological & Pharmaceutical Bulletin* 2006;29(7) 1521-1523.

[79] Li S, Rizzo MA, Bhattacharya S, Huang L. Characterization of cationic lipid-protamine-DNA (LPD) complexes for intravenous gene delivery. *Gene Therapy* 1998;5(7) 930-937.

[80] Goula D, Remy JS, Erbacher P, Wasowicz M, Levi G, Abdallah B, Demeneix BA. Size, diffusibility and transfection performance of linear PEI/DNA complexes in the mouse central nervous system. *Gene Therapy* 1998;5(5) 712-717.

[81] Sato A, Takagi M, Shimamoto A, Kawakami S, Hashida M. Small interfering RNA delivery to the liver by intravenous administration of galactosylated cationic liposomes in mice. *Biomaterials* 2007;28(7) 1434-1442.

[82] Semple SC, Akinc A, Chen J, Sandhu AP, Mui BL, Cho CK, Sah DW, Stebbing D, Crosley EJ, Yaworski E, Hafez IM, Dorkin JR, Qin J, Lam K, Rajeev KG, Wong KF, Jeffs LB, Nechev L, Eisenhardt ML, Jayaraman M, Kazem M, Maier MA, Srinivasulu M, Weinstein MJ, Chen Q, Alvarez R, Barros SA, De S, Klimuk SK, Borland T, Kosovrasti V, Cantley WL, Tam YK, Manoharan M, Ciufolini MA, Tracy MA, de Fougerolles A, MacLachlan I, Cullis PR, Madden TD, Hope MJ. Rational design of cationic lipids for siRNA delivery. *Nature Biotechnology* 2010;28(2) 172-176.

[83] Fumoto S, Kawakami S, Shigeta K, Higuchi Y, Yamashita F, Hashida M. Interaction with blood components plays a crucial role in asialoglycoprotein receptor-mediated in vivo gene transfer by galactosylated lipoplex. *Journal of Pharmacology and Experimental Therapeutics* 2005;315(2) 484-493.

[84] Yoshikawa N, Sakamoto K, Mizuno S, Sakaguchi J, Miyamoto H, Mine T, Sasaki H, Fumoto S, Nishida K. Multiple components in serum contribute to hepatic transgene expression by lipoplex in mice. *Journal of Gene Medicine* 2011;13(11) 632-643.

[85] Wolff JA, Malone RW, Williams P, Chong W, Acsadi G, Jani A, Felgner PL. Direct gene transfer into mouse muscle in vivo. *Science* 1990;247(4949 Pt. 1) 1465-1468.

[86] Li K, Welikson RE, Vikstrom KL, Leinwand LA. Direct gene transfer into the mouse heart. *Journal of Molecular and Cellular Cardiology* 1997;29(5) 1499-1504.

[87] Su H, Lu R, Kan YW. Adeno-associated viral vector-mediated vascular endothelial growth factor gene transfer induces neovascular formation in ischemic heart. *Proceedings of the National Academy of Science of the United States of America* 2000;97(25) 13801-13806.

[88] Hickman MA, Malone RW, Lehmann-Bruinsma K, Sih TR, Knoell D, Szoka FC, Walzem R, Carlson DM, Powell JS. Gene expression following direct injection of DNA into liver. *Human Gene Therapy* 1994;5(12) 1477-1483.

[89] Gusella GL, Fedorova E, Hanss B, Marras D, Klotman ME, Klotman PE. Lentiviral gene transduction of kidney. *Human Gene Therapy* 2002;13(3) 407-414.

[90] White SA, LoBuglio AF, Arani RB, Pike MJ, Moore SE, Barlow DL, Conry RM. Induction of anti-tumor immunity by intrasplenic administration of a carcinoembryonic antigen DNA vaccine. *Journal of Gene Medicine* 2000;2(2) 135-140.

[91] Takehara T, Hayashi N, Yamamoto M, Miyamoto Y, Fusamoto H, Kamada T. In vivo gene transfer and expression in rat stomach by submucosal injection of plasmid DNA. *Human Gene Therapy* 1996;7(5) 589-593.

[92] DeMatteo RP, Raper SE, Ahn M, Fisher KJ, Burke C, Radu A, Widera G, Claytor BR, Barker CF, Markmann JF. Gene transfer to the thymus. A means of abrogating the immune response to recombinant adenovirus. *Annals of Surgery* 1995;222(3) 229-239.

[93] Yang JP, Huang L. Direct gene transfer to mouse melanoma by intratumor injection of free DNA. *Gene Therapy* 1996;3(6) 542-548.

[94] Nomura T, Nakajima S, Kawabata K, Yamashita F, Takakura Y, Hashida M. Intratumoral pharmacokinetics and in vivo gene expression of naked plasmid DNA and its cationic liposome complexes after direct gene transfer. *Cancer Research* 1997;57(13) 2681-2686.

[95] Nomura T, Yasuda K, Yamada T, Okamoto S, Mahato RI, Watanabe Y, Takakura Y, Hashida M. Gene expression and antitumor effects following direct interferon (IFN)-gamma gene transfer with naked plasmid DNA and DC-chol liposome complexes in mice. *Gene Therapy* 1999;6(1) 121-129.

[96] Mathiesen I. Electropermeabilization of skeletal muscle enhances gene transfer in vivo. *Gene Therapy* 1999;6(4) 508-514.

[97] Dai H, Jiang X, Leong KW, Mao HQ. Transient depletion of kupffer cells leads to enhanced transgene expression in rat liver following retrograde intrabiliary infusion of plasmid DNA and DNA nanoparticles. *Human Gene Therapy* 2011;22(7) 873-878.

[98] Gau P, Rodriguez S, De Leonardis C, Chen P, Lin DM. Air-assisted intranasal instillation enhances adenoviral delivery to the olfactory epithelium and respiratory tract. *Gene Therapy* 2011;18(5) 432-436.

[99] Eliyahu H, Joseph A, Schillemans JP, Azzam T, Domb AJ, Barenholz Y. Characterization and in vivo performance of dextran-spermine polyplexes and DOTAP/cholesterol lipoplexes administered locally and systemically. *Biomaterials* 2007;28(14) 2339-2349.

[100] Mohri K, Okuda T, Mori A, Danjo K, Okamoto H. Optimized pulmonary gene transfection in mice by spray-freeze dried powder inhalation. *Journal of Controlled Release* 2010;144(2) 221-226.

[101] Deroose CM, Reumers V, Gijsbers R, Bormans G, Debyser Z, Mortelmans L, Baekelandt V. Noninvasive monitoring of long-term lentiviral vector-mediated gene expression in rodent brain with bioluminescence imaging. *Molecular Therapy* 2006;14(3) 423-431.

[102] Gaffal E, Schweichel D, Tormo D, Steitz J, Lenz J, Basner-Tschakarjan E, Limmer A, Tüting T. Comparative evaluation of CD8+CTL responses following gene gun immunization targeting the skin with intracutaneous injection of antigen-transduced dendritic cells. *European Journal of Cell Biology* 2007;86(11-12) 817-26.

[103] Akiyama M, Thorne S, Kirn D, Roelvink PW, Einfeld DA, King CR, Wickham TJ. Ablating CAR and integrin binding in adenovirus vectors reduces nontarget organ transduction and permits sustained bloodstream persistence following intraperitoneal administration. *Molecular Therapy* 2004;9(2) 218-230.

[104] Kawakami S, Hirayama R, Shoji K, Kawanami R, Nishida K, Nakashima M, Sasaki H, Sakaeda T, Nakamura J. Liver- and lobe-selective gene transfection following the instillation of plasmid DNA to the liver surface in mice. *Biochemical and Biophysical Research Communications* 2002;294(1) 46-50.

[105] Hirayama R, Kawakami S, Nishida K, Nakashima M, Sasaki H, Sakeda T, Nakamura J. Development of the liver- and lobe-selective nonviral gene transfer following the instillation of naked plasmid DNA using catheter on the liver surface in mice. *Pharmaceutical Research* 2003;20(2) 328-332.

[106] Fumoto S, Furukawa H, Nakamura J, Nishida K. Safety of liver surface instillation of plasmid DNA in normal and carbon tetrachloride-induced hepatitis mice. *Journal of Pharmacy & Pharmaceutical Sciences* 2011;14(2) 274-282.

[107] Nishida K, Sato N, Sasaki H, Nakamura J. Absorption of organic anions as model drugs following application to rat liver surface in-vivo. *Journal of Pharmacy and Pharmacology* 1994;46(11) 867-870.

[108] Hirayama R, Nishida K, Fumoto S, Nakashima M, Sasaki H, Nakamura J. Liver site-specific gene transfer following the administration of naked plasmid DNA to the liver surface in mice. *Biological & Pharmaceutical Bulletin* 2004;27(10) 1697-1699.

[109] Hirayama R, Fumoto S, Nishida K, Nakashima M, Sasaki H, Nakamura J. Effect of solution composition of plasmid DNA on gene transfection following liver surface administration in mice. *Biological & Pharmaceutical Bulletin* 2005;28(11) 2166-2169.

[110] Zuhorn IS, Kalicharan R, Hoekstra D. Lipoplex-mediated transfection of mammalian cells occurs through the cholesterol-dependent clathrin-mediated pathway of endocytosis. *Journal of Biological Chemistry* 2002;277(20) 18021-18028.

[111] Rejman J, Bragonzi A, Conese M. Role of clathrin- and caveolae-mediated endocytosis in gene transfer mediated by lipo- and polyplexes. *Molecular Therapy* 2005;12(3) 468-474.

[112] Rejman J, Conese M, Hoekstra D. Gene transfer by means of lipo- and polyplexes: role of clathrin and caveolae-mediated endocytosis. *Journal of Liposome Research* 2006;16(3) 237-247.

[113] von Gersdorff K, Sanders NN, Vandenbroucke R, De Smedt SC, Wagner E, Ogris M. The internalization route resulting in successful gene expression depends on both cell line and polyethylenimine polyplex type. *Molecular Therapy* 2006;14(5) 745-753.

[114] Fumoto S, Nishi J, Ishii H, Wang X, Miyamoto H, Yoshikawa N, Nakashima M, Nakamura J, Nishida K. Rac-mediated macropinocytosis is a critical route for naked plasmid DNA transfer in mice. *Molecular Pharmaceutics* 2009;6(4) 1170-1179.

[115] Hirayama R, Nishida K, Fumoto S, Nakashima M, Sasaki H, Nakamura J. Unilateral kidney-selective gene transfer following the administration of naked plasmid DNA to the kidney surface in mice. *Biological & Pharmaceutical Bulletin* 2005;28(1) 181-184.

[116] Nakamura J, Fumoto S, Ariyoshi K, Kodama Y, Nishi J, Nakashima M, Sasaki H, Nishida K. Unilateral lung-selective gene transfer following the administration of naked plasmid DNA onto the pulmonary pleural surface in mice. *Biological & Pharmaceutical Bulletin* 2007;30(4) 729-732.

[117] Nakamura J, Fumoto S, Kawanami R, Kodama Y, Nishi J, Nakashima M, Sasaki H, Nishida K. Spleen-selective gene transfer following the administration of naked plasmid DNA onto the spleen surface in mice. *Biological & Pharmaceutical Bulletin* 2007;30(5) 941-945.

[118] Nakamur, J, Fumoto S, Shoji K, Kodama Y, Nishi J, Nakashima M, Sasaki H, Nishida K. Stomach-selective gene transfer following the administration of naked plasmid DNA onto the gastric serosal surface in mice. *Biological & Pharmaceutical Bulletin* 2006;29(10) 2082-2086.

[119] Fumoto S, Nishi J, Nakamura J, Nishida K. Gene therapy for gastric diseases. *Current Gene Therapy* 2008;8(3) 187-200.

[120] Nishi J, Fumoto S, Ishii H, Kodama Y, Nakashima M, Sasaki H, Nakamura J, Nishida K. Highly stomach-selective gene transfer following gastric serosal surface instillation of naked plasmid DNA in rats. *Journal of Gastroenterology* 2008;43(12) 912-919.

[121] Fumoto S, Tsuchimochi M, Nishi J, Ishii H, Kodama Y, Nakashima M, Sasaki H, Nakamura J, Nishida K. Liver- and lobe-specific gene transfer following the continuous

microinstillation of Plasmid DNA onto the liver surface in mice: effect of instillation speed. *Biological & Pharmaceutical Bulletin* 2009;32(7) 1298-302.

[122] Berraondo P, Crettaz J, Ochoa L, Pañeda A, Prieto J, Trocóniz IF, González-Aseguinolaza G. Intrahepatic injection of recombinant adeno-associated virus serotype 2 overcomes gender-related differences in liver transduction. *Human Gene Therapy* 2006;17(6) 601-610.

[123] Mohr L, Yoon SK, Eastman SJ, Chu Q, Scheule RK, Scaglioni PP, Geissler M, Heintges T, Blum HE, Wands JR. Cationic liposome-mediated gene delivery to the liver and to hepatocellular carcinomas in mice. *Human Gene Therapy* 2001;12(7) 799-809.

[124] Crettaz J, Berraondo P, Mauleón I, Ochoa-Callejero L, Shankar V, Barajas M, van Rooijen N, Kochanek S, Qian C, Prieto J, Hernández-Alcoceba R, González-Aseguinolaza G. Intrahepatic injection of adenovirus reduces inflammation and increases gene transfer and therapeutic effect in mice. *Hepatology* 2006;44(3) 623-632.

[125] Liu F, Huang L. Electric gene transfer to the liver following systemic administration of plasmid DNA. *Gene Therapy* 2002;9(16) 1116-1169.

[126] Sakai M, Nishikawa M, Thanaketpaisarn O, Yamashita F, Hashida M.. Hepatocyte-targeted gene transfer by combination of vascularly delivered plasmid DNA and in vivo electroporation. *Gene Therapy* 2005;12(7) 607-616.

[127] Thanaketpaisarn O, Nishikawa M, Yamashita F, Hashida M. Tissue-specific characteristics of in vivo electric gene: transfer by tissue and intravenous injection of plasmid DNA. *Pharmaceutical Research* 2005;22(6) 883-891.

[128] Taniyama Y, Tachibana K, Hiraoka K, Aoki M, Yamamoto S, Matsumoto K, Nakamura T, Ogihara T, Kaneda Y, Morishita R. Development of safe and efficient novel nonviral gene transfer using ultrasound: enhancement of transfection efficiency of naked plasmid DNA in skeletal muscle. *Gene Therapy* 2002;9(6) 372-380.

[129] Lu QL, Liang HD, Partridge T, Blomley MJ. Microbubble ultrasound improves the efficiency of gene transduction in skeletal muscle in vivo with reduced tissue damage. *Gene Therapy* 2003;10(5) 396-405.

[130] Shen ZP, Brayman AA, Chen L, Miao CH. Ultrasound with microbubbles enhances gene expression of plasmid DNA in the liver via intraportal delivery. *Gene Therapy* 2008;15(16) 1147-1155.

[131] Xenariou S, Griesenbach U, Liang HD, Zhu J, Farley R, Somerton L, Singh C, Jeffery PK, Ferrari S, Scheule RK, Cheng SH, Geddes DM, Blomley M, Alton EW. Use of ultrasound to enhance nonviral lung gene transfer in vivo. *Gene Therapy* 2007;14(9) 768-774.

[132] Suzuki R, Takizawa T, Negishi Y, Hagisawa K, Tanaka K, Sawamura K, Utoguchi N, Nishioka T, Maruyama K. Gene delivery by combination of novel liposomal bubbles with perfluoropropane and ultrasound. *Journal of Controlled Release* 2007;117(1) 130-136.

[133] Un K, Kawakami S, Suzuki R, Maruyama K, Yamashita F, Hashida M. Enhanced transfection efficiency into macrophages and dendritic cells by a combination method using mannosylated lipoplexes and bubble liposomes with ultrasound exposure. *Human Gene Therapy* 2010;21(1) 65-74.

[134] Un K, Kawakami S, Suzuki R, Maruyama K, Yamashita F, Hashida M. Development of an ultrasound-responsive and mannose-modified gene carrier for DNA vaccine therapy. *Biomaterials* 2010;31(30) 7813-7826.

[135] Un K, Kawakami S, Suzuki R, Maruyama K, Yamashita F, Hashida M. Suppression of melanoma growth and metastasis by DNA vaccination using an ultrasound-responsive and mannose-modified gene carrier. *Molecular Pharmaceutics* 2011;8(2) 543-554.

[136] Un K, Kawakami S, Yoshida M, Higuchi Y, Suzuki R, Maruyama K, Yamashita F, Hashida M. The elucidation of gene transferring mechanism by ultrasound-responsive unmodified and mannose-modified lipoplexes. *Biomaterials* 2011;32(20) 4659-4669.

[137] Un K, Kawakami S, Higuchi Y, Suzuki R, Maruyama K, Yamashita F, Hashida M. Involvement of activated transcriptional process in efficient gene transfection using unmodified and mannose-modified bubble lipoplexes with ultrasound exposure. *Journal of Controlled Release* 2011;156(3) 355-363.

[138] Liu F, Song Y, Liu D. Hydrodynamics-based transfection in animals by systemic administration of plasmid DNA. *Gene Therapy* 1999;6(7) 1258-1266.

[139] Zhang G, Budker V, Wolff JA. High levels of foreign gene expression in hepatocytes after tail vein injections of naked plasmid DNA. *Human Gene Therapy* 1999;10(10) 1735-1737.

[140] Fabre JW, Grehan A, Whitehorne M, Sawyer GJ, Dong X, Salehi S, Eckley L, Zhang X, Seddon M, Shah AM, Davenport M, Rela M. Hydrodynamic gene delivery to the pig liver via an isolated segment of the inferior vena cava. *Gene Therapy* 2008;15(6) 452-462.

[141] Zhang G, Gao X, Song YK, Vollmer R, Stolz DB, Gasiorowski JZ, Dean DA, Liu D. Hydroporation as the mechanism of hydrodynamic delivery. *Gene Therapy* 2004;11(8) 675-682.

[142] Kobayashi N, Nishikawa M, Takakura Y. The hydrodynamics-based procedure for controlling the pharmacokinetics of gene medicines at whole body, organ and cellular levels. *Advanced Drug Delivery Reviews* 2005;57(5) 713-731.

[143] Nishikawa M, Nakayama A, Takahashi Y, Fukuhara Y, Takakura Y. Reactivation of silenced transgene expression in mouse liver by rapid, large-volume injection of isotonic solution. *Human Gene Therapy* 2008;19(10) 1009-1020.

[144] Takiguchi N, Takahashi Y, Nishikawa M, Matsui Y, Fukuhara Y, Oushiki D, Kiyose K, Hanaoka K, Nagano T, Takakura Y. Positive correlation between the generation of reactive oxygen species and activation/reactivation of transgene expression after hydrodynamic injections into mice. *Pharmaceutical Research* 2011;28(4) 702-711.

[145] Liu F, Huang L. Noninvasive gene delivery to the liver by mechanical massage. *Hepatology* 2002;35(6) 1314-1319.

[146] Mukai H, Kawakami S, Hashida M. Renal press-mediated transfection method for plasmid DNA and siRNA to the kidney. *Biochemical and Biophysical Research Communications* 2008;372(3) 383-387.

[147] Mukai H, Kawakami S, Kamiya Y, Ma F, Takahashi H, Satake K, Terao K, Kotera H, Yamashita F, Hashida M. Pressure-mediated transfection of murine spleen and liver. *Human Gene Therapy* 2009;20(10) 1157-1167.

[148] Mukai H, Kawakami S, Takahashi H, Satake K, Yamashita F, Hashida M. Key physiological phenomena governing transgene expression based on tissue pressure-mediated transfection in mice. *Biological & Pharmaceutical Bulletin* 2010;33(9) 1627-1632.

[149] Fang J, Nakamura H, Maeda H. The EPR effect: Unique features of tumor blood vessels for drug delivery, factors involved, and limitations and augmentation of the effect. *Advanced Drug Delivery Reviews* 2011;63(3) 136-151.

[150] Gjetting T, Arildsen NS, Christensen CL, Poulsen TT, Roth JA, Handlos VN, Poulsen HS. In vitro and in vivo effects of polyethylene glycol (PEG)-modified lipid in DOTAP/cholesterol-mediated gene transfection. *International Journal of Nanomedicine* 2010;5 371-383.

[151] Suzuki-Kouyama E, Katayama K, Sakurai F, Yamaguchi T, Kurachi S, Kawabata K, Nakagawa S, Mizuguchi H. Hexon-specific PEGylated adenovirus vectors utilizing avidin-biotin interaction. *Biomaterials* 2011;32(6) 1724-1730.

[152] Hatakeyama H, Akita H, Kogure K, Oishi M, Nagasaki Y, Kihira Y, Ueno M, Kobayashi H, Kikuchi H, Harashima H. Development of a novel systemic gene delivery system for cancer therapy with a tumor-specific cleavable PEG-lipid. *Gene Therapy* 2007;14(1), 68-77.

[153] Simões S, Slepushkin V, Pires P, Gaspar R, Pedroso de Lima MC, Düzgüneş N. Human serum albumin enhances DNA transfection by lipoplexes and confers resistance to inhibition by serum. *Biochimica et Biophysica Acta -Biomembranes* 2000;1463(2) 459-469.

[154] Arangoa MA, Düzgüneş N, Tros de Ilarduya C. Increased receptor-mediated gene delivery to the liver by protamine-enhanced-asialofetuin-lipoplexes. *Gene Therapy* 2003;10(1) 5-14.

[155] Tros de Ilarduya C, Arangoa MA, Moreno-Aliaga MJ, Düzgüneş N. Enhanced gene delivery in vitro and in vivo by improved transferrin-lipoplexes. *Biochimica et Biophysica Acta -Biomembranes* 2002;1561(2) 209-221.

[156] Hattori Y, Maitani Y. DNA/Lipid complex incorporated with fibronectin to cell adhesion enhances transfection efficiency in prostate cancer cells and xenografts. *Biological, Pharmaceutical Bulletin* 2007;30(3) 603-607.

[157] Tan Y, Liu F, Li Z, Li S, Huang L. Sequential injection of cationic liposome and plasmid DNA effectively transfects the lung with minimal inflammatory toxicity. *Molecular Therapy* 2001;3(5, Pt. 1) 673-682.

[158] Zhang JS, Liu F, Conwell CC, Tan Y, Huang L. Mechanistic studies of sequential injection of cationic liposome and plasmid DNA. *Molecular Therapy* 2006;13(2) 429-437.

[159] Conwell CC, Liu F, Huang L. Several serum proteins significantly decrease inflammatory response to lipid-based non-viral vectors. *Molecular Therapy* 2008;16(2) 370-377.

[160] Fumoto S, Kawakami S, Ito Y, Shigeta K, Yamashita F, Hashida M. Enhanced hepatocyte-selective in vivo gene expression by stabilized galactosylated liposome/plasmid DNA complex using sodium chloride for complex formation. *Molecular Therapy* 2004;10(4) 719-729.

[161] Kawakami S, Ito Y, Fumoto S, Yamashita F, Hashida M. Enhanced gene expression in lung by a stabilized lipoplex using sodium chloride for complex formation. *Journal of Gene Medicine* 2005;7(12) 1526-1533.

[162] Miyamoto H, Baba S, Nakajima S, Mine T, Yoshikawa N, Fumoto S, Nishida K. Pretreatment with Epidermal Growth Factor Enhances Naked Plasmid DNA Transfer onto Gastric Serosal Surface in Mice. *Biological and Pharmaceutical Bulletin* 2012;35(6) 903-908.

[163] Mine T, Ishii H, Nakajima S, Yoshikawa N, Miyamoto H, Nakashima M, Nakamura J, Fumoto S, Nishida K. Rubbing gastric serosal surface enhances naked plasmid DNA transfer in rats and mice. *Biological & Pharmaceutical Bulletin* 2011;34(9) 1514-1517.

[164] Fumoto S, Nakajima S, Mine T, Yoshikawa N, Kitahara T, Sasaki H, Miyamoto H, Nishida K. Efficient in Vivo Gene Transfer by Intraperitoneal Injection of Plasmid DNA and Calcium Carbonate Microflowers in Mice. *Molecular Pharmaceutics* 2012;9(7) 1962-1970.

[165] Morishita R, Makino H, Aoki M, Hashiya N, Yamasaki K, Azuma J, Taniyama Y, Sawa Y, KanedaY, Ogihara T. Phase I/IIa clinical trial of therapeutic angiogenesis using hepatocyte growth factor gene transfer to treat critical limb ischemia. *Arteriosclerosis, Thrombosis, and Vascular Biology* 2011;31(3) 713-720.

[166] Tripathy SK, Svensson EC, Black HB, Goldwasser E, Margalith M, Hobart PM, Leiden JM. Long-term expression of erythropoietin in the systemic circulation of mice after intramuscular injection of a plasmid DNA vector. *Proceedings of the National Academy of Science of the United States of America* 1996;93(20) 10876-10880.

[167] Bonini C, Bondanza A, Perna SK, Kaneko S, Traversari C, Ciceri F, Bordignon C. The suicide gene therapy challenge: how to improve a successful gene therapy approach. *Molecular Therapy* 2007;15(7) 1248-1252.

[168] Matsuno Y, Iwata H, Umeda Y, Takagi H, Mori Y, Kosugi A, Matsumoto K, Nakamura, T., Hirose, H. Hepatocyte growth factor gene transfer into the liver via the portal vein using electroporation attenuates rat liver cirrhosis. *Gene Therapy* 2003;10(18) 1559-1566.

[169] Wilson JM, Grossman M, Wu CH, Chowdhury NR, Wu GY, Chowdhury JR. Hepatocyte-directed gene transfer in vivo leads to transient improvement of hypercholesterolemia in low density lipoprotein receptor-deficient rabbits. *Journal of Biological Chemistry* 1992;267(2) 963-967.

[170] Miranda PS, Bosma PJ. Towards liver-directed gene therapy for Crigler-Najjar syndrome. *Current Gene Therapy* 2009;9(2) 72-82.

[171] Kasinrerk W, Moonsom S, Chawansuntati K. Production of antibodies by single DNA immunization: comparison of various immunization routes. *Hybridoma and Hybridomics* 2002;21(4) 287-293.

[172] Guan X, Nishikawa M, Takemoto S, Ohno Y, Yata T, Takakura Y. Injection site-dependent induction of immune response by DNA vaccine: comparison of skin and spleen as a target for vaccination. *Journal of Gene Medicine* 2010;12(3) 301-309.

[173] Alvarez D, Harder G, Fattouh R, Sun J, Goncharova S, Stämpfli MR, Coyle AJ, Bramson JL, Jordana M. Cutaneous antigen priming via gene gun leads to skin-selective Th2 immune-inflammatory responses. *Journal of Immunology* 2005;174(3) 1664-1674.

[174] Ettinger M, Gratz IK, Gruber C, Hauser-Kronberger C, Johnson TS, Mahnke K, Thalhamer J, Hintner H, Peckl-Schmid D, Bauer JW. Targeting of the hNC16A collagen domain to dendritic cells induces tolerance to human type XVII collagen. *Experimental Dermatology* 2012;21(5) 395-398.

[175] Hattori Y, Kawakami S, Lu Y, Nakamura K, Yamashita F, Hashida M. Enhanced DNA vaccine potency by mannosylated lipoplex after intraperitoneal administration. *Journal of Gene Medicine* 2006;8(7) 824-834.

[176] Hattori Y, Kawakami S, Nakamura K, Yamashita F, Hashida M. Efficient gene transfer into macrophages and dendritic cells by in vivo gene delivery with mannosylated lipoplex via the intraperitoneal route. *Journal of Pharmacology and Experimental Therapeutics* 2006;318(2) 828-834.

[177] Hattori Y, Kawakami S, Suzuki S, Yamashita F, Hashida M. Enhancement of immune responses by DNA vaccination through targeted gene delivery using mannosylated cationic liposome formulations following intravenous administration in mice. *Biochemical and Biophysical Research Communications* 2004;317(4) 992-999.

Chapter 2

Solid Lipid Nanoparticles: Tuneable Anti-Cancer Gene/Drug Delivery Systems

Tranum Kaur and Roderick Slavcev

Additional information is available at the end of the chapter

1. Introduction

With the advent of multifunctional nano delivery systems, simultaneous imaging and therapy aspires to detect and treat tumors at a very early stage with promising outcomes. In this context, numerous anti-cancer drug/gene delivery systems have been explored with the primary aim to increase the treatment efficacy without compromising safety. Secondary goals include enhancing bioavailability, specific targeting, apart from the enhanced stability of the formulation [1]. The multifaceted applications of nanoparticles are the direct result of their ability to deliver high pay loads of drugs or biomarkers to the desired sites within the body. Design and development of tumor specific nanoparticles could significantly amplify the delivering capacity to a specific target of interest, without affecting healthy cells [2]. Technological advances in nanomaterials and nanotechnology have paved the way for several carriers such as liposomes [3], dendrimers [4], and micelles [5], solid lipid nanoparticles (SLN) [6] and recently nanostructured lipid carriers [1, 7]. Polymeric micelles, or nanosized (~10–100 nm) supramolecular constructs composed of amphiphilic block-copolymers, are emerging as powerful drug delivery vehicles for hydrophobic drugs. Liposomes are currently the most popular nanosized drug delivery systems, with one or several lipid bilayers enclosing an aqueous core. Liposome-encapsulated formulations of doxorubicin earlier approved for the treatment of Kaposi's sarcoma, are now used against breast cancer and refractory ovarian cancer. Breast cancer in particular has been the focus of many studies involving liposome-based chemotherapeutics, in part due to the clinical success of various drugs such as Doxil, which is a liposomal formulation currently used to treat recurrent breast cancer [7]. The anthracycline doxorubicin is the active cytotoxic agent and is contained within the internal aqueous core of the liposome. The encapsulation of doxorubicin within liposomes significantly reduces the cardiotoxicity that commonly results from the use of unencapsulated anthracyclines by decreasing the amount of the drug being delivered to the heart [7]. As such, patients can receive much higher doses of the chemotherapeutic in the liposomal formulation compared to unencapsulated, thereby allowing tumor tissue to potentially be exposed to a lethal dose of the drug while minimizing deleterious side effects. This inherent advantage associated with the use of liposomes as drug delivery vehicles also serves to minimize the many other toxic side effects associated with doxorubicin including gastrointestinal toxicity and complications arising from myelosuppression.

Each delivery system however, has its advantages and limitations. Advantages afforded for drug delivery include the presence of an inner core for lipophilic drug entrapment, as well as a hydrophilic outer shell that prevents particle aggregation and opsonisation [8]. This complexation prevents uptake by the reticuloendothelial system (RES), thereby improving circulation times which, combined with nanoscale sizing, confers preferential accumulation in tumor tissue. In general, nanovectors can be targeted to tumors by passive and active targeting approaches, where a passive strategy takes advantage of a nanvector's small size permitting it to penetrate and accumulate in the tumor. Most solid tumors are sustained by extensive angiogenesis leading to hypervascular tissue with an incomplete vascular architecture. They also have an impaired lymphatic drainage and an increased production of permeability factors resulting in the accumulation and inefficient clearance of nanoparticles leading to the enhanced permeability and retention effect [9]. The hyperpermeable nature of tumor vasculature is characterized by a pore cut off size ranging between 380 and 780 nm allowing particles less than 780 nm to extravasate into the tumor interstitium [10]. In addition, active targeting to various tissues may be achieved *via* utilization of ligands on the surface of nanoparticles, reducing the side effects to the normal tissue by limiting drug/gene distribution to the target organ [11]. An excellent example is Abraxane, an albumin bound nanoparticle formulation of Paclitaxel (PTX), approved by FDA in January 2005 for the treatment of metastatic breast cancer. Abraxane has been shown to outperform standard PTX in the treatment of breast cancer [12]. Utility of this drug was initially limited due to its poor aqueous solubility [13], requiring use of an excipient, Cremophor, which is satisfied by novel engineered nanovectors. A recent Gynecologic Oncology Group Phase II evaluation of albumin-bound paclitaxel nanoparticles to treat recurrent or persistent platinum-resistant ovarian, fallopian tube, or primary peritoneal cancer, concluded that these nanoparticles are as effective and tolerable in their cohort of refractory ovarian cancer patients previously treated with paclitaxel [14]. Nanoparticles fabricated with albumin [15], poly(lactic-co-glycolic acid) [16] and poly lactic acid have also been loaded with PTX and used to passively target tumors. Albumin has been shown to be nontoxic, non-immunogenic, biocompatible and biodegradable making it an ideal candidate to fabricate nanoparticles for drug delivery. Site-specific drug delivery allows for the clinical translation of chemotherapeutic agents with safer targeted cell killing, that are otherwise abandoned due to insolubility, toxicity and safety concerns. Moreover, these new delivery devices can preferentially confine treatments to tumors within the nodal space while sparing healthy tissues.

2. Solid lipid nanoparticles

Solid lipid nanoparticles [17] or lipospheres are rapidly emerging as new class of safer and efficient gene/drug delivery vectors. SLNs are sub-micron colloidal carriers, ranging from 50 nm to 1 μm, that are composed of physiological lipid dispersed in water or in aqueous surfactant solution (Figure 1). SLNs function as an alternative drug carrier system to other novel delivery approaches such as emulsions, liposomes, and polymeric nanoparticles. SLNs offer several advantages conferred by their colloidal dimensions including: i) feasibility of incorporation of lipophilic and hydrophilic drugs; ii) improved physical stability; iii) controlled release; iv) improved biocompatibility; v) potential for site specific drug delivery; vi) improved drug stability; vii) better formulation stability; viii) the ability to freeze dry and reconstitute; ix) high drug payload; x) controllable particle size; xi) the avoidance of carrier toxicity; xii) low production cost; and xiii) easy scale-up and manufacturing [18]. In addition, significant toxicity and acidity associated with a number of biodegradable polymeric materials are not observed with SLNs. And, in contrast to emulsions and liposomes, the particle matrix of SLNs is composed of solid lipids. SLNs can be prepared using wide variety of lipids including lipid acids, mono- (glycerol monostearate), di- (glycerol bahenate) or triglycerides (tristearin), glyceride mixtures or waxes (e.g. cetyl palmitate) and stabilized by the biocompatible surfactants(s) of choice (non-ionic or ionic). Lipids most commonly used are triglyceride esters of hydrogenated fatty acids, including hydrogenated cottonseed oil (Lubritab™ or Sterotex™), hydrogenated palm oil (Dynasan™ P60 or Softisan™ 154), hydrogenated castor oil (Cutina™ HR), and hydrogenated soybean oil (Sterotex™ HM, or Lipo™) as typical examples [19]. Various emulsifiers and their combination (Pluronic F 68, F 127) have also been added to stabilize the lipid dispersion by more efficiently preventing particle agglomeration.

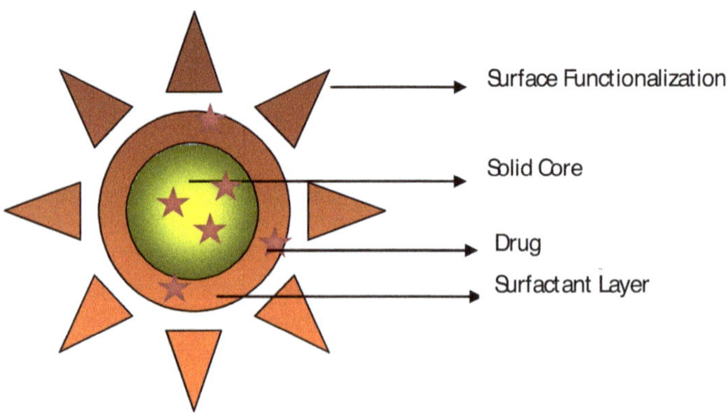

Figure 1. Schematics of Functionalized Solid Lipid Nanoparticles

The disavantages associated with SLNs relate mostly to their preparation, which generally involves high pressure and rapid temperature changes that can lead to high pressure-induced drug degradation, lipid crystallization, gelation phenomena and the co-existence of several colloidal species [20]. The drug loading capacity of a conventional SLN is limited by the solubility of drug in the lipid melt, the structure of the lipid matrix and the polymeric state of the lipid matrix. If the lipid matrix consists of highly similar molecules (i.e. tristearin or tripalmitin), a perfect crystal with few imperfections is formed. Since incorporated drugs are located between fatty acid chains, between the lipid layers and also in crystal imperfections, a highly ordered crystal lattice cannot accommodate large amounts of drug. This may also lead to the fast release of a large dose of drug initially, generally known as "burst effect", followed by slow and incomplete release of drug. Since high lipid crystallinity is the major cause of burst release of drug from SLNs, this undesirable phenomenon may be minimized by choosing lipids that do not form good crystals, including mono- or di-glycerides, or triglycerides with chains of different lengths. For this reason, in formulation design use of more complex lipids is recommended for higher drug loading. Nanostructured lipid carriers or NLCs were designed to overcome these disadvantages with the main goal to increase drug loading and prevent drug expulsion [21]. For NLCs, the highest drug load could be achieved by mixing solid lipids with small amounts of liquid lipids (oils). These types of NLCs are called multiple types NLC, and are analogous to w/o/w emulsions since it is an oil-in-solid lipid-in-water dispersion.

3. SLN preparation methods

There are two main established SLN synthesis techniques, namely, the high-pressure homogenisation technique described by Müller and Lucks [21], and the microemulsion-based technique described by Gasco [22, 23]. SLNs are prepared from lipid, emulsifier and water/solvent using different methods, discussed below.

3.1. High Pressure Homogenization (HPH)

High Pressure Homogenization (HPH) is a very reliable technique in the production of SLNs. High pressure homogenizers are employed to push a liquid with high pressure (100–2000 bar) and the fluid accelerates on a very short distance to very high velocity (>1000 Km/h).. Very high shear stress and cavitation forces disrupt the particles down to the submicron range. Generally 5-10% lipid content is used but up to 40% lipid content has also been investigated. Typical SLNs production conditions are 500 bar and two or three homogenisation cycles. Two general approaches of HPH are hot and cold homogenization, both working on the same concept of mixing the drug in bulk of lipid melt.

3.1.1. Hot homogenization

Hot homogenization is carried out at temperatures above the melting point of the lipid and can therefore be regarded as the homogenization of an emulsion (Figure 2). A pre-emulsion of the drug loaded lipid melt and the aqueous emulsifier phase (same temperature) is obtained by high-shear mixing device. The quality of the pre-emulsion affects the quality of the final product to a great extent and it is desirable to obtain droplets in the size range of a few micrometers. HPH of the pre-emulsion is carried out at temperatures above the melting point of the lipid. Usually, lower particle sizes are obtained at higher processing temperatures because of lowered viscosity of the lipid phase [24].

Hot homogenisation is the most frequently applied technique in which even temperature sensitive compounds can be processed because of the short exposure time to the elevated temperatures [25]. However, high temperatures increase the degradation rate of the drug and the carrier. Increasing the homogenization pressure or the number of cycles often results in an increase of the particle size due to high kinetic energy of the particles. The cold homogenisation technique is therefore recommended for extremely temperature sensitive compounds and hydrophilic compounds, which might partition from the liquid lipid phase to the water phase during the hot homogenisation.

3.1.2. Cold homogenization

During cold homogenization, the drug containing lipid melt is cooled and, after solidification, the lipidic mass is ground to yield lipid microparticles [26]. The lipid microparticles are dispersed in cold surfactant solution by stirring, yielding a macro-suspension. This suspension is then passed through a high-pressure homogeniser at or below room temperature, where the microparticles are broken down to solid lipid nanoparticles. However, compared to hot homogenization, larger particle sizes and a broader size distribution are typical of cold homogenized samples.

3.1.3. Ultrasonication or high speed homogenization

SLNs are also developed by high speed stirring or sonication [27]. The ultrasonic dispersion may offer an appropriate alternative for laboratory scale productions due to its rapid nature and the relatively low cost of required apparatus. So far, its suitability has only been evaluated for SLN [17, 28]. The primary disadvantage of this method is the broader particle size distribution that is yielded, ranging into the micrometer range. Potential metal contamination due to ultrasonication is another issue presented by this method. To generate more stable formulations, high speed stirring and ultrasonication may be used in combination at high temperature.

3.2. Solvent emulsification/evaporation

In this method, the lipidic material, such as glyceride is dissolved in an organic solvent (e.g. chloroform, cyclohexane) and the solution is emulsified in an aqueous phase [29]. After evaporation of the solvent the lipid precipitates to form nanoparticles with a mean diameter of around 30 nm using cholesterol acetate as a model drug and lecithin/sodium glycocholate blend as an emulsifier [30]. The solution is emulsified in an aqueous phase by high pressure homogenization and the organic solvent is removed from the emulsion by evaporation under reduced pressure (40–60 mbar).

3.3. Supercritical fluid

This platform technology, with several variations for powder and nanoparticle preparation, is a relatively new technique for SLN production and offers the advantage of solvent-less processing [31]. SLNs can be prepared by the rapid expansion of supercritical carbon dioxide solutions (RESS) method, where carbon dioxide (99.99%) is a good choice as solvent.

4. Microemulsion method

This method is based on the dilution of microemulsions that are two-phase systems composed of an inner and outer phase (e.g. o/w microemulsions) [32]. They are made by stirring an optically transparent mixture at 65-70°C, which typically composed of a low melting fatty acid (e.g. stearic acid), an emulsifier (e.g. polysorbate 20), co-emulsifiers (e.g. butanol) and water. The hot microemulsion is dispersed in cold water (2-3°C) with stirring. SLN dispersion can be used as granulation fluid for transferring into solid product (tablets, pellets) by granulation process, but in case of low particle content, excess water must first be removed. High-temperature gradients facilitate rapid lipid crystallization and prevent aggregation. Due to the dilution step, achievable lipid contents are considerably lower compared with the HPH based formulations.

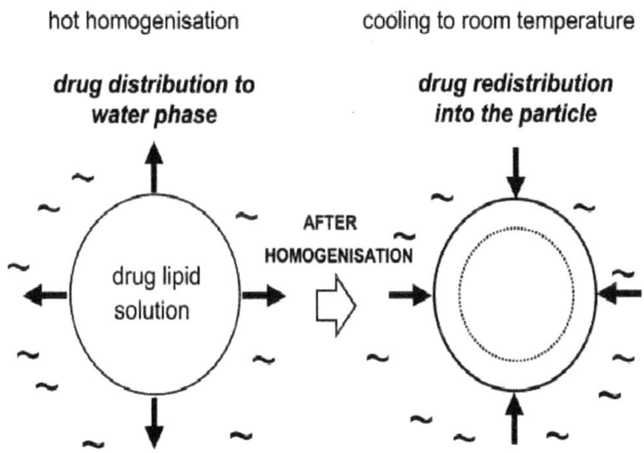

Figure 2. Partitioning effects on drug during the hot homogenization technique production of SLNs. *Left:* Partitioning of drug from the lipid phase to the water phase at increased temperature. *Right:* Re-partitioning of the drug to the lipid phase during cooling of the produced O/W nanoemulsion. Source: Muller RH et al. Solid lipid nanoparticles (SLN) for controlled drug delivery - a review of the state of the art. European Journal of Pharmaceutics and Biopharmaceutics 50: (2000) 161-177.

4.1. Spray drying method

Spray drying is an alternative procedure to lyophilization in the transformation of an aqueous SLN dispersion into a solid drug product. This method results in particle aggregation due to high temperature, shear forces and partial melting of the particle. The use of lipid with melting point >70°C for spray drying is recommended [33]. Best results are obtained with an SLN concentration of 1% in a solution of trehalose in water or 20% trehalose in ethanol-water mixtures (10/90 v/v).

4.2. Double emulsion method

For the preparation of hydrophilic loaded SLN, double emulsion method, a novel approach based on solvent emulsification-evaporation can be employed. Here, the drug is encapsulated with a stabilizer to prevent drug partitioning to external water phase during solvent evaporation in the external water phase of w/o/w double emulsion [34]

5. SLNs cellular uptake, pharmacokinetics and bio-distribution

Research on cellular uptake mechanisms has repeatedly demonstrated that endocytosis is the preferred route of internalization of non-viral gene vectors via a number of distinct endocytic processes. The most studied mechanisms include macropinocytosis, circular dorsal ruffles, clathrin-mediated endocytosis and several clathrin-independent endocytic pathways [35]. Endocytic uptake mechanisms are highly dependent on cell type and on the nature of gene vectors [36]. Clathrin-mediated processes are limited to particles under 200 nm in size, whereas caveolae-dependent uptake prevails for particles between 200 and 500 nm [37]. The prevalent pathway for the cell internalization of PEI polyplexes is however, clathrin-dependent [38].

Apart from overcoming cellular barriers of uptake, an **anticancer** drug must be specifically targeted to the tumor in order to maximize its therapeutic effect, and therefore biodistribution studies are critical to assess the safety of a nanomedicine. However, since most groups work on healthy instead of tumor-bearing animals, it is difficult to confirm whether SLNs can lead to increased tumor drug concentrations by way of enhanced permeability and retention [9]. Recently, Zhang *et al.* (2010) evaluated antitumor efficacy of docetaxel-loaded **solid lipid nanoparticles** (DSN) in a murine ovarian **cancer** model [39]. In this study, SLN biodistribution from RES more toward the circulation system was observed. Moreover, SLNs in comparison to the free drug demonstrated more potent *in vivo* anti-ovarian **cancer** activity with improved pharmacokinetics. In contrast, paclitaxel loaded in pegylated **solid lipid** nanoparticles were mainly taken up by the RES after intravenous administration in rats, showing 8-fold and 3-fold higher levels in liver and spleen, respectively, 8 h after administration compared to paclitaxel in Taxol® [40]. Moreover, paclitaxel levels in kidney, heart and lung were indistinguishable between the two formulations. The difference in biodistribution of SLNs reported in literature may be due to several factors including variations in size, surface functionalization and composition.

The biodistribution of an anticancer drug delivered by SLN may be further manoeuvred by route of injection to achieve the desired therapeutic goal. Harivardhan Reddy *et al.* (2005) compared the biodistribution of free ^{99m}Technetium-labeled etoposide and radio-labeled etoposide loaded SLNs in Dalton's lymphoma tumor-bearing mice [41]. They showed that administration via the subcutaneous route resulted in high tumor uptake of etoposide and etoposide loaded tripalmitin nanoparticles and was the preferred route as compared to intravenous or intraperitoneal administration. However, elevated tumor drug concentrations were also found with intravenously administered etoposide loaded SLN in comparison to the free drug, (approximately 67% increase 1 h post-injection, 30% increase 24 h post-injection). In yet another study by Zara *et al.* (2002) duodenal administration of idarubicin-loaded SLN led to higher bioavailability than intravenously administered SLNs [42]. Also, idarubicin and its main metabolite, idarubicinol, were detected in the brain after IDA-SLN administration, indicating that the SLNs were able to pass the blood-brain barrier; an attractive attribute in the tratement of brain tumors. Thus, the route of administration of SLN formulation is a key consideration in the design of animal or clinical anti-cancer drug delivery studies.

6. SLNs as anti-cancer gene/drug delivery vectors: Challenges and successes

Solid lipid nanoparticles have rapidly established themselves during the past decade as stable, reliable and easy to produce vectors. SLN advantages over other existing transfection vectors include safety, good storage stability, possibility of lyophilization and a high degree of flexibility in design and optimization [25]. Cationic SLNs can efficiently bind DNA directly *via* ionic interaction and mediate gene transfection. However, as with all non-viral vectors, many cellular obstacles have to be overcome to achieve satisfactory levels of transfection activity: i) binding to the cell surface; ii) cellular internalization; iii) escape from the endolysosomal compartment; and iv) translocation through the nuclear envelope. In order to surmount these barriers, cationic SLNs are designed as multifunctional "smart" carriers for efficient gene expression [43]. Components such as chitosan [44] and surface functionalization moieties e.g. poly(styrene-4 sodium sulfonate) (PSS) and poly(L-lysine hydrochloride) (PLL) [45], folate–chitosan and cholesterol derivative (CHETA) [46], cetyltrimethyl ammonium bromide (CTAB) [47] and a phyto-ceramide [48] and TAT peptides [49], may each individually assist in overcoming the barriers of efficient transfection. In addition, protamine a cationic small protein rich in arginine exerts both DNA condensation activity and proton sponge effect facilitating endosomal escape as well as assisting nanovectors to enter the nucleus owing to its nuclear localization signal (NLS) [50]. Table 1 lists some of the successful SLN formulations evaluated as anti-cancer agents in various cancers.

SLN Composition	Characterization	Indication	Drug/Gene	Reference
Stearic acid, DOTAP, Pluronic F68 and dioleoylphosphatidylethanolamine (DOPE)	Size, Zeta Potential	Prostate Cancer	Plasmid DNA	[s51]
Tricaprin as a core, 3beta[N-carbamoyl] cholesterol (DC-Chol), DOPE and Tween 80	Size, Zeta Potential, Differential Scanning Calorimetry	Lung Cancer	Plasmid DNA	[52]
Stearic acid, Lecithin and PS	Transmission electron microscopy	Lung Cancer	Phospho-Sulindac	[53]
Poloxamer 188 and Tween 80	Size, Zeta potential	Breast Cancer	Emodin	[54]
Precirol, Compritol, soybean Phosphatidylcholine, Tween 80	Size, Zeta Potential	Breast Cancer	Tryptanthrin	[55]
Myristic acid, Stearic acid, Palmitic acid, lauric acid, poly(ethylene glycol)-100-stearate (PEG100SA), poly(ethylene glycol)-40-stearate (PEG40SA), Hydrolyzed polymer of epoxidized soybean oil, Pluronic F68 (PF68) (non-ionic block copolymer)	Size, Zeta Potential, Transmission Electron Microscopy	Breast Cancer	Doxorubicin and Mitomycin -C	[56]
Stearyl alcohol and cetyltrimethylammonium bromide (CTAB), Ceramide VI, polysorbate 60	Size, Zeta Potential	Ovarian Cancer	Doxorubicin and mixed-backbone GCS antisense oligonucleotides (MBO-asGCS)	[57]
1,2-Dioleoyl-sn-glycero-3-ethylphosphocholine 1,2-diphytanoyl-sn-glycero-3-phosphatidylethanolamine (DPhPE), 3â[N-(N′,N′-dimethylaminoethane)-carbamoyl] cholesterol (DC-Chol), 1,2-Dioleoyl-sn-glycero-3-ethylphosphocholine (EDOPC), and methoxypolyethylene glycol 2000-distearoyl phosphatidylethanolamine (mPEG-DSPE), glyceryl trioleate.	Zeta potential and Gel retardation	Epithelial Cancer	Paclitaxel and siRNA	[58]
Cholesteryl oleate, glyceryl trioleate, DOPE, Chol , and DC-Chol	Size, Zeta Potential	Brain Cancer (glioblastomas)	c-Met siRNA	[59]
Stearic acid, Glyceryl behenate	Size, Zeta Potential	Skin Cancer	Doxorubicin	[60]

Table 1. Solid Lipid Nanoparticles loaded with DNA/ Drug as anti-cancer delivery systems in various cancers.

Nanovectors offer the potential to both detect and treat cancer at a very early stage, thereby maximizing survival rates. The NCI (National Cancer Institute) Alliance for Nanotechnology in Cancer provides up-to-date information in nano-cancer research and its promise for cancer diagnosis and treatment (http://nano.cancer.gov/). Using siRNA molecules loaded in nano-vectors, early proof-of-principle experiments in various tumor cells suggest that RNA silencing may have great potential as a strategy for treating cancer. However, siRNA therapeutics are hindered by poor intracellular uptake, limited blood stability and undesirable non-specific immune stimulation [61]. An interesting strategy used to target the vector employs three-amino-acid peptide, arginine-glycine-aspartic acid (known by its amino acid code RGD) that binds to integrins, which in turn are involved in angiogenesis, tumor cell growth, metastasis, and inflammation. Intravenous administration into tumor-bearing mice of nanoparticles combined with a dual strategy of siRNA inhibiting vascular endothelial growth factor receptor-2 and RGD peptide ligand attached at the distal end of the polyethylene glycol [40], conferred selective tumor uptake, and inhibition of both tumor angiogenesis and growth rate, achieving both tissue and gene selectivity [62]. In February 2012, Calando Pharmaceuticals, in Pasadena, Canada, and the National Cancer Institute (NCI) entered into a collaborative development program for a nanoparticle-based siRNA therapeutic aimed at treating neuro-blastoma, the most common extracranial solid tumor in children less than five years of age. Previous attempts to develop targeted nanoparticles were unsuccessful due to the inherent difficulties of designing and scaling up a particle capable of targeting, long-circulating via immune-response evasion and controlled drug release. Very recently, Hrkach *et al.* (2012) reported the preclinical development and clinical translation of a docetaxel nanoparticle with prostate-specific membrane antigen, a clinically validated tumor antigen expressed on prostate cancer cells and on the neovasculature of most non-prostate solid tumors including breast, head, lung, neck, prostate and stomach [63]. This targeted nanoparticle-based compound called "BIND-014" is currently the first one to enter clinical trial, although with small number of only 17 patients. Patients with advanced or metastatic cancer receive an injection of the nano-drug once every three weeks and are showing signals of efficacy even at relatively low doses. This initial but positive result shows promise and the potential impact of nanomedicines as a paradigm shift in the treatment of cancer.

Very recently, Vighi E *et al.* (2012) developed a multicomponent cationic SLN as a pDNA delivery vehicle. The formulations were prepared using stearic acid as the main component in the lipid phase, stearylamine, the main component in the aqueous phase, as cationic agent and protamine as transfection promoter along with the phosphatidylcholine (SLN–PC), cholesterol (SLN–Chol) or both (SLN–PC–Chol). Transfection results on various cell lines in this study revealed the best transfection for SLN–PC–Chol on COS-1 cells (African green monkey kidney cell line) [64]. However, lower transfection levels than poly [62] were observed on HepG2 cells (human hepatocellular liver carcinoma cell line), regardless of the SLN composition. Using COS-1 monkey kidney fibroblast-like cells, SLNs and liposomes formu-lated from the same cationic lipids, demonstrated equipotent *in vitro* transfection efficiencies [65]. This study suggests that only the lipid composition in the tested lipid-based formulations affected transfection efficiencies. The intrinsic toxicity that is common in cationic gene delivery vehicles may also be minimized, while maintaining high transfection efficiency, by selecting good combinations of two-tailed cationic lipids and matrix lipids. Hence, structural or compositional design changes of nanovectors may influence the outcome in relation with cell physiology, cell internalization pathways and transfection efficiency. The above results support the use of SLNs to serve as nano/microcarriers for anti-cancer gene therapies.

Under optimised conditions SLNs can be designed to incorporate lipophilic or hydrophilic drugs and seem to fulfil the requirements for an optimum particulate carrier system. Stability studies were performed on SLNs loaded with all-*trans* retinoic acid (ATRA), another compound that is sensitive to light, heat and oxidants, and quickly degrades into less active products such as isotretinoin and all-*trans*-4-oxo [66]. After 3 months of storage at 4 °C, more than 90% of the ATRA drug molecules in SLN remained chemically intact. This can be compared to approximately 50% drug degradation when stored at the same temperature in the form of methanol solution or 1% polysorbate-80 solution for only 1 month. Hence, SLNs are useful for the protection of anticancer compounds that are sensitive to light, and probably heat and oxidants as well. In a study conducted by our group, modulatory effects of encapsulated and free forms of sesamol (anti-oxidant and anti-cancer compound) were evaluated by the topical delivery systems in a skin cancer mice model. Both free sesamol and SLN dispersion were applied as gels (using 1% w/v of Carbopol 934P®) on the skin of mice. Encapsulated or nanosesamol was found to safely exert chemopreventive effects by decreasing the lipid peroxidation levels and increasing the anti-oxidant levels, thereby decreasing the development and promotion of skin tumors. Immunofluorescence studies of pro- and anti-apoptotic markers, bcl-2 and bax protein expression revealed higher expression of anti-apoptotic protein, bcl-2, in the tissue sections of tumor bearing mice in comparison to their control counterparts and groups which received sesamol treatment, reinforcing the role of bcl-2 in skin carcinogenesis. Higher expression of bax was also observed in sesamol treated animals as compared to the tumor bearing mice. Up-regulation of bax in the control and sesamol treated groups suggests that it follows the intrinsic pathway of apoptosis (unpublished results).

Ongoing work by our group compared neutraceutical curcumin-loaded SLNs to the free form as a chemopreventive topical delivery system in 7,12-dimethylbenz [*a*]anthracene (DMBA) induced skin cancer model mice. In order to understand the molecular events underlying nanocurcumin-mediated chemoprevention, protein expression of various biomolecules e.g. anti and pro inflammatory cytokines (Il-4 and Il-1β) were analyzed by Western immunoblotting and immunoflourscence. For cancer induction, male Balb/c mice were subcutaneously injected with 30 mg/Kg body weight of DMBA (in olive oil) once a week for three weeks. DMBA skin cancer induced mice were topically applied free and encapsulated curcumin (50mg/Kg b.w) as a chemopreventive agent from one week before DMBA injection to the experiment's end (18 weeks). We found that free and nanocurcumin treatment of DMBA treated mice reduced the levels of malondialdehyde, a by-product of lipid degradation (Figure 3). Antioxidant analysis revealed increased levels of enzymes (SOD, Catalase, Reduced Glutathione, Total Glutathione) in encapsulated nanocurcumin treated group as compared to free curcumin group (Figure 4-7). Immunofluorscence studies and western blot analysis of Il-4 and Il-1β suggest enhanced anti-inflammatory potential of encapsulated curcumin in comparison to mice treated with free curcumin. Mice bearing skin tumors showed increased expression of pro-inflammatory interleukins when compared to the control, which was decreased on treatment with curcumin (Figure 8). Furthermore, the immunoflourscence assay of anti-inflammatory interleukin (IL-4) showed a far greater increase in IL-4 expression by topical treatment with encapsulated curcumin as compared to the free curcumin in mice bearing skin tumors (Figure 9).

7. Conclusion

Solid Lipid Nanoparticles serve as efficient and safe DNA/ drug loaded nanosystems in both the imaging and treatment of cancer. Traditional drug delivery systems are often hindered by their low bioavailabilty, low solubility, toxicity and rapid clearance. In future, clinicians and researchers will be able to "**tune and time**" the amount of DNA/Drug delivery by controlling the release at specific location thereby minimizing their toxicity and side- effects.

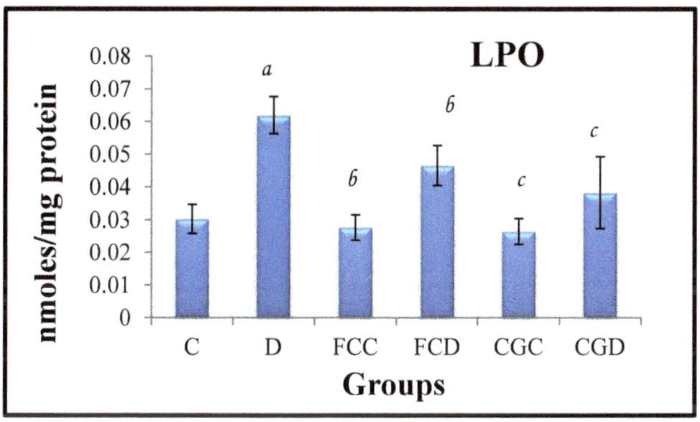

The value are presented as Mean ± SEM., N=8-10

Statistical significance : Control vs DMBA $p \leq 0.001^{a}$

:DMBA vs FCD and FCC $p \leq 0.001^{b}$

:DMBA vs CGD and CGC $p \leq 0.001^{c}$

Figure 3. Effect of encapsulated and free curcumin on lipid peroxidation (LPO) in control and experimental groups. Control (C), DMBA (D), Free Curcumin (FCC), Free Curcumin + DMBA (FCD), Encapsulated Curcumin (CGC), Encapsulated Curcumin + DMBA (CGD).

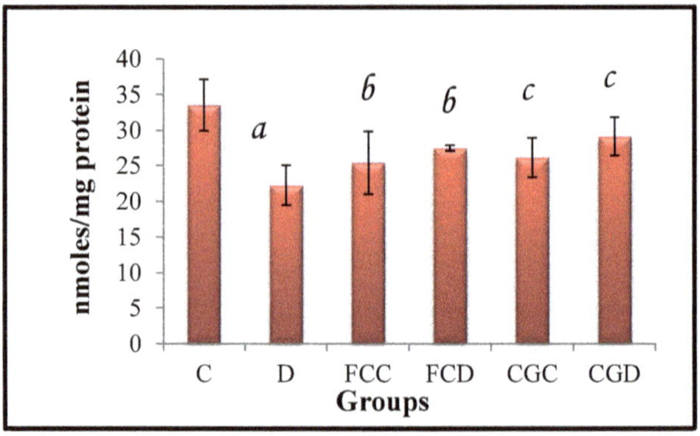

The value are presented as Mean ± SEM., N=8-10

Statistical significanc: Control vs DMBA $p \leq 0.001$[a]

:DMBA vs FCD and FCC $p \leq 0.001$[b]

:DMBA vs CGD and CGC $p \leq 0.001$[c]

Figure 4. Effect of encapsulated and free curcumin on reduced glutathione in control and experimental groups. Control (C), DMBA (D), Free Curcumin (FCC), Free Curcumin + DMBA (FCD), Encapsulated Curcumin (CGC), Encapsulated Curcumin + DMBA (CGD).

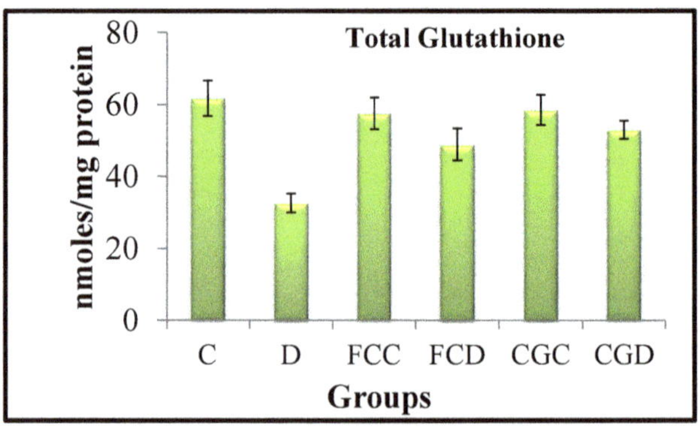

The value are presented as Mean ± SEM., N=8-10

Statistical significance: Control vs DMBA $p \leq 0.001$[a]

:DMBA vs FCD and FCC $p \leq 0.001$[b]

:DMBA vs CGD and CGC $p \leq 0.001$[c]

Figure 5. Effect of encapsulated and free curcumin on total glutathione in control and experimental groups. Control (C), DMBA (D), Free Curcumin (FCC), Free Curcumin + DMBA (FCD), Encapsulated Curcumin (CGC), Encapsulated Curcumin + DMBA (CGD).

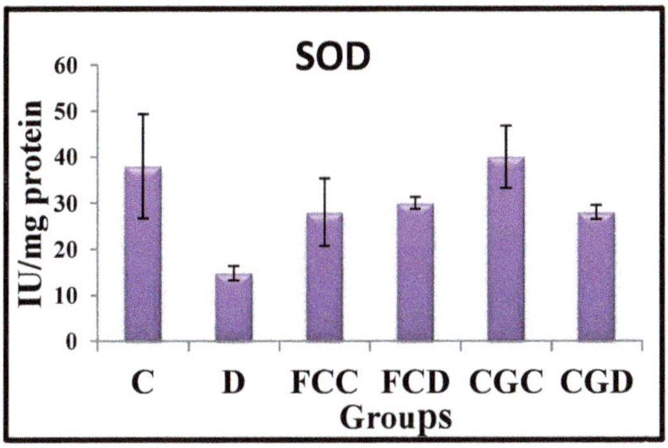

The value are presented as Mean± SEM., N=8-10

Statistical significance: Control vs DMBA $p \leq 0.05^a$

:DMBA vs FCD and FCC $p \leq 0.01^b$

:DMBA vs CGD and CGC $p \leq 0.01^c$

Figure 6. Effect of encapsulated and free curcumin on superoxide dismutase in control and experimental groups. Control (C), DMBA (D), Free Curcumin (FCC), Free Curcumin + DMBA (FCD), Encapsulated Curcumin (CGC), Encapsulated Curcumin + DMBA (CGD).

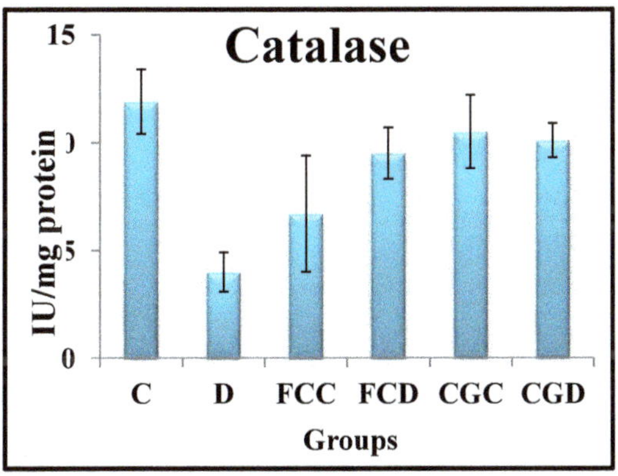

The value are presented as Mean± SEM., N=8-10

Statistical significance: Control vs DMBA $p \leq 0.05^a$

:DMBA (D) vs FCD and FCC $p \leq 0.05^b$

:DMBA (D) vs CGD and CGC $p \leq 0.01^c$

Figure 7. Effect of encapsulated and free curcumin on Catalase in control and experimental groups. Control (C), DMBA (D), Free Curcumin (FCC), Free Curcumin DMBA (FCD), Encapsulated Curcumin (CGC), Encapsulated Curcumin + DMBA (CGD).

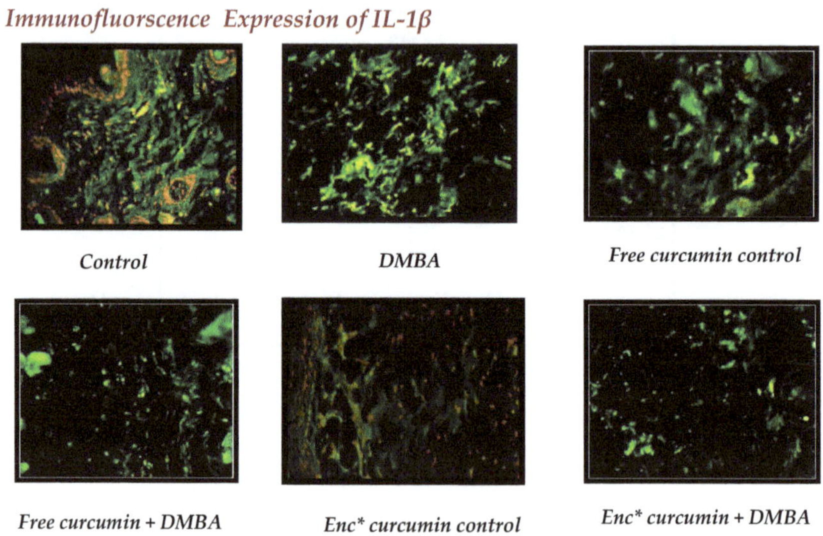

Figure 8. Photomicrographs (20X) showing expression of IL-1Beta in paraffin sections by immunofluoroscence after 18 weeks of treatment.

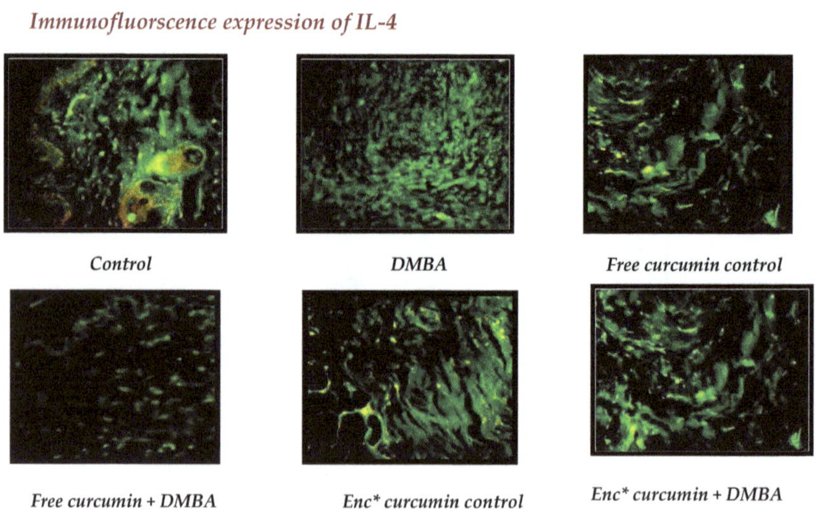

Figure 9. Photomicrographs (20X) showing expression of IL-4 in paraffin sections by immunofluoroscence after 18 weeks of treatment.

Author details

Tranum Kaur[1] and Roderick Slavcev[2*]

*Address all correspondence to: slavcev@uwaterloo.ca

1 Department of Biophysics, Panjab University, Chandigarh, India

2 School of Pharmacy, University of Waterloo, Kitchener, Ontario, Canada

References

[1] Petkar, K. C, Chavhan, S. S, Gatonovik-kustrin, S, & Sawant, K. K. Nanostructured materials in drug and gene delivery: a review of the state of the art. Crit Rev Ther Drug Carrier Syst (2011). , 28(2), 101-64.

[2] Arias, J. L, Clares, B, Morales, M. E, Gallardo, V, & Ruiz, M. A. Lipid-based drug delivery systems for cancer treatment. Curr Drug Targets (2011). Jul;, 12(8), 1151-65.

[3] Kozako, T, Arima, N, Yoshimitsu, M, Honda, S. I, & Soeda, S. Liposomes and nanotechnology in drug development: focus on oncotargets. Int J Nanomedicine (2012). doi:IJN.S30726. Epub;%2012 Sep 14.:4943-51., 7, 4943-51.

[4] Pearson, R. M, Sunoqrot, S, Hsu, H. J, Bae, J. W, & Hong, S. Dendritic nanoparticles: the next generation of nanocarriers? Ther Deliv (2012). Aug;, 3(8), 941-59.

[5] Blanco, E, Kessinger, C. W, Sumer, B. D, & Gao, J. Multifunctional micellar nanomedicine for cancer therapy. Exp Biol Med (Maywood) (2009). Feb;, 234(2), 123-31.

[6] Mehnert, W, & Mader, K. Solid lipid nanoparticles Production, characterization and applications. Adv Drug Deliv Rev (2012). Sep;(12):10.

[7] Prados, J, Melguizo, C, Ortiz, R, Velez, C, Alvarez, P. J, Arias, J. L, Ruiz, M. A, Gallardo, V, & Aranega, A. Doxorubicin-Loaded Nanoparticles: New Advances in Breast Cancer Therapy. Anticancer Agents Med Chem (2012). Feb.

[8] Torchilin, V. P. Structure and design of polymeric surfactant-based drug delivery systems. J Control Release (2001). Jun;73(2-3):137-72.

[9] Greish, K. Enhanced permeability and retention (EPR) effect for anticancer nanomedicine drug targeting. Methods Mol Biol (2010). , 624, 25-37.

[10] Hobbs, S. K, Monsky, W. L, Yuan, F, Roberts, W. G, Griffith, L, Torchilin, V. P, & Jain, R. K. Regulation of transport pathways in tumor vessels: role of tumor type and microenvironment. Proc Natl Acad Sci U S A (1998). Apr;, 95(8), 4607-12.

[11] Brigger, I, Dubernet, C, & Couvreur, P. Nanoparticles in cancer therapy and diagnosis. Adv Drug Deliv Rev (2012). Sep;(12):10.

[12] Miele, E, Spinelli, G. P, Miele, E, Tomao, F, & Tomao, S. Albumin-bound formulation of paclitaxel (Abraxane ABI-007) in the treatment of breast cancer. Int J Nanomedicine (2009). Epub;%2009 Apr;%20.:99-105., 4, 99-105.

[13] Liggins, R. T, Hunter, W. L, & Burt, H. M. Solid-state characterization of paclitaxel. J Pharm Sci (1997). Dec;, 86(12), 1458-63.

[14] Coleman, R. L, Brady, W. E, Mcmeekin, D. S, Rose, P. G, Soper, J. T, Lentz, S. S, Hoffman, J. S, & Shahin, M. S. A phase II evaluation of nanoparticle, albumin-bound (nab) paclitaxel in the treatment of recurrent or persistent platinum-resistant ovarian, fallopian tube, or primary peritoneal cancer: a Gynecologic Oncology Group study. Gynecol Oncol (2011). Jul;, 122(1), 111-5.

[15] Ibrahim, N. K, Desai, N, Legha, S, Soon-shiong, P, Theriault, R. L, Rivera, E, Esmaeli, B, Ring, S. E, Bedikian, A, Hortobagyi, G. N, Ellerhorst, J. A, & Phase, I. and pharmacokinetic study of ABI-007, a Cremophor-free, protein-stabilized, nanoparticle formulation of paclitaxel. Clin Cancer Res (2002). May;, 8(5), 1038-44.

[16] Su, W. P, Cheng, F. Y, Shieh, D. B, Yeh, C. S, & Su, W. C. PLGA nanoparticles codeliver paclitaxel and Stat3 siRNA to overcome cellular resistance in lung cancer cells. Int J Nanomedicine (2012). Epub;%2012 Aug 3.:4269-83., 7, 4269-83.

[17] Dasgupta, S, Mazumder, B, Ghosh, S. K, & Kaurav, S. S. Solid lipid nanoparticles (SLNs) for topical delivery of aceclofenac by using xanthan gum: Ex vivo and in vivo evaluation. Curr Drug Deliv (2012). Sep.

[18] Mukherjee, S, Ray, S, & Thakur, R. S. Solid lipid nanoparticles: a modern formulation approach in drug delivery system. Indian J Pharm Sci (2009). Jul;, 71(4), 349-58.

[19] Weyhers, H, Ehlers, S, Hahn, H, Souto, E. B, & Muller, R. H. Solid lipid nanoparticles (SLN)--effects of lipid composition on in vitro degradation and in vivo toxicity. Pharmazie (2006). Jun;, 61(6), 539-44.

[20] Mehnert, W, & Mader, K. Solid lipid nanoparticles: production, characterization and applications. Adv Drug Deliv Rev (2001). Apr;47(2-3):165-96.

[21] Iqbal, M. A, Md, S, Sahni, J. K, Baboota, S, Dang, S, & Ali, J. Nanostructured lipid carriers system: Recent advances in drug delivery. J Drug Target (2012). Aug.

[22] Mu, R. H. Èller, J.S.Lucks. ArzneistofftraÈger aus festen Lipidteilchen, Feste LipidnanosphaÈren (SLN). European Patent (1996). Ref Type: Journal (Full)(0605497)

[23] Ugazio, E, Cavalli, R, & Gasco, M. R. Incorporation of cyclosporin A in solid lipid nanoparticles (SLN). Int J Pharm (2002). Jul;, 241(2), 341-4.

[24] Lander, R, Manger, W, Scouloudis, M, Ku, A, Davis, C, & Lee, A. Gaulin homogenization: a mechanistic study. Biotechnol Prog (2000). Jan;, 16(1), 80-5.

[25] Muller, R. H, Mader, K, & Gohla, S. Solid lipid nanoparticles (SLN) for controlled drug delivery- a review of the state of the art. Eur J Pharm Biopharm (2000). Jul;, 50(1), 161-77.

[26] Muller, R. H, Schwarz, C, Mehnert, W, & Lucks, J. S. Production of solid lipid nanoparticles (SLN) for controlled drug delivery. Proc.Int.Symp.Control.Release Bioact.Mater. (1993). Ref Type: Journal (Full), 20, 480-481.

[27] Eldem, T, Speiser, P, & Hincal, A. Optimization of spray-dried and-congealed lipid micropellets and characterization of their surface morphology by scanning electron microscopy. Pharm Res (1991). Jan;, 8(1), 47-54.

[28] Julia, C. Schwarz AWEPMLGPRCV. Nanocarriers for dermal drug delivery: Influence of preparation method, carrier type and rheological properties. International Journal of Pharmaceutics 437 [(2012). Ref Type: Journal (Full), 1-2.

[29] Sjostrom, B, & Bergenstahl, B. Preparation of submicron drug particles in lecithin-stabilized o/w emulsions: I: Model studies of the precipitation of cholesteryl acetate. Int J Pharm. (1992). Ref Type: Journal (Full), 88, 53-62.

[30] Siekmann, B, & Westesen, K. Investigations on solid lipid nanoparticles prepared by precipitation in o/w emulsions. Eur J Pharm Biopharm (1996). Ref Type: Journal (Full), 43, 104-109.

[31] Chen, Y. J, Jin, R. X, Zhou, Y. Q, Zeng, J, Zhang, H, & Feng, Q. R. Preparation of solid lipid nanoparticles loaded with Xionggui powder-supercritical carbon dioxide fluid extraction and their evaluation in vitro release]. Zhongguo Zhong Yao Za Zhi (2006). Mar;, 31(5), 376-9.

[32] Gasco, M. R. Method for producing solid lipid microspheres having narrow size distribution. United State Patent.US 188837. (1993). Ref Type: Journal (Full)

[33] Freitas, C, & Mullera, R. H. Spray-drying of solid lipid nanoparticles (SLN TM). Eur J Pharm Biopharm (1998). Sep;, 46(2), 145-51.

[34] Yang, R, Gao, R, Li, F, He, H, & Tang, X. The influence of lipid characteristics on the formation, in vitro release, and in vivo absorption of protein-loaded SLN prepared by the double emulsion process. Drug Dev Ind Pharm (2011). Feb;, 37(2), 139-48.

[35] Garaiova, Z, Strand, S. P, Reitan, N. K, Lelu, S, Storset, S. O, Berg, K, Malmo, J, Folasire, O, & Bjorkoy, A. de LD. Cellular uptake of DNA-chitosan nanoparticles: The role of clathrin- and caveolae-mediated pathways. Int J Biol Macromol (2012). Aug;, 51(5), 1043-51.

[36] Pichon, C, Billiet, L, & Midoux, P. Chemical vectors for gene delivery: uptake and intracellular trafficking. Curr Opin Biotechnol (2010). Oct;, 21(5), 640-5.

[37] Rejman, J, Oberle, V, Zuhorn, I. S, & Hoekstra, D. Size-dependent internalization of particles via the pathways of clathrin- and caveolae-mediated endocytosis. Biochem J (2004). Jan;377(Pt 1):159-69.

[38] Midoux, P, Breuzard, G, Gomez, J. P, & Pichon, C. Polymer-based gene delivery: a current review on the uptake and intracellular trafficking of polyplexes. Curr Gene Ther (2008). Oct;, 8(5), 335-52.

[39] Zhang, P, Chen, L, Zhang, Z, Lin, L, & Li, Y. Pharmacokinetics in rats and efficacy in murine ovarian cancer model for solid lipid nanoparticles loading docetaxel. J Nanosci Nanotechnol (2010). Nov;, 10(11), 7541-4.

[40] Li, R, Eun, J. S, & Lee, M. K. Pharmacokinetics and biodistribution of paclitaxel loaded in pegylated solid lipid nanoparticles after intravenous administration. Arch Pharm Res (2011). Feb;, 34(2), 331-7.

[41] Harivardhan, R. L, Sharma, R. K, Chuttani, K, Mishra, A. K, & Murthy, R. S. Influence of administration route on tumor uptake and biodistribution of etoposide loaded solid lipid nanoparticles in Dalton's lymphoma tumor bearing mice. J Control Release (2005). Jul;%20;, 105(3), 185-98.

[42] Zara, G. P, Bargoni, A, Cavalli, R, Fundaro, A, Vighetto, D, & Gasco, M. R. Pharmacokinetics and tissue distribution of idarubicin-loaded solid lipid nanoparticles after duodenal administration to rats. J Pharm Sci (2002). May;, 91(5), 1324-33.

[43] Vighi, E, Leot, E, Montanari, M, Mucci, A, Hanuskova, M, & Iannuccelli, V. Structural investigation and intracellular trafficking of a novel multicomposite cationic solid lipid nanoparticle platform as a pDNA carrier. Ther Deliv (2011). Nov;, 2(11), 1419-35.

[44] Sandri, G, Bonferoni, M. C, Gokce, E. H, Ferrari, F, Rossi, S, Patrini, M, & Caramella, C. Chitosan-associated SLN: in vitro and ex vivo characterization of cyclosporine A loaded ophthalmic systems. J Microencapsul (2010). , 27(8), 735-46.

[45] Jayagopal, A, Sussman, E. M, & Shastri, V. P. Functionalized solid lipid nanoparticles for transendothelial delivery. IEEE Trans Nanobioscience (2008). Mar;, 7(1), 28-34.

[46] Liu, Z, Zhong, Z, Peng, G, Wang, S, Du, X, Yan, D, Zhang, Z, He, Q, & Liu, J. Folate receptor mediated intracellular gene delivery using the charge changing solid lipid nanoparticles. Drug Deliv (2009). Aug;, 16(6), 341-7.

[47] Doktorovova, S, Shegokar, R, Rakovsky, E, Gonzalez-mira, E, Lopes, C. M, Silva, A. M, Martins-lopes, P, Muller, R. H, & Souto, E. B. Cationic solid lipid nanoparticles (cSLN): structure, stability and DNA binding capacity correlation studies. Int J Pharm (2011). Nov;, 420(2), 341-9.

[48] Siddiqui, A, Patwardhan, G. A, Liu, Y. Y, & Nazzal, S. Mixed backbone antisense glucosylceramide synthase oligonucleotide (MBO-asGCS) loaded solid lipid nanoparticles: in vitro characterization and reversal of multidrug resistance in NCI/ADR-RES cells. Int J Pharm (2010). Nov;400(1-2):251-9.

[49] Musacchio, T, & Torchilin, V. P. Recent developments in lipid-based pharmaceutical nanocarriers. Front Biosci (2011). Jan;, 16, 1388-412.

[50] Vighi, E, Ruozi, B, Montanari, M, Battini, R, & Leo, E. pDNA condensation capacity and in vitro gene delivery properties of cationic solid lipid nanoparticles. Int J Pharm (2010). Apr;389(1-2):254-61.

[51] De Jesus, M. B, & Ferreira, C. V. de PE, Hoekstra D, Zuhorn IS. Design of solid lipid nanoparticles for gene delivery into prostate cancer. J Control Release (2010). Nov; %20;148(1):ee90., 89.

[52] Choi, S. H, Jin, S. E, Lee, M. K, Lim, S. J, Park, J. S, Kim, B. G, Ahn, W. S, & Kim, C. K. Novel cationic solid lipid nanoparticles enhanced gene transfer to lung cancer cells. Eur J Pharm Biopharm (2008). Mar;68(3):545-54., 53.

[53] Zhu, R, Cheng, K. W, Mackenzie, G, Huang, L, Sun, Y, Xie, G, Vrankova, K, Constantinides, P. P, & Rigas, B. Phospho-Sulindac (OXT-328) Inhibits the Growth of Human Lung Cancer Xenografts in Mice: Enhanced Efficacy and Mitochondria Targeting by its Formulation in Solid Lipid Nanoparticles. Pharm Res (2012). Jun.

[54] Wang, S, Chen, T, Chen, R, Hu, Y, Chen, M, & Wang, Y. Emodin loaded solid lipid nanoparticles: preparation, characterization and antitumor activity studies. Int J Pharm (2012). Jul;430(1-2):238-46.

[55] Fang, Y. P, Lin, Y. K, Su, Y. H, & Fang, J. Y. Tryptanthrin-loaded nanoparticles for delivery into cultured human breast cancer cells, MCF7: the effects of solid lipid/liquid lipid ratios in the inner core. Chem Pharm Bull (Tokyo) (2011). Feb;, 59(2), 266-71.

[56] Shuhendler, A. J, Cheung, R. Y, Manias, J, Connor, A, Rauth, A. M, & Wu, X. Y. A novel doxorubicin-mitomycin C co-encapsulated nanoparticle formulation exhibits anti-cancer synergy in multidrug resistant human breast cancer cells. Breast Cancer Res Treat (2010). Jan;, 119(2), 255-69.

[57] Siddiqui, A, Gupta, V, Liu, Y. Y, & Nazzal, S. Doxorubicin and MBO-asGCS oligonucleotide loaded lipid nanoparticles overcome multidrug resistance in adriamycin resistant ovarian cancer cells (NCI/ADR-RES). Int J Pharm (2012). Jul;431(1-2):222-9.

[58] Yu, Y. H, Kim, E, Park, D. E, Shim, G, Lee, S, Kim, Y. B, Kim, C. W, & Oh, Y. K. Cationic solid lipid nanoparticles for co-delivery of paclitaxel and siRNA. Eur J Pharm Biopharm (2012). Feb;, 80(2), 268-73.

[59] Jin, J, Bae, K. H, Yang, H, Lee, S. J, Kim, H, Kim, Y, Joo, K. M, Seo, S. W, Park, T. G, & Nam, D. H. In vivo specific delivery of c-Met siRNA to glioblastoma using cationic solid lipid nanoparticles. Bioconjug Chem (2011). Dec;, 22(12), 2568-72.

[60] Taveira, S. F, & Araujo, L. M. de S, Nomizo A, de Freitas LA, Lopez RF. Development of cationic solid lipid nanoparticles with factorial design-based studies for topical administration of doxorubicin. J Biomed Nanotechnol (2012). Apr;, 8(2), 219-28.

[61] Schiffelers, R. M. siRNA based approaches in medicinal chemistry and drug discovery. Curr Top Med Chem (2012). , 12(2), 67-8.

[62] Schiffelers, R. M, Ansari, A, Xu, J, Zhou, Q, Tang, Q, Storm, G, Molema, G, Lu, P. Y, Scaria, P. V, & Woodle, M. C. Cancer siRNA therapy by tumor selective delivery with ligand-targeted sterically stabilized nanoparticle. Nucleic Acids Res (2004). Nov; 32(19):e149.

[63] Hrkach, J. Von HD, Mukkaram AM, Andrianova E, Auer J, Campbell T, De WD, Figa M, Figueiredo M, Horhota A, Low S, McDonnell K, Peeke E, Retnarajan B, Sabnis A, Schnipper E, Song JJ, Song YH, Summa J, Tompsett D, Troiano G, Van Geen HT, Wright J, LoRusso P, Kantoff PW, Bander NH, Sweeney C, Farokhzad OC, Langer R, Zale S. Preclinical development and clinical translation of a PSMA-targeted docetaxel nanoparticle with a differentiated pharmacological profile. Sci Transl Med (2012). Apr; 4(128):128ra39.

[64] Vighi, E, Montanari, M, Hanuskova, M, Iannuccelli, V, Coppi, G, & Leo, E. Design flexibility influencing the in vitro behavior of cationic SLN as a nonviral gene vector. Int J Pharm (2012). Sep;(12):10.

[65] Ho Lun Wong RBAMRYLXYWChemotherapy with anticancer drugs encapsulated in solid lipid nanoparticles. Advanced Drug Delivery Reviews 59 [6], (2007). Ref Type: Journal (Full), 491-504.

[66] Lim, S. J, Lee, M. K, & Kim, C. K. Altered chemical and biological activities of all-trans retinoic acid incorporated in solid lipid nanoparticle powders. J Control Release (2004). Nov;, 100(1), 53-61.

Chapter 3

Extracellular and Intracellular Barriers to Non-Viral Gene Transfer

Lynn F. Gottfried and David A. Dean

Additional information is available at the end of the chapter

1. Introduction

Non-viral gene therapy vectors are highly desirable tools for the introduction of DNA into cells; they have better safety profiles than viral methods of delivery and are more amenable to repeated administration. Non-viral vectors include naked DNA, cationic lipid-DNA complexes (lipoplex), polymer-DNA complexes (polyplex) or combinations of lipids and polymers. Successful gene delivery depends upon the ability of the vector of choice to target a specific cell type, enter the cell and obtain sufficient levels of gene expression. This is not a simple task since there are several barriers encountered by both viral and non-viral vectors that make this process difficult. First, the vector must have a method by which to target a specific cell type, while also avoiding extracellular insults including nucleases and the immune system. Next, once the vector has reached its particular target, it must traverse the plasma membrane and/or escape the endosome, and pass through the dense cytoskeletal network en route to the nucleus. The nuclear envelope presents a final barrier, since DNA must enter the nucleus in order to be transcribed. While viruses have evolved mechanisms to enter target cells, deliver their genetic material and continue to propagate, non-viral systems lack these innate mechanisms. Consequently, there has been much work aimed at characterizing and overcoming these barriers in order to improve the efficacy of these vectors.

2. Extracellular barriers

Regardless of the method by which a non-viral vector is administered *in vivo* (e.g., by inhalation, intramuscular injection, gavage, intravascular injection, etc), it will unavoidably come into contact with the extracellular environment. Within the extracellular milieu, multiple factors exist which can result in rapid clearance and/or degradation of the vector before it ever reaches its targeted organ. Intravenously delivered naked DNA has been shown to have a very short half-life within serum, on the range of 1.2 to 21 minutes depending upon the topoform of the DNA [1]. This is believed to be the result of both endo and exonuclease activity in the plasma. Similar degradation has been observed in plasmid DNA delivered intramuscularly [2]. Strategies to protect DNA from nuclease activity include the use of cationic lipids, such as DOTAP:DOPE, to encapsulate the plasmid and shield it from the enzymatic environment outside the cell [1]. In addition, the use of PEGylated lipids and polymers has been demonstrated to enhance the stability of complexes in serum, greatly lengthening the vectors' half-life [3].

DNA that does evade nucleases, however, also comes into contact with proteins and cells within the extracellular environment. Serum contains a variety of proteins which have the ability to bind to non-viral vectors and, as a result, inhibit the biological activity of the vector or sequester it for degradation and/or removal. For example, negatively charged serum proteins form connections between cationic liposomes, which results in the aggregration of the delivery vehicles. When this happens, the vectors are quickly removed from circulation by the reticuloendothelial system. Some of the key blood proteins that have been identified to associate with non-viral vectors include albumin, complement, immunoglobulins, fibronectin, apolipoproteins, C-reactive protein, and b2-glycoprotein I [4]. PEGylation of both lipolexes and polyplexes as well as the use of cholesterol as a helper lipid have shown promise in the prevention of this type of aggregation [3].

It is important to note that DNA delivery vehicles also come into contact with blood cells. These cells, which include erythrocytes, leukocytes, macrophages, and platelets, have a negative surface charge, thereby allowing for electrostatic interactions to occur between cells and cationic vectors. In particular, the interaction of lipoplexes with erythrocytes has been shown to be a significant factor in *in vivo* gene delivery, as binding occurs within minutes of *in vivo* intravenous gene transfer [5]. The vector is then able to directly associate (in the case of DOTMA/cholesterol complexes) and/or fuse (in the case of DOTMA/DOPE complexes) with erythrocytes, thereby decreasing transfection efficiency and encouraging removal of the delivery vehicle by way of the liver and spleen [5]. (Since erythrocytes have no nuclei, entry of vectors into these cells represents a dead end.) In the lung, the alveolar macrophage is regarded as a major barrier to both viral and non-viral delivery since this professional phagocytic cell "eats" up delivery agents before they can transfect any other cell type [6].

Another extracellular barrier to consider is activation of the immune system. While immune activation has been most associated with viral gene delivery, some non-viral methods have been shown to induce an immune response. For example, intravenously injected cationic lipoplexes can induce an inflammatory response involving the release of TNFα and IFNγ into the serum [7]. This is believed to be a result of unmethylated CpG motifs on the plasmid DNA and the subsequent recognition by Toll-like receptors [8, 9]. Thus, the removal of these CpG motifs is important for successful gene delivery [10]. The cationic polymer, PEI, has also been shown to activate the immune system through complement and activation of both a Th1 and Th2 response [11] Finally, as previously discussed, PEGylation of non-viral vectors is a common technique used for avoiding some extracellular barriers, however the production of anti-PEG IgM has the potential to interfere with repeated administration of the vector [12-17]. Thus, much care and consideration must be put into the selection of the proper non-viral vector for specific disease therapeutics.

3. The plasma membrane

Once the delivery vehicle has reached a cell, it then encounters a second significant barrier: the plasma membrane. Successful transfection relies on the ability of the vector to enter the cell of interest. In the absence of a delivery vehicle, naked DNA does not efficiently associate with the plasma membrane due to the negative charge density on both the DNA and the cell surface. Delivery vehicles help circumvent this problem through the use of polycations to neutralize the negative charge of the DNA, thereby increasing association with the plasma membrane. This non-specific electrostatic association is mediated largely by heparin sulfate proteoglycans on the cell surface that trigger endocytosis of the delivery vehicle and entry into the cell.

While most chemical transfection methods require endocytosis for transport across the plasma membrane into the cytoplasm, more recently, several short peptides have been reported to facilitate cell entry in an endocytosis-independent manner [18-20]. These have been termed cell-penetrating peptides (CPPs) and include peptides from proteins such as Tat, antennapedia, and penetratin as well as polyarginine peptides. Depending upon the CPP used, different internalization mechanisms are used to access the cytoplasm including direct transduction through the lipid bilayer as well as energy-dependent macropinocytosis [21]. Regardless of the mechanism for cell entry, these peptides may prove very useful in delivery of small DNAs and synthetic RNAs.

Physical methods of gene delivery, such as the gene gun, electroporation (electric fields), sonoporation (ultrasound) and hydrodynamic (high pressure) delivery can also facilitate delivery of DNA across the plasma membrane. The gene gun utilizes metal particles coated with plasmid DNA that are accelerated and bombard a tissue of interest [22]. This technique, however is limited by the superficial penetration of the DNA into the tissue and is therefore most successful for percutaneous delivery of DNA. Electroporation is a more versatile technique that has been used on a variety of tissues with success. During this process, a series of electrical pulses are delivered that result in destabilization of the cell membrane. Transient pores are then created which allow the passage of plasmid DNA into the cell. Blood vessels, skin, muscle, heart, liver, and lung have all been successfully transfected with electroporation [23-27]. Sonoporation has seen most success in soft tissues and it's use deep within the body is a major potential strength. This technique uses ultrasound to enhance cell permeability through acoustic cavitation and subsequent gene transfer through passive diffusion of DNA across pores in the cell membranes. A number of in vivo studies have demonstrated successful gene transfer in skeletal muscle, cardiac muscle, kidney, carotid artery, pancreas and liver of mice and rats [28-37]. Finally, hydrodynamic gene delivery is a highly efficient method for gene transfer to highly perfused organs such as the liver or muscle in peripheral limbs. A large volume of DNA injected into the tail vein of a mouse has been shown to result in transient membrane changes in hepatocytes, resulting in direct transfer of DNA into the cytoplasm [38, 39]. Like electroporation and sonoporation, pores within the plasma membrane are thought to be formed allowing entry of plasmids, in this case by the rapid change in hydrostatic pressure [40]. Modifications of this technique using balloon catheters in larger animals has suggested potential for ultimate success in humans as well [41-43].

While all of these approaches facilitate endocytosis or direct entry into the cytoplasm of any cell type, one of the goals of gene therapy is often cell-specific targeting. Thus, the development of delivery vehicles that only interact with specific cell types is highly desirable. In most cases, cell-specificity is acheived by specific interactions between ligands on the vector and receptors on the cell surface. For example, as many tumor cells overexpress receptors for nutrients, such as folate and transferrin, this phentoype has been exploited for the development of DNA and drug delivery vehicles carrying either folic acid or transferrin as ligands. Recently, a transferrin-PEG-PE conjugated cationic lipid carrier and a PEG-transferrin-PEI nanocomplex were developed, which exhibited increased transfection efficiency in vitro as well as in vivo [44, 45]. Similar results have been obtained using folate linked nanoparticles as well [46]. Delivery of DNA to specific cell types has also been achieved through the use of glycosylated carriers, specifically cationic liposomes [47]. Mannosylated and galactose conjugated liposomes have demonstrated efficacy as delivery agents for macrophages and hepatocytes [48, 49].

4. Vector release and cytoplasmic trafficking

Gene delivery vectors that utilize endocytosis to access the cytoplasm are then moved through the endocytic compartment. Thus, another major barrier to successful gene delivery is the release of the DNA from the endosome before it is degraded at the lysosomal level. There are several mechanisms employed to increase the likelihood of endosomal escape including membrane fusion, the proton-sponge effect and incorporation of fusogenic and pore-forming peptides.

Lipoplexes are able to escape the endosome through fusion of the liposome with the endosomal membrane. In particular, inclusion of dioleoylphosphatidylethanolamine (DOPE) has been shown to enhance endosomal escape due to its ability to transition from bilayer to inverted hexagonal structures [50, 51]. The instability of this type of structure increases fusion with endosomes and subsequently releases the DNA [52]. This is not common across all lipids as a similar phospholipid, dioleoylphosphatidylcholine (DOPC), does not exhibit similar activity [53, 54]. Therefore, complex structure plays an important role in enhancement of endosomal escape.

In contrast to lipoplexes, cationic polymers such as PEI achieve endosomal escape through a 'proton sponge' mechanism. PEI possesses a very high buffering capacity due to the presence of amino nitrogen at every third atom, which can be protonated within the acidifying endosomes. Consequently, an accumulation of protons causes an influx of chloride ions thereby resulting in osmotic swelling and lysis of the endosome. Therefore, use of cationic polymers with this type of buffering capacity increases the amount of time before passage of DNA to lysosomes, which therefore increases the likelihood of the DNA getting transferred to the cytoplasm.

Finally, many fusogenic and pore-forming peptides have been discovered and incorporated into gene delivery vehicles. The influenza-derived peptides GALA and KALA undergo pH-dependent conformational changes that result in disruption of endosomal membranes [55-58]. Several bacteria derived and animal derived peptides with membrane disruptive properties have also been developed and appear to increase endosomal escape and transfection efficiency [59].

Once DNA has successfully been released into the cytoplasm, it must then traffic to the nucleus in order for gene expression to occur. This step represents another significant barrier to gene delivery. First, the cytoplasm contains nucleases that will degrade free DNA. Studies have demonstrated that plasmid DNA is degraded in the cytoplasm of HeLa and COS cells with a half-life of 50 to 90 minutes [60]. This poses a big problem for delivery of naked DNA and DNA-lipid complexes that are believed to dissociate prior to nuclear entry. Additionally, the cytoplasm itself poses a diffusional barrier as well. The cytoplasm is a viscous environment crowded with molecules, which results in decreased mobility of macromolecules [61-63]. Thus, if DNA is released from an endosome at a distant site from the nucleus, the DNA cannot simply diffuse toward its desired location. This has been demonstrated in the case of liposome transfections where some DNA is left free in the cytoplasm and never reaches the nucleus [64, 65]. Although it has been shown that lipoplex-containing endosomes themselves traffic toward the nucleus and the interior of the cell, there is still quite a lot of distance for the free DNA following endosomal release to move before it reaches the nucleus. We and others have shown that DNA in the cytoplasm utilizes the microtubule network and the molecular motor, dynein [66-68] for its trafficking to the nucleus. Since DNA does not directly bind to dynein, the mechanism of this interaction was investigated and was found to involve a multiprotein complex that bridges the DNA and dynein. Our laboratory has shown that transcription factors are key proteins in this complex, and they are involved in the movement of DNA along microtubules [69]. Furthermore, the velocity of plasmid DNA movement can be increased through addition of specific transcription factor binding sites in the plasmid, such as CREB [69] or by inducing acetylation of the microtubules themselves [70]. The acetylation status is largely controlled by histone deacetylase 6 (HDAC6), and studies have shown that modulation of this enzyme can increase the efficiency of gene transfer [70]. Thus, despite the fact that the cytoplasm poses as a significant barrier to gene transfer, many techniques for overcoming this problem are being revealed.

5. Nuclear import

DNA that has successfully navigated all of the barriers previously discussed finally comes into contact with the nuclear envelope. However, depending upon cell type, DNA dose and detection method, only 1 to 10% of transfected plasmid can be found within the nucleus [71, 72]. This suggests that an overwhelming proportion of DNA that enters the cytoplasm will never successfully enter the nucleus. It has been appreciated for over 30 years that the nuclear envelope is a major barrier to DNA delivery [73]. Our laboratory has shown in microinjection experiments using non-dividing cells that 30 to 100 times more plasmid must be injected into the cytoplasm of a cell to equal levels of gene expression of plasmid injected directly into the nucleus [74]. While it is true that DNA delivery to the nucleus is greater within dividing cells, even breakdown of the nuclear envelope does not completely eliminate nuclear import as a barrier to transfer [75]. Therefore, studies aimed at understanding how DNA is imported into the nucleus as well as development of strategies to improve this process have been key to enhancing the efficiency of non-viral gene delivery.

A number of studies have shown that the vast majority of transfected DNA enters the nucleus during mitosis when the nuclear envelope has broken down [76, 77]. While plasmids can enter the nucleus in the absence of cell division, the process is slow and highly inefficient, resulting in very low levels of nuclear entry. However, our laboratory has shown that the delivery of plasmid DNA into the nucleus can be greatly increased by the addition of specific DNA sequences. We have demonstrated that plasmids containing only 72bp of the SV40 enhancer are able to target the nucleus of non-dividing cells within a few hours [78]. This sequence, termed a DNA nuclear targeting sequence (DTS), functions to enhance nuclear import in all cell types tested. It is the presence of ubiquitously expressed transcription factor binding sites within the SV40 DTS that mediate this effect. Since these transcription factors contain nuclear localization signals (NLS) to allow their targeting to the nucleus, nuclear import of the DNA is controlled by the interaction of these proteins with the NLS-receptors importin-α and importin-β, that then transport cargo through the nuclear pore complex (NPC). Thus, when NLS-containing transcription factors bind to the SV40 DTS on a plasmid, the plasmid utilizes this system to enter the nucleus [79, 80]. We have shown that these DTS sequences act not only in microinjected cells, but in transfected cells as well to increase DNA nuclear uptake and gene expression as well as in tissues in living animals [81-83].

We have also identified several cell-specific DTSs, in which nuclear import of a plasmid is regulated by the presence of cell-specific transcription factor binding sites within the DTS. DTSs specific for smooth muscle cells, osteoblasts, endothelial cells, alveolar epithelial type I cells and alveolar epithelial type II cells have been identified and large studies are underway to screen hundreds of DNA sequences for the potential to act as cell-specific DTSs [83-86]. In all of these cases, the cell-specific DTS contains binding sites for cell specific transcription factors that are expressed in unique cell types. Thus, if the plasmid is delivered to a cell that expresses those transcription factors, it will be transported into the nucleus and gene expression will ensue; if, however, the plasmid enters any other cell type that does not express the specific transcription factor, the DNA will remain in the cytoplasm until cell division or until it is degraded by cytoplasmic nucleases. Again, as for the SV40 DTS, these cell-specific DTSs work in cultured cells and in animal tissues to increase gene expression in a cell-restricted manner [83, 86].

A number of other methods for enhancing nuclear import have been studied, all of which center around exploiting the cells protein nuclear import machinery. These approaches include complexing plasmid DNA with NLS peptides, nuclear proteins or small molecule ligands. The success of NLS peptides has been variable, likely due to the fact that the NLS must be visible to the importin proteins for nuclear import to occur [87]. However, in vivo studies using DNA with conjugated NLS peptides have demonstrated increased gene expression in muscle as well as increased immune response against the expressed antigen [88]. Also, more recently, analysis of a bipartite NLS construct as a non-viral gene carrier has revealed the potential success of this type of method over traditional monopartite peptides [89]. Due to the varied success of NLS peptides at promotion of nuclear import, it is still unclear if this will be a promising approach for gene therapy.

As an alternative to NLS peptides, some work has tested direct conjugation of importins to plasmid DNA. The importin-β-binding domain of importin-α was covalently coupled to plasmid DNA, but this also failed to enhance nuclear import [90]. In a separate study, a plasmid DNA/importin-β conjugate was made via binding of biotinylated plasmid DNA and recombinant streptavidin-importin-β chimeric protein. While this did enhance nuclear import, gene expression was very low due to the highly modified plasmid [91].

6. Conclusion

To maximize non-viral gene delivery, levels of expression must be improved. Unfortunately, many extracellular and intracellular barriers (including the extracellular environment, immune scavengers, the cell membrane, endosomal escape, the cytoskeletal network and the nuclear membrane) preclude efficient gene transfer. In this review, we have focused on these barriers and various means to overcome them. The goal of all gene therapy approaches is to target enough DNA to the nuclei of cells to obtain sufficient expression for a therapeutic effect. By characterizing and understanding these barriers, we can overcome our relative inability to target substantial amounts of DNA to the nucleus and increase transfection efficiency and ultimately gene therapy.

Author details

Lynn F. Gottfried and David A. Dean

Department of Pediatrics, University of Rochester Medical Center, Rochester, NY, USA

References

[1] Houk, B. E, Hochhaus, G, & Hughes, J. A. Kinetic modeling of plasmid DNA degradation in rat plasma. AAPS PharmSci. (1999). E9.

[2] Mumper, R. J, Duguid, J. G, Anwer, K, Barron, M. K, Nitta, H, & Rolland, A. P. Polyvinyl derivatives as novel interactive polymers for controlled gene delivery to muscle. Pharm Res. (1996). May;, 13(5), 701-9.

[3] Sternberg, B, Hong, K, Zheng, W, & Papahadjopoulos, D. Ultrastructural characterization of cationic liposome-DNA complexes showing enhanced stability in serum and high transfection activity in vivo. Biochim Biophys Acta. (1998). Oct 15;1375(1-2):23-35.

[4] Cullis, P. R, Chonn, A, & Semple, S. C. Interactions of liposomes and lipid-based carrier systems with blood proteins: Relation to clearance behaviour in vivo. Adv Drug Deliv Rev. (1998). Jun 8;32(1-2):3-17.

[5] Sakurai, F, Nishioka, T, Saito, H, Baba, T, Okuda, A, Matsumoto, O, et al. Interaction between DNA-cationic liposome complexes and erythrocytes is an important factor in systemic gene transfer via the intravenous route in mice: the role of the neutral helper lipid. Gene Ther. (2001). May;, 8(9), 677-86.

[6] Mccray, P. B. Jr., Wang G, Kline JN, Zabner J, Chada S, Jolly DJ, et al. Alveolar macrophages inhibit retrovirus-mediated gene transfer to airway epithelia. Hum Gene Ther. (1997). Jun 10;, 8(9), 1087-93.

[7] Dow, S. W, Fradkin, L. G, Liggitt, D. H, Willson, A. P, Heath, T. D, & Potter, T. A. Lipid-DNA complexes induce potent activation of innate immune responses and antitumor activity when administered intravenously. J Immunol. (1999). Aug 1;, 163(3), 1552-61.

[8] Zhao, H, Hemmi, H, Akira, S, Cheng, S. H, Scheule, R. K, & Yew, N. S. Contribution of Toll-like receptor 9 signaling to the acute inflammatory response to nonviral vectors. Mol Ther. (2004). Feb;, 9(2), 241-8.

[9] Yasuda, K, Ogawa, Y, Yamane, I, Nishikawa, M, & Takakura, Y. Macrophage activation by a DNA/cationic liposome complex requires endosomal acidification and TLR9-dependent and-independent pathways. J Leukoc Biol. (2005). Jan;, 77(1), 71-9.

[10] Hyde, S. C, Pringle, I. A, Abdullah, S, Lawton, A. E, Davies, L. A, Varathalingam, A, et al. CpG-free plasmids confer reduced inflammation and sustained pulmonary gene expression. Nat Biotechnol. (2008). May;, 26(5), 549-51.

[11] Regnstrom, K, Ragnarsson, E. G, Koping-hoggard, M, Torstensson, E, Nyblom, H, & Artursson, P. PEI- a potent, but not harmless, mucosal immuno-stimulator of mixed T-helper cell response and FasL-mediated cell death in mice. Gene Ther. (2003). Sep;, 10(18), 1575-83.

[12] Dams, E. T, Laverman, P, Oyen, W. J, Storm, G, Scherphof, G. L, Van Der Meer, J. W, et al. Accelerated blood clearance and altered biodistribution of repeated injections of sterically stabilized liposomes. J Pharmacol Exp Ther. (2000). Mar;, 292(3), 1071-9.

[13] Laverman, P, Carstens, M. G, Boerman, O. C, Dams, E. T, Oyen, W. J, Van Rooijen, N, et al. Factors affecting the accelerated blood clearance of polyethylene glycol-liposomes upon repeated injection. J Pharmacol Exp Ther. (2001). Aug;, 298(2), 607-12.

[14] Semple, S. C, Harasym, T. O, Clow, K. A, Ansell, S. M, Klimuk, S. K, & Hope, M. J. Immunogenicity and rapid blood clearance of liposomes containing polyethylene glycol-lipid conjugates and nucleic Acid. J Pharmacol Exp Ther. (2005). Mar;, 312(3), 1020-6.

[15] Ishida, T, Ichihara, M, Wang, X, Yamamoto, K, Kimura, J, Majima, E, et al. Injection of PEGylated liposomes in rats elicits PEG-specific IgM, which is responsible for rapid elimination of a second dose of PEGylated liposomes. J Control Release. (2006). May 1;, 112(1), 15-25.

[16] Ishida, T, Wang, X, Shimizu, T, Nawata, K, & Kiwada, H. PEGylated liposomes elicit an anti-PEG IgM response in a T cell-independent manner. J Control Release. (2007). Oct 8;, 122(3), 349-55.

[17] Wang, X, Ishida, T, & Kiwada, H. Anti-PEG IgM elicited by injection of liposomes is involved in the enhanced blood clearance of a subsequent dose of PEGylated liposomes. J Control Release. (2007). Jun 4;, 119(2), 236-44.

[18] Thoren, P. E, Persson, D, Isakson, P, Goksor, M, Onfelt, A, & Norden, B. Uptake of analogs of penetratin, Tat(48-60) and oligoarginine in live cells. Biochem Biophys Res Commun. (2003). Jul 18,, 307(1), 100-7.

[19] Vives, E, Brodin, P, & Lebleu, B. A truncated HIV-1 Tat protein basic domain rapidly translocates through the plasma membrane and accumulates in the cell nucleus. J Biol Chem. (1997). Jun 20;, 272(25), 16010-7.

[20] Luedtke, N. W, Carmichael, P, & Tor, Y. Cellular uptake of aminoglycosides, guanidinoglycosides, and poly-arginine. J Am Chem Soc. (2003). Oct 15;, 125(41), 12374-5.

[21] Raagel, H, Saalik, P, & Pooga, M. Peptide-mediated protein delivery-which pathways are penetrable? Biochim Biophys Acta. Dec;(2240). , 1798(12), 2240-8.

[22] Yang, N. S, Burkholder, J, Roberts, B, Martinell, B, & Mccabe, D. In vivo and in vitro gene transfer to mammalian somatic cells by particle bombardment. Proc Natl Acad Sci U S A. (1990). Dec;, 87(24), 9568-72.

[23] Heller, R, Jaroszeski, M, Atkin, A, Moradpour, D, Gilbert, R, Wands, J, et al. In vivo gene electroinjection and expression in rat liver. FEBS Lett. (1996). Jul 8;, 389(3), 225-8.

[24] Heller, R, Schultz, J, Lucas, M. L, Jaroszeski, M. J, Heller, L. C, Gilbert, R. A, et al. Intradermal delivery of interleukin-12 plasmid DNA by in vivo electroporation. DNA Cell Biol. (2001). Jan;, 20(1), 21-6.

[25] Hargrave, B, Downey, H, & Strange, R. Jr., Murray L, Cinnamond C, Lundberg C, et al. Electroporation-mediated gene transfer directly to the swine heart. Gene Ther. Mar 29.

[26] Dean, D. A, Machado-aranda, D, Blair-parks, K, Yeldandi, A. V, & Young, J. L. Electroporation as a method for high-level nonviral gene transfer to the lung. Gene Ther. (2003). Sep;, 10(18), 1608-15.

[27] Mir, L. M, Bureau, M. F, Gehl, J, Rangara, R, Rouy, D, Caillaud, J. M, et al. High-efficiency gene transfer into skeletal muscle mediated by electric pulses. Proc Natl Acad Sci U S A. (1999). Apr 13;, 96(8), 4262-7.

[28] Akowuah, E. F, Gray, C, Lawrie, A, Sheridan, P. J, Su, C. H, Bettinger, T, et al. Ultrasound-mediated delivery of TIMP-3 plasmid DNA into saphenous vein leads to increased lumen size in a porcine interposition graft model. Gene Ther. (2005). Jul;, 12(14), 1154-7.

[29] Pislaru, S. V, Pislaru, C, Kinnick, R. R, Singh, R, Gulati, R, Greenleaf, J. F, et al. Optimization of ultrasound-mediated gene transfer: comparison of contrast agents and ultrasound modalities. Eur Heart J. (2003). Sep;, 24(18), 1690-8.

[30] Guo, D. P, Li, X. Y, Sun, P, Tang, Y. B, Chen, X. Y, Chen, Q, et al. Ultrasound-targeted microbubble destruction improves the low density lipoprotein receptor gene expression in HepG2 cells. Biochem Biophys Res Commun. (2006). May 5;, 343(2), 470-4.

[31] Sakakima, Y, Hayashi, S, Yagi, Y, Hayakawa, A, Tachibana, K, & Nakao, A. Gene therapy for hepatocellular carcinoma using sonoporation enhanced by contrast agents. Cancer Gene Ther. (2005). Nov;, 12(11), 884-9.

[32] Azuma, H, Tomita, N, Kaneda, Y, Koike, H, Ogihara, T, Katsuoka, Y, et al. Transfection of NFkappaB-decoy oligodeoxynucleotides using efficient ultrasound-mediated gene transfer into donor kidneys prolonged survival of rat renal allografts. Gene Ther. (2003). Mar;, 10(5), 415-25.

[33] Chen, S, Shohet, R. V, Bekeredjian, R, Frenkel, P, & Grayburn, P. A. Optimization of ultrasound parameters for cardiac gene delivery of adenoviral or plasmid deoxyribonucleic acid by ultrasound-targeted microbubble destruction. J Am Coll Cardiol. (2003). Jul 16;, 42(2), 301-8.

[34] Kondo, I, Ohmori, K, Oshita, A, Takeuchi, H, Fuke, S, Shinomiya, K, et al. Treatment of acute myocardial infarction by hepatocyte growth factor gene transfer: the first demonstration of myocardial transfer of a "functional" gene using ultrasonic microbubble destruction. J Am Coll Cardiol. (2004). Aug 4;, 44(3), 644-53.

[35] Zhigang, W, Zhiyu, L, Haitao, R, Hong, R, Qunxia, Z, Ailong, H, et al. Ultrasound-mediated microbubble destruction enhances VEGF gene delivery to the infarcted myocardium in rats. Clin Imaging. (2004). Nov-Dec;, 28(6), 395-8.

[36] Chen, S, Ding, J. H, Bekeredjian, R, Yang, B. Z, Shohet, R. V, Johnston, S. A, et al. Efficient gene delivery to pancreatic islets with ultrasonic microbubble destruction technology. Proc Natl Acad Sci U S A. (2006). May 30;, 103(22), 8469-74.

[37] Miao, C. H, Brayman, A. A, Loeb, K. R, Ye, P, Zhou, L, Mourad, P, et al. Ultrasound enhances gene delivery of human factor IX plasmid. Hum Gene Ther. (2005). Jul;, 16(7), 893-905.

[38] Liu, F, Song, Y, & Liu, D. Hydrodynamics-based transfection in animals by systemic administration of plasmid DNA. Gene Ther. (1999). Jul;, 6(7), 1258-66.

[39] Zhang, G, Budker, V, & Wolff, J. A. High levels of foreign gene expression in hepatocytes after tail vein injections of naked plasmid DNA. Hum Gene Ther. (1999). Jul 1;, 10(10), 1735-7.

[40] Zhang, G, Gao, X, Song, Y. K, Vollmer, R, Stolz, D. B, Gasiorowski, J. Z, et al. Hydroporation as the mechanism of hydrodynamic delivery. Gene Ther. (2004). Apr;, 11(8), 675-82.

[41] Eastman, S. J, Baskin, K. M, Hodges, B. L, Chu, Q, Gates, A, Dreusicke, R, et al. Development of catheter-based procedures for transducing the isolated rabbit liver with plasmid DNA. Hum Gene Ther. (2002). Nov 20;, 13(17), 2065-77.

[42] Alino, S. F, Herrero, M. J, Noguera, I, Dasi, F, & Sanchez, M. Pig liver gene therapy by noninvasive interventionist catheterism. Gene Ther. (2007). Feb;, 14(4), 334-43.

[43] Yoshino, H, Hashizume, K, & Kobayashi, E. Naked plasmid DNA transfer to the porcine liver using rapid injection with large volume. Gene Ther. (2006). Dec;, 13(24), 1696-702.

[44] Wang, W, Zhou, F, Ge, L, Liu, X, & Kong, F. Transferrin-PEG-PE modified dexamethasone conjugated cationic lipid carrier mediated gene delivery system for tumor-targeted transfection. Int J Nanomedicine., 7, 2513-22.

[45] Lee, K. M, Lee, Y. B, & Oh, I. J. Evaluation of PEG-transferrin-PEI nanocomplex as a gene delivery agent. J Nanosci Nanotechnol. Aug;, 11(8), 7078-81.

[46] Hofland, H. E, Masson, C, Iginla, S, Osetinsky, I, Reddy, J. A, Leamon, C. P, et al. Folate-targeted gene transfer in vivo. Mol Ther. (2002). Jun;, 5(6), 739-44.

[47] Hashida, M, Nishikawa, M, Yamashita, F, & Takakura, Y. Cell-specific delivery of genes with glycosylated carriers. Adv Drug Deliv Rev. (2001). Nov 19;, 52(3), 187-96.

[48] Irache, J. M, Salman, H. H, Gamazo, C, & Espuelas, S. Mannose-targeted systems for the delivery of therapeutics. Expert Opin Drug Deliv. (2008). Jun;, 5(6), 703-24.

[49] Wu, J, Nantz, M. H, & Zern, M. A. Targeting hepatocytes for drug and gene delivery: emerging novel approaches and applications. Front Biosci. (2002). Mar 1;7:d, 717-25.

[50] Koltover, I, Salditt, T, Radler, J. O, & Safinya, C. R. An inverted hexagonal phase of cationic liposome-DNA complexes related to DNA release and delivery. Science. (1998). Jul 3;, 281(5373), 78-81.

[51] Allen, T. M, Hong, K, & Papahadjopoulos, D. Membrane contact, fusion, and hexagonal (HII) transitions in phosphatidylethanolamine liposomes. Biochemistry. (1990). Mar 27;, 29(12), 2976-85.

[52] Noguchi, A, Furuno, T, Kawaura, C, & Nakanishi, M. Membrane fusion plays an important role in gene transfection mediated by cationic liposomes. FEBS Lett. (1998). Aug 14;433(1-2):169-73.

[53] Farhood, H, Serbina, N, & Huang, L. The role of dioleoyl phosphatidylethanolamine in cationic liposome mediated gene transfer. Biochim Biophys Acta. (1995). May 4;, 1235(2), 289-95.

[54] Mok, K. W, & Cullis, P. R. Structural and fusogenic properties of cationic liposomes in the presence of plasmid DNA. Biophys J. (1997). Nov;, 73(5), 2534-45.

[55] Wyman, T. B, Nicol, F, Zelphati, O, Scaria, P. V, Plank, C, & Szoka, F. C. Jr. Design, synthesis, and characterization of a cationic peptide that binds to nucleic acids and permeabilizes bilayers. Biochemistry. (1997). Mar 11;, 36(10), 3008-17.

[56] Lee, H, Jeong, J. H, & Park, T. G. A new gene delivery formulation of polyethylenimine/ DNA complexes coated with PEG conjugated fusogenic peptide. J Control Release. (2001). Sep 11;76(1-2):183-92.

[57] Min, S. H, Lee, D. C, Lim, M. J, Park, H. S, Kim, D. M, Cho, C. W, et al. A composite gene delivery system consisting of polyethylenimine and an amphipathic peptide KALA. J Gene Med. (2006). Dec;, 8(12), 1425-34.

[58] Parente, R. A, Nir, S, & Szoka, F. C. Jr. Mechanism of leakage of phospholipid vesicle contents induced by the peptide GALA. Biochemistry. (1990). Sep 18;, 29(37), 8720-8.

[59] Varkouhi, A. K, Scholte, M, Storm, G, & Haisma, H. J. Endosomal escape pathways for delivery of biologicals. J Control Release. May 10;, 151(3), 220-8.

[60] Lechardeur, D, Sohn, K. J, Haardt, M, Joshi, P. B, Monck, M, Graham, R. W, et al. Metabolic instability of plasmid DNA in the cytosol: a potential barrier to gene transfer. Gene Ther. (1999). Apr;, 6(4), 482-97.

[61] Kao, H. P, Abney, J. R, & Verkman, A. S. Determinants of the translational mobility of a small solute in cell cytoplasm. J Cell Biol. (1993). Jan;, 120(1), 175-84.

[62] Lukacs, G. L, Haggie, P, Seksek, O, Lechardeur, D, Freedman, N, & Verkman, A. S. Size-dependent DNA mobility in cytoplasm and nucleus. J Biol Chem. (2000). Jan 21;, 275(3), 1625-9.

[63] Dauty, E, & Verkman, A. S. Actin cytoskeleton as the principal determinant of size-dependent DNA mobility in cytoplasm: a new barrier for non-viral gene delivery. J Biol Chem. (2005). Mar 4;, 280(9), 7823-8.

[64] Gao, X, & Huang, L. Cytoplasmic expression of a reporter gene by co-delivery of T7 RNA polymerase and T7 promoter sequence with cationic liposomes. Nucleic Acids Res. (1993). Jun 25;, 21(12), 2867-72.

[65] Zabner, J, Fasbender, A. J, Moninger, T, Poellinger, K. A, & Welsh, M. J. Cellular and molecular barriers to gene transfer by a cationic lipid. J Biol Chem. (1995). Aug 11;, 270(32), 18997-9007.

[66] Mesika, A, Kiss, V, Brumfeld, V, Ghosh, G, & Reich, Z. Enhanced intracellular mobility and nuclear accumulation of DNA plasmids associated with a karyophilic protein. Hum Gene Ther. (2005). Feb;, 16(2), 200-8.

[67] Vaughan, E. E, & Dean, D. A. Intracellular trafficking of plasmids during transfection is mediated by microtubules. Mol Ther. (2006). Feb;, 13(2), 422-8.

[68] Salman, H, Abu-arish, A, Oliel, S, Loyter, A, Klafter, J, Granek, R, et al. Nuclear localization signal peptides induce molecular delivery along microtubules. Biophys J. (2005). Sep;, 89(3), 2134-45.

[69] Badding, M. A, Vaughan, E. E, & Dean, D. A. Transcription factor plasmid binding modulates microtubule interactions and intracellular trafficking during gene transfer. Gene Ther. Mar;, 19(3), 338-46.

[70] Vaughan, E. E, Geiger, R. C, Miller, A. M, Loh-marley, P. L, Suzuki, T, Miyata, N, et al. Microtubule acetylation through HDAC6 inhibition results in increased transfection efficiency. Mol Ther. (2008). Nov;, 16(11), 1841-7.

[71] Cohen, R. N, Van Der Aa, M. A, Macaraeg, N, Lee, A. P, & Szoka, F. C. Jr. Quantification of plasmid DNA copies in the nucleus after lipoplex and polyplex transfection. J Control Release. (2009). Apr 17;, 135(2), 166-74.

[72] Glover, D. J, Leyton, D. L, Moseley, G. W, & Jans, D. A. The efficiency of nuclear plasmid DNA delivery is a critical determinant of transgene expression at the single cell level. J Gene Med. Jan;, 12(1), 77-85.

[73] Cappechi, M. R. High efficiency transformation by direct microinjection of DNA into cultured mammalian cells. Cell. (1980). , 22, 479-88.

[74] Dean, D. A, Dean, B. S, Muller, S, & Smith, L. C. Sequence requirements for plasmid nuclear import. Exp Cell Res. (1999). Dec 15;, 253(2), 713-22.

[75] Ludtke, J. J, Sebestyen, M. G, & Wolff, J. A. The effect of cell division on the cellular dynamics of microinjected DNA and dextran. Mol Ther. (2002). May;5(5 Pt 1):579-88.

[76] Tseng, W. C, Haselton, F. R, & Giorgio, T. D. Transfection by cationic liposomes using simultaneous single cell measurements of plasmid delivery and transgene expression. J Biol Chem. (1997). Oct 10;, 272(41), 25641-7.

[77] Brunner, S, Sauer, T, Carotta, S, Cotten, M, Saltik, M, & Wagner, E. Cell cycle dependence of gene transfer by lipoplex, polyplex and recombinant adenovirus. Gene Ther. (2000). Mar;, 7(5), 401-7.

[78] Dean, D. A. Import of plasmid DNA into the nucleus is sequence specific. Exp Cell Res. (1997). Feb 1;, 230(2), 293-302.

[79] Wilson, G. L, Dean, B. S, Wang, G, & Dean, D. A. Nuclear import of plasmid DNA in digitonin-permeabilized cells requires both cytoplasmic factors and specific DNA sequences. J Biol Chem. (1999). Jul 30;, 274(31), 22025-32.

[80] Miller, A. M, Munkonge, F. M, Alton, E. W, & Dean, D. A. Identification of protein cofactors necessary for sequence-specific plasmid DNA nuclear import. Mol Ther. (2009). Nov;, 17(11), 1897-903.

[81] Vacik, J, Dean, B. S, Zimmer, W. E, & Dean, D. A. Cell-specific nuclear import of plasmid DNA. Gene Ther. (1999). Jun;, 6(6), 1006-14.

[82] Young, J. L, Benoit, J. N, & Dean, D. A. Effect of a DNA nuclear targeting sequence on gene transfer and expression of plasmids in the intact vasculature. Gene Ther. (2003). Aug;, 10(17), 1465-70.

[83] Young, J. L, Zimmer, W. E, & Dean, D. A. Smooth muscle-specific gene delivery in the vasculature based on restriction of DNA nuclear import. Exp Biol Med (Maywood). (2008). Jul;, 233(7), 840-8.

[84] Miller, A. M, & Dean, D. A. Tissue-specific and transcription factor-mediated nuclear entry of DNA. Adv Drug Deliv Rev. (2009). Jul 2;61(7-8):603-13.

[85] Miller, A. M, & Dean, D. A. Cell-specific nuclear import of plasmid DNA in smooth muscle requires tissue-specific transcription factors and DNA sequences. Gene Ther. (2008). Aug;, 15(15), 1107-15.

[86] Degiulio, J. V, Kaufman, C. D, & Dean, D. A. The SP-C promoter facilitates alveolar type II epithelial cell-specific plasmid nuclear import and gene expression. Gene Ther. Apr;, 17(4), 541-9.

[87] Sebestyen, M. G, Ludtke, J. J, Bassik, M. C, Zhang, G, Budker, V, Lukhtanov, E. A, et al. DNA vector chemistry: the covalent attachment of signal peptides to plasmid DNA. Nat Biotechnol. (1998). Jan;, 16(1), 80-5.

[88] (Choi Y, Jeon YH, Kang JH, Chung JK, Schmidt M, Kim AC. MIDGE/hNIS vaccination generates antigen-associated CD8+IFN-gamma+ T cells and enhances protective antitumor immunity. Int J Cancer. 2007 May 1;120(9):1942-50). 120(9), 1942-50.

[89] Matschke, J, Bohla, A, Maucksch, C, Mittal, R, Rudolph, C, & Rosenecker, J. Characterization of KuNLS as bipartite nuclear localization sequence for non-viral gene delivery. PLoS One.7(2):e24615., 70(2)

[90] Carriere, M, Escriou, V, Savarin, A, & Scherman, D. Coupling of importin beta binding peptide on plasmid DNA: transfection efficiency is increased by modification of lipoplex's physico-chemical properties. BMC Biotechnol. (2003). Sep 12;3:14.

[91] Nagasaki, T, Kawazu, T, Tachibana, T, Tamagaki, S, & Shinkai, S. Enhanced nuclear import and transfection efficiency of plasmid DNA using streptavidin-fused importin-beta. J Control Release. (2005). Mar 2;, 103(1), 199-207.

Chapter 4

Electrically Mediated Gene Delivery : Basic and Translational Concepts

J. Teissié

Additional information is available at the end of the chapter

1. Introduction

Naked plasmid (pDNA) electrotransfer is an approach for gene transfer that is very efficient for in vitro studies since its introduction in 1982. It was extended for a use in vivo in a perspective for clinical gene therapy.

This chapter is a review on the state of the art. The molecular processes bringing the pDNA transfer and expression will be described. A critical view of the barriers preventing an efficient level of expression is given. This gives the tools to design the relevant protocols for the use on animals and the potential clinical trials.

Delivery of naked plasmids (pDNA) in tissue to obtain gene expression was facing the limit of a poor level of expression [1]. But the clinical advantage was that it was a safe approach for the patient. Improvement of the delivery and the resulting expression was known to be obtained at the cellular level by applying electric field pulses to the cell-pDNA mixture [2]. It was shown that this boost in expression could be obtained on tissues [3]. During the last 15 years, many developments in this approach have been performed and Electrotransfection is now considered as a perspective for gene therapies [4-9]. A Phase I clinical trial using gene therapy by electrically mediated delivery has been performed (www.clinicaltrials.gov identifier NCT00323206)[10]. More recent data showed that the delivery and expression can be obtained on very sensitive organs [11-13]. Electropulsation mediated gene delivery appears now to be one of the effective contributors for the success of gene therapy

2. Basic processes

2.1. Electropermeabilization

Biological membrane cohesion is known for almost 40 years to be affected by external electric field pulses [14]. A transient and reversible membrane permeabilization (Electropermeabilization) results from a controlled application of electric pulses to cells [15]. This can be induced not only in vitro but on living tissues as well. The key feature is that the structural transition is obtained only when the external field is larger than a critical value. A physical targeting of the effect is therefore present in tissues. This improves the safety of the approach as only a limited volume of the tissue is affected. This metastable membrane structural organization remains poorly understood. New properties are brought to the cell plasma membrane that, besides being permeabilized, becomes fusogenic and allows exogenous proteins to be inserted in it. Electropermeabilization is used to introduce a large variety of molecules into many different cells *in vitro* [16, 17]. The molecular transports, that result, are either due to an electrophoretic drift or/and to a concentration driven diffusion [18, 19]. The practical use for drug delivery remains rather empirical but results from more than 20 years of trials. Clinical applications of the method are now routinely used in many oncology centers (more than 100 in Europe only) as results from the EU funded Cliniporator and ESOPE programs. A local antitumoral drug delivery to patients (electrochemotherapy) results from the direct application of electric pulses to the patient [20-27]. In Europe, the treatment has been approved and patients can be reimbursed,

2.2. Electrotransfection

The most frequent application of electric field induced membrane permeabilization is the transfer and expression of gene into mammalian cells. Plasmid DNA (pDNA) can be transferred and expressed in mammalian cells when electropermeabilization is triggered [2]. This a complex process that involves not only the transport of pDNA into the cytoplasm, but also depends on subsequent cellular processes [27]. The transfer of naked DNA plasmid and the expression of the gene of interest are enhanced by electropulsation into different tissues, including the skeletal muscle [28, 29], liver [3,30], skin [31, 32], lungs [33] and tumors [34, 35]. The transfection efficiency of this physical method *in vivo* must still be improved compared to the viral vectors. But it is obtained with naked pDNA avoiding the biological risks associated to the viral methods. Furthermore there is no theoretical restriction on the size of the pDNA to transfer. As a result, due to its easiness to perform, to the very fast expression after electric pulse delivery, reproducibility, limited costs (of the technology and logistics) and safety, gene electrotransfer is an attractive technology of gene therapy for clinical application. This is well illustrated by the increasing number of reviews covering the pre-clinical developments of the approach [4-9, 36].

As mentioned above, one of main limits of the widespread use of electropermeabilization is that very few is known on the biophysical mechanisms supporting the reorganization of the cell membrane (pore, electropore, defects?). The molecular target of the field effect remains unclear [15]. The other main limit in gene electrotransfer is that the transport is not only across the plasma membrane but must target the nucleus volume.

The present review focuses on the processes supporting gene electrotransfer in vitro and their implications for the clinical applications. The events occurring before, during, after pulse application leading to gene electrotransfer will be described. Theoretical considerations about membrane structures involved in the plasmid uptake will be described in a (very) critical manner as very few direct experimental data are available.

3. Theories of DNA plasmid electroentry

Although the first pioneering report on gene electrotransfer in cells was published 30 years ago by E. Neumann, the molecular basis behind the process of gene electrotransfer is still highly debated.

3.1. The sliding model

Most theories are based on the DNA sliding model [37]. Several steps are predicted: entry, electrophoretic translocation as long as the field was present, diffusion after the pulse delivery. An interesting simulation with predictive conclusions has just been published [38]. The DNA translocation was through a putative "electropore" assuming that the DNA was double stranded but linear (i.e open) meaning that the length was 2.4 μm. Indeed the sliding model needs the DNA to be linear to allow the "binding" of one end to the "electropore" entry. Experimental results just showed that the closed form was more effective for expression [39]. One speculative hypothesis in the simulation was that it always assumed that the binding step (entry) of the DNA to the "electropore" was present before the simulation started. De Gennes predicted that it was a very limiting step in the process (a crucial moment) when a chain end faces the electropore and enters it against the strong friction coefficient against the "pore" sides. A black box remains the "electropore".

3.2. The electropore

The major hypothesis in the sliding model is that "pores" must be present. Krassowska's model supports the simplest mechanism, in which plasmid enters the 5 nm thick membrane through stable electropores (up to 20 nm in diameter)[40, 41]. The electrically induced defects result from the field associated membrane potential changes. It predicts a post-pulse growth of "macropores" on the sub-second time scale fairly consistent with experimental evidence on pure lipid vesicles [42]. This model predicts "electropores" large enough to permit the plasmid uptake (under a linear form). These "electropores" are supposed to remain open for the entire duration of electrotransfer providing adequate time for the plasmid to enter the cell [43]. Indeed in Lin's simulation [38], they may remain present on a much longer duration than the pulse as a diffusion might follow a partial electrotransfer.

This model remains very attractive in spite of the existence of many experimental contradictions. Indeed, until now, no study made it possible to visualize these membrane pores. This validation appears impossible [27]. Moreover, the resealing time of pores appears to be shorter in this lipidic model than in experiments on cells (e.g. seconds rather than minutes) [44-47]. The conclusion is that pDNA transport across the membrane is always very fast. To date, theoretical models could predict stable pores of only a few nanometers in radius; larger pores are unstable while they are needed for the sliding pDNA transfer [48, 49]. These models are confirmed by some experiments, in which high-voltage pulses a few microseconds long are used that are supposed to have created a large number of very small pores (radii of about 1 nm, i.e. the size of a few phospholipids cluster) [50]. To reconcile these results with the experimental evidence of plasmid translocation after electropulsation, some researchers postulated that plasmid entry into cells relies on the plasmid/membrane interactions, which may be facilitated by a coalescence of many small, 1 nm defects [51-54, 43]. The slow transport of DNA across the electropermeabilized membrane reflects a highly interactive electrotransfer, where many small lipid defects coalesced into large DNA-lipids assemblies where the transmembrane transport occurs [55].

3.3. Electrophoresis across the micellar structures

Other data report that gene electrotransfer through lipid bilayer could be mediated by transient complexes between plasmid and specific lipids in the edges of elongated, electropercolated hydrophilic membrane associated micellar structures [56]. The plasmid association with a lipid bilayer results in a facilitated transport of small ions. A locally conductive plasmid/lipid interaction zone is induced where parts of the plasmid may be inserted in the bilayer. Plasmid is transiently inserted in, and then electrophoretically pulled through the permeabilized zones onto the other membrane side [57]. With such a model, in the case of mammalian cells, the resting potential difference should be the driving force for plasmid translocation after the pulse induced insertion. The external field is only used to electrophoretically accumulate the pDNA on the cell surface. This has not been checked yet.

3.4. An electrophoretic transfer

Previous works suggested that electric pulses induce the membrane permeabilization, then plasmid molecules are concentrated near the membrane surface and pushed through by electrophoretic forces [58-60, 54]. The plasmid may interact with electropermeabilized membrane by three possible ways: (a) the plasmid coil is aligned in an electric field, and at the appropriate pulse polarity it moves toward the permeabilized membrane. Transfer is dependent on electrophoretic forces and is complete at the end of the pulse. Post pulse cell treatment should not affect the efficiency of transfer.

If the electrophoretic forces are the only driving forces of the plasmid transfer into the cell, similar transfection efficiencies should be obtained for equal E.T values (i.e. E, field strength and T, pulse duration). This is not supported by the experiments [61] When the E.N.T value is constant, transfection rate depends preferentially on T [52]. Therefore, the electrophoretic migration cannot be the only driving force of the plasmid transfer into the cells but clearly supports the formation of aggregates. Trypsin treatment of cells at 10 min post electrotransfection stripped off membrane-bound pDNA and resulted in a significant reduction in transfection, indicating that the time period for complete cellular uptake of pDNA (between 10 and 40 min) far exceeded the lifetime of electric field-induced transient pores (10 msec) in the cell membrane [62]. In addition, in the case of CHO cells, plasmid remains accessible to DNAase I in the minute, which follows the end of electropulsation. This shows that the plasmid transfer inside the cell occurs after the electropulsation [17].

3.5. In silico electrotransfer

A molecular dynamic approach gives a mechanism, in which plasmids do not translocate across the membrane during the electropulsation [63]. The DNA/lipid system simulation was undertaken starting from a well-equilibrated 12bp-DNA duplex placed near a model POPC bilayer. The perturbation of the system under a 1.0 V.nm^{-1} transverse electric field (i.e. a transmembrane voltage of 5 V !) is followed during 2 ns. Under this high electric field, the DNA duplex diffuses towards the interior of the bilayer only after the creation of a pore beneath it, and within the same timescale, it remains at the interfacial region when no pore is present. Diffusion of the strand toward the interior of the membrane leads to a DNA/lipid complex in which the lipid head groups encapsulate the strand. The dipole carried by the zwitterionic phosphatidylcholine groups of the lipids is known to be efficient for neutralizing the charges carried by the DNA [64]. Such interactions between the plasmid and the lipids contribute to the effective screening of DNA charges and therefore to the stabilization of the complex. One should not forget that electropulsation-mediated gene delivery concerns much larger super-coiled plasmids than the 12 bp construct considered in the MD simulation.

3.6. Endocytosis

Most methods for chemically mediated gene transfer described the transport as an endocytotic complex formation between the DNA vesicles and the cell surface. Several studies investigated if this can occur in electrotransfection. Treatment of cells with three endocytic inhibitors (chlorpromazine, genistein, dynasore) yielded substantial and statistically significant reductions in the electrotransfection mediated expression [62]. These findings suggest that electro-transfection depends on endocytosis of membrane-bound pDNA. [65]. Colocalization studies with endocytotic markers under a microscope showed that pDNA is internalized with concomitant clathrin- and caveolin/raft-mediated endocytosis [66]. But this cannot explain how the pDNA is released from the endocytic vesicles and why free PDNA was observed in the cytoplasm a few minutes after the pulse delivery [67]. A direct assay of the formation of endocytic vesicles brought the conclusion that endocytosis was not stimulated by applying electric pulses with intensities above the threshold value for gene electrotransfer. The conclusion was that electro-endocytosis is not a crucial mechanism for gene electrotransfer [68].

3.7. The multistep model

PDNA electrotransfer was observed at the single cell level by digitized high resolution fluorescence microscopy [67]. The introduction of DNA only occurs in the part of the membrane facing the cathode and requires a number of consecutive steps: electrophoretic migration of DNA towards the cell, DNA insertion into the membrane, translocation across the membrane, migration of DNA towards the nucleus and, finally, transfer of DNA across the nuclear envelope. Only localized parts of the cell membrane brought to the permeabilized state are competent for transfer. The transport of plasmid follows an "anchoring step", connecting the plasmid to the permeabilized membrane, that takes place during the pulse. During the first pulsation, plasmids are electrophoretically drifted and interact with a limited number of sites on the membrane. These sites become highly conductive and attract the field lines giving an electrophoretic local accumulation [69]. PDNAs form a limited number of aggregates on the cell surface. Their sizes increase during the pulses or with successive pulses but not their number [70]. Transfer of membrane bound plasmids is certainly a complex process, that is not occurring during but after the pulse delivery. Two classes of DNA/membrane interactions result from the pulse: (i) a metastable DNA/membrane complex from which the DNA can leave and return to external medium and (ii) a stable DNA/membrane. Only DNA belonging to the second class may be effective for transmembrane transport and the resulting gene expression [71]. Nevertheless this model shows that the plasmid is stabilized in the millisecond following the pulse in the membrane core after electropulsation (in agreement with the overall experimentally observed process of DNA translocation).

4. The cytoplasmic transfer

Transfer from the membrane to the nucleus is mediated by the cell (cytoskeleton with molecular motors?). The final step should take place through the nuclear pore complex [72-74]. No direct biophysical method to alter the nuclear envelope or pore has been reported (yet). But imaging methods [75, 76] support the occurrence of a direct effect of the field on organelles [77].

For non-viral gene delivery to be successful, plasmids must move through the cytoplasm to the nucleus in order to be transcribed. 2 steps are therefore present involving 2 classes of barriers. The cytoskeletal meshwork prevents pDNA (larger than 1 kb) movement in the cytoplasm. Actin patches colocalizing with the DNA at the plasma membrane were observed several minutes after pulse delivery with characteristics similar to those of the DNA aggregates, that are formed during the early stages of electrotransfection [78]. The microtubule network is required for directed plasmid trafficking to the nucleus [79]. Microtubule–DNA interactions can be enhanced due to sequence specificity with promoters containing binding sites for cyclic AMP response-element binding protein (CREB), such as the cytomegalovirus immediate early promoter (CMViep). Insertion of cytoplasmic adapter proteins transcription factors (TFs) binding sites within plasmids permits cytoplasmic trafficking of plasmids and an effective expression.

NLS sequences can help for the transfer inside the nucleus. In non-dividing cells, the nuclear envelope is an especially problematic hurdle to gene transfer. A successful approach is in modifying plasmid (pDNA) vectors to enhance nuclear import through the Nuclear Pore Complex [80]. Proteomics tools have been used to study DNA nuclear entry telling that Transcription factor-binding sites promote DNA nuclear translocation and Cell-specific transcription factors drive cell-specific DNA nuclear entry [81]. NLS peptides or nuclear proteins complexed with plasmids may enhance DNA nuclear translocation.

5. PDNA under electrotransfection conditions

5.1. Complexities in the determination of pDNA size evaluation

The size of the plasmid can be a significant modulator of the efficiency of transfer. The sliding model assumed that the pDNA was linear. This is not relevant of the experiments where a closed form was used in almost all reported cases. The gyration volume appears more appropriated. It is known that this diameter is highly sensitive to the compaction factors that are present. A tightly packed form is found in viral capsids. During the last 20 years, biotechnologists have been playing with chemical additives to obtain more compact forms. Indeed adding NaCl and/or MgCl2 is affecting the diameters. In [82] the authors wrote: "conformational and thermodynamic properties of supercoiled DNA depend strongly on ionic conditions. The effective double-helix diameter increases from 3 to 15 nm as the salt concentration is reduced from 1.00 to 0.01 M.". It was later observed with pUC18 (2686 bp), in dilute aqueous solution at salt concentrations between 0 and 1.5 M Na+ in 10 mM Tris, that the superhelix diameter from the simulated conformations decreased from 18.0 +/- 1.5 nm at 10 mM to 9.4 +/- 1.5 nm at 100 mM salt concentration[83]. This value did not significantly change to lower values at higher Na+ concentration. And in [84] upon addition of 0.122 M NaCl, the radius of gyration (RG) decreased substantially, which indicates that p30 delta adopts a more compact structure. When 4 mM Mg2+ was added to native supercoiled p30 delta in 0.1 M NaCl, Rg decreased.

Using Polymethacrylate monoliths,[85], size evaluations are described on a model plasmid, consisting of 4.9 kbp, Under physiological conditions, a 45 nm radius was evaluated. But the pore size distributions in these samples (see below) are broad: as such, the changes in the median pore diameter measured by mercury intrusion porosimetry reflect general shifts in the position of the pore distribution envelope, rather than the position of a well-defined, sharp peak [86](in http://www.liv.ac.uk/~aicooper/AKH_monolith.pdf).In [87] it was found for covalently closed supercoiled ColE1-plasmid DNA in 0.2 M NaCl, 0.002 M NaPO4 pH 7.0,0.002 M EDTA, a gyration radius about 100 nm but with EDTA meaning with no divalent ions but in 0.2 M NaCl. Finally, in [88] for pGem1a plasmids (3730 base pairs) in the relaxed circular (nicked) and supercoiled forms, RG = 90 +/- 3 nm,, and RG = 82 +/- 2.5 nm were obtained.

As a conclusion, a large distribution of gyration radii is described in the literature but, they are all larger that the compact form reported by Krassowska and that she used to predict the need of "electropores" of about 10 nm for DNA translocation during the pulse. Even larger sizes are requested with linearized form, that are known to be effective for expression after their electrotransfer [39]. For a closed form (highly effective for expression after the electrotransfer), in a condensed form under physiological conditions (Na> 20 mM, MgCl2 about 1 mM), the diameter of the structures supporting a free transmembrane transfer needs to be at least 100 nm.

Simulations give shapes of supercoiled closed form of PDNA (7 kb) [89]

As NaCl concentration decreases, the superhelix becomes less regular and more compact. In the presence of just 10 mM $MgCl_2$, supercoiled DNA adopts essentially the same set of conformations as in moderate to high concentrations of NaCl.

The size of a supercoiled plasmid is difficult to access. As shown in [89], the bulk size is large. This explains why many reports are giving data around 100 nm. But in fact, it is not a sphere (a coil) but a rather elongated thread-like shape that is more relevant. The DNA topology is described quantitatively by the twist of double helix and by the number of times the helix crosses over on itself (plectoneme). Plectonemic structures are typically formed by bacterial plasmids. Then in one direction we got a cross section close to the 20 nm used by Krassowska. A larger value is indeed observed under the low salt (Mg free) solution [90, 91].

The final conclusion is that the general conformation of pDNA used for electrotransfection is "complex" and do not support the model used for the sliding model. The lack of knowledge on the theoretical processes supporting the transmembrane transport brings the need of a rather empirical approach in the optimization of the technology for gene therapy.[92].

5.2. Smaller plasmids are more effective

The basic protocols are using Naked plasmid DNA under a Double strand closed form. No advantage is brought by preparing the linear form by restriction enzymes digestion.

As size controls the efficiency of transfer, minicircle forms (MC) are more efficient [93]. Minicircle DNA lacks the bacterial backbone sequence consisting of an antibiotic resistance gene, an origin of replication, and inflammatory sequences intrinsic to bacterial DNA that represent a potential risk for safe clinical application and reduce gene transfer rates as well as transgene expression. Expression following electrotransfer is improved with MC constructs over full-length plasmid (same promoter, same coding cassette) with different reporter genes. This great efficiency of MC was correlated to more efficient vector uptake by cells. Nevertheless, one should keep in mind that huge pDNA have been transferred and that decreasing the size of the plasmid is just bringing improvement but is not needed [94].

5.3. Field effect on pDNA conformation

Under electrotransfection protocols, besides the ionic content of the buffer that can be easily adjusted under in vitro protocols (but remains poorly controlled for gene therapy) [95], a critical parameter is present. An electric field is present that may affect the conformation of the pDNA.

Concerning DNA in electric fields, conflicting observations and predictions are present in the literature. Low DC field do not greatly perturb the conformation of large DNA. In [96], it is reported that larger fields give rise to chain orientation and stretching. This is in agreement with a simulation [97]. In fact, at high concentrations, strong intermolecular aggregation was observed even under 100V/cm [98, 99]. This can be considered as an explanation for the formation of the stable spots that we observed as an early stage in the multistep process.

6. Physical controls in optimizing the protocols

6.1. Electrical pulse parameters

Cell electropermeabilization must occur and an efficient electrophoretic accumulation of pDNA must be applied. This means that the field strength must be larger than a critical value (permeabilizing threshold at the level of the target in the tissue). Again the advantage of a targeted effect in tissues is present. But a modulation of transfer in this well defined volume by the cumulated pulse duration is present[100, 101].

The pulse duration can be short (0.1 ms) but longer pulses are more efficient as they are associated to a longer and therefore more efficient electrophoresis of the pDNA [102, 104]. The electrical parameters must be chosen to preserve the cell viability.

A double pulse method (a short high voltage pulse followed after a short delay by a long low voltage one)(HV LV) was therefore described [105]. The electrophoretic drift can be delayed from the permeabilizing pulse. This protocol is better to preserve the viability.

A destructive Joule effect can be present bringing limits in the parameters of the protocol. Intra pulse delay choice in a train of pulses can help to reduce this damaging effect by allowing a inter-pulse cooling of the pulsed sample.

6.2. Electrodes

Getting an optimized field distribution of the field intensities at the level of the target in the tissue is controlled by the geometry of the electrodes [106].

Most trials are performed by using needle electrodes that are penetrating inside the target tissues. Many designs have been reported (number of needles, diameters, distances, number, depth of penetration (see [107]). One major concern with these systems (that allow a deep penetration of the field) is the damaging effects of the electrodes (not only due to the perforation of the tissue but linked to the local effects at the electrode surface (local heating [108], electrochemical reactions [109]). Contact electrodes appear less destructive as the skin to electrodes contact is due to a conductive gel [110] but the field penetration remains rather limited

7. Cellular responses and controls

7.1. Reactive Oxygen Species (ROS)

Cellular responses are present under electrotransfection. The field induced membrane reorganization is a stress for the molecular assembly. A defense mechanism is present as shown by the generation of reactive oxygen species at the surface of the permeabilized cell [111-113]. ROS are highly destructive for DNA and reduce the number of copies that remains intact and therefore effective for expression. Protective effects are brought by the addition of antioxydants as long as they are not interfering with the transport.[114, 115]. There is a need to find biocompatible additive to reduce the ROS generation. Co-block polymers appear as a promising pathway.It was shown that postshock poloxamer administration reduced tissue inflammation and damage in comparison with dextran-treated or control tissues [116].

7.2. Extracellular matrix (ECM)

Uniform DNA distribution in tumors is a prerequisite step for an homogeneous transfection efficiency in solid tumors. This is of course valid for other target tissues (skin, muscles). The interstitial space is a rate limiting physiological barrier to non-viral gene delivery. External pulsed electric fields have been proposed to increase DNA transport in the interstitium, thereby improving non-viral gene delivery. The characteristic electromobility behavior, under most electrotransfection pulsing conditions, consisted of three distinct phases: stretching, reptation, and relaxation. Electromobility depended strongly on the field magnitude, pulse duration, but a decisive role is played by the pore size of the fibrous matrix (the extracellular matrix in tumors) through which the DNA migrated [117, 118]. The intratumoral field, which determines the efficiency of electric field-mediated gene delivery, can differ significantly from the applied field at the surface of the tumor.[119]. This local field is under the control of the geometry of the electrodes as described above. The field strengths in tumor tissues were significantly lower (down to 50%) than the applied field due to the multicellular organization. But when the external field was uniform (plate parallel electrodes) the electric fields in the center region of tumors were macroscopically uniform on ex Vivo slices.

Indeed tumor histological properties strongly affected transfection efficiency. Soft tumors with larger spherical cells, low proteoglycan and collagen content, and low cell density are more effectively transfected than rigid tumors with high proteoglycan and collagen content, small spindle-shaped cells and high cell density [120].

Electrotransfection in tissue can be improved by modulation of the extracellular matrix, using collagenase and/or hyaluronidase in tumors [121] as well as in muscles, a major target organ for DNA vaccination, a great topic for gene therapy [122].

8. Conclusion

Even if our knowledge on the molecular mechanisms governing the transfer of pDNA due to the delivery of pulsed electric field remains limited, it gives recommandations for an optimal choice of the protocols.

Pulse generators should provide the largest flexibility in the choice of the electrical parameters (voltage, duration, delay, number, current intensity, sharpness of the pulse onset) and offer an internal monitoring of the delivered pulse. Very few products on the market meet these specifications.

The local field on the tissue target is a complex function of the choice of the electrodes and on the electrical changes of the tissue due to the electrical treatment. This last parameter is highly dynamic and takes place during the pulse delivery. This remains under technical investigations by using simulations in electrical engineering [123, 124]. This time dependence of the electrical properties of the pulse tissue is an important parameter for the proper choice of the sequence of electrical pulses that must be delivered [125].

But clearly the biotechnological contributions cannot be neglected. Optimization in the plasmid constructs is strongly needed. The use of minicircles is promising to get a better transfer. But a key problem remains the design of the promoter that is shown to be an active partner in the cytoplasmic traffic to the nuclear volume.

Acknowledgements

The work was supported by grants from the seventh framework programme OncomiR (# 201102) and from the region Midi-Pyrénées (#11052700). The author wants to thank Dr JM Escoffre for many discussions.

Author details

J. Teissié[1,2*]

Address all correspondence to: justin.teissie@ipbs.fr

1 CNRS;IPBS (Institut de Pharmacologie et de Biologie Structurale), Toulouse, France

2 Université de Toulouse, Toulouse, France

References

[1] Wolff, J. A, Malone, R. W, Williams, P, Chong, W, Acsadi, G, & Jani, A. Felgner PL Direct gene transfer into mouse muscle in vivo. Science. (1990). 247(4949 Pt 1), 1465-8.

[2] Neumann, E, Shaefer-ridder, M, & Wang, Y. Hofschneider PH Gene transfer into mouse lyoma cells by electroporation in high electric fields. EMBO J (1982). , 1, 841-845.

[3] Heller, R, Jaroszeski, M, Atkin, A, Moradpour, D, Gilbert, R, Wands, J, & Nicolau, C. In vivo gene electroinjection and expression in rat liver.FEBS Lett. (1996). , 389(3), 225-8.

[4] Satkauskas, S, Ruzgys, P, & Venslauskas, M. S. Towards the mechanisms for efficient gene transfer into cells and tissues by means of cell electroporation. Expert Opin Biol Ther. (2012). , 12(3), 275-86.

[5] Gothelf, A, & Gehl, J. Gene electrotransfer to skin; review of existing literature and clinical perspectives.Curr Gene Ther. (2010). , 10(4), 287-99.

[6] Kee, S. T, & Gehl, J. Lee EW Editors, Clinical aspects of Electroporation, Springer (New York), (2011).

[7] Andre, F. M, & Mir, L. M. Nucleic acids electrotransfer in vivo: mechanisms and practical aspects.Curr Gene Ther. (2010). , 10(4), 267-80.

[8] Hojman, P. Basic principles and clinical advancements of muscle electrotransfer. Curr Gene Ther. (2010). , 10(2), 128-38.

[9] Cemazar, M. Sersa G Electrotransfer of therapeutic molecules into tissues.Curr Opin Mol Ther. (2007). , 9(6), 554-62.

[10] Daud, A. I, Deconti, R. C, Andrews, S, Urbas, P, Riker, A. I, Sondak, V. K, Munster, P. N, Sullivan, D. M, Ugen, K. E, Messina, J. L, & Heller, R. Phase I trial of interleukin-12 plasmid electroporation in patients with metastatic melanoma. J Clin Oncol. (2008). , 26(36), 5896-903.

[11] Eigeldinger-berthou, S, Buntschu, P, Flück, M, Frobert, A, Ferrié, C, Carrel, T. P, Tevaearai, H. T, & Kadner, A. Electric pulses augment reporter gene expression in the beating heart. J Gene Med. (2012). doi:jgm.2603., 14(3), 191-203.

[12] Ayuni, E. L, Gazdhar, A, Giraud, M. N, Kadner, A, Gugger, M, Cecchini, M, Caus, T, Carrel, T. P, Schmid, R. A, & Tevaearai, H. T. In vivo electroporation mediated gene delivery to the beating heart. PLoS One. (2010). e14467.

[13] Hargrave, B, & Downey, H. Strange R Jr, Murray L, Cinnamond C, Lundberg C, Israel A, Chen YJ, Marshall W Jr, Heller R Electroporation-mediated gene transfer directly to the swine heart.. Gene Ther. (2012). doi:gt.2012.15.

[14] Neumann, E, Sowers, A. E, & Jordan, C. A. Electroporation and electrofusion in cell biology. York:Plenum press; (1989).

[15] Teissié, J, & Golzio, M. Rols MP Mechanisms of cell membrane electropermeabilization: a minireview of our present (lack of?) knowledge. Biochim Biophys Acta (2005). , 1724, 270-280.

[16] Orlowski, S. Mir LM Cell electropermeabilization: a new tool for biochemical and pharmacological studies. Biochim. Biophys Acta (1993). , 1154, 51-63.

[17] Eynard, N, Rols, M. P, Ganeva, V, Galutzov, B, & Sabri, N. Teissie J Electrotransformation pathways of prokaryotic and eukaryotic cells: recents developments. Bioelectrochem Bioenerg (1997). , 44, 103-10.

[18] Li, J, & Lin, H. Numerical simulation of molecular uptake via electroporation Bioelectrochemistry, (2011). , 82(1), 10-21.

[19] Pucihar, G, Kotnik, T, Miklavcic, D, & Teissié, J. Kinetics of transmembrane transport of small molecules into electropermeabilized cells. Biophys. J. (2008). , 95, 2837-2848.

[20] Mir, L. M, Roth, C, & Orlowski, S. Quintin Colonna F, Fradelizi D, et al. Systemic antitumor effects of electrochemotherapy combined with histocompatible cells secreting interleukin-2. J Immunother Emphasis Tumor Immunol (1995). , 17, 30-38.

[21] Sersa, G, Miklavcic, D, Cemazar, M, Rudolf, Z, & Pucihar, G. Snoj M Electrochemotherapy in treatment of tumours. Eur J Surg Oncol (2008). , 34, 232-240.

[22] Mir, L. M, Gehl, J, Sersa, G, Collins, C. G, Garbay, J. R, Billard, V, et al. Standard operating procedures of the electrochemotherapy: Instructions for the use of bleomycin or cisplatin administrated either systemically or locally and electric pulses delivered by the cliniporatorTM by means of invasive or non-invasive electrodes. Eur J Cancer (2006). suppl 4):14-25

[23] Mir, L. M, Glass, L. F, Sersa, G, Teissie, J, Domenge, C, Miklavcic, D, et al. Effective treatment of cutaneaous and subcutaneaous malignant tumours by electrochemotherapy. Br J Cancer (1998). , 77, 2336-2342.

[24] Testori, A, Rossi, C. R, & Tosti, G. Utility of electrochemotherapy in melanoma treatment. Curr Opin Oncol. (2012). , 24(2), 155-61.

[25] Campana, L. G, Mocellin, S, Basso, M, Puccetti, O, De Salvo, G. L, Chiarion-sileni, V, Vecchiato, A, Corti, L, Rossi, C. R, & Nitti, D. Bleomycin-based electrochemotherapy: clinical outcome from a single institution's experience with 52 patients.Ann Surg Oncol. (2009). , 16(1), 191-9.

[26] Hampton T Electric Pulses Help With ChemotherapyMay Open New Paths for Other Agents,JAMA, (2011). , 305, 549-51.

[27] Weaver, J. C. Chizmadzhev YA Theory of electroporation: A review. Bioelectrochem Bioenerg (1996). , 41, 135-160.

[28] Aihara, H. Miyazaki JI Gene transfer into muscle by electroporation in vivo. Nature Biotechnol (1998). , 16, 867-870.

[29] Mir, L. M, Bureau, M. F, Gehl, J, Rangara, R, Rouy, D, Caillaud, J. M, Delaere, P, Branellec, D, & Schwartz, B. Scherman D High-efficiency gene transfer into skeletal muscle mediated by electric pulses. Proc Natl Acad Sci USA (1999). , 96, 4262-4267.

[30] Liu, F. Huang L Electric gene transfer to the liver following systemic administration of plasmid DNA. Gene Ther (2002). , 9, 1116-1119.

[31] Titomirov, A. V, & Sukharev, S. Kistanova E In vivo electroporation and stable transformation of skin cells of newborn mice by plasmid DNA. Biochim Biophys Acta Report (1991). , 1088, 131-134.

[32] Vandermeulen, G, Staes, E, Vanderhaeghen, M. L, Bureau, M. F, & Scherman, D. Préat V Optimisation of intradermal DNA electrotransfer for immunisation. J Control Res (2007). , 124, 81-87.

[33] Kaufman, C. D, Geiger, R. C, & Dean, D. A. Electroporation- and mechanical ventilation-mediated gene transfer to the lung. Gene therapy. (2010). , 17(9), 1098-104.

[34] Rols, M. P, Delteil, C, Golzio, M, Dumond, P, & Cros, S. Teissie J In vivo electrically mediated protein and gene transfer in murine melanoma. Nat Biotechnol (1998). , 16, 168-171.

[35] Bettan, M, Ivanov, M. A, Mir, L. M, Boissiere, F, & Delaere, P. Scherman D Efficient DNA electrotransfer into tumors Bioelectrochemistry (2000).

[36] Tevz, G, Pavlin, D, Kamensek, U, Kranjc, S, Mesojednik, S, Coer, A, Sersa, G, & Cemazar, M. Gene electrotransfer into murine skeletal muscle: a systematic analysis of parameters for long-term gene expression Technol Cancer Res Treat. (2008). , 7(2), 91-101.

[37] De Gennes, P. G. Passive entry of a DNA molecule into a small pore Proc. Natl. Acad. Sci. USA (1999). , 96, 7262-7264.

[38] Yu, M, Tan, W, & Lin, H. A stochastic model for DNA translocation through an electropore BBA Biomembranes (2012). , 1818(11), 2494-2501.

[39] Escoffre, J. M, Nikolova, B, Mallet, L, Henri, J, Favard, C, Golzio, M, Teissié, J, & Tsoneva, I. Rols MP New insights in the gene electrotransfer process: Evidence for the involvement of the plasmid DNA topology. Curr Gene Ther. (2012). Epub ahead of print]

[40] Smith, K. C, & Neu, J. C. Krassowska W Model of creation and evolution of stables electropores for DNA delivery. Biophys J (2004). , 86, 2813-2826.

[41] Krassowska, W. Filev PD Modeling electroporation in a single cell. Biophys J (2007). , 92, 404-417.

[42] Neu, J. C. Krassowska W Modeling postshock evolution of large electropores. Phys Rev E Stat Nonlin Soft Matter Phys (2003).

[43] Sukharev, S. I, & Titomirov, A. V. Klenchin VA Electrically induced DNA transfer into cells. Electroporation in vivo. In Gene Therapeutics: Methods and Applications of Direct Gene Transfer. JA Wolff, editor. Birkhäuser, Boston, MA. 210-232,(1994).

[44] Bier, M, Hammer, S. M, & Canaday, D. J. Lee RC Kinetics of resealing for transient electropores in isolated mammalian skeletal muscle cells. Bioelectromagnetics (1999). , 20, 194-201.

[45] Golzio, M, Mora, M. P, Raynaud, C, Delteil, C, & Teissie, J. Rols MP Control by osmotic pressure of voltage-induced permeabilization and gene transfer in mammalian cells. Biophys J (1998). , 74, 3015-3022.

[46] Satkauskas, S, Bureau, M. F, Puc, M, Mahfoudi, A, Scherman, D, & Miklavcic, D. Mir LM Mechanisms of in vivo DNA electrotransfer: respective contributions of cell electropermeabilization and DNA electrophoresis. Mol Ther (2002). , 5, 133-140.

[47] Tekle, E, & Astumian, R. D. Chock PB Electroporation by using bipolar oscillating electric field: an improved method for DNA transfection of NIH 3T3 cells. Proc Natl Acad Sci USA (1991). , 88, 4230-4234.

[48] Freeman, S. A, & Wang, M. A. Weaver JC Theory of electroporation of planar bilayer membranes: predictions of the aqueous area, change in capacitance, and pore-pore separation. Biophys J (1994)., 67, 42-56.

[49] Joshi, R. P. Schoenbach KH Electroporation dynamics in biological cells subjected to ultrafast electrical pulses: a numerical simulation study. Phys Rev E (2000). , 62, 1025-1033.

[50] Kakorin, S, & Neumann, E. Ionic conductivity of electroporated lipid bilayer membranes. Bioelectrochem (2002)., 56, 163-166.

[51] Neumann, E, Kakorin, S, Tsoneva, I, & Nikolova, B. Tomov T Calcium-mediated DNA adsorption to yeast cells and kinetics of cell transformation by electroporation. Biophys J (1996)., 71, 868-877.

[52] Rols, M. P. Teissie J Electropermeabilization of mammalian cells to macromolecules: control by pulse duration. Biophys J (1998)., 75, 1415-1423.

[53] Rols, M. P, & Delteil, C. Teissie J Control by ATP and ADP of voltage-induced mammalian-cell-membrane permeabilization, gene transfer and resulting expression. Eur J Biochem (1998)., 254, 382-388.

[54] Sukharev, S. I, Klenchin, V. A, Serov, S. M, & Chernomordik, L. V. Chizmadzhev, Yu A Electroporation and electrophoretic DNA transfer into cells. The effect of DNA interaction with electropores. Biophys J (1992)., 63, 1320-1327.

[55] Neumann, E, & Kakorin, S. Toensing K Fundamentals of electroporative delivery of drugs and genes. Bioelectrochem Bioenerg (1999)., 48, 3-16.

[56] Hristova, N. I, & Tsoneva, I. Neumann E Sphingosine-mediated electroporative DNA transfer through lipid bilayers. FEBS Lett (1997)., 415, 81-86.

[57] Spassova, M, Tsoneva, I, Petrov, A. G, & Petkova, J. I. Neumann E Dip patch clamp currents suggest electrodiffusive transport of the polyelectrolyte DNA through lipid bilayers. Biophys Chem (1994)., 52, 267-274.

[58] Winterbourne, D. J, Thomas, S, Hermon-taylor, J, & Hussain, I. Johnstone AP Electric-shock-mediated transfection of cells. Biochem J (1988)., 251, 427-434.

[59] Klenchin, V. A, Sukharev, S. I, Serov, S. M, & Chernomordik, L. V. Chizmadzev YuA Electrically induced DNA uptake by cells is a fast process involving DNA electrophoresis. Biophys J (1991)., 60, 804-811.

[60] Tekle, E, & Astumian, R. D. Chock PB Selective and asymmetric molecular transport across electroporated cell membranes. Proc Natl Acad Sci USA (1994)., 91, 11512-11516.

[61] Hui SW Effects of pulse length and strength on electroporation efficiencyMethods Mol Biol (1995)., 55, 29-40.

[62] Wu, M. Yuan F Membrane Binding of Plasmid DNA and Endocytic Pathways Are Involved in Electrotransfection of Mammalian Cells. PLoS ONE (2011). e20923. doi: 10.1371/journal.pone.0020923

[63] Tarek M Membrane electroporation: a molecular dynamics simulationBiophys J (2005). , 88, 4015-4053.

[64] Bandyopadhyay, S, Tarek, M, & Klein, M. L. (1999). Molecular dynamics study of lipid-DNA complexes. J Phys Chem B 1999; , 103, 10075-10080.

[65] Lin, R, & Chang, D. C. Lee YK Single-cell electroendocytosis on a micro chip using in situ fluorescence microscopy. Biomed Microdevices. (2011). , 13(6), 1063-73.

[66] Rosazza, C, Phez, E, Escoffre, J. M, Cézanne, L, Zumbusch, A, & Rols, M. P. Cholesterol implications in plasmid DNA electrotransfer: Evidence for the involvement of endocytotic pathways. Int J Pharm. (2012). , 423(1), 134-43.

[67] Golzio, M, & Teissié, J. Rols MP Direct visualization at the single-cell level of electrically mediated gene delivery. Proc Natl Acad Sci USA (2002). , 99, 1292-1297.

[68] Pavlin, M, & Pucihar, G. Kandušer M The role of electrically stimulated endocytosis in gene electrotransferBioelectrochemistry (2012). , 83, 38-45.

[69] Pavlin, M, Flisar, K, & Kandušer, M. The role of electrophoresis in gene electrotransfer. J. Membrane Biol. (2010). , 236, 75-79.

[70] Escoffre, J. M, Portet, T, Favard, C, Teissié, J, Dean, D. S, & Rols, M. P. Electromediated formation of DNA complexes with cell membranes and its consequences for gene delivery.Biochim Biophys Acta. (2011). , 1808(6), 1538-43.

[71] Faurie, C, Rebersek, M, Golzio, M, Kanduser, M, Escoffre, J. M, Pavlin, M, Teissie, J, & Miklavcic, D. Rols MP Electro-mediated gene transfer and expression are controlled by the life-time of DNA/membrane complex formation. J Gene Med. (2010). , 12(1), 117-25.

[72] Van Der Aa, M. A, Mastrobattista, E, Oosting, R. S, Hennik, W. E, Koning, G. A, & Crommelin, D. J. The nuclear pore complex: the gateway to successful nonviral gene delivery. Pharm Res (2006). , 23, 447-459.

[73] Van Der Aa, M. A, Mastrobattista, E, Oosting, R. S, Hennink, W. E, & Koning, G. A. Crommelin DJ The nuclear pore complex: the gateway to successful nonviral gene delivery. Adv Drug Deliv Rev (2007). , 59, 698-717.

[74] Pouton, C. W, Wagstaff, K. M, Roth, D. M, & Moseley, G. W. Jans DA Targeted delivery to the nucleus. Adv Drug Deliv Rev (2007). , 59, 698-717.

[75] Bellard, E. Teissie J Double-Pulse Approach of Electrogenotherapy: An Analysis at the Single Cell Level- IEEE Trans Plasma Sci, (2009)., 37(4), 538-44.

[76] Bellard, E. Teissié J Double pulse approach of electropulsation: a fluorescence analysis of the nucleus perturbation at the single cell level IEEE Trans Dielect Electr In, (2009). , 16, 1267-1272.

[77] Esser, A. T, Smith, K. C, Gowrishankar, T. R, Vasilkoski, Z, & Weaver, J. C. Mechanisms for the intracellular manipulation of organelles by conventional electroporation. Biophys J. (2010)., 98(11), 2506-14.

[78] Rosazza, C, Escoffre, J. M, Zumbusch, A, & Rols, M. P. The actin cytoskeleton has an active role in the electrotransfer of plasmid DNA in mammalian cells. Mol Ther. (2011)., 19(5), 913-21.

[79] Badding, M. A, & Vaugham, E. E. Dean DA Transcription factor plasmid binding modulates microtubule interactions and intracellular trafficking during gene transfer Gene Therapy (2012)., 19, 338-346.

[80] Miller, A. M. Dean DA Tissue-specific and transcription factor-mediated nuclear entry of DNA. Adv Drug Deliv Rev (2009)., 61, 603-613.

[81] Lam, A. P. Dean DA Progress and prospects: nuclear import of nonviral vectors Gene Therapy (2010)., 17, 439-447.

[82] Vologodskii, A. V, & Cozzarelli, N. R. Conformational and thermodynamic properties of supercoiled DNA. Annu Rev Biophys Biomol Struct. (1994)., 23, 609-43.

[83] Hammermann, M, Brun, N, Klenin, K. V, May, R, & Tóth, K. Langowski JSalt-dependent DNA superhelix diameter studied by small angle neutron scattering measurements and Monte Carlo simulations. Biophys J. (1998)., 75(6), 3057-63.

[84] Gebe, J. A, Delrow, J. J, Heath, P. J, Fujimoto, B. S, & Stewart, D. W. Schurr JM Effects of Na+ and Mg2+ on the structures of supercoiled DNAs: comparison of simulations with experiments. J Mol Biol. (1996)., 262(2), 105-28.

[85] Zöchling, A, Hahn, R, Ahrer, K, Urthaler, J, & Jungbauer, A. Mass transfer characteristics of plasmids in monoliths. J Sep Sci. (2004)., 27(10-11), 819-27.

[86] http://wwwliv.ac.uk/~aicooper/AKH_monolith.pdf

[87] Voordouw, G, Kam, Z, & Borochov, N. Eisenberg H Isolation and physical studies of the intact supercoiled, the open circular and the linear forms of ColE1-plasmid DNA. Biophys Chem. (1978)., 8(2), 171-89.

[88] Fishman, D. M, & Patterson, G. D. Light scattering studies of supercoiled and nicked DNA. Biopolymers. (1996)., 38(4), 535-52.

[89] Rybenkov, V, & Vologodskii, A. V. Cozzarelli NR The effect of ionic conditions on the conformations of supercoiled DNA. I. sedimentation analysis1 Journal of Molecular Biology (1997)., 267, 299-311.

[90] Rybenkov, V, & Vologodskii, A. V. Cozzarelli NR The effect of ionic conditions on DNA helical repeat,effective diameter and free energy of supercoiling Nucleic Acids Research, (1997)., 25, 1412-8.

[91] Baranello, L, Levens, D, & Guptaa, A. Kouzine F The importance of being supercoiled: How DNA mechanics regulate dynamic processes Biochimica et Biophysica Acta

(BBA)- Gene Regulatory Mechanisms (2012). Chromatin in time and space, 1819, 632-638.

[92] Golzio, M, Escoffre, J. M, Portet, T, Mauroy, C, Teissié, J, Dean, D. S, & Rols, M. P. Observations of the mechanisms of electromediated DNA uptake--from vesicles to tissues. Curr Gene Ther. (2010). , 10(4), 256-66.

[93] Kobelt, D, Schleef, M, Schmeer, M, Aumann, J, & Schlag, P. M. Walther W Performance of High Quality Minicircle DNA for In Vitro and In Vivo Gene Transfer Mol Biotechnol (2012). on line DOIs12033-012-9535-6).

[94] Chabot, S, Orio, J, Schmeer, M, Schleef, M, Golzio, M, & Teissié, J. Minicircle DNA electrotransfer for efficient tissue-targeted gene delivery. Gene Ther. (2013)., 20(1), 62-8 doi:gt.2011.215

[95] Lee, M. J, Cho, S. S, Jang, H. S, Lim, Y. S, You, J. R, Park, J, Suh, H, Kim, J. A, Park, J. S, & Kim, D. K. Optimal salt concentration of vehicle for plasmid DNA enhances gene transfer mediated by electroporation. Exp Mol Med. (2002). , 34(4), 265-72.

[96] Jonsson, M, Jacobsson, U, & Takahashi, M. Nordén B Orientation of large DNA during free solution electrophoresis studied by linear dichroism J Chem Soc Faraday trans (1993), 89, 2791–2798

[97] Netz RR Nonequilibrium Unfolding of Polyelectrolyte Condensates in Electric Fields Phys Rev Lett 2003; 90:128104

[98] Magnúsdóttir, S, Isambert, H, Heller, C, & Viovy, J. L. Electrohydrodynamically induced aggregation during constant and pulsed field capillary electrophoresis of DNA. Biopolymers (1999)., 49, 385–401

[99] Mitnik, L, Heller, C, & Prost, J. Viovy JL Segregation in DNA solutions induced by electric fields. Science. (1995). , 267(5195), 219-22.

[100] Cemazar, M, Golzio, M, Sersa, G, Rols, M. P, & Teissié, J. Electrically-assisted nucleic acids delivery to tissues in vivo: where do we stand? Curr Pharm Des. (2006). , 12(29), 3817-25.

[101] Miklavcic, D, Beravs, K, Semrov, D, Cemazar, M, Demsar, F, & Sersa, G. The importance of electric field distribution for effective in vivo electroporation of tissues.Biophys J. (1998). , 74(5), 2152-8.

[102] Satkauskas, S, Bureau, M. F, Puc, M, Mahfoudi, A, Scherman, D, Miklavcic, D, & Mir, L. M. Mechanisms of in vivo DNA electrotransfer: respective contributions of cell electropermeabilization and DNA electrophoresis. Mol Ther. (2002). , 5(2), 133-40.

[103] Satkauskas, S, André, F, Bureau, M. F, Scherman, D, Miklavcic, D, & Mir, L. M. Electrophoretic component of electric pulses determines the efficacy of in vivo DNA electrotransfer. Hum Gene Ther. (2005). , 16(10), 1194-201.

[104] Cemazar, M, Golzio, M, Sersa, G, Hojman, P, Kranjc, S, Mesojednik, S, Rols, M. P, & Teissie, J. Control by pulse parameters of DNA electrotransfer into solid tumors in mice. Gene Ther. (2009). , 16(5), 635-44.

[105] André, F. M, Gehl, J, Sersa, G, Préat, V, Hojman, P, Eriksen, J, Golzio, M, Cemazar, M, Pavselj, N, Rols, M. P, Miklavcic, D, Neumann, E, Teissié, J, & Mir, L. M. Efficiency of high- and low-voltage pulse combinations for gene electrotransfer in muscle, liver, tumor, and skin.Hum Gene Ther. (2008). , 19(11), 1261-71.

[106] Gothelf, A, Mahmood, F, Dagnaes-hansen, F, & Gehl, J. Efficacy of transgene expression in porcine skin as a function of electrode choice. Bioelectrochemistry. (2011). , 82(2), 95-102.

[107] Guo, S, Donate, A, Basu, G, Lundberg, C, Heller, L, & Heller, R. Electro-gene transfer to skin using a noninvasive multielectrode array. J Control Release. (2011). , 151(3), 256-62.

[108] Davalos, R. V, Rubinsky, B, & Mir, L. M. Theoretical analysis of the thermal effects during in vivo tissue electroporation. Bioelectrochemistry. (2003)., 61, 99–107

[109] Turjanski, P, Olaiz, N, Maglietti, F, Michinski, S, Suárez, C, Molina, F. V, & Marshall, G. The role of pH fronts in reversible electroporation. PLoS One. (2011). e17303

[110] Golzio, M, Mazeres, S, & Teissie, J. Electrodes for in vivo localised subcutaneous electropulsation and associated drug and nucleic acid delivery. Expert Opin Drug Deliv. (2009). , 6(12), 1323-31.

[111] Gabriel, B, & Teissié, J. Control by electrical parameters of short- and long-term cell death resulting from electropermeabilization of Chinese hamster ovary cells.Biochim Biophys Acta. (1995). , 1266(2), 171-8.

[112] Bonnafous, P, Vernhes, M, Teissié, J, & Gabriel, B. The generation of reactive-oxygen species associated with long-lasting pulse-induced electropermeabilisation of mammalian cells is based on a non-destructive alteration of the plasma membrane.Biochim Biophys Acta. (1999). , 1461(1), 123-34.

[113] Pakhomova, O. N, Khorokhorina, V. A, Bowman, A. M, Rodaite-riševiciene, R, Saulis, G, Xiao, S, & Pakhomov, A. G. Oxidative effects of nanosecond pulsed electric field exposure in cells and cell-free media.Arch Biochem Biophys. (2012). Aug 15. [Epub ahead of print]).

[114] Markelc, B, Tevz, G, Cemazar, M, Kranjc, S, Lavrencak, J, Zegura, B, Teissie, J, & Sersa, G. Muscle gene electrotransfer is increased by the antioxidant tempol in mice. Gene Ther. (2012). , 19(3), 312-20.

[115] Sabri, N, Pelissier, B, & Teissie, J. Ascorbate increases electrotransformation efficiency of intact maize cells. Anal Biochem. (1998). , 264(2), 284-6.

[116] Lee, R. C, River, L. P, Pan, F. S, & Ji, L. Wollmann RL Surfactant-induced sealing of electropermeabilized skeletal muscle membranes in vivo. Proc Natl Acad Sci U S A. (1992). , 89(10), 4524-8.

[117] Henshaw, J. W, Zaharoff, D. A, Mossop, B. J, & Yuan, F. A single molecule detection method for understanding mechanisms of electric field-mediated interstitial transport of genes Bioelectrochemistry. (2006). , 69(2), 248-53.

[118] Henshaw, J. W, Zaharoff, D. A, & Mossop, B. J. Yuan F Electric field-mediated transport of plasmid DNA in tumor interstitium in vivo Bioelectrochemistry (2007). , 71, 233-242.

[119] Mossop, B. J, Barr, R. C, Henshaw, J. W, & Zaharoff, D. A. YuanF Electric Fields in Tumors Exposed to External Voltage Sources: Implication for Electric Field-Mediated Drug and Gene Delivery Annals of Biomedical Engineering, (2006). C 2006):1564-1572

[120] Mesojednik, S, Pavlin, D, Sersa, G, Coer, A, Kranjc, S, Grosel, A, & Tevz, G. Cemazar M The effect of the histological properties of tumors on transfection efficiency of electrically assisted gene delivery to solid tumors in mice. Gene Ther. (2007). , 14(17), 1261-9.

[121] Cemazar, M, Golzio, M, Sersa, G, Escoffre, J. M, Coer, A, Vidic, S, & Teissie, J. Hyaluronidase and collagenase increase the transfection efficiency of gene electrotransfer in various murine tumors. Hum Gene Ther. (2012). , 23(1), 128-37.

[122] Mcmahon, J. M, Signori, E, Wells, K. E, Fazio, V. M, & Wells, D. J. Optimisation of electrotransfer of plasmid into skeletal muscle by pretreatment with hyaluronidase--increased expression with reduced muscle damage. Gene Ther. (2001). , 8(16), 1264-70.

[123] Zupanic, A, & Kos, B. Miklavcic D Treatment planning of electroporation-based medical interventions: electrochemotherapy, gene electrotransfer and irreversible electroporation. Phys Med Biol. (2012). , 57(17), 5425-40.

[124] Zupanic, A, Corovic, S, Miklavcic, D, & Pavlin, M. Numerical optimization of gene electrotransfer into muscle tissue. Biomed Eng Online. (2010)., 9():66.

[125] Cukjati, D, Batiuskaite, D, André, F, & Miklavcic, D. Mir LM Real time electroporation control for accurate and safe in vivo non-viral gene therapy. Bioelectrochemistry. (2007). , 70(2), 501-7.

Section 2

Gene Therapy Using Viral Vectors

Chapter 5

Viral Vectors for Vaccine Development

Qiana L. Matthews, Linlin Gu,
Alexandre Krendelchtchikov and Zan C. Li

Additional information is available at the end of the chapter

1. Introduction

Recombinant vectors can be used to deliver antigens and to stimulate immune responses in humans. Viral vectors possess various intrinsic properties which may lend to advantages and disadvantages for usage for a given therapeutic application [reviewed by Larocca and Schlom] [1]. The safety and flexibility of recombinant viral vectors have lead to their usage in gene therapy, virotherapy, and vaccine applications. In this chapter, we will discuss the utility and importance of recombinant vectors as vaccine agents. This chapter will highlight some of the uses of recombinant viral vectors for therapeutic vaccines; and will mostly focus on the application of a range of recombinant viral vectors for prophylactic vaccines against infectious agents. More specifically, this chapter will focus in depth on the use of recombinant adenovirus (Ad) for vaccine development against infectious agents.

2. Gene therapy vectors and oncolytic vectors

Viruses can be used as gene delivery tools for a variety of diseases and conditions [1]. Most viruses are naturally immunogenic and can be engineered to express genes that modulate the immune system or express tumor antigen transgenes. Human Ad vectors have been widely used as vehicles for gene therapy [2]. Replication-defective Ads were the first vectors to be evaluated for *in vivo* gene transfer in a wide variety of preclinical models. For instance, Stratford-Perricaudet, and group reported efficient, long-term *in vivo* gene transfer throughout mouse skeletal and cardiac muscles after intravenous administration of a recombinant Ad vector [3]. This study focused on the transfer of the report gene, *β-galactosidase*; however, studies similar to this lead to the delivery of therapeutic genes by means of recombinant vectors. Routinely, viral vectors such as human Ad vectors have been engineered to express

[4–6] or display [7–9] herpes simplex virus type 1 thymidine kinase which kills proliferating tumor cells in the presence of the prodrug gancyclovir. This strategy is commonly referred to as cancer gene therapy. Concerning non-cancerous diseases, viral vectors have been utilized to deliver genes to a multitude of cells types ranging from dental cells [10], islets cells [11], and many other cell types. In these instances, viral vectors transduce cells to deliver genes which may lead to an overexpression or knock down of protein, leading to a corrective phenomenon or destruction of damaged cells.

Viruses can also be used as oncolytic agents. Oncolytic viruses which have been identified or engineered belong to several viral families. They include herpes simplex viruses, adenovirus, retroviruses, paramyxoviruses, and poxviruses [12]. These viruses can be categorized into four major groups on the basis of their oncolytic restriction: (1) mutation/deletion derived viruses, (2) transcriptionally targeted oncolytic viruses, (3) transductionally targeted oncolytic vectors, and (4) "naturally smart" viruses [13]. Oncolytic viruses for cancer exploit the difference of the molecular makeup between the tumor cells and their normal counterparts; they also utilize recombinant DNA technology to engineer viral vectors to selectively replicate in the tumor cells and destroy them. Conditionally replicative Ads (CRAds) [14,15], measles virus [16,17], herpes simplex virus [18], and vesicular stomatitis virus [reviewed in [1]], have been shown to preferentially infect and propagate in tumor cells. It has been demonstrated that these vectors not only have direct cytopathic effect on tumor cells but in addition, these oncolytic vectors are likely to enhance immune-mediated killing of tumor cells likely through the release of tumor antigens. Tumor antigens have been demonstrated to be more immunogenic when delivered as transgenes in a viral vector, compared with employing tumor antigens used as a peptide or protein vaccine [19,20].

However, some oncolytic vectors are unlikely to be used as cancer vaccines due to the short duration of transgene expression in infected cells given the onset of lysis; this might limit their ability to elicit a robust immune response against the transgene. Many types of recombinant vectors can infect antigen presenting cells (APC), specifically dendritic cells (DCs). Once engineered recombinant vectors infect APCs and then express antigens or transgenes which are then presented to the immune system [21–26]. However, some oncolytic vectors have a limited tropism for DCs. Ads or CRAds do not infect DCs well due to the fact that DCs possess limited expression of the primary Ad5 docking receptor, Cosxackie-Adenovirus Receptor (CAR). Naturally, DCs are virtually resistant to Ad5 infection, presenting a challenge for effective transduction of DCs by Ad [27]. Direct *in vivo* administration of untargeted Ad5 may result in cytopathic effects due to ectopic gene transfer to CAR expressing bystander cells rather than DCs. Moreover, additional antigen presentation by these transduced non-processional APCs may lead to suboptimal T cell activation, or even tolerance induction [28]. Despite these caveats, DCs are key orchestrators of the adaptive immune system. DCs have an exceptional ability to capture, process, and present antigens to activate naïve T cells. DCs have the ability to regulate the nature of the T cell response by providing appropriate co-stimulatory signals that dictate immunogenic or tolerogenic T cell stimulation. These unique features make targeted manipulation of DCs an attractive approach for modulating immune response against cancer [29]. Therapeutic strategies related to DCs, cancer vaccination, and oncolytic vectors are summarized in the following reviews [17,29–31].

3. Viral vectors for vaccine development

Each viral vector has its own distinct advantage and disadvantage. The most extensively studied viral vectors are from the poxviridae family. They include derivatives of vaccinia virus from the orthopoxvirus genera, and members of the avipoxvirus genera, such as fowlpox and canarypox (ALVAC). Poxviruses have a long and successful track record related to vaccination. In particular, vaccinia virus was used to vaccinate over one billion people against smallpox, leading to the eradication of the disease in 1978. Poxviruses are double stranded DNA viruses with a linear genome. Poxviruses have the ability to accept large inserts of foreign DNA, and therefore can accommodate multiple genes. Vaccinia virus has a genome of ~190 kilobases (kb), which encodes for ~250 genes [32]. Fowlpox viruses have a ~260 kb to 309 kb genome with approximately 260 recognized genes. Attenuated canarypox strain ALVAC has an approximate 330 kb genome with ~320 putative genes [33].

Viral replication and transcription of the poxvirus genome is limited to the cytoplasm of the host cell. This extranuclear replication eliminates the risk of insertional mutagenesis, the random insertion of viral genetic sequences into host cell genomic DNA [34]. Vaccinia virus infects mammalian cells, and expresses recombinant genes for about 7 days before the infected cell are eliminated by the immune system [21]. Avipoxviruses infect mammalian cells and express their transgenes for 14 to 21 days [35,36]. Despite the attractive features of poxviruses, replication competent viruses like vaccinia should not be administered to severely immunocompromised patients. To circumvent this problem, an attenuated vaccinia virus called modified vaccinia virus Ankara (MVA) was developed for high-risk individuals. MVA was developed by over 500 serial passages of a smallpox vaccine from Ankara, Turkey, in chicken embryo fibroblasts (CEF). This technique resulted in over 15% loss of the vaccinia virus genome [37]. MVA can infect mammalian cells and express transgenes, but it cannot produce infectious viral particles. Similarly, fowlpox and canarypox, which are pathogenic in some avian species, are unable to productively infect humans because they cannot complete their life cycle and form infectious particles [38]. As a result, mammalian poxviruses generate a stronger immune response compared to avipoxviruses. Unfortunately, MVA and vaccinia virus vectors can only be given once or twice to vaccinia immune or vaccinia naïve patients due to the development of host neutralizing antibodies against these vectors [39]. Neutralizing antibodies (NAbs) are not developed against the avipoxvirus vectors, allowing them to be given several times to patients as booster vaccinations [40]. Similarly, alphaviruses, like avipox viruses, are also desirable vectors because infected hosts do not develop neutralizing antibodies to the vectors, allowing for multiple administrations.

In 2010, adenovirus-based vectors accounted for 23.9% of gene-therapy clinical trials [41]. The broad utility of these vectors is derived from several key characteristics: (a) the recombinant viral genome is readily manipulated; (b) replication-defective Ads can be propagated in complementing cell lines; (c) Ads infect a broad range of target cells, [42,43] and (d) Ads can achieve high levels of *in vivo* gene transfer with concomitantly high levels of transgene expression [44]. Adenovirus is a non-enveloped double stranded DNA virus. The 36 kb genome can accommodate cDNA sequences of up to 7.5 kb. Replication of the adenovirus occurs in the nucleus but remains extrachromosomal, minimizing the risk associated with insertional mutagenesis. The majority of Ad vectors are replication- incompetent because of a deletion of the viral gene, E1. This limits the vectors' pathogenicity, while still allowing for humoral and cellular responses to the transgene. Most Ad vectors are E3-deleted [E1-, E3-], for the potential to have increased cloning capacity. However, retainment of the E3 gene-encoding regions within an [E1-, E3+] Ad vector would given an optimal effect related to vector characteristics. There has been some speculation that E3 gene promoters are dependent primarily upon the trans-activation capabilities of the E1 gene products. There have been various studies where the E3 region (or selected genes from E3) is re-introduced into the Ad vector under appropriate control of E1 independent promoters. These studies have shown some improvement in small animal models, including reduced humoral and CD8 T cell responses to the vector, and/or long-term transgene expression [45–47]. Oncolytic vectors have, in some cases, the E1 regions intact and, therefore, could potentially benefit from expression of these immune evasion proteins [48]. Most importantly, Ad vectors can be easily manipulated in the laboratory setting, which allows researchers to easily modify these vectors. This includes retargeting the viral tropism to infect DCs which are usually resistant to Ad infection. These properties have also led to Ads being used as molecular vaccine agents.

4. Adenoviral vectors as vaccine agents

Traditionally, Ad vaccination embodies the concept that the vector uses the host-cell machinery to express antigens that are encoded as transgenes within the viral vector, specifically within the E1 and/or the E3 regions. Cellular and humoral immune responses are generated against these antigens for a vaccine effect. Several preclinical successes have used this approach in animal model systems. In one example, an Ad serotype 5 (Ad5) vector encoding Ebola surface glycoprotein generated neutralizing antibodies and protected monkeys after a single administration of Ebola [49]. In murine models protection against malaria has also been observed using Ad vectors that express the circumsporozite antigen in *Plasmodium yoelii* [50–52] or *Plasmodium berghei [53]*. Ad vectors are currently being used in clinical trials for vaccine development against tuberculosis [54], HIV [55–57], and malaria [58–60]. Ad5-based HIV and malaria vaccines were well tolerated and induced antigen-specific CD4+ T cell, CD8+ T cell, and antibody responses in volunteers [55,59,60].

However, in some instances, these conventional Ad-based vaccines have yielded suboptimal clinical results. These suboptimal results are attributed, in part, to preexisting Ad5 immunity. It is estimated that 50% to 90% of the adult population has preexisting immunity (PEI) to Ad serotype 2 (Ad2) or Ad5 [61–65]; and this Ad PEI can limit efficacy of Ad based vaccinations due to Ad clearance by the immune system. In this regard, innovative strategies have been developed to circumvent drawbacks associated with Ad5 PEI, some of these strategies include the "antigen capsid-incorporation" strategy, vector chimeras, covalent modifications (i.e. such as polyethylene glycol, PEGylation) [66–68], and Gutless (helper-dependent) Ad vectors. Gutless vectors are devoid of the majority of viral genes. Therefore, they avoid cellular immunity to Ad viral genes and diminish liver toxicity, thus promoting long-term transgene expression [67,69,70].

5. Antigen capsid-incorporation strategies for vaccination schemes

The "antigen capsid-incorporation" or "capsid-display of antigen" strategies are currently being used to circumvent drawbacks associated with conventional transgene expression of antigens by viral vectors. Initially, the "capsid-display" strategy had been developed and utilized to present ligands [8,71,72], imaging motifs [7–9,73–75], and more recently immunomodulatory inhibitors and/or activators ligands [76–78]. More recently, the capsid-display of antigen strategy has been used to present antigens for vaccination applications. The antigen capsid-incorporation strategy embodies the incorporation of antigenic peptides within the capsid structure of viral vectors. The human rhinovirus has been utilized for HIV vaccination in the context of the antigen capsid-incorporation strategy. Researchers have constructed human rhinovirus: HIV chimeras to stimulate immunity against HIV-1 [79]. As well, researchers have designed combinatorial libraries of human rhinovirus capsid incorporated HIV-1 glycoprotein 41 (gp41) epitope, eliciting antibodies whose activity can mimic the NAb effect [80]. Commercial and clinical development of Ad-based HIV vaccines has progressed faster than the development of vector systems such as human rhinovirus because the tremendous flexibility of Ad generally exceeds that of current rhinovirus systems. For instance, since human rhinovirus is a relatively small RNA virus, the human rhinovirus platform can only display 60 copies of a single HIV-1 epitope [79]. In contrast, the Ad vector capsid platform could allow incorporation of HIV-1 epitopes into 4 structurally distinct domains including hexon [81], fiber, penton base, and protein IX (pIX), similar to the illustration depicted in Figure 1 [82,83].

Fiber, penton base, and pIX have been used for antigen capsid-incorporation strategies [84]. However, the major capsid protein hexon has been involved in the majority of antigen capsid-incorporation strategies. Hexon is the most plentiful of the capsid's structural proteins, accounting for 63% of the total protein mass [85,86]. Current hexon sequence analysis from different species revealed that, in addition to the conserved regions, there were 9 discrete hypervariable regions (HVRs). The HVRs of hexon contain serotype-specific epitopes [85,87]. The loops at the top of the HVRs are the most amenable to modification by genetic engineering. Some research groups have shown that short heterologous peptides can be incorporated within the HVRs of the hexon without affecting the virion's stability or function. Of note, a subset of these modifiable loops were exposed on the surface of the capsid [88,89]. HVRs1, 2, and 5 have been utilized respectively for peptide or antigen incorporation [84,88–94].

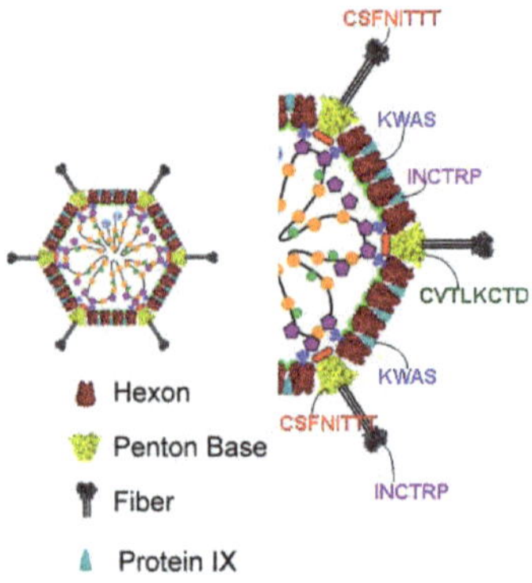

Figure 1. Antigen Capsid-Incorporation within Adenovirus Structural Proteins. Adenoviral capsid protein consists of: Hexon (II), Penton Base (III), Fiber (IV), and protein IX (pIX). Antigenic epitopes can be incorporated into these capsid structural proteins to induce antigen-specific immune responses. For example, this figure depicts the incorporation of HIV antigens from the variable region 2 (CSFNITTT), glycoprotein 41(KWAS) and glycoprotein 120 (INCTRP). This figure is adapted from Nemerow et al., 2009. Virology 384 (2009) 380–388, copyright Elsevier.

One drawback associated with conventional transgene expression of antigen is the inability of Ad-based vectors to produce a potent humoral immune response against certain antigens (as seen in the case of some malaria antigens) [95]. The antigen capsid-incorporation strategy may circumvent this drawback because this strategy embodies the incorporation of antigenic peptides within the capsid structure of viral vectors. By incorporating antigens directly into the capsid proteins, the capsid-incorporated antigen is processed through the exogenous pathway leading to strong humoral response, similar to the response generated by native Ad capsid proteins. Incorporating immunogenic peptides into the Ad capsid offers potential advantages. This strategy may allow vectors to circumvent Ad5 PEI allowing a more robust immune response to either the antigen presented on the vector capsid or the antigen that is expressed as a transgene. Additionally, because anti-Ad capsid responses are augmented by administering the vector repeatedly, immune responses against antigenic epitopes that are part of the Ad capsid should be increased by this approach as well, thus allowing boosting of the response [96–98]. This strategy may also allow for cross-priming [99,100] and activation of CD8+ T cells by means of incorporating T cell helper epitopes into the Ad capsid proteins [90]. Therefore, this antigen capsid-incorporation approach offers feasible opportunities to create Ad-based vaccine vector strategies that circumvent the major limitations associated with traditional Ad-based vaccine vectors.

Preclinically, incorporating antigens into viral capsid structures has been used as a vaccination approach for several diseases [84,90,91,93,94,101]. In 1994, Crompton and colleagues used this strategy for the first time in the context of Ad [101]. Crompton's group genetically incorporated an 8 amino acid sequence of the VP1 capsid protein of poliovirus type 3 into 2 regions of the adenovirus serotype 2 hexon. One of the chimeric vectors produced was able to grow well in tissue culture, and antiserum raised against the Ad with the polio antigen specifically recognized the VP1 capsid of the polio virus [89]. More recently, similar studies have been performed by other research groups. For example, Worgall and colleagues used the antigen capsid-incorporation strategy to vaccinate against *Pseudomonas aeruginosa* (*pseudomonas*), a Gram-negative bacterium that causes respiratory tract infections in individuals who are immunocompromised or who have cystic fibrosis [102]. Because *pseudomonas* is an extracellular pathogen, anti-*pseudomonas* humoral immunity should be sufficient to provide protective immunity. Therefore, *pseudomonas* can be a candidate agent for vaccine development. Several immunogenic peptides have been identified in the outer membrane protein F (OprF) of *pseudomonas*, including the immunodominant 14-mer peptide Epi8. This study characterizes genetic incorporations of a neutralizing epitope from the *pseudomonas* Epi8 into Ad5 HVR5 (AdZ.Epi8) [90]. BALB/c mice immunized with the capsid-modified vectors showed an increase in antibody response consisting of both anti-*pseudomonas* IgG1 and IgG2a subtypes. In addition, mice immunized with the vector containing the OprF epitope were subjected to pulmonary challenge with *pseudomonas*, 60% to 80% of them survived. This group also performed additional studies where they attempted DC targeting in combination with the antigen capsid-incorporation strategy [103].

To expand on knowledge gained from previous antigen capsid-incorporation studies, our group set out to create novel vaccine vectors that would yield optimal vaccine efficacy by maximizing the size of antigens which could be incorporated within the capsid protein, hexon. Our 2008 manuscript evaluated the use of Ad5 HVR2 or HVR5 vectors containing identical antigenic epitopes in either region. To compare the capacities and flexibility of Ad5 HVR2 to those of HVR5, we genetically incorporated identical epitopes of increasing size within HVR2 or HVR5 of the Ad5 hexon. The epitopes ranged in size from 33-83 amino acids. Stable vectors were produced with incorporations of 33 amino acids plus a 12 amino acid linker at HVR2 or HVR5. In addition, stable vectors were produced with incorporations up to 53 amino acids plus a 12 amino acid linker in HVR5. With respect to the selected antigens, HVR5 was more permissive, allowing an epitope incorporation of 65 amino acids. Whole virus enzyme-linked immunosorbent assay (ELISA) analysis revealed that the model antigens were virion surface-exposed, and *in vivo* immunization with these vectors elicited antigen-specific immune responses [93].

In our most recent published study we evaluated the antigen capsid-incorporation strategy further by using novel vectors that were constructed to provide cellular and humoral HIV immunity [104]. Our study was the first of its kind to genetically incorporate an HIV antigen within the Ad5 hexon's HVR2, alone or in combination with the genomic/E1 incorporation of the HIV Gag gene (Ad5/HVR2-MPER-L15(Gag)). In this study, we incorporated a 24 amino acid epitope of HIV within Ad5 HVR2. The HIV region selected was the membrane proximal ectodomain region (MPER) derived from HIV gp41. When the MPER epitope was incorporated within HVR2 in combination with transgene incorporation, we observed growth kinetics and thermostability changes similar to those observed in other studies after using antigen capsid-incorporated vectors [7,105], indicating that incorporation of the MPER epitope within HVR2 was not substantially detrimental to vector characteristics [9,105]. In this study we demonstrated for the first time that a disease-specific antigen could be incorporated within HVR2 of

Ad5. Also, we demonstrated that the MPER epitope is surface exposed within HVR2. Most importantly, we observed a humoral anti-HIV response in mice immunized with the hexon-modified vector. Immunization with the MPER-modified vector allows boosting when compared to that of immunization with AdCMVGag vector, possibly because the Ad5/HVR2-MPER-L15(Gag) vector elicits less of an anti-Ad5 immune response. It is plausible that the MPER epitope which is incorporated within this vector reduces the immunogenicity of the Ad5 vector. This finding is notable because HVR2 has not been fully explored for its potential use in antigen capsid-incorporation strategies.

While many studies have examined the efficacy of targeting genetic vector based vaccines to DCs to enhance cellular immune responses, our group will examine a novel question. How does DC targeting affect the vector capsid antigenicity with respect to focusing humoral immune responses to finite amounts of capsid-incorporated HIV antigen? Specifically, we are interested in evaluating how DC targeting impacts the quality and potency of humoral responses generated from our capsid-incorporated antigen approach. As previously mentioned, in our 2010 manuscript, we illustrated that immunizations with Ad5/HVR2-MPER-L15(Gag) and Ad5/HVR2-MPER-L15ΔE1 yielded MPER-specific humoral responses in BALB/c mice [104]. However, we eventually plan to use the antigen-capsid incorporation system in combination with DCs activation. The C57BL/6 mouse model will allow us to better evaluate the antigen capsid-incorporation strategy in combination with DC targeting. Our initial data illustrates (data not shown) that there are substantially more DCs available for targeting in C57BL/6 mice as compared to BALB/c mice. Therefore, it was necessary to evaluate our antigen capsid-incorporation strategy in C57BL/6 mice. In brief, C57BL/6 mice were immunized with Ad5/HVR2-MPER-L15(G/L) (green fluorescent protein/ luciferase) and Ad5/HVR2-MPER-L15(Gag), respectively. 17 days later these mice were boosted in a similar manner with the same vectors. This data indicates that there is MPER-specific humoral response produced after immunizations with both vectors in C57BL/6 mice (Figure 2). In summary, we observed a similar outcome with our antigen capsid-incorporated vectors in C57BL/6 mice; therefore, we can continue with our DC targeted antigen capsid-incorporated studies. These experiments are likely to be very informative because DCs represent a unique junction for intervention by antigen-specific vaccination strategies.

With the vast diversity of many bacterial pathogens and viral pathogens, such as HIV, the need remains for vaccine vectors that yield a broad immune response. Successful HIV vaccination remains a tremendous challenge because HIV-1 vaccine strategies must contend with the enormous global sequence diversity of HIV-1. To attempt to overcome this obstacle, mosaic vectors and Ad vectors schemes that utilize "heterologous inserts" in prime-boost regimens have been developed in order to increase the breadth and depth of cellular immune responses in nonhuman primate models [106,107]. These vectors have shown promise; however, these constructs focused primarily on cellular immunity. It is likely that the most successful prophylactic HIV-1 vaccine will elicit a broad and robust cellular and humoral response. In order to create vectors that could provide a varied humoral response we generated multivalent proof-of-concept vectors. Our definition of a multivalent vector is, a vector that has the ability to vaccinate against several strains of an organism or vaccinate against two or more distinct organisms. In this regard, our current unpublished data herein demonstrates for the first time ever that multiple antigens can be incorporated in combination at two sites within the major capsid protein, hexon (Figures 3, 4 and 5). In order to create a multivalent vaccine vector, we created vectors that display antigens within HVR1 and HVR2 or HVR1 and HVR5. Our unpublished findings focus on the generation of proof-of-concept vectors that can ultimately result in the development of multivalent vaccine vectors displaying dual antigens within the hexon of one Ad virion particle. These novel vectors utilize HVR1 as an incorporation site for a seven amino acid region (ELDKWAS) (called KWAS in this chapter) derived from HIV gp41; in combination with a six Histidine (His6) incorporation within HVR2 or HVR5. After these vectors were rescued they were designated as Ad5/H5-HVR1-KWAS-HVR2-His6 and Ad5/H5-HVR1-KWAS-HVR5-His6. In order to determine the quality of these vectors, we determined the viral particle (VP)/infectious particle (IP) ratios for the hexon-modified vectors. We compared these parameters to unmodified Ad5. Importantly, we observed similar VP/IP ratios for Ad5/H5-HVR1-KWAS-HVR2-His6 and Ad5/H5-HVR1-KWAS-HVR5-His6 as compared to Ad5 (Figure 3). These values are similar to what we observed in our previous 2008 study [93].

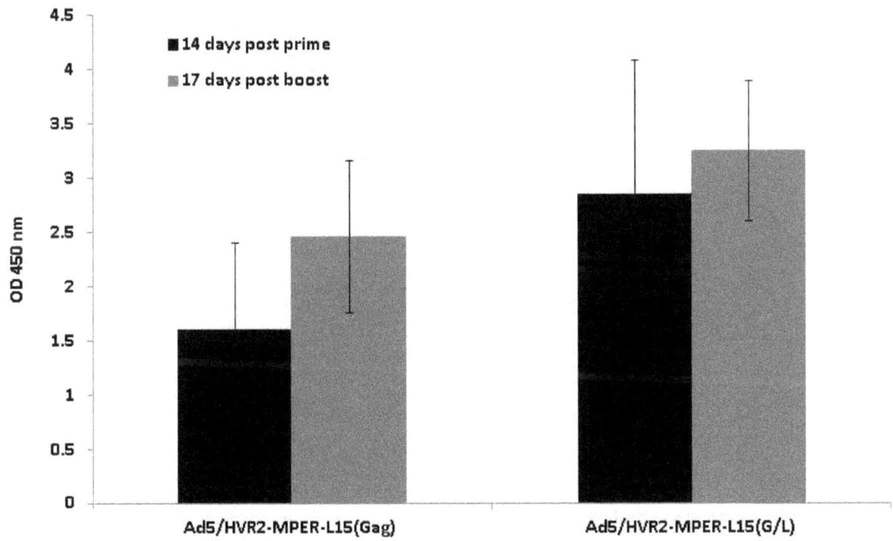

Figure 2. Adenovirus Presenting Capsid-Incorporated HIV Antigen Elicits an HIV Humoral Immune Response in C57BL/6 Mice. C57BL/6 mice (n=8) were primed and boosted with 1 x 10^{10} VP of Ad vectors. Post-prime and post-boost sera was collected at various time points for ELISA binding assays. 10 μM of purified MPER (EKNEKELLELDKWASLWNWFDITN) antigenic peptide was bound to ELISA plates. Residual unbound peptide was washed from the plates. The plates were then incubated with immunized mice sera and the binding was detected with HRP conjugated secondary antibody. OD absorbance at 450 nm represents MPER antibody levels in sera.

Modified Vectors	Viral Particles (VP)	Infectious Particles (IP)	VP/IP
Ad5	3.1 x 10^{12} VP/ml	1.0 x10^{11} IP/ml	31
Ad5/H5-HVR1-KWAS-HVR2-His_6	2.0 X 10^{12} VP/ml	3.5 x 10^{10} IP/ml	57
Ad5/H5-HVR1-KWAS-HVR5-His_6	1.3 x 10^{11} VP/ml	1.4 x 10^{9} IP/ml	92

Figure 3. Virological Characterization of Multivalent Vaccine Vectors Displaying Dual Antigens.

After the successful rescue of the multivalent vectors we next sought to verify expression of genetic incorporations at the protein level by Western blot analysis. In order to determine if the dual hexon-modified vectors were presenting His6 tag within HVR2 or HVR5, the vectors were subjected to Western blot analysis. The His6 tag was detected as a 117 kilodalton (kDa) protein band associated with Ad5/H5-HVR1-KWAS-HVR2-His6 and Ad5/H5-HVR1-KWAS-HVR5-His6. Figure 4, lanes 2 and 3, respectively. The size of the 117 kDa band corresponds to the expected size of the Ad5 hexon protein with His6 peptide genetically incorporated into the HVR2 or HVR5 region. As expected, there was no His6 protein detected on Ad5 wild type particles (Figure 4, lane 1). Similar results were observed when these vectors were analyzed in order to verify expression of KWAS incorporations within the HVR1 locale of our dual hexon-modified vectors (Figure 5, lanes 2 and 3, respectively).

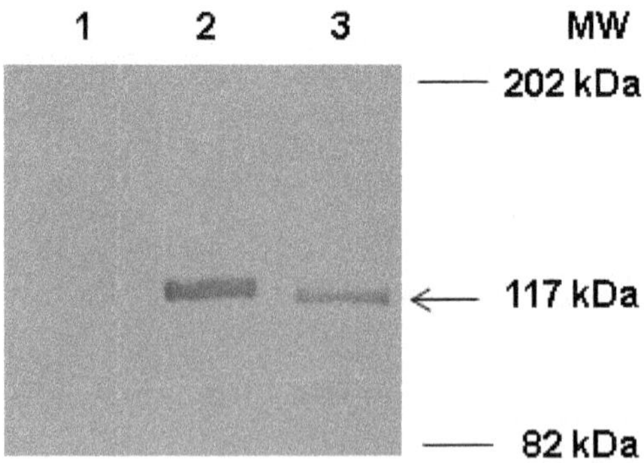

Figure 4. Western Blotting Confirms the Presence of His6 on Multivalent Vaccine Vectors Displaying Dual Antigens. Western blotting confirmed the presence of His6 incorporation within the dual modified vectors. In this assay, 1 x 10^{10} VP of Ad5 (lane 1), Ad5/H5-HVR1-KWAS-HVR2-His6 (lane 2), and Ad5/H5-HVR1-KWAS-HVR5-His6 (lane 3) were separated on 4 to 15% polyacrylamide gradient SDS-PAGE gel. The proteins were transferred to polyvinylidene fluoride membrane then blotted with anti-His antibody. The arrow indicates the His tag is genetically incorporated into the hexon protein.

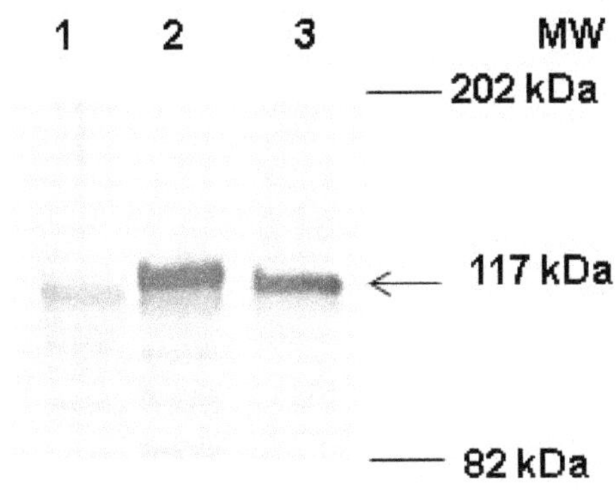

Figure 5. Western Blotting Confirms the Presence of KWAS on Multivalent Vaccine Vectors Displaying Dual Antigens. Western blotting confirmed the presence of KWAS incorporation within the dual modified vectors. In this assay, 1 x 10^{10} VP of Ad5 (lane 1), Ad5/H5-HVR1-KWAS-HVR2-His6 (lane 2), and Ad5/H5-HVR1-KWAS-HVR5-His6 (lane 3) were separated on 4 to 15% polyacrylamide gradient SDS-PAGE gel. The proteins were transferred to polyvinylidene fluoride membrane then blotted with anti-gp41 antibody (NIH AIDS Reagent Program). The arrow indicates KWAS/gp41 protein genetically incorporated into the hexon.

The size of the 117 kDa band corresponds to the expected size of the Ad5 hexon protein with KWAS peptide genetically incorporated into the HVR1 region. There was a slight KWAS protein detected on Ad5 wild type particles, we attribute this to a cross reactive sequence within the Ad vector (Figure 5, lane 1). Most importantly, Figures 4 and 5 illustrate that KWAS and His6 proteins were incorporated at comparable levels within HVR1 and HVR2 or HVR5.

We also performed a series of ELISA assays to verify that the KWAS and His6 motifs were surface accessible on the hexon double-modified virions. These results indicated that the His6 epitope was properly exposed on the virion surfaces when incorporated within HVR2 or HVR5 (data not shown). In addition, the HIV-specific ELISA also illustrated that that the HIV motif was accessible on the virion surface within the HVR1 region. Our results showed significant binding of the anti-HIV antibody to the Ad5/H5-HVR1-KWAS-HVR2-His6 and Ad5/H5-HVR1-KWAS-HVR5-His6, whereas no binding was seen in response to Ad5 control (data not shown). Currently, we are in the process of testing these vectors *in vivo*. Our initial findings lead us to believe that these vectors can have tremendous impact for multivalent vaccine development.

6. Chimeric serotype Ad vectors and rare serotype vectors for vaccine usage

In the near future, it is possible that viral vector-based vaccination will become a common clinical intervention; therefore, it has become increasingly necessary to design vectors that can overcome Ad5 pre-existing immunity [108,109]. In order to overcome Ad5 pre-existing immunity rare and non-human Ad serotypes have been used. Chimeric Ad vectors consist of either a sub-portion of the Ad5 vector genome that is replaced with genomic portions of another alternative serotype, thus creating "chimeric" Ad vectors, or, in a more drastic approach, the entire Ad vector genome is composed of proteins solely derived from alternative Ad serotypes [27,109–114]. Ad hexon and fiber have been the proteins manipulated genetically in chimeric strategies, primarily because these proteins are known to be the target of vector neutralizing antibodies [115–118]. Several chimeric fiber and hexon strategies have been endeavored [109]. Specifically, NAbs generated against hexon HVRs account for 80-90% of the Anti-Ad NAb response. These antibodies appear to be most critical for vector clearance, therefore, diminishing therapeutic efficacy of the vaccine vector administered [119]. The importance of the seven HVRs as NAbs epitopes remains unclear as it relates to Ad5 and other serotypes [120]. Therefore, exact mapping of the NAb epitopes in these HVRs, maybe necessary to obtain improved chimeric Ad5-based vectors [121].

One of the first reports of Ad5-based chimeric vectors generated was performed in 1998. This was done by replacing Ad serotype 5 hexon gene with sequences from Ad2 [122]. This study was the launching point for other chimeric vectors, such as experiments performed in 2002 by Wu and group. They constructed a chimeric adenoviral vector, Ad5/H3, by replacing the Ad5 hexon gene with the hexon gene of serotype Ad3. The chimeric vector was successfully rescued in 293 cells. Ad5/H3 had a significantly lower growth profile as compared to Ad5/H5. Indicating that the Ad3 hexon could encapsidate the Ad5 genome, but with less efficiency than the Ad5 hexon. The gene transfer efficiency of Ad5H3 in HeLa cells was also lower than that of Ad5/H5. They also tested the host neutralization responses against the two vectors after immunizing C57BL/6 mice. The neutralizing antibodies against Ad5/H3 and Ad5/H5 generated by the immunized mice did not cross-neutralize each other in the context of *in vitro* infection of HeLa cells. Preimmunization of C57BL/6 mice with one of the two types of vectors also did not prevent subsequent infection of the other type. These data suggest that replacing the Ad5 hexon with the Ad3 hexon can circumvent the host neutralization response to Ad5 [117]. Along these same lines, another research group constructed a chimeric Ad vector, Ad3/H7. This construction was generated by replacing the Ad3 hexon gene (H3) with the hexon gene (H7) of Ad7. The chimeric vectors were successfully rescued in HEp-2 cells, and the Ad7 hexon was able to encapsidate the Ad3 genome, and functioned as efficiently as the Ad3 hexon. In addition, this group tested the host neutralization responses against the vectors using BALB/c mice. Up to 97% of the NAbs produced by mice that were infected with these vectors were specific for the hexon protein *in vitro*. Preimmunization of mice with one of Ad7 and Ad3/H7 significantly prevented subsequent intranasal infection of the other vector *in vivo*. In contrast, preimmunization of mice with either Ad3 or Ad3/H7 did not remarkably prevent subsequent infection of the other vector [123].

Roberts et. al, previously demonstrated that replacing seven of the HVRs in Ad5 with that of rare serotype, Ad48, resulted in a chimeric vector, Ad5HVR48 (1-7). Ad5HVR48 (1-7) was able to evade the majority of Ad5 pre-existing immunity in preclinical studies in mice and rhesus monkeys, [112] Ad5 chimeric vectors in which all seven HVRs were exchanged induced the same level of anti-antigen immune responses in mice with Ad5 PEI as in naïve mice. However, replacing only one HVR provided little improvement over non-chimeric Ad5 vectors. Since the role of the seven individual HVRs as NAb epitopes remains unclear, there are several studies which are currently underway. Recent studies suggested that Ad5 responses maybe focused on one specific HVR, such as HVR1 or HVR5 [81,124]. Bradley and group attempted to answer some of these issues; in their study they characterized the contribution of the individual hexon HVRs as Ad5 NAb epitopes. They constructed chimeric Ad5 vectors in which subsets of Ad5 HVRs were exchanged for Ad48 HVRs. These partial HVR-chimeric vectors were evaluated by NAb assays and immunogenicity studies with and without baseline Ad5 immunity. Through a series of complex and thorough experiments they demonstrated that Ad5-specific NAbs are targeted against several of the HVRs. This data suggest that it is necessary to replace all HVRs to optimize evasion of Anti-Ad5 immunity [125]. Along those same lines, another group evaluated Ad5-based vectors where the hexon HVRs are replaced with that of the HVRs of rare serotypes, Ad43 and Ad34. Ad43 and 34 are group D and B viruses, each of these have low prevalence of neutralizing antibodies in humans. They demonstrated that these hexon-modified Ad vectors are not neutralized efficiently by Ad5 neutralizing antibodies *in vitro* using sera from mice, rabbits, and human volunteers. This research yielded significant findings related to malaria antigen expression, in combination with hexon-modified vectors. Their data also demonstrates that hexon-modified vectors can be highly immunogenic in the presence of Ad5 pre-existing immunity. The authors comment that these hexon-modified vectors may have useful applications in places such as sub-Saharan Africa where there is high prevalence of pre-existing Ad5 immunity [126].

Liver sequestration of Ad5-based vectors is another major drawback that hinders Ad5-based therapies. Previous studies illustrate that human coagulation factor X (FX) binds Ad5 hexon through an interaction between HVRs and the FX Gla domain leading to liver infection after systemic delivery [127,128]. The binding affinities for FX vary among vector serotypes, and may explain differences in heptaocyte transduction *in vivo* previously observed between serotypes. Although, some differences in binding affinities were noted in this report, overall, Ad2 and Ad5 bound factor X with the highest affinity, however, weak or no binding was detected with Ad9, Ad35, Ad48, and Ad51. This interaction has been observed in multiple human adenovirus serotypes and shows diversity and affinity. The domains and amino acid sequences in the HVRs are integral for high-affinity interaction with FX, however, several aspects of this binding and mechanism remain unclear [121]. In recent studies, Yu and colleagues evaluated the role of chimeric hexon HVRs with FX binding and affinity. In this study they constructed and expressed several chimeric HVR proteins and demonstrated that the native proteins were oligomers and had consistent structure and function with that of the virus. Their data demonstrated that HVR5 and HVR7 had only a fraction of hexon activity to NAbs compared to a group of HVRs, 1 through 7. In addition, they demonstrated a differential high-affinity interaction of the HVR proteins with FX and indicated that the HVRs had similar binding activity with corresponding Ad vector serotypes. This study highlighted some properties of chimeric HVR proteins and exposed the influences on the structure and function of hexon proteins and Ad vectors resulting from the incorporations of these HVRs [129].

The use of vectors derived completely from alternative human serotypes (including Ad26 and Ad35) have also shown great promise, in particular, in terms of ability to deliver transgenes [110,113,130,131]. The development of vectors based on Ads which normally infect nonhuman species have also shown a great deal of promise. These nonhuman Ad vectors have been developed from multiple species, including, bovine, canine, chimpanzee and porcine [67]. Vectors derived from chimpanzee Ads C1 or C8 (AdC), have been recently developed, initially these vectors gained popularity since it was demonstrated that human sera does not significantly neutralize AdC vectors [132]. Importantly, unlike some other serotypes, the E1-deleted version of AdC7 is easily propagated [133]. An AdC7 vector expressing the SARS-coronavirus antigen elicited higher T-and B-cell responses than an Ad5 vector in mice with Ad5 PEI [134]. Importantly, a single injection of AdC7 encoding the Ebola glycoprotein provided protection from a lethal challenge, unlike the corresponding Ad5 vector [133].

It is essential to note that several Ad epitopes recognized by T cells are conserved among a broad range of human and nonhuman primate-derived Ads, making it possible that the T cells in patient with Ad5 PEI will also recognize vectors derived from these viruses [135–138]. Bovine Ads have been examined, since NAbs to bovine Ad3 (BAd3) have not been reported in humans. In a mouse model, a single immunization of BAd3 encoding the hemagglutination antigen of H5N1 influenza induced greater levels of cellular immunity than Ad5 vectors, and this was not diminished by Ad5 PEI [139]. It is important to note that, mice which had Ad5 PEI and received a prime-boost regimen of BAd3-Ad5 vectors encoding HA were fully protected from lethal influenza virus challenge. However, those receiving a homologous Ad5-Ad5 regimen were not. Therefore, Ad vectors that normally infect nonhuman species may induce responses and offer protection comparable or superior to Ad5, while maintaining protection in the presence of Ad5 PEI. The use of alternative serotype Ads allow for improved induction of immune responses to vector re-administration in host that have Ad5 PEI [110,113,140]. As a result of these earlier studies, alternative serotypes vectors have been tested in patient populations for HIV vaccine development [141]. In addition, human clinical trials utilizing Ad26 as a HIV vaccine agent have been initiated.

There are benefits to using alternative serotype vectors, however, the use of alternative serotypes vectors can also have limitations as well as potential side effects for human use. One limitation of alternative serotype usage is that, some alternative serotypes do not afford the same benefits of Ad5 because they are unable to induce high levels of transgene expression and are less amenable to large scale purification [108]. Humans have evolved with previous exposure to human Ad vectors, and have not been exposed to Ads derived from other species. Consequently, it may be predicted that the human innate immune system may react to the capsid proteins of alternative serotype Ads in a way that is different from that of human Ad vectors. It is also possible that the human immune system may have a response which is more robust when challenged with alternative serotypes as compared with human serotypes Ads. Recently, it has been demonstrated that the innate immune response to capsid proteins of alternative serotypes Ads have not only been shown to be significantly more robust as compared to Ad5, but in some cases toxic in animal models [110,142–144]. Alternative serotype vectors have different tropism than Ad5; therefore the biodistribution of these vectors could be quite different than that of Ad5-based vectors. Ad5 vectors have been proven to be safe in humans and animals over the last decade and the knowledge gained from this experimentation must be applied and tested as it relates to alternative serotype vectors.

7. Conclusion

Recombinant viral vectors have been utilized as therapeutic agents to prevent or cure disease because of their tremendous capacity to deliver antigens and to stimulate immune responses in humans. Viral vectors are generally more immunogenic than antigen administered adjuvant [19,145]. In addition, it is easier to generate recombinant vectors as compared to tumor cell or DC-based vaccines. Tumor cell or DC-based vaccines can be complex to acquire. They are often time consuming to produce and costly because they are customized treatments. Whereas, on the other hand, recombinant vectors are thought to be "off the shelf" treatments because they are relatively easy to produce, purify, and store. One major advantage of utilizing viral vectors for vaccination in multi-center clinical trials is the relatively low cost of vector production. However, the paramount factor to overcome when using viral vectors for gene therapy, virotherapy, and vaccine applications is the development of host-induced neutralizing antibodies to the vector itself which limits continued usage.

The past few years have bought forward exciting technical advances, along with critical structure/function analyses of viral vectors which have allowed for better understanding of the interaction of recombinant vector and host immune systems. It has become increasingly more obvious that there are many factors which must be evaluated to optimize each specific vaccine. In order to achieve optimal therapeutic outcomes when treating patients with vector PEI, careful consideration must be given to determine prime-boost schemes, epitope-capsid incorporation (monovalent versus polyvalent), transgene selection (homologous versus heterologous), vector dosing, and serotype selection.

Acknowledgements

This work was supported by a grant from the National Institutes of Health: 5R01AI089337-02 (Matthews). I would like to thank Dr. Phoebe L. Stewart for allowing me to reproduce her figure (Nemerow et al. Virology 2009, 384, 380-388), copyright Elsevier. I would also like to thank Dr. Glenn C. Rowe for his thoughtful insight and review of this chapter. We would also like to thank the NIH AIDS Reagent Program, for providing HIV-1 gp41 monoclonal antibody (2F5), Cat # 1475.

Author details

Qiana L. Matthews*, Linlin Gu, Alexandre Krendelchtchikov and Zan C. Li

Department of Medicine, Division of Infectious Diseases, The University of Alabama, Birmingham, AL, USA

References

[1] Larocca C, Schlom J (2011) Viral vector-based therapeutic cancer vaccines. Cancer J 17: 359-371.

[2] Benihoud K, Yeh P, Perricaudet M (1999) Adenovirus vectors for gene delivery. Curr Opin Biotechnol 10: 440-447.

[3] Stratford-Perricaudet LD, Makeh I, Perricaudet M, Briand P (1992) Widespread long-term gene transfer to mouse skeletal muscles and heart. J Clin Invest 90: 626-630.

[4] Puntel M, Muhammad AK, Candolfi M, Salem A, Yagiz K, Farrokhi C, Kroeger KM, Xiong W, Curtin JF, Liu C, Bondale NS, Lerner J, Pechnick RN, Palmer D, Ng P, Lowenstein PR, Castro MG (2010) A novel bicistronic high-capacity gutless adenovirus vector that drives constitutive expression of herpes simplex virus type 1 thymidine kinase and tet-inducible expression of Flt3L for glioma therapeutics. J Virol 84: 6007-6017.

[5] Li N, Zhou J, Weng D, Zhang C, Li L, Wang B, Song Y, He Q, Lin D, Chen D, Chen G, Gao Q, Wang S, Xu G, Meng L, Lu Y, Ma D (2007) Adjuvant adenovirus-mediated delivery of herpes simplex virus thymidine kinase administration improves outcome of liver transplantation in patients with advanced hepatocellular carcinoma. Clin Cancer Res 13: 5847-5854.

[6] Lopez M, Matthews Q, Curiel D, Borovjagin A (2010) Imaging in Vector Development. In: Weissleder, Gambhir, Ross, Rehemtulla, editors. Molecular Imaging: Principles and Practice. BC Decker Inc.

[7] Matthews QL, Sibley DA, Wu H, Li J, Stoff-Khalili MA, Waehler R, Mathis JM, Curiel DT (2006) Genetic incorporation of a herpes simplex virus type 1 thymidine kinase and firefly luciferase fusion into the adenovirus protein IX for functional display on the virion. Mol Imaging 5: 510-519.

[8] Tang Y, Le LP, Matthews QL, Han T, Wu H, Curiel DT (2008) Derivation of a triple mosaic adenovirus based on modification of the minor capsid protein IX. Virology 377: 391-400. S0042-6822(08)00263-8 [pii];10.1016/j.virol.2008.04.023 [doi].

[9] Li J, Le L, Sibley DA, Mathis JM, Curiel DT (2005) Genetic incorporation of HSV-1 thymidine kinase into the adenovirus protein IX for functional display on the virion. Virology 338: 247-258.

[10] Borovjagin AV, Dong J, Passineau MJ, Ren C, Lamani E, Mamaeva OA, Wu H, Keyser E, Murakami M, Chen S, MacDougall M (2011) Adenovirus gene transfer to amelogenesis imperfecta ameloblast-like cells. PLoS One 6: e24281.

[11] Wu H, Yoon AR, Li F, Yun CO, Mahato RI (2011) RGD peptide-modified adenovirus expressing HGF and XIAP improves islet transplantation. J Gene Med .

[12] Guo ZS, Thorne SH, Bartlett DL (2008) Oncolytic virotherapy: molecular targets in tumor-selective replication and carrier cell-mediated delivery of oncolytic viruses. Biochim Biophys Acta 1785: 217-231.

[13] Ahmed AU, Ulasov IV, Mercer RW, Lesniak MS (2012) Maintaining and loading neural stem cells for delivery of oncolytic adenovirus to brain tumors. Methods Mol Biol 797: 97-109.

[14] Curiel DT (2000) The development of conditionally replicative adenoviruses for cancer therapy. Clin Cancer Res 6: 3395-3399.

[15] Sonabend AM, Ulasov IV, Lesniak MS (2006) Conditionally replicative adenoviral vectors for malignant glioma. Rev Med Virol 16: 99-115.

[16] Myers R, Greiner S, Harvey M, Soeffker D, Frenzke M, Abraham K, Shaw A, Rozenblatt S, Federspiel MJ, Russell SJ, Peng KW (2005) Oncolytic activities of approved mumps and measles vaccines for therapy of ovarian cancer. Cancer Gene Ther 12: 593-599.

[17] Russell SJ, Peng KW (2009) Measles virus for cancer therapy. Curr Top Microbiol Immunol 330: 213-241.

[18] Lou E (2003) Oncolytic herpes viruses as a potential mechanism for cancer therapy. Acta Oncol 42: 660-671.

[19] Kass E, Schlom J, Thompson J, Guadagni F, Graziano P, Greiner JW (1999) Induction of protective host immunity to carcinoembryonic antigen (CEA), a self-antigen in CEA transgenic mice, by immunizing with a recombinant vaccinia-CEA virus. Cancer Res 59: 676-683.

[20] Arlen PM, Kaufman HL, DiPaola RS (2005) Pox viral vaccine approaches. Semin Oncol 32: 549-555.

[21] Moss B (1996) Genetically engineered poxviruses for recombinant gene expression, vaccination, and safety. Proc Natl Acad Sci U S A 93: 11341-11348.

[22] Brown M, Davies DH, Skinner MA, Bowen G, Hollingsworth SJ, Mufti GJ, Arrand JR, Stacey SN (1999) Antigen gene transfer to cultured human dendritic cells using recombinant avipoxvirus vectors. Cancer Gene Ther 6: 238-245.

[23] Drillien R, Spehner D, Bohbot A, Hanau D (2000) Vaccinia virus-related events and phenotypic changes after infection of dendritic cells derived from human monocytes. Virology 268: 471-481.

[24] Bonini C, Lee SP, Riddell SR, Greenberg PD (2001) Targeting antigen in mature dendritic cells for simultaneous stimulation of CD4+ and CD8+ T cells. J Immunol 166: 5250-5257.

[25] Hodge JW, Chakraborty M, Kudo-Saito C, Garnett CT, Schlom J (2005) Multiple costimulatory modalities enhance CTL avidity. J Immunol 174: 5994-6004.

[26] Yang S, Tsang KY, Schlom J (2005) Induction of higher-avidity human CTLs by vector-mediated enhanced costimulation of antigen-presenting cells. Clin Cancer Res 11: 5603-5615.

[27] Noureddini SC, Curiel DT (2005) Genetic targeting strategies for adenovirus. Mol Pharm 2: 341-347.

[28] Aichele P, Brduscha-Riem K, Zinkernagel RM, Hengartner H, Pircher H (1995) T cell priming versus T cell tolerance induced by synthetic peptides. J Exp Med 182: 261-266.

[29] Hangalapura BN, Timares L, Oosterhoff D, Scheper RJ, Curiel DT, de Gruijl TD (2012) CD40-targeted adenoviral cancer vaccines: the long and winding road to the clinic. J Gene Med .

[30] Lech PJ, Russell SJ (2010) Use of attenuated paramyxoviruses for cancer therapy. Expert Rev Vaccines 9: 1275-1302.

[31] Schlom J (2012) Therapeutic cancer vaccines: current status and moving forward. J Natl Cancer Inst 104: 599-613.

[32] Jacobs BL, Langland JO, Kibler KV, Denzler KL, White SD, Holechek SA, Wong S, Huynh T, Baskin CR (2009) Vaccinia virus vaccines: past, present and future. Antiviral Res 84: 1-13.

[33] Tulman ER, Afonso CL, Lu Z, Zsak L, Kutish GF, Rock DL (2004) The genome of canarypox virus. J Virol 78: 353-366.

[34] Roberts KL, Smith GL (2008) Vaccinia virus morphogenesis and dissemination. Trends Microbiol 16: 472-479.

[35] Somogyi P, Frazier J, Skinner MA (1993) Fowlpox virus host range restriction: gene expression, DNA replication, and morphogenesis in nonpermissive mammalian cells. Virology 197: 439-444.

[36] Aarts WM, Schlom J, Hodge JW (2002) Vector-based vaccine/cytokine combination therapy to enhance induction of immune responses to a self-antigen and antitumor activity. Cancer Res 62: 5770-5777.

[37] Sutter G, Staib C (2003) Vaccinia vectors as candidate vaccines: the development of modified vaccinia virus Ankara for antigen delivery. Curr Drug Targets Infect Disord 3: 263-271.

[38] Pastoret PP, Vanderplasschen A (2003) Poxviruses as vaccine vectors. Comp Immunol Microbiol Infect Dis 26: 343-355.

[39] Kundig TM, Kalberer CP, Hengartner H, Zinkernagel RM (1993) Vaccination with two different vaccinia recombinant viruses: long-term inhibition of secondary vaccination. Vaccine 11: 1154-1158.

[40] Taylor J, Paoletti E (1988) Fowlpox virus as a vector in non-avian species. Vaccine 6: 466-468.

[41] [Anonymous]www.wiley.co.uk/genetherapy/clinical. Journal Gene Therapy Worldwide web site .

[42] Kay MA, Glorioso JC, Naldini L (2001) Viral vectors for gene therapy: the art of turning infectious agents into vehicles of therapeutics. Nat Med 7: 33-40.

[43] Barnett BG, Crews CJ, Douglas JT (2002) Targeted adenoviral vectors. Biochim Biophys Acta 1575: 1-14.

[44] Curiel DT (1999) Strategies to adapt adenoviral vectors for targeted delivery. Ann N Y Acad Sci 886: 158-171.

[45] Wold WS, Doronin K, Toth K, Kuppuswamy M, Lichtenstein DL, Tollefson AE (1999) Immune responses to adenoviruses: viral evasion mechanisms and their implications for the clinic. Curr Opin Immunol 11: 380-386.

[46] Hayder H, Mullbacher A (1996) Molecular basis of immune evasion strategies by adenoviruses. Immunol Cell Biol 74: 504-512.

[47] Bruder JT, Jie T, McVey DL, Kovesdi I (1997) Expression of gp19K increases the persistence of transgene expression from an adenovirus vector in the mouse lung and liver. J Virol 71: 7623-7628.

[48] Ribacka C, Pesonen S, Hemminki A (2008) Cancer, stem cells, and oncolytic viruses. Ann Med 40: 496-505.

[49] Sullivan NJ, Geisbert TW, Geisbert JB, Xu L, Yang ZY, Roederer M, Koup RA, Jahrling PB, Nabel GJ (2003) Accelerated vaccination for Ebola virus haemorrhagic fever in non-human primates. Nature 424: 681-684.

[50] Gilbert SC, Schneider J, Hannan CM, Hu JT, Plebanski M, Sinden R, Hill AV (2002) Enhanced CD8 T cell immunogenicity and protective efficacy in a mouse malaria model using a recombinant adenoviral vaccine in heterologous prime-boost immunisation regimes. Vaccine 20: 1039-1045.

[51] Ophorst OJ, Radosevic K, Havenga MJ, Pau MG, Holterman L, Berkhout B, Goudsmit J, Tsuji M (2006) Immunogenicity and protection of a recombinant human adenovirus serotype 35-based malaria vaccine against Plasmodium yoelii in mice. Infect Immun 74: 313-320.

[52] Rodrigues EG, Claassen J, Lee S, Wilson JM, Nussenzweig RS, Tsuji M (2000) Interferon-gamma-independent CD8+ T cell-mediated protective anti-malaria immunity elicited by recombinant adenovirus. Parasite Immunol 22: 157-160.

[53] Sridhar S, Reyes-Sandoval A, Draper SJ, Moore AC, Gilbert SC, Gao GP, Wilson JM, Hill AV (2008) Single-dose protection against Plasmodium berghei by a simian adenovirus vector using a human cytomegalovirus promoter containing intron A. J Virol 82: 3822-3833.

[54] Abel B, Tameris M, Mansoor N, Gelderbloem S, Hughes J, Abrahams D, Makhethe L, Erasmus M, de KM, van der ML, Hawkridge A, Veldsman A, Hatherill M, Schirru G,

Pau MG, Hendriks J, Weverling GJ, Goudsmit J, Sizemore D, McClain JB, Goetz M, Gearhart J, Mahomed H, Hussey GD, Sadoff JC, Hanekom WA (2010) The novel tuberculosis vaccine, AERAS-402, induces robust and polyfunctional CD4+ and CD8+ T cells in adults. Am J Respir Crit Care Med 181: 1407-1417.

[55] Catanzaro AT, Koup RA, Roederer M, Bailer RT, Enama ME, Moodie Z, Gu L, Martin JE, Novik L, Chakrabarti BK, Butman BT, Gall JG, King CR, Andrews CA, Sheets R, Gomez PL, Mascola JR, Nabel GJ, Graham BS (2006) Phase 1 safety and immunogenicity evaluation of a multiclade HIV-1 candidate vaccine delivered by a replication-defective recombinant adenovirus vector. J Infect Dis 194: 1638-1649.

[56] Buchbinder SP, Mehrotra DV, Duerr A, Fitzgerald DW, Mogg R, Li D, Gilbert PB, Lama JR, Marmor M, Del RC, McElrath MJ, Casimiro DR, Gottesdiener KM, Chodakewitz JA, Corey L, Robertson MN (2008) Efficacy assessment of a cell-mediated immunity HIV-1 vaccine (the Step Study): a double-blind, randomised, placebo-controlled, test-of-concept trial. Lancet 372: 1881-1893. S0140-6736(08)61591-3 [pii];10.1016/S0140-6736(08)61591-3 [doi].

[57] McElrath MJ, De Rosa SC, Moodie Z, Dubey S, Kierstead L, Janes H, Defawe OD, Carter DK, Hural J, Akondy R, Buchbinder SP, Robertson MN, Mehrotra DV, Self SG, Corey L, Shiver JW, Casimiro DR (2008) HIV-1 vaccine-induced immunity in the test-of-concept Step Study: a case-cohort analysis. Lancet 372: 1894-1905. S0140-6736(08)61592-5 [pii];10.1016/S0140-6736(08)61592-5 [doi].

[58] Sedegah M, Kim Y, Peters B, McGrath S, Ganeshan H, Lejano J, Abot E, Banania G, Belmonte M, Sayo R, Farooq F, Doolan DL, Regis D, Tamminga C, Chuang I, Bruder JT, King CR, Ockenhouse CF, Faber B, Remarque E, Hollingdale MR, Richie TL, Sette A (2010) Identification and localization of minimal MHC-restricted CD8+ T cell epitopes within the Plasmodium falciparum AMA1 protein. Malar J 9: 241.

[59] Sedegah M, Tamminga C, McGrath S, House B, Ganeshan H, Lejano J, Abot E, Banania GJ, Sayo R, Farooq F, Belmonte M, Manohar N, Richie NO, Wood C, Long CA, Regis D, Williams FT, Shi M, Chuang I, Spring M, Epstein JE, Mendoza-Silveiras J, Limbach K, Patterson NB, Bruder JT, Doolan DL, King CR, Soisson L, Diggs C, Carucci D, Dutta S, Hollingdale MR, Ockenhouse CF, Richie TL (2011) Adenovirus 5-vectored P. falciparum vaccine expressing CSP and AMA1. Part A: safety and immunogenicity in seronegative adults. PLoS One 6: e24586.

[60] Tamminga C, Sedegah M, Regis D, Chuang I, Epstein JE, Spring M, Mendoza-Silveiras J, McGrath S, Maiolatesi S, Reyes S, Steinbeiss V, Fedders C, Smith K, House B, Ganeshan H, Lejano J, Abot E, Banania GJ, Sayo R, Farooq F, Belmonte M, Murphy J, Komisar J, Williams J, Shi M, Brambilla D, Manohar N, Richie NO, Wood C, Limbach K, Patterson NB, Bruder JT, Doolan DL, King CR, Diggs C, Soisson L, Carucci D, Levine G, Dutta S, Hollingdale MR, Ockenhouse CF, Richie TL (2011) Adenovirus-5-vectored P. falciparum vaccine expressing CSP and AMA1. Part B: safety, immunogenicity and protective efficacy of the CSP component. PLoS One 6: e25868.

[61] Chirmule N, Propert K, Magosin S, Qian Y, Qian R, Wilson J (1999) Immune responses to adenovirus and adeno-associated virus in humans. Gene Ther 6: 1574-1583. 10.1038/sj.gt.3300994 [doi].

[62] Kass-Eisler A, Falck-Pedersen E, Elfenbein DH, Alvira M, Buttrick PM, Leinwand LA (1994) The impact of developmental stage, route of administration and the immune system on adenovirus-mediated gene transfer. Gene Ther 1: 395-402.

[63] Kass-Eisler A, Leinwand L, Gall J, Bloom B, Falck-Pedersen E (1996) Circumventing the immune response to adenovirus-mediated gene therapy. Gene Ther 3: 154-162.

[64] Wohlfart C (1988) Neutralization of adenoviruses: kinetics, stoichiometry, and mechanisms. J Virol 62: 2321-2328.

[65] Schagen FH, Ossevoort M, Toes RE, Hoeben RC (2004) Immune responses against adenoviral vectors and their transgene products: a review of strategies for evasion. Crit Rev Oncol Hematol 50: 51-70. 10.1016/S1040-8428(03)00172-0 [doi];S1040842803001720 [pii].

[66] Campos SK, Barry MA (2007) Current advances and future challenges in Adenoviral vector biology and targeting. Curr Gene Ther 7: 189-204.

[67] Bangari DS, Mittal SK (2006) Current strategies and future directions for eluding adenoviral vector immunity. Curr Gene Ther 6: 215-226.

[68] Wagner E (2008) Converging paths of viral and non-viral vector engineering. Mol Ther 16: 1-2.

[69] Brown BD, Shi CX, Rawle FE, Tinlin S, McKinven A, Hough C, Graham FL, Lillicrap D (2004) Factors influencing therapeutic efficacy and the host immune response to helper-dependent adenoviral gene therapy in hemophilia A mice. J Thromb Haemost 2: 111-118. 552 [pii].

[70] Kim IH, Jozkowicz A, Piedra PA, Oka K, Chan L (2001) Lifetime correction of genetic deficiency in mice with a single injection of helper-dependent adenoviral vector. Proc Natl Acad Sci U S A 98: 13282-13287.

[71] Wickham TJ, Roelvink PW, Brough DE, Kovesdi I (1996) Adenovirus targeted to heparan-containing receptors increases its gene delivery efficiency to multiple cell types. Nat Biotechnol 14: 1570-1573. 10.1038/nbt1196-1570 [doi].

[72] Kimball KJ, Rivera AA, Zinn KR, Icyuz M, Saini V, Li J, Zhu ZB, Siegal GP, Douglas JT, Curiel DT, Alvarez RD, Borovjagin AV (2009) Novel infectivity-enhanced oncolytic adenovirus with a capsid-incorporated dual-imaging moiety for monitoring virotherapy in ovarian cancer. Mol Imaging 8: 264-277.

[73] Le LP, Le HN, Dmitriev IP, Davydova JG, Gavrikova T, Yamamoto S, Curiel DT, Yamamoto M (2006) Dynamic monitoring of oncolytic adenovirus in vivo by genetic capsid labeling. J Natl Cancer Inst 98: 203-214. 98/3/203 [pii];10.1093/jnci/djj022 [doi].

[74] Meulenbroek RA, Sargent KL, Lunde J, Jasmin BJ, Parks RJ (2004) Use of adenovirus protein IX (pIX) to display large polypeptides on the virion--generation of fluorescent virus through the incorporation of pIX-GFP. Mol Ther 9: 617-624. 10.1016/j.ymthe. 2004.01.012 [doi];S1525001604000450 [pii].

[75] Borovjagin AV, McNally LR, Wang M, Curiel DT, MacDougall MJ, Zinn KR (2010) Noninvasive monitoring of m. Mol Imaging 9: 59-75.

[76] Jerry LB, Hui L, Jesus G, Igor D, Victor K, Christy AR, Denise RS, Ronald DA, David TC, Theresa VS (2000) Using a Tropism-Modified Adenoviral Vector to Circumvent Inhibitory Factors in Ascites Fluid. Human Gene Therapy 11: 1657-1669.

[77] Seregin SS, Hartman ZC, Appledorn DM, Godbehere S, Jiang H, Frank MM, Amalfitano A (2010) Novel adenovirus vectors 'capsid-displaying' a human complement inhibitor. J Innate Immun 2: 353-359.

[78] Seregin SS, Aldhamen YA, Appledorn DM, Hartman ZC, Schuldt NJ, Scott J, Godbehere S, Jiang H, Frank MM, Amalfitano A (2010) Adenovirus capsid-display of the retro-oriented human complement inhibitor DAF reduces Ad vector-triggered immune responses in vitro and in vivo. Blood 116: 1669-1677.

[79] Smith AD, Resnick DA, Zhang A, Geisler SC, Arnold E, Arnold GF (1994) Use of random systematic mutagenesis to generate viable human rhinovirus 14 chimeras displaying human immunodeficiency virus type 1 V3 loop sequences. J Virol 68: 575-579.

[80] Arnold GF, Velasco PK, Holmes AK, Wrin T, Geisler SC, Phung P, Tian Y, Resnick DA, Ma X, Mariano TM, Petropoulos CJ, Taylor JW, Katinger H, Arnold E (2009) Broad neutralization of human immunodeficiency virus type 1 (HIV-1) elicited from human rhinoviruses that display the HIV-1 gp41 ELDKWA epitope. J Virol 83: 5087-5100. JVI. 00184-09 [pii];10.1128/JVI.00184-09 [doi].

[81] Abe S, Okuda K, Ura T, Kondo A, Yoshida A, Yoshizaki S, Mizuguchi H, Klinman D, Shimada M (2009) Adenovirus type 5 with modified hexons induces robust transgene-specific immune responses in mice with pre-existing immunity against adenovirus type 5. J Gene Med 11: 570-579. 10.1002/jgm.1332 [doi].

[82] Matthews QL (2011) Capsid-incorporation of antigens into adenovirus capsid proteins for a vaccine approach. Mol Pharm 8: 3-11.

[83] Nemerow GR, Pache L, Reddy V, Stewart PL (2009) Insights into adenovirus host cell interactions from structural studies. Virology 384: 380-388. S0042-6822(08)00658-2 [pii]; 10.1016/j.virol.2008.10.016 [doi].

[84] Krause A, Joh JH, Hackett NR, Roelvink PW, Bruder JT, Wickham TJ, Kovesdi I, Crystal RG, Worgall S (2006) Epitopes expressed in different adenovirus capsid proteins induce different levels of epitope-specific immunity. J Virol 80: 5523-5530. 80/11/5523 [pii]; 10.1128/JVI.02667-05 [doi].

[85] Rux JJ, Kuser PR, Burnett RM (2003) Structural and phylogenetic analysis of adenovirus hexons by use of high-resolution x-ray crystallographic, molecular modeling, and sequence-based methods. J Virol 77: 9553-9566.

[86] van OJ, Burnett RM (1985) Molecular composition of the adenovirus type 2 virion. J Virol 56: 439-448.

[87] Crawford-Miksza L, Schnurr DP (1996) Analysis of 15 adenovirus hexon proteins reveals the location and structure of seven hypervariable regions containing serotype-specific residues. J Virol 70: 1836-1844.

[88] Wu H, Han T, Belousova N, Krasnykh V, Kashentseva E, Dmitriev I, Kataram M, Mahasreshti PJ, Curiel DT (2005) Identification of sites in adenovirus hexon for foreign peptide incorporation. J Virol 79: 3382-3390. 79/6/3382 [pii];10.1128/JVI. 79.6.3382-3390.2005 [doi].

[89] Vigne E, Mahfouz I, Dedieu JF, Brie A, Perricaudet M, Yeh P (1999) RGD inclusion in the hexon monomer provides adenovirus type 5-based vectors with a fiber knob-independent pathway for infection. J Virol 73: 5156-5161.

[90] Worgall S, Krause A, Rivara M, Hee KK, Vintayen EV, Hackett NR, Roelvink PW, Bruder JT, Wickham TJ, Kovesdi I, Crystal RG (2005) Protection against P. aeruginosa with an adenovirus vector containing an OprF epitope in the capsid. J Clin Invest 115: 1281-1289. 10.1172/JCI23135 [doi].

[91] McConnell MJ, Danthinne X, Imperiale MJ (2006) Characterization of a permissive epitope insertion site in adenovirus hexon. J Virol 80: 5361-5370. 80/11/5361 [pii]; 10.1128/JVI.00256-06 [doi].

[92] Worgall S, Krause A, Qiu J, Joh J, Hackett NR, Crystal RG (2007) Protective immunity to pseudomonas aeruginosa induced with a capsid-modified adenovirus expressing P. aeruginosa OprF. J Virol 81: 13801-13808. JVI.01246-07 [pii];10.1128/JVI.01246-07 [doi].

[93] Matthews QL, Yang P, Wu Q, Belousova N, Rivera AA, Stoff-Khalili MA, Waehler R, Hsu HC, Li Z, Li J, Mountz JD, Wu H, Curiel DT (2008) Optimization of capsid-incorporated antigens for a novel adenovirus vaccine approach. Virol J 5: 98. 1743-422X-5-98 [pii];10.1186/1743-422X-5-98 [doi].

[94] Palma C, Overstreet MG, Guedon JM, Hoiczyk E, Ward C, Karen KA, Zavala F, Ketner G (2011) Adenovirus particles that display the Plasmodium falciparum circumsporozoite protein NANP repeat induce sporozoite-neutralizing antibodies in mice. Vaccine 29: 1683-1689.

[95] Shiratsuchi T, Rai U, Krause A, Worgall S, Tsuji M (2010) Replacing adenoviral vector HVR1 with a malaria B cell epitope improves immunogenicity and circumvents preexisting immunity to adenovirus in mice. J Clin Invest 120: 3688-3701. 39812 [pii]; 10.1172/JCI39812 [doi].

[96] Yang Y, Li Q, Ertl HC, Wilson JM (1995) Cellular and humoral immune responses to viral antigens create barriers to lung-directed gene therapy with recombinant adenoviruses. J Virol 69: 2004-2015.

[97] Jooss K, Chirmule N (2003) Immunity to adenovirus and adeno-associated viral vectors: implications for gene therapy. Gene Ther 10: 955-963.

[98] Sette A, Fikes J (2003) Epitope-based vaccines: an update on epitope identification, vaccine design and delivery. Curr Opin Immunol 15: 461-470.

[99] Heath WR, Carbone FR (2001) Cross-presentation, dendritic cells, tolerance and immunity. Annu Rev Immunol 19: 47-64. 19/1/47 [pii];10.1146/annurev.immunol.19.1.47 [doi].

[100] Carbone FR, Heath WR (2010) Cross-priming: its beginnings. J Immunol 185: 1353-1354. 185/3/1353 [pii];10.4049/jimmunol.1090065 [doi].

[101] Crompton J, Toogood CI, Wallis N, Hay RT (1994) Expression of a foreign epitope on the surface of the adenovirus hexon. J Gen Virol 75 (Pt 1): 133-139.

[102] Garau J, Gomez L (2003) Pseudomonas aeruginosa pneumonia. Curr Opin Infect Dis 16: 135-143. 10.1097/01.aco.0000065080.06965.86 [doi].

[103] Worgall S, Busch A, Rivara M, Bonnyay D, Leopold PL, Merritt R, Hackett NR, Rovelink PW, Bruder JT, Wickham TJ, Kovesdi I, Crystal RG (2004) Modification to the capsid of the adenovirus vector that enhances dendritic cell infection and transgene-specific cellular immune responses. J Virol 78: 2572-2580.

[104] Matthews QL, Fatima A, Tang Y, Perry BA, Tsuruta Y, Komarova S, Timares L, Zhao C, Makarova N, Borovjagin AV, Stewart PL, Wu H, Blackwell JL, Curiel DT (2010) HIV antigen incorporation within adenovirus hexon hypervariable 2 for a novel HIV vaccine approach. PLoS One 5: e11815. 10.1371/journal.pone.0011815 [doi].

[105] Li J, Fatima A, Komarova S, Ugai H, Uprety P, Roth JC, Wang M, Oster RA, Curiel DT, Matthews QL (2010) Evaluation of adenovirus capsid labeling versus transgene expression. Virol J 7: 21. 1743-422X-7-21 [pii];10.1186/1743-422X-7-21 [doi].

[106] Barouch DH, O'Brien KL, Simmons NL, King SL, Abbink P, Maxfield LF, Sun YH, La PA, Riggs AM, Lynch DM, Clark SL, Backus K, Perry JR, Seaman MS, Carville A, Mansfield KG, Szinger JJ, Fischer W, Muldoon M, Korber B (2010) Mosaic HIV-1 vaccines expand the breadth and depth of cellular immune responses in rhesus monkeys. Nat Med 16: 319-323. nm.2089 [pii];10.1038/nm.2089 [doi].

[107] Kaufman DR, Li F, Cruz AN, Self SG, Barouch DH (2012) Focus and breadth of cellular immune responses elicited by a heterologous insert prime-boost vaccine regimen in rhesus monkeys. Vaccine 30: 506-509.

[108] Thacker EE, Timares L, Matthews QL (2009) Strategies to overcome host immunity to adenovirus vectors in vaccine development. Expert Rev Vaccines 8: 761-777. 10.1586/erv.09.29 [doi].

[109] Seregin SS, Amalfitano A (2009) Overcoming pre-existing adenovirus immunity by genetic engineering of adenovirus-based vectors. Expert Opin Biol Ther 9: 1521-1531.

[110] Abbink P, Lemckert AA, Ewald BA, Lynch DM, Denholtz M, Smits S, Holterman L, Damen I, Vogels R, Thorner AR, O'Brien KL, Carville A, Mansfield KG, Goudsmit J, Havenga MJ, Barouch DH (2007) Comparative seroprevalence and immunogenicity of six rare serotype recombinant adenovirus vaccine vectors from subgroups B and D. J Virol 81: 4654-4663.

[111] Youil R, Toner TJ, Su Q, Chen M, Tang A, Bett AJ, Casimiro D (2002) Hexon gene switch strategy for the generation of chimeric recombinant adenovirus. Hum Gene Ther 13: 311-320. 10.1089/10430340252769824 [doi].

[112] Roberts DM, Nanda A, Havenga MJ, Abbink P, Lynch DM, Ewald BA, Liu J, Thorner AR, Swanson PE, Gorgone DA, Lifton MA, Lemckert AA, Holterman L, Chen B, Dilraj A, Carville A, Mansfield KG, Goudsmit J, Barouch DH (2006) Hexon-chimaeric adenovirus serotype 5 vectors circumvent pre-existing anti-vector immunity. Nature 441: 239-243. nature04721 [pii];10.1038/nature04721 [doi].

[113] Liu J, O'Brien KL, Lynch DM, Simmons NL, La PA, Riggs AM, Abbink P, Coffey RT, Grandpre LE, Seaman MS, Landucci G, Forthal DN, Montefiori DC, Carville A, Mansfield KG, Havenga MJ, Pau MG, Goudsmit J, Barouch DH (2009) Immune control of an SIV challenge by a T-cell-based vaccine in rhesus monkeys. Nature 457: 87-91.

[114] McCoy K, Tatsis N, Korioth-Schmitz B, Lasaro MO, Hensley SE, Lin SW, Li Y, Giles-Davis W, Cun A, Zhou D, Xiang Z, Letvin NL, Ertl HC (2007) Effect of preexisting immunity to adenovirus human serotype 5 antigens on the immune responses of nonhuman primates to vaccine regimens based on human- or chimpanzee-derived adenovirus vectors. J Virol 81: 6594-6604. JVI.02497-06 [pii];10.1128/JVI.02497-06 [doi].

[115] Molinier-Frenkel V, Lengagne R, Gaden F, Hong SS, Choppin J, Gahery-Segard H, Boulanger P, Guillet JG (2002) Adenovirus hexon protein is a potent adjuvant for activation of a cellular immune response. J Virol 76: 127-135.

[116] Roy S, Shirley PS, McClelland A, Kaleko M (1998) Circumvention of immunity to the adenovirus major coat protein hexon. J Virol 72: 6875-6879.

[117] Wu H, Dmitriev I, Kashentseva E, Seki T, Wang M, Curiel DT (2002) Construction and characterization of adenovirus serotype 5 packaged by serotype 3 hexon. J Virol 76: 12775-12782.

[118] Gall J, Kass-Eisler A, Leinwand L, Falck-Pedersen E (1996) Adenovirus type 5 and 7 capsid chimera: fiber replacement alters receptor tropism without affecting primary immune neutralization epitopes. J Virol 70: 2116-2123.

[119] Sumida SM, Truitt DM, Lemckert AA, Vogels R, Custers JH, Addo MM, Lockman S, Peter T, Peyerl FW, Kishko MG, Jackson SS, Gorgone DA, Lifton MA, Essex M, Walker BD, Goudsmit J, Havenga MJ, Barouch DH (2005) Neutralizing antibodies to adenovi-

rus serotype 5 vaccine vectors are directed primarily against the adenovirus hexon protein. J Immunol 174: 7179-7185.

[120] Yuan X, Qu Z, Wu X, Wang Y, Liu L, Wei F, Gao H, Shang L, Zhang H, Cui H, Zhao Y, Wu N, Tang Y, Qin L (2009) Molecular modeling and epitopes mapping of human adenovirus type 3 hexon protein. Vaccine 27: 5103-5110.

[121] Alba R, Bradshaw AC, Parker AL, Bhella D, Waddington SN, Nicklin SA, van RN, Custers J, Goudsmit J, Barouch DH, McVey JH, Baker AH (2009) Identification of coagulation factor (F)X binding sites on the adenovirus serotype 5 hexon: effect of mutagenesis on FX interactions and gene transfer. Blood 114: 965-971.

[122] Gall JG, Crystal RG, Falck-Pedersen E (1998) Construction and characterization of hexon-chimeric adenoviruses: specification of adenovirus serotype. J Virol 72: 10260-10264.

[123] Tian X, Su X, Li H, Li X, Zhou Z, Liu W, Zhou R (2011) Construction and characterization of human adenovirus serotype 3 packaged by serotype 7 hexon. Virus Res 160: 214-220.

[124] Crawford-Miksza LK, Schnurr DP (1996) Adenovirus serotype evolution is driven by illegitimate recombination in the hypervariable regions of the hexon protein. Virology 224: 357-367.

[125] Bradley RR, Maxfield LF, Lynch DM, Iampietro MJ, Borducchi EN, Barouch DH (2012) Adenovirus serotype 5-specific neutralizing antibodies target multiple hexon hypervariable regions. J Virol 86: 1267-1272.

[126] Bruder JT, Semenova E, Chen P, Limbach K, Patterson NB, Stefaniak ME, Konovalova S, Thomas C, Hamilton M, King CR, Richie TL, Doolan DL (2012) Modification of Ad5 hexon hypervariable regions circumvents pre-existing Ad5 neutralizing antibodies and induces protective immune responses. PLoS One 7: e33920.

[127] Waddington SN, McVey JH, Bhella D, Parker AL, Barker K, Atoda H, Pink R, Buckley SM, Greig JA, Denby L, Custers J, Morita T, Francischetti IM, Monteiro RQ, Barouch DH, van RN, Napoli C, Havenga MJ, Nicklin SA, Baker AH (2008) Adenovirus serotype 5 hexon mediates liver gene transfer. Cell 132: 397-409. S0092-8674(08)00116-5 [pii]; 10.1016/j.cell.2008.01.016 [doi].

[128] Kalyuzhniy O, Di Paolo NC, Silvestry M, Hofherr SE, Barry MA, Stewart PL, Shayakhmetov DM (2008) Adenovirus serotype 5 hexon is critical for virus infection of hepatocytes in vivo. Proc Natl Acad Sci U S A 105: 5483-5488. 0711757105 [pii];10.1073/pnas.0711757105 [doi].

[129] Yu B, Wang C, Dong J, Zhang M, Zhang H, Wu J, Wu Y, Kong W, Yu X (2012) Chimeric hexon HVRs protein reflects partial function of adenovirus. Biochem Biophys Res Commun 421: 170-176.

[130] Barouch DH, Pau MG, Custers JH, Koudstaal W, Kostense S, Havenga MJ, Truitt DM, Sumida SM, Kishko MG, Arthur JC, Korioth-Schmitz B, Newberg MH, Gorgone DA,

Lifton MA, Panicali DL, Nabel GJ, Letvin NL, Goudsmit J (2004) Immunogenicity of recombinant adenovirus serotype 35 vaccine in the presence of pre-existing anti-Ad5 immunity. J Immunol 172: 6290-6297.

[131] Liu J, Ewald BA, Lynch DM, Denholtz M, Abbink P, Lemckert AA, Carville A, Mansfield KG, Havenga MJ, Goudsmit J, Barouch DH (2008) Magnitude and phenotype of cellular immune responses elicited by recombinant adenovirus vectors and heterologous prime-boost regimens in rhesus monkeys. J Virol 82: 4844-4852.

[132] Roy S, Gao G, Lu Y, Zhou X, Lock M, Calcedo R, Wilson JM (2004) Characterization of a family of chimpanzee adenoviruses and development of molecular clones for gene transfer vectors. Hum Gene Ther 15: 519-530. 10.1089/10430340460745838 [doi].

[133] Kobinger GP, Feldmann H, Zhi Y, Schumer G, Gao G, Feldmann F, Jones S, Wilson JM (2006) Chimpanzee adenovirus vaccine protects against Zaire Ebola virus. Virology 346: 394-401. S0042-6822(05)00654-9 [pii];10.1016/j.virol.2005.10.042 [doi].

[134] Zhi Y, Figueredo J, Kobinger GP, Hagan H, Calcedo R, Miller JR, Gao G, Wilson JM (2006) Efficacy of severe acute respiratory syndrome vaccine based on a nonhuman primate adenovirus in the presence of immunity against human adenovirus. Hum Gene Ther 17: 500-506.

[135] Calcedo R, Vandenberghe LH, Roy S, Somanathan S, Wang L, Wilson JM (2009) Host immune responses to chronic adenovirus infections in human and nonhuman primates. J Virol 83: 2623-2631.

[136] Leen AM, Sili U, Vanin EF, Jewell AM, Xie W, Vignali D, Piedra PA, Brenner MK, Rooney CM (2004) Conserved CTL epitopes on the adenovirus hexon protein expand subgroup cross-reactive and subgroup-specific CD8+ T cells. Blood 104: 2432-2440.

[137] Tang J, Olive M, Pulmanausahakul R, Schnell M, Flomenberg N, Eisenlohr L, Flomenberg P (2006) Human CD8+ cytotoxic T cell responses to adenovirus capsid proteins. Virology 350: 312-322.

[138] Joshi A, Tang J, Kuzma M, Wagner J, Mookerjee B, Filicko J, Carabasi M, Flomenberg N, Flomenberg P (2009) Adenovirus DNA polymerase is recognized by human CD8+ T cells. J Gen Virol 90: 84-94. 90/1/84 [pii];10.1099/vir.0.002493-0 [doi].

[139] Singh N, Pandey A, Jayashankar L, Mittal SK (2008) Bovine adenoviral vector-based H5N1 influenza vaccine overcomes exceptionally high levels of pre-existing immunity against human adenovirus. Mol Ther 16: 965-971.

[140] McCoy K, Tatsis N, Korioth-Schmitz B, Lasaro MO, Hensley SE, Lin SW, Li Y, Giles-Davis W, Cun A, Zhou D, Xiang Z, Letvin NL, Ertl HC (2007) Effect of preexisting immunity to adenovirus human serotype 5 antigens on the immune responses of nonhuman primates to vaccine regimens based on human- or chimpanzee-derived adenovirus vectors. J Virol 81: 6594-6604.

[141] Barouch DH, Kik SV, Weverling GJ, Dilan R, King SL, Maxfield LF, Clark S, Ng'ang'a D, Brandariz KL, Abbink P, Sinangil F, de BG, Gray GE, Roux S, Bekker LG, Dilraj A,

Kibuuka H, Robb ML, Michael NL, Anzala O, Amornkul PN, Gilmour J, Hural J, Buchbinder SP, Seaman MS, Dolin R, Baden LR, Carville A, Mansfield KG, Pau MG, Goudsmit J (2011) International seroepidemiology of adenovirus serotypes 5, 26, 35, and 48 in pediatric and adult populations. Vaccine 29: 5203-5209.

[142] Appledorn DM, Kiang A, McBride A, Jiang H, Seregin S, Scott JM, Stringer R, Kousa Y, Hoban M, Frank MM, Amalfitano A (2008) Wild-type adenoviruses from groups A-F evoke unique innate immune responses, of which HAd3 and SAd23 are partially complement dependent. Gene Ther 15: 885-901.

[143] Hartman ZC, Appledorn DM, Serra D, Glass O, Mendelson TB, Clay TM, Amalfitano A (2008) Replication-attenuated Human Adenoviral Type 4 vectors elicit capsid dependent enhanced innate immune responses that are partially dependent upon interactions with the complement system. Virology 374: 453-467.

[144] Hensley SE, Cun AS, Giles-Davis W, Li Y, Xiang Z, Lasaro MO, Williams BR, Silverman RH, Ertl HC (2007) Type I interferon inhibits antibody responses induced by a chimpanzee adenovirus vector. Mol Ther 15: 393-403.

[145] Kantor J, Irvine K, Abrams S, Kaufman H, DiPietro J, Schlom J (1992) Antitumor activity and immune responses induced by a recombinant carcinoembryonic antigen-vaccinia virus vaccine. J Natl Cancer Inst 84: 1084-1091.

Chapter 6

Replicating Retroviral Vectors for Gene Therapy of Solid Tumors

Matthias Renner and Juraj Hlavaty

Additional information is available at the end of the chapter

1. Introduction

Despite recent progress in the treatment of solid tumours by conventional therapeutic options including surgery, chemotherapy, and radiotherapy, development of more efficient strategies is urgently needed due to delimited efficacy and occurrence of severe side effects in current treatment regimens. Cancer gene therapy can be defined as the introduction of genetic material into the patient's body for the purpose of reducing tumour burden, increasing life expectancy, and improving the quality of life of the treated individual. It is most commonly intended to either initiate tumour self-destruction, down-regulate angiogenesis and/or metastasis, enhance anti-tumour activity of the immune system, suppress function of an activated oncogene, or restore expression and/or function of tumour suppressor genes [1-4].

Viral vectors are the most widely used tools for the delivery of therapeutic genetic material into host cells in a clinical setting. More than 65 % of gene therapy clinical trials worldwide are making use of viral vectors (http://www.wiley.com). With almost 370 trials (~20 % of all gene therapy clinical trials), gamma-retroviruses and in particular the murine leukaemia virus (MLV)-based vectors are the second most used gene transfer system employed in recent years. These vectors are able to transduce most cell types, as long as they are actively dividing. However, most of these retroviral vectors are designed to be replication-deficient, resulting in poor transduction efficiencies in vivo. This might be one, if not the reason for the poor therapeutic success observed so far in clinical trials for cancer [5–7]. Thus, nowadays, replication-deficient retroviral vectors are mainly used in ex vivo gene transfer for the treatment of inherited monogenic disorders [8–10], rather than for in vivo tumour therapy.

However, to increase in vivo transduction efficiency and the poor therapeutic outcome observed using replication-deficient retroviral (RDR) vectors, replication-competent retroviral (RCR) vectors were created which allow vector production in the infected tumour cell and thus, as a consequence, efficient delivery of the therapeutic gene eventually to almost all target cells (for review see [11-13]). Several research groups were involved in the design and construction of such MLV-based RCR vectors and were able to show that these vectors are well suited for efficient transduction of tumour cells and thus represent an efficacious treatment option for tumour therapy.

In the following sections we will provide an overview on MLV-derived RCR vectors and their therapeutic principle. Emphasis will be put on the different vector designs available and their influence on vector spread kinetics, vector genome stability, and transgene expression levels. Furthermore, strategies to target the vector by either selective infection of distinct cell types or selective expression and replication of the vector genome and expression of the delivered transgene in distinct cell types will be presented. Data from in vivo studies employing a set of different therapeutic genes and targeting different tumour types in various animal models will be reviewed and the therapeutic efficacy in these indications discussed. Finally issues regarding the safety of these vectors such as data from biodistribution and toxicological studies as well as potential risks associated with such a therapy are addressed in the following.

2. Biology of the murine leukaemia virus

The murine leukaemia virus belongs to the genus of gamma-retroviruses which are small, enveloped viruses carrying two copies of a single-stranded RNA genome within an icosaedric core. The unique feature of retroviruses is their replication cycle, as their RNA genome is reverse transcribed into DNA, which then integrates into the host DNA before being transcribed to give rise to new virus genomes and viral proteins. MLV is a so-called simple retrovirus carrying only 3 genes in its genome, encoding the viral Gag, Pol and Env polyproteins. The group-specific antigen Gag is processed by the viral protease (PR) to the matrix (MA), capsid (CA) and nucleocapsid (NC) proteins which all form the viral core. The surface (SU) and transmembrane (TM) proteins are processed from the Env protein and are embedded in the host-cell derived lipid-bilayer. The pol gene encodes the viral PR, the reverse transcriptase (RT) and the integrase (IN), which are delivered in the virus particle to the cell to be transduced. After release of the virus core in the cytoplasm of an infected cell, reverse transcription of the single-stranded RNA into double-stranded DNA takes place and the pre-integration complex (PIC) consisting of virus DNA and viral and cellular proteins assembles [14]. As the MLV PIC, in contrast to lentiviruses such as HIV, is not able to cross the nuclear membrane, productive infection only occurs when the nuclear membrane is disrupted, as in dividing cells. Integration of the viral DNA into the host genome occurs randomly, however an integration preference of MLV-based vectors into the 5′-proximity of transcriptionally active genes was observed [15].

During reverse transcription identical long terminal repeats (LTRs) consisting of the so-called U3, R, and U5 region and flanking the viral genes are created which carry the viral promoter in the U3 region and the poly(A) site downstream of the R region. Expression from this promoter leads to two RNA species, a genomic one also encoding the viral proteins Gag and Pol, and the subgenomic env coding message. The Gag and Pol proteins assemble together with the genomic RNA which is recognized by Gag via a packaging signal present immediately downstream of the 5′-LTR. Newly synthesized virus particles exit the cell via budding through Env protein-rich regions of the host cell membrane without lysis of the cell.

Thus, due to its non-lytic nature retroviruses per se cannot be used as so-called oncolytic viruses, which are able to kill tumour cells by their productive infection only, but require additional gene sequences to exert a tumour destroying effect. Such therapeutic replication-competent MLV vectors can only be generated by adding therapeutic sequences in addition to the viral genes, which are all essential for virus replication, making the design of such vectors challenging and their genomic stability critical due to genomic overlength.

3. Replicating MLV vectors

3.1. Vector designs, spread kinetics and genome stability

Early attempts to produce replication-competent retroviral vectors have been already made in the late 80′s of the last century, when various groups inserted a transgene expression cassette into the 3′-LTR of replicating MLV to generate a research tool for analyses in whole-animal models [16-18]. During infection and reverse transcription of the proviral mRNA message, the transgene expression cassette was duplicated and, now present in the 5′- and 3′-LTR, independently expressed from the respective heterologous promoter. An RCR containing a mutant form of the dihydrofolate reductase (DHFR) gene was shown to stably transmit methotrexate resistance to infected fibroblasts upon multiple rounds of virus replication in vitro in the absence of drug selection and was produced at high titres by fibroblast cells [16].

Later, the group of Finn Skou Pedersen adopted this concept and inserted the transgene within the U3 region of the 3′-LTR of the Akv strain of MLV, mediating expression of the eGFP-transgene via an internal ribosomal entry site (IRES) of the encephalomyocarditis virus (EMCV) (Figure 1, (B)) [19]. This design again resulted in doubling of the IRES-transgene cassette in the infected cell, albeit, only the eGFP gene located in the 3′-LTR, but not the transgene present in the 5′-LTR, was expressed from the regulatory elements in the MLV 5′-LTR. Intraperitoneal injection of this vector at a concentration of 10e4 colony forming units into 3-4 days old mice led to more than 50 % eGFP-expressing spleen cells 4 days after injection. The level of eGFP-positive cells remained constant till day 7, but dramatically dropped from day 12 onwards, most likely to genetic instability of the vector and reversion to wild-type (wt) virus lacking the marker gene [20].

Due to the highly compact nature of the MLV genome, however, the positions into which heterologous sequences can be inserted without impacting on viral replication are limited. Thus, up to now only few vector designs in which the transgene is located at different positions and/or its expression is facilitated by different mechanism have been created and are currently under in-depth evaluation.

Kasahara and colleagues favoured insertion of the transgene right downstream of the envelope reading frame, as well linked via an ECMV IRES element (Figure 1, (C)) [21,22].

These RCR vectors are based on the Moloney strain of MLV and are equipped with the amphotropic MLV envelope gene, both of which are features allowing infection of human and other mammalian cells. The effect of insert size and sequence on the genetic stability and spread efficacy of the vector revealed a strong negative correlation between insert size and deletion of the introduced sequence. Insertion of 1.6 kb in length led to greatly attenuated replication kinetics relative to wild-type virus and loss of the insert within a single infection cycle, whereas inserts up to 1.3 kb were well tolerated with slightly attenuated replication kinetics. In addition, the genomic integrity was maintained over multiple serial infection cycles [21,22].

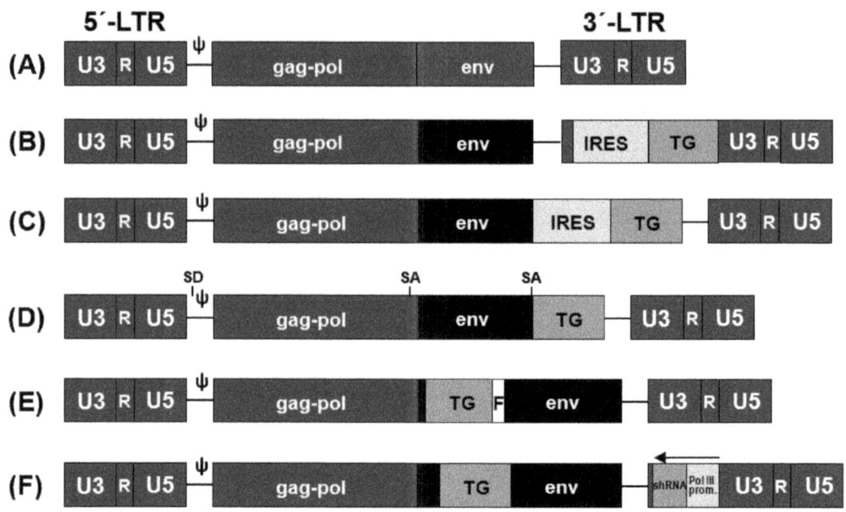

Figure 1. Schematic depiction of the different RCR vector designs ((B) – (F)). The inserted transgene is located at different positions in the viral vector and expression is facilitated by different means. (A) represents the genomic organisation of the wt-MLV provirus. LTR = long terminal repeat; gag = viral group specific antigen gene; pol = viral polymerase gene; env = viral envelope gene; IRES = internal ribosomal entry site; TG = transgene; F = protein cleavage site; SD = splice donor; SA = splice enhancer; ψ = psi packaging site; Pol III Prom = Polymerase III dependent promoter.

To further unravel the effects of viral strain and transgene position in the vector, as well as the impact the target cell type might have on spread kinetics and on the genetic stability of the virus vector in particular, we have independently compared the different parameters in serial rounds of infection in different cultured cell types as well as in vivo in tumour bearing animals [23]. To this end, various cell lines have been inoculated with RCR vectors based on the Akv and Moloney strain of MLV and carrying an IRES-EGFP transgene cassette either in the U3 region of the 3´-LTR or immediately downstream of the env gene, and passaged and monitored over time. Supernatant of the infected cells was also used to infected fresh cells for a further round of infection to allow exponential spread of virus vector until a maximum of EGFP-expressing cells was reached. Supernatant of the freshly infected cells was then used for a next round of infection to finally end up with more than 20 rounds of infection, and virus propagation for up to 100 days. The obtained data revealed a clear advantage of the Moloney-MLV strain over the Akv-MLV strain in respect to spread kinetics, transgene expression and vector stability and demonstrated that location of the transgene immediately downstream of the env gene is preferred in respect to genomic stability of the vector. These observations have been confirmed in spread and stability analyses after virus injection in tumour xenografts of mice [23]. Unexpectedly, our results also indicated that the host cell can influence the ability of MLV-based RCR vectors to stably propagate the expression of heterologous genes, since all vectors, regardless of design, lost the ability to express eGFP in NIH-3T3 cells much more rapidly than in HEK-293 cells [23]. Differences in vector genome stability between infected cell lines seem to be dependent neither on species nor on different replication kinetics of the vector in the respective cell lines. It rather might be due to differences in other virus and/or host-cell features including fidelity of the virus reverse transcriptase linked with the p53 status of the infected cells, expression of the anti-viral mechanisms such as APOBEC and TRIM family members, availability and balance of intracellular dNTP pools, and in general, due to an overall genetic instability of certain cell types and cell lines [24].

Employing this design in which the heterologous sequences are located in the 3′-untranslated region immediately downstream of the env reading frame, expression of the transgene could also be facilitated by introducing, instead of the IRES, a splice acceptor site upstream of the transgene, which would result in a transgene specific mRNA message (Figure 1 (D)) [25]. Propagation of such vectors in cell culture however, revealed a much slower vector spread as compared to the IRES-carrying vector, which led to almost 100% infected cells after 3 days after infection [25].

RCR vectors based on Mo-MLV carrying a therapeutic gene in the 3′-untranslated region resemble currently the most advanced RCR vector design for tumour therapy and are already employed in the first clinical trial for the treatment of cancer.

A different approach in the design of RCR vectors has been pursued by the group of Christian Buchholz from the Paul-Ehrlich-Institut, as they inserted heterologous sequences including a 3′-terminally located furin cleavage site in frame into the envelope gene of the virus between the signal peptide and surface protein domain coding region (Figure 1, (E)) [26,27]. During production of the Env protein in virus vector transduced cells, the heterologous amino acid sequence will be cleaved off while the Env protein is processed through the secretory pathway and eventually will be secreted from the infected cell. Proof-of-concept for this vector design was shown with the immune stimulatory cytokine GM-CSF and the laminin-specific or T-cell specific single-chain antibody variable region fragment (scFv) [27]. The resulting viruses infected a variety of human cell lines and infectious virus particles were detected in supernatants of infected cells. Moreover, these cells were able to efficiently process the encoded Env-fusion proteins and to release reasonable amounts of protein molecules of GM-CSF, laminin-specific or T-cell specific scFvs into the cell culture media. Furthermore, the replicating viruses were genetically stable for at least 12 serial cycles of propagation. Thus, these vectors are ideally suited for production of therapeutic factors which need to be secreted, but less suitable in case the protein produced is intended to be active in the infected cell.

An additional site for integration of foreign sequences into the vector genome without impairing virus life cycle is the proline-rich region tract within the Env protein (Figure 1, (F)). Insertion of the eGFP marker gene into this site in a Mo-MLV-based RCR vector resulted in spread through almost 100% of cultured NIH-3T3 cells within one week after initial transfection with virus sequences [28,29]. PCR analysis of integrated virus vector DNA from chronically infected cells indicated no genetic recombination in the modified env gene region. An additional insertion of a Pol III promoter-shRNA expression cassette in antisense orientation into the 3′-untranslated region of the virus vector resulted in only slightly reduced spread kinetics as compared to the parental vector and in delivery and functional expression of the shRNA in most of the cells [30]. Again PCR analysis did not reveal any recombination events over 4 infection cycles.

3.2. Targeting of infection and expression

MLV-based RCR vectors can be accounted for being intrinsically tumour-selective due to the specific nature of MLV to replicate in dividing cells only. Nevertheless, it would be desirable to further improve the vector safety profile. This can be achieved by introducing transcriptional control elements that restrict RCR gene expression and subsequent virus vector replication to tumour cells - so-called transcriptional targeting; or by modulating the interaction of the RCR vector with host cells at the very early step of the infection process, known as physical targeting, via adaptation of the virus envelope glycoprotein to selectively bind to surface molecules exclusively or predominantly present on cancer cells. Alternatively, initial targeting could also be enabled by the use of delivery vehicles to facilitate transport or homing of the RCR vectors to the tumour site.

3.2.1. Transcriptional targeting

To allow transcriptional targeting of MLV-based RCR vectors, the most reasonable approach is the exchange of the ubiquitously active viral promoter located in the U3 region of the viral LTR by a tissue- or tumour-specific promoter delimiting its activity and thus virus vector replication to a specific cell type. Due to the particularities of retroviral reverse transcription, modifications of this promoter must be introduced into the U3 region of the 3′-LTR. This allows, after initial vector production and infection, duplication of the regulatory elements into the 5′-LTR (Figure 2). This strategy has been successfully employed previously in conventional replication-defective retroviral vectors to direct transgene expression to a particular cell type [31–33]. In RCR vectors however, not only expression of the transgene sequences is mediated by these regulatory elements, but also expression of viral genes which are needed to ensure efficient RCR vector replication in infected target cells and which have to be produced in an ample but well balanced manner. Moreover, as the LTR contains regulatory elements important for reverse transcription, RNA processing, and virus genome integration, modifications in this area may interfere with or may disrupt these elements and may thus negatively affect virus replication kinetics. This altogether renders the transcriptional targeting approach for RCR vectors rather complex.

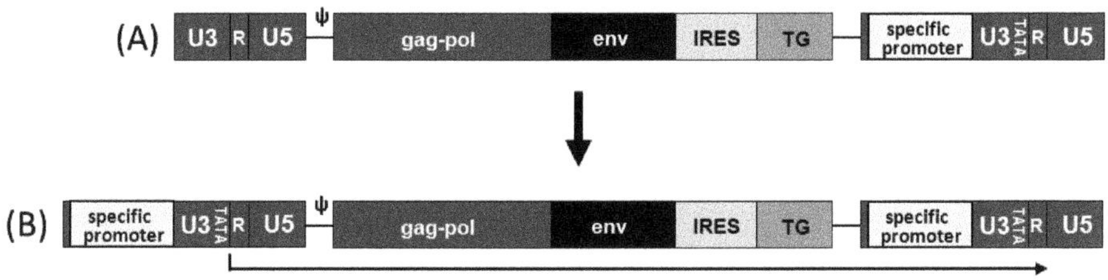

Figure 2. Principle of transcriptional targeting of RCR vectors. (A) schematically depicts the RCR proviral genome as present in a virus producer cell. The tumour- or tissue-specific regulatory sequence (specific promoter) is located in the 3′-LTR of the viral vector. After infection and reverse transcription of the virus genome, the 3′-LTR U3 region is duplicated to the 5′-LTR and is thus able to drive expression of the viral genes and of the inserted transgene (B). For abbreviations please see legend to Figure 1.

In early studies, the murine liver-specific transthyretin promoter/enhancer was inserted into the LTR U3 region, lacking the endogenous enhancer, of a replication-competent MLV [34]. When compared to wt-MLV however, the recombinant virus did not reveal an improved rate of infectivity of hepatocytes in vitro or a restricted tissue tropism in vivo [34].

Transcriptional targeting of MLV-based RCR vectors harbouring modifications in the U3 region by insertion of a heterologous promoter was demonstrated initially by Kasahara and colleagues [35]. In these vectors, hybrid LTRs were constructed by replacement of the MLV 3′-LTR U3 region from the very 5′ end to either the CAAT box, the TATA box, or the transcriptional start site (TSS) by a heterologous promoter complementing the deleted boxes, respectively. Using a highly prostate-specific rat probasin (PB) proximal promoter and a synthetic variant of this promoter containing several copies of the androgen responsive region (ARR_2PB), respectively, virus gene expression and virus production was shown to be restricted to prostate cancer cells in vitro [35]. Replication of vectors in which the heterologous promoter was fused directly to the MLV TSS was greatly impaired relative to that of vectors in which the viral CAAT and TATA box, or the viral TATA box only, was retained. The configuration in which the MLV TATA box was preserved, but all upstream elements had been replaced by heterologous regulatory sequences was found to be ideal in respect to transgene expression, vector spread and specificity [35]. The use of the stronger ARR_2PB promoter resulted in a greatly improved efficacy of vector replication [35]. Moreover, results from biodistribution studies in immunocompetent and immunodeficient mice indicated that this targeting strategy prevents the productive spread of RCR vectors to spleen and bone marrow of systemically infected mice [12].

Using a different set of promoter/enhancer elements, Metzl et al. were able to demonstrate that MLV-based RCR vectors can also be targeted to liver cancer cells and to tumour cells harbouring a deregulated ß-catenin signalling pathway [36]. Vectors equipped with a chimeric promoter consisting of the hepatitis B virus enhancer II fused to the human α1-antitrypsin promoter (EIIPa1AT promoter) revealed a substantial spread in the liver cancer cell lines HepG2, AKH12, AKH13, but replicated only scarcely in the colon carcinoma cell lines SW480 and DLD-1, the cervical cancer cell line HeLa and the human embryonic kidney cell line

HEK-293 [36]. Similarly, vectors equipped with the synthetic beta-catenin/T-cell factor dependent CTP4 promoter replicated in the ß-catenin deregulated cancer cell lines HepG2, SW480, and DLD-1, but not in the cell lines AKH12, AKH13, HeLa, and HEK-293, which revealed a normal ß-catenin signalling pathway. When the heterologous promoters were used to replace almost the entire U3 region, including the MLV TATA box and TSS (TATA-replacement (TR) design), vector replication was inefficient as virus particle production from infected cells was clearly reduced by factor 100 as compared to a vector harbouring the wt-MLV 3′-LTR. On the contrary, fusion of the heterologous promoter lacking the TATA box to the MLV TATA box (TATA-fusion (TF) design) generated vectors which replicated with almost wt-MLV kinetics throughout permissive cells despite the fact that virion production from infected cells was reduced by 10-fold as compared to the prototype vector ACE-GFP. As expected, these TF-vectors exhibited low or negligible spread in non-permissive cells. The genomic stability of the TF-vectors, however, was shown to be comparable to those containing wt-MLV LTRs [36].

Both studies indicated that the precise manner in which the heterologous promoters are inserted into the U3 region of the 3′-LTR is of paramount importance. Only vectors retaining the MLV TATA box in its natural position exhibited both regulated gene expression and rapid replication kinetics [35,36].

3.2.2. *Physical targeting*

For decades it was generally accepted, that with MLV, and as a consequence, with MLV-based vectors, infection can only take place in dividing cells. Therefore, such vectors can be *a priori* accounted as intrinsically tumour-selective in the appropriate environment. However, very recently Liu et al. reported infection of neurons and growth arrested neuroendocrine cells with MLV-based RCR and RDR vectors harbouring an amphotropic envelope at efficiency similar to that of lentiviral vectors, which are known to infect also non-dividing cells [37]. This new and unexpected observation, if confirmed, will further raise the need for retrovirus vectors with a specific and/or targeted infection and/or replication range.

Retroviruses are unique among viral vectors in their capacity to incorporate a wide range of envelope proteins from other retroviruses and even from completely unrelated virus types. Insertion of heterologous envelope proteins into the outer shell of viral particles, so called pseudotyping, to exert an infection targeting approach has already been demonstrated in RDR vectors for a variety of envelope molecules [38–40]. The MLV-based RCR vectors used in cancer gene therapy applications to date are mostly based on the Moloney strain of MLV, which naturally expresses the ecotropic MLV envelope and thus are able to only infect rodent cells. To allow infection of human cells, the vectors are pseudotyped with the amphotropic envelope gene from the 4070A strain of MLV, which can infect most mammalian cell types via the ubiquitously-expressed Pit-2 receptor [41]. Logg and colleagues also replaced the native env sequence with that of the gibbon ape leukaemia virus (GALV) retaining a short portion of the signal peptide coding sequence of the MLV Env to avoid alteration of the MLV polymerase reading frame which is overlapping with the 5′-end of the envelope reading frame [42]. This env gene replacement greatly attenuated viral replication, most probably by a large clearance in splicing of the viral RNA. However, employing an in vitro evolution strategy, extended passaging of cells exposed to the chimeric virus resulted in selection of virus mutants with rapid replication kinetics. Different variants arose from different sets of infection experiments. None of the revertants exhibited mutations in the GALV env gene itself, but rather in other areas of the virus to retain the ratio of spliced to unspliced viral messages which had been pertubated by the substitution of the env gene [42].

An alternative strategy for changing the tropism of MLV-based RCR vectors is via direct engineering of the specific targeting ligand sequence within the env gene. Again, several strategies have been demonstrated for RDR vectors, including the incorporation of ligands or single chain antibodies into the env gene to allow targeting to an alternative receptor [43-45]. However, these approaches were of limited success in respect to transciptional targeting, as, although retargeting of the vector was achieved, infection efficiency was greatly reduced, since the conformational change in the envelope protein necessary for proper virus-cell fusion failed to happen subsequently to the binding of the modified envelope to the alternate receptor [46].

In another approach to allow the physical targeting of RCR vectors, two tandem repeats of the immunoglobulin G-binding Z-domains of Staphylococcus protein A were inserted into the proline-rich region of amphotropic or ecotropic MLV envelope proteins present in MLV-based RCR vector particles, respectively [47]. This approach should allow virus particles to be conjugated to an antibody of choice, which can then be used for the selective binding of virus to cells (over)-expressing the chosen antibody target. Modified envelopes were efficiently expressed and incorporated into virions, while infectivity was markedly reduced by this pseudotyping [47].

For RCR vectors the most efficient physical targeting system up to now is based on protease-activatable envelope proteins [48]. Rather than attempting to redirect infection to target cells by incorporation of specific binding domains into the envelope protein, here, the virus remains non-infectious until the Env proteins become activated by cleavage by a secreted or membrane-bound cellular protease recognizing the protease target site present in the engineered Env molecule. A directed evolution-based approach was employed for the selection of retroviruses activatable by matrix metalloproteinases (MMPs) which are specifically expressed by tumour cells [26,49,50]. RCR vectors generated to express either the epidermal growth factor (EGF) or the CD40 ligand, linked via MMP cleavage sites as fusion to the N-terminal of the MLV 4070A envelope protein, were sequestered by the EGF receptor or the CD40 receptor, which are ubiquitously-expressed on potential host cells. By that the envelope protein was prevented from interacting with its natural Pit-2 receptor resulting in poor infection efficiencies and thus de-targeting of the RCR vectors from non-tumour cells [49,50]. Infection efficiency however, is restored in cells which express high levels of MMPs, such as many tumour cell types, due to Env-ligand cleavage and interaction of the Env protein with its natural receptor [50]. In a comparative study Duerner and colleagues analysed the spread of targeted and non-targeted MLV RCR variants in s.c. tumours derived from HT1080 and U-87MG cells, respectively, and in extratumoral organs after systemic tail vein injection of the vector into SCID mice [48]. Both virus types were able to efficiently infect tumour cells however, the non-targeted virus efficiently infected also extratumoral organs such as bone marrow, spleen, and liver. Quantitative analyses revealed an up to 500-fold higher selective infection of tumour tissue with the targeted viruses than with the non-targeted counterpart [50].

3.2.3. Alternative ways for RCR vector targeting

Recently, a fully functional chimeric vector system that uses a helper-dependent adenovirus 5 (Ad) vector as a first stage carrier to express and deliver a fully functional RCR vector has been described [51]. The RCR vectors are produced *in situ* from initially adenovirus-transduced cells, thereby combining benefits of both vector systems – high titers reached with adenoviruses and stable integration of retroviruses. At equivalent initial transduction levels, more secondary RCR progeny were produced from Ad-RCR-transduced cells as compared to RCR-transduced cells, resulting in further acceleration of RCR replication kinetics [51]. In pre-established *s.c.* human breast cancer xenografts in mice, suicide gene therapy with high titre chimeric Ad-RCR vectors achieved, in a dose dependent manner, an enhanced efficacy compared to delivery of respective RCR-only vectors [52]. As the target cell binding tropism of adenoviral vectors can be altered by modifications to the fibre knob [53], the strategy of employing a chimeric Ad-RCR vector system might represent a promising step forward towards a targeted and efficacious cancer gene therapy.

As a future option, delivery of RCR vectors to tumours could also be facilitated by the use of tumour-homing cells as vector carriers. Mesenchymal stromal cells, for example, which have been shown to be able to home to malignant areas, have been loaded with replicating adenoviral vectors to deliver them to the tumour tissue to execute their oncolytic potential [54], an approach which might be also applicable to RCR vectors.

3.3. Therapeutic application of MLV-based RCR vectors

Despite the fact that the first experiments employing MLV-based RCR vectors have been commenced more than 20 years ago, the utilization of these vectors for cancer gene therapy is still at an early stage. The vectors are not oncolytic *per se* and the choice of therapeutic genes which can be used is limited, as large heterologous sequences cannot be inserted into the MLV genome without impairing vector stability and replication efficiency. Nonetheless a number of therapeutic sequences such as those encoding suicide genes, cytokines and interfering RNAs have been demonstrated to be stably propagated over several infection cycles by MLV-based RCR vectors.

3.3.1. Suicide genes

Suicide genes, also called prodrug-converting genes, encode proteins which are not toxic *per se*, but which are able to catalyse the formation of toxic metabolite(s) from a non-toxic or low-toxic prodrug. By the delivery of suicide genes to and their expression in tumour cells, conversion of a systemically administered prodrug by the respective suicide gene product results in a highly specific and effective anti-tumor therapy [55]. Although the toxic metabolites generated are quite often identical to those of classical chemotherapy, here, the local production of metabolites in the tumour cells results in a more contained and specific effect as compared to the, in most cases, systemically given chemotherapy.

Initial data demonstrating therapeutic efficacy of an RCR vector mediated suicide therapy approach have been shown using the yeast cytosine deaminase (yCD) gene in a mouse model of human glioma [56]. In cells infected with the yCD expressing RCR vector ACE-CD, the non-toxic prodrug 5-fluorocytosine (5-FC) was converted into the toxic component 5-fluorouracil (5-FU), leading to cell death not only in infected cells but also in surrounding non-infected dividing cells due to intercellular diffusion of 5-FU. Stereotactic intratumoral injection of only 1x10e4 infectious ACE-CD particles into pre-established intracranial U-87MG human glioma xenografts in nude mice followed by daily intraperitoneal (*i.p.*) administration of 500 mg 5-FC per kg body weight eight days later for 15 days (ACE-CD + 5-FC) led to survival of all treated animals for a follow up period of 60 days, whereas mice of both control groups, vector only (ACE-CD + PBS) and prodrug only (PBS + 5-FC), died within 40 days [56]. Subsequent studies, however, revealed that this treatment regimen is insufficient to get complete eradication of U-87MG tumours in the treated animals, resulting in death of the animals after 70 and more days [57]. Retrospective immunohistochemical analyses showed that in most of the treated animals still small areas of tumour tissue were present indicating an ectopic spread of glioma cells in the brain. Despite the fact that all of the surviving tumour cells stained positive for viral envelope protein, these tumour cells had not been killed by the administration of 5-FC. This suggests that these cells either have been infected with a suicide gene deletion variant of the vector or the therapeutic gene, although present, is not expressed in these cells or that the cells are refractory to chemotherapy [57]. Tai et al. also examined whether the efficacy of this treatment could be increased by administering multiple cycles of 5-FC [57]. To this end, after injection of 1x10e4 transducing units of vector ACE-CD into preformed intracranial tumours, mice received multiple cycles of 5-FC for 8 consecutive days with 3-week intervals between the treatment periods [57]. Again, all control animals receiving virus vector only and prodrug only, respectively, died within 40 days, whereas all mice treated with vector and prodrug survived for more than 100 days, demonstrating that the multi-cycle strategy provides a significant therapeutic benefit compared to a single cycle of prodrug administration [57].

To investigate the effect of the immune system on the effectiveness of the RCR vector-mediated glioma therapy, the rat glioma cell line RG2 was used to establish syngeneic intracranial tumours in Fischer 344 rats [58]. Three days after tumour implantation, 1x10e6 infectious ACE-CD virus particles were stereotactically injected into the growing tumours. Ten days after virus injection, 5-FC at 500 mg/kg body weight was administered *i.p.* for 7 consecutive days and after a 10 days interval the treatment cycle was repeated. Animals treated with vector ACE-CD and 5-FC survived for up to 35 days, whereas control animals (ACE-CD + PBS) died within 21 days. Despite the higher initial virus vector load injected into the tumour and the shorter intervals between the treatment cycles a significantly shorter survival time of treated Fischer 344 rats was observed as compared to data of vector/prodrug treated U-87MG tumour bearing nude mice [58]. This observation might be, to a certain extent, due to reduced spread kinetics in the RG2 tumour as compared to the U-87MG tumours, as only 65 % of RG2 tumour cells got transduced after 21 days after initial virus infection. On the other hand, animals with tumours derived from pre-infected and 100 % CD-expressing cells treated with 5-FC died due to tumour burden at a significantly later time point, however still within 50 days [58]. This indicates that other factors might contribute to the poorer treatment efficacy, such as insufficient levels of 5-FC/5-FU in the tumour, differences in resistance to 5-FU, or effects triggered by the immune system. Regarding this latter point, however, no immune response against the RCR vector in the brain has been detected [58].

Recently, we have critically analysed a panel of 15 different human and rodent glioma and glioblastoma cell lines in respect to spread of RCR vectors derived from vector ACE-CD to their sensitivity towards the 5-FC/5-FU suicide system, and to their orthotopic growth characteristics in mice to identify suitable preclinical animal models as test bed for the development and evaluation of RCR vector mediated treatment of glioblastoma [59]. Rapid virus spread was observed in eight out of nine human cell lines tested in vitro. As expected, only CD-expressing cells became sensitive to 5-FC. All LD_{50} values were within the range of concentrations obtained in human body fluids after conventional 5-FC administration. In addition, a significant bystander effect was observed in all human glioma cell lines tested, supporting the potential of this suicide gene therapy for the treatment of brain tumours [59].

This therapeutic concept has also been experimentally employed to subcutaneous and orthotopic liver metastasis of colorectal cancer in an immunocompetent rodent model [60,61]. To this end, murine CT26 cells pre-transduced with vector ACE-CD were mixed with non-transduced CT26 cells at a ratio of 1:200 prior to implantation into BALB/c mice. Twelve days later, daily 5-FC treatment at 500 mg/kg, given *i.p.* twice a day, was started and continued until the end of the experiment. 5-FC treated animals showed significant inhibition of tumour growth resulting in an average tumour size of approx. 100 mm^3 at day 24, whereas in animals whose drinking water was supplemented with 0.4 mg/ml of azidothymidine (AZT) to prevent MLV vector replication, tumour growth was inhibited only moderately with an average tumour size of approx. 500 mm^3 at day 24 [61]. Tumour size in untreated animals reached more than 800 mm^3 at day 24 [61]. The effect on tumour size observed in the AZT-treated group most probably was due to the presence of a bystander effect, in which toxic metabolites produced by the CD-positive cells can freely diffuse into neighbouring, CD-negative cells to cause cell death and thereby eventually lead to a delay in tumour growth. These observations clearly indicate that the efficacy of the ACE-CD/5-FC treatment is dependent on a sustained vector spread. Proof-of-concept of this therapy was also shown in a multifocal hepatic metastasis model [61]. Here, CT26 cells stably expressing the firefly luciferase marker gene were infused into the portal system via intrasplenic injection, became trapped within the hepatic microcirculation, and seeded metastases. Three days later, 2x10e4 ACE-CD virus vector particles were instilled into tumour-bearing mice, again via intrasplenic injection, followed by daily 5-FC administration at 500 mg/kg given *i.p.* twice a day, initiated 14 days after tumour cells inoculation [61]. In contrast to untreated animals or animals which received vector and PBS only, and which revealed increasing bioluminescence throughout the 28 day experiment, 5 out of 7 animals treated with both vector ACE-CD and 5-FC showed stable or decreased levels of bioluminescence, indicating that the development of metastases was inhibited [61]. The locoregional delivery of the CD suicide gene by RCR vectors infused into the portal circulation thus resulted in progressive transduction of multiple tumour foci in the liver without evidence of spread to adjacent normal parenchyma or extrahepatic tissues as shown by qPCR analyses of MLV-specific sequences in the DNA of liver tumour tissue, normal liver, and bone marrow cells [61].

For proof-of-concept in a further indication, Kikuchi and colleagues evaluated the transduction and therapeutic efficacy of intravesically administered RCR vectors in orthotopic bladder tumours in mice [62]. Tumours were established by implantation of either MBT-2 murine bladder cancer cells into immunocompetent syngeneic C3H/HeJ mice or of KU-19-19 human bladder cancer cells into nude mice. RCR vector particles carrying the eGFP transgene were delivered intravesically *via* a catheter inserted into the bladder 5 days after tumour formation. Upon injection of 3.2x10e5 infectious virus particles, vector spread in the human xenograft model reached almost all of the tumour cells within 35 days post infection [62]. In the orthotopic syngeneic model, vector spread resulted in, on average, 30 % of infected tumour cells 27 days after vector instillation, as revealed by immunohistochemical analyses of transgene expression [62]. The effects of the respective therapeutic vector ACE-CD were demonstrated in the MBT-2 bladder cancer model, whereby 3.2x10e5 infectious virus particles were instilled intravesically into the bladder of mice containing preformed tumours. Twelve days following infection, animals received daily 5-FC at 500 mg/kg given *i.p.* for 15 days [62]. A single course of 5-FC treatment led to significantly reduced tumour growth and 50 % of the animals survived for more than 70 days. In contrast, all of the animals in vector only or vehicle control groups died within 40 days. Again, the locoregional delivery of intravesically administered RCR vectors was shown to achieve significant tumour growth inhibition by efficient delivery of the therapeutic gene into the orthotopic bladder tumour cells without any evidence of spread to adjacent distant organs [62].

Recently, Kawasaki et al. investigated RCR vector mediated gene therapy for the treatment of human malignant mesothelioma [63]. Cells of this tumour type were found to be highly permissive for RCR infection [63]. After a single intratumoral injection of 1x10e4 ACE-CD virus vector particles into pre-established subcutaneous MSTO-211H human mesothelioma tumour xenografts in nude mice, followed by daily 5-FC administration at 500 mg/kg body weight given *i.p.* from day 12 to day 32 post-infection, significant inhibition of tumour growth was observed in ACE-CD/5-FC treated mice compared to control groups as indicated by a tumour volume of 200 mm^3 *vs.* 800 mm^3, respectively, at day 32 after infection. Efficacy of the treatment was also investigated in a peritoneally disseminated human mesothelioma xenograft model [63]. Here, MSTO-211H cells stably expressing the mCherry fluorescence protein and transduced with vector ACE-CD were mixed at a ratio of 1:100 with non-transduced mCherry expressing MSTO-211H cells and the mixture was injected i.p. into nude mice. After confirmation of tumour formation by in vivo imaging, daily 5-FC administration was initiated (500 mg/kg *i.p.*) for 15 consecutive days. In 4 out of 9 mice of the vector/5-FC receiving group no visible tumours were observed and mice survived until day 100 after cell injection. On the contrary, all non-treated mice had died at day 61 at the latest. In summary, the 5-FC treated group showed a significantly prolonged median survival time as compared to the control group (81 days *vs.* 34 days) [63].

Beside the CD/5-FC suicide gene/prodrug combination, which is the most prominent and extensively studied system in context of RCR vectors, other therapeutic genes have been introduced in this vector system and have been analysed. The bacterial purine nucleoside phosphorylase (PNP) gene, for example, converts the prodrugs fludarabine phosphate (F-araAMP) or 6-methylpurine 2′-deoxyriboside (MeP-dR) into its toxic metabolites and represents a reasonable alternative to the CD/5-FC suicide system. Kikuchi et al. demonstrated the therapeutic efficacy of vector ACE-PNP, an MLV-based RCR vector expressing the *E.*coli PNP gene, in a subcutaneous model of KU-19-19 human bladder cancer cells in nude mice [64]. Five days following tumour cell implantation, 3.2x10e5 infectious virus particles were injected directly into the tumour and 10 days later F-araAMP at 75 mg/m^2 body surface was administered *i.p.* every other day for a total of seven injections. Significant tumour growth inhibition could be demonstrated with a tumour mass of 600 mm^3 *vs.* ≥ 2,200 mm^3 at day 26 post virus injection in treated mice *vs.* vector and vehicle control groups [64]. These results indicate that the PNP-RCR system is a reasonable alternative to the use of CD-expressing RCR vectors, in particular as enzymatic products generated by PNP seem to be more cytotoxic than 5-FU [65,66].

In in vitro experiments using human U-87MG glioma cells, Tai and colleagues were able to show that transduction of even only 1 % of cells with the ACE-PNP vector and subsequent systemic prodrug administration is sufficient to achieve significant cell killing over time [67]. Thereby, the rapidity of cell killing is highly dependent on the initial level of transduction. Treatment of pre-established *s.c.* U-87MG tumour xenografts with 1x10e5 ACE-PNP vector particles followed by F-araAMP prodrug administration 14 days after virus injection at a concentration of 80 mg/kg given *i.p.* once every other day for five times resulted in significantly inhibited tumour growth [67]. A second cycle of prodrug administration reduced tumour growth even further. The potential of an ACE-PNP RCR vector-based therapy to improve survival of nude mice bearing intracranial U-87MG tumours was evaluated by inoculating pre-established xenografts with 1x10e4 vector particles 7 days after tumour onset. Eight days later, the mice received F-araAMP (40 mg/kg given i.p. once every other day) for a total of eight treatments. The median survival time was 59 days *vs.* 30 and 28 days in treated *vs.* control groups [67]. In a second experiment, the same experimental setting was employed, but a second round of F-araAMP treatment was done after a 14 days recovery period. The median survival time of treated mice was further improved to 73 days *vs.* 33 days in the control groups [67]. This data again demonstrated the potential for additional survival benefit from multiple cycles of prodrug administration.

In summary, the published data of non-preclinical studies using suicide gene-expressing MLV-based RCR vectors have demonstrated that such vectors are therapeutically efficacious in solid tumours and/or metastases of a range of different tumour types (glioma, colorectal and bladder cancer, mesothelioma) in both immunodeficient and immunocompetent mouse and rat models, and using different therapeutic genes (yCD and PNP). On grounds of these non-clinical data the therapeutic concept of replicating retroviral vectors was moved towards clinical application. To this end, based on the design of the extensively evaluated vector ACE-

CD, a lead clinical candidate (vocimagene amiretrorepvec, Tocagen Inc., San Diego, CA) has been constructed carrying a human codon-optimised thermostable yeast CD gene [68]. Comparison with the prototype vector ACE-CD harbouring the wildtype yeast CD gene revealed a three-fold increased CD-specific conversion of 5-FC to 5-FU in infected cells and a markedly higher genetic stability of the clinical vector candidate Toca 511 [68]. To further support the production of toxic metabolites in infected cells, the modified CD gene was further linked as fusion to the gene encoding the yeast uracil phosphoribosyl transferase (UPRT) or, alternatively, to the human orotate phosphoribosyltransferase (OPRT) gene. It has been reported that expression of the UPRT gene in the CD-expressing cells leads to increased sensitivity to 5-FC, as the UPRT converts 5-FU directly to 5-FUMP, from which the active metabolites 5-FdUMP and 5-FUTP are formed [69,70]. The human OPRT protein, as part of a multifunctional UMP synthase, is a human analogue of the UPRT, converting 5-FU directly to 5-FUMP with direct impact on the cellular sensitivity towards 5-FU, since downregulation of this endogenous enzyme was found in tumour cells resistant to 5-FU [71,72]. Moreover, exogenous expression of the OPRT gene led to increased 5-FU sensitivity in cancer cell lines in vitro [73]. Despite better individual in vitro cell killing with vectors carrying these fusion genes, it remains unclear, whether this would be beneficial for therapy, as the highly efficient 5-FC salvage to phosphorylated nucleotides may diminish 5-FU diffusion and thereby the effects exerted by the bystander mechanism. Furthermore, initial killing of most of the infected cells might hinder vector spread during the 5-FC-rest period, leading to a reduced antitumor activity in vivo [68,74]. In addition, serial passaging of these infectious viruses on human U-87MG glioma cells revealed a decreased genomic stability of vectors containing fusion constructs as compared to Toca 511, probably due to the size and nature of the inserted transgene(s) sequences (~500 bp in Toca 511 *vs.* ~1250 bp in the fusion constructs) [68].

The therapeutic potential of Toca 511 was evaluated in two different intracranial brain tumour models in immune competent mice (CT26-BALB/c and Tu-2449-B6C3F1) [75]. Treatment of CT26 brain metastases with three different virus doses (1x10e6, 1x10e5, 1x10e4 transforming units (TU)/g brain weight) plus 5-FC administration initiated nine days after intratumoral virus injection at 500 mg/kg given *i.p.* twice a day for always 7 days, followed by 10 days off until termination of the study, revealed a statistically significant prolongation in median survival of mice treated with the mid (1x10e5) and high (1x10e6) vector dose as compared to their PBS-treated counterparts [75]. In a similar experiment mouse Tu-2449 gliomas were treated using different virus doses (1x10e6, 1x10e5, 1x10e4 and 1x10e3 TU/g brain weight) and 5-FC doses (500 mg/kg and 50 mg/kg body weight) [75]. 5-FC treatment or PBS treatment as control was initiated 9 days after vector injection and was given twice a day for 4 days, followed by a 10 day recovery phase. Cycles were repeated until termination of the study [75]. All vector doses in combination with 5-FC treatment at 500 mg/kg resulted in prolonged survival, as compared to PBS controls. Mice treated with vector doses of 1x10e4 and 1x10e5 and high dose 5-FC revealed a significantly prolonged survival when compared to the PBS controls [75]. However, even the 1x10e5 vector dose level with a rather low prodrug dose of 50 mg/kg 5-FC resulted in a survival advantage when compared to control. Histological analyses of Tu-2449 tumours taken before the first, second, and fourth treatment cycle with 500 mg/kg 5-FC revealed tumour growth between the first and the second dosing. Most of the tumour tissue however, was no longer visible and gliosis was evident by the start of the fourth treatment [75].

Currently, Toca 511 is being investigated in clinical trials in the United States in subjects with recurrent high-grade glioma either as a direct intratumoral vector injection (Phase I/II Study; NCT01156584; http://www.clinicaltrials.gov) or vector injection at the time of tumour removal (Phase I Study; NCT01470794 http://www.clinicaltrials.gov).

3.3.2. *Secreted therapeutic molecules*

Beside direct killing of tumour cells mediated by suicide gene products, different other therapeutic approaches, e.g. based on the secretion of therapeutic molecules such as cytokines or single chain antibodies (scFv) directed against specific tumour antigens could be facilitated by RCR vectors.

To allow secretion of therapeutic molecules from infected cells, a replicating retroviral vector was constructed by inserting specific transgene sequences to the first codon of the MLV env gene via a furin cleavage site sequence [26]. The respective fusion protein will be cleaved by furin proteases in the Golgi and the scFv will be secreted upon release of the new virus particles from infected cells (for details see above). The resulting vectors were capable of efficiently transducing susceptible cells, were genetically stable for more than 12 passages and were able to efficiently mediate intracellular production and secretion of the GM-CSF cytokine and the functional laminin-specific or T-cell-specific scFv antibody, respectively [27].

Sun and colleagues demonstrated the potential of the human chemokine interferon-gamma-inducible protein 10 (IP10) gene, delivered and expressed from a MLV-based RCR vectors, to inhibit tumour growth *in vivo* [76]. IP10 is known to be a potent inhibitor of angiogenesis, tumour growth, and metastasis [77,78]. Using human fibrosarcoma HT1080 cells transduced with the IP10 RCR vector designed as described above in an *s.c.* xenograft tumour model in nude mice, significant tumour growth inhibition and a marked reduction in microvessel density was observed as compared to non-infected HT1080 control mice (tumour volume 190 mm^3 *vs.* 510 mm^3) [76]. In addition, both, growth of *s.c.* tumour xenografts established from pre-infected murine Lewis lung carcinoma (LLC) cells as well as the formation of lung metastases from pre-infected murine melanoma B16F10 cells in immunocompetent C57BL/6 mice was significantly reduced [76].

3.3.3. *RNA interference*

In cancer gene therapy applications, RNAi-expressing RCR vectors can be used to inhibit tumour growth, invasion and metastasis. The length of the RNA duplex required for efficient RNAi is not longer than 21-23 bp. Therefore, the insertion of RNAi expression cassettes into RCR vectors should be well tolerated in respect to genetic stability and spread kinetics of the vector. The expression of duplex RNA is usually achieved using an expression cassette consisting of the RNA Pol III promoter transcribing a sequence designed to form a short hairpin RNA structure (shRNA). MLV-based RCR vectors were constructed encompassing a transcription cassette consisting of an H1-RNA Pol III promoter inserted in antisense orientation into the 3′ UTR of the vector backbone to drive expression of an shRNA sequence targeted against the epidermal growth factor receptor (EGFR) gene or the STAT3 gene [30]. To allow monitoring of infection efficiency, these vectors also contain the eGFP gene fused into the virus envelope gene. Insertion of both expression cassettes did not interfere significantly with virus fitness, and the receptor specificity of the Env protein was not impaired by the introduced eGFP sequences [28]. The modified vectors replicated rapidly and were genetically stable over several infection cycles. In addition, silencing of EGFR and STAT3 target gene expression in cells infected to levels of 80 – 95 % was shown to be highly efficient [30].

An improved, second generation MLV-based RNAi transfer vector suitable for in vivo application was recently described [79]. This RCR vector encodes miRNA modified shRNA sequences specifically targeting the eGFP and luciferase reporter genes under control of the small nuclear U6 promoter inserted in antisense orientation into the 3′ UTR of the vector. In HT1080 cells stably expressing eGFP or luciferase, marker gene expression was suppressed by more than 80 %, even when only 0.1 % of the cells were initially infected with the RCR vectors [79]. In vivo systemic tail vein administration of 2.9x10e7 of shLuc expressing vector particles in animals with pre-established subcutaneous HT1080-Luc tumours led to more than 80 % reduction in luciferase activity compared to uninfected tumours at day 25 post infection [79]. To investigate the effects of downregulation of tumour-promoting proteins, PLK1- and MMP14-specific shRNA expression cassettes were inserted into the vector. Upon infection of target cells, PLK1 and MMP14 mRNA and protein levels were reduced [79]. MLV-shPLK-infected cells were trapped in the G2-phase of the cell cycle at day 3 post infection, followed by induction of apoptosis at day 5 post infection. MLV-shMMP14 infected cells showed reduced MMP2 activity consistent with a reduced invasion capacity by ~75 % as compared to non-infected cells [79]. Tumour growth of MLV-shMMP14 infected HT1080-Rec-1 cells in immunodeficient mice was significantly and substantially reduced in comparison to controls. Similarly, direct intratumoral application of 1x10e6 of shPLK1 expressing vector particles in animals with pre-established subcutaneous HT1080 xenografts led to a significantly reduced tumour growth in comparison to the controls [79].

3.4. Safety of MLV-based RCR vectors

Up to now, a variety of different therapeutic approaches have been utilized in context of RCR vectors. High levels of vector spread, infection efficiency, and therapeutic gene expression have been detected leading to an efficacious therapeutic option for the treatment of cancer. From data on the eradication of tumour mass in animal models existing so far, a clear benefit of the RCR mediated tumour therapy is indicated. However, the use of replicating retroviral vectors also bears a number of risks which have to be identified and analysed.

In particular, 3 major concerns directly related to the use of RCR vectors have to be taken into consideration: (i) the risk of insertional mutagenesis due to integration of the vector genome into the host cell DNA, a step that can trigger the transformation of normal cells into tumour cells, (ii) the spread of viral vectors throughout the body of the patient causing viraemia, and (iii) the infection of dividing non-tumour cells and their loss due to therapeutic intervention leading to severe side effects.

The risk of insertional oncogenesis is an issue associated with the use of retroviral vectors in general, irrespective if they are replication-deficient or replication-competent. With RCR vectors this concern might be more substantial as due to the replicating nature more cells might be affected and multiple infections of the single cell might occur. On the other hand, in tumour therapy it is intended to kill the infected cells. Hence, due to this, insertional oncogenesis should not be an issue unless infected cells are resistant to treatment or got infected with an RCR vector which is reverted to wild-type due to genetic instability and thus is not able to exert its therapeutic potential.

The use of replication-competent retroviral vectors might also bear the risk of uncontrolled spread of vectors throughout the human body, resulting in infection of dividing cells other than the tumour cells itself. Non-dividing cells should not be infected as MLV-based vectors are thought to transduce dividing cells only, and, as most cells in the adult human body are non-dividing, virus spread should be limited. Moreover, some cell types, such as dividing human primary T-lymphocytes have only a low capacity to produce MLV-based RCR and, in addition, the produced virions are largely non-infectious [80]. Nevertheless, in case of unintended virus spread and high risk of viraemia, an early systemic intervention with antiretroviral drug(s) could be implemented to limit viral load [81]. Recent findings, on the other hand, suggest that the host range of MLV-based RCR vectors might include also post-mitotic and other growth-arrested cells in mammals [37]. Therefore, the issue of RCR-vector dissemination outside of the tumor mass is of particular concern in clinical studies employing RCR vectors and thus should be addressed in respective biodistribution studies.

For RCR biodistribution studies, sensitivity of the analysis is of utmost importance. Techniques based on conventional PCR, real-time PCR, flow-cytometry and immunohistochemical detection were employed so far to analyse the infection range of RCR vectors in animal models. In an early report, Logg and colleagues analysed the presence of the eGFP transgene in the DNA extracted from tumour tissue as well as from a variety of extratumoral tissues including spleen, lung, kidney, liver, and heart obtained from *nu/nu* BALB/c mice harbouring *s.c.* xenografts 7 weeks after intratumoral application of 6x10e3 RCR vector particles [22]. A PCR assay detecting 140 copies of GFP in a background of 100,000 equivalents of untransduced genomic DNA (transduction level 0.14 %) was employed [22]. Transgene sequences have been detected in tumour samples only. These data were further supported by flow cytometric analysis of the same tissues [22]. By improving this PCR assay, Wang et al. were able to detect as few as 35 copies of proviral DNA in 0.5 μg of genomic DNA. In an orthotopic glioma model in nude mice, in which animals were intratumorally inoculated with 1.2x10e4 virus particles, proviral sequences have been detected in tumour tissue, but not in contralateral brain parenchyma, bone marrow, GI tract, liver, kidney, spleen, lung, and skin [56]. Using a PCR driven detection method, eGFP transgene sequences could not be observed in normal tissues surrounding the injected tumours in a *s.c.* bladder tumour xenograft model in *nu/nu* BALB/c mice [62, 64]. No signals have been obtained in distant organs such as brain, liver, spleen, lung, bladder, kidney, heart, ovary, uterus, and stomach in an orthotopic model of bladder cancer, when RCR vectors were administered intravesically [62, 64].

By detection of CD gene-specific sequences by PCR at a detection limit of 400 copies per 100,000 cell genomes (600 ng of gDNA, transduction level 0.4 %), Tai and co-workers were able to determine proviral sequences in the transduced glioma tissue, but observed no extratumoral spread to and in any of the tissue examined (lung, liver, oesophagus and stomach, intestine, spleen, kidney, skin, bone marrow, contralateral normal brain) in an orthotopic glioma model in nude mice intratumorally injected with 1.2x10e4 virus particles [57]. However, all of these studies had been based on the detection of the non-viral transgene (e.g. GFP, CD, PNP, etc.). Hence, putative spread of vectors which have lost the transgene or parts of it will not be considered in these analyses.

In an immunocompetent intracranial RG2-glioma model performed in Fischer 344 rats, tumours were injected with 1x10e6 of CD expressing RCR vector particles followed by 5-FC or PBS treatment initiated 10 days later [58]. Organs from moribund animals were collected and quantitative real-time PCR targeting the MLV env gene was performed [58]. There was no evidence of presence of the env gene from the RCR vector in systemic tissues carrying highly mitotic cells such as lung, liver, kidney, spleen, bone marrow, skin, oesophagus, intestine, and testis [58]. Using this highly sensitive technique which enables detection of 20-35 copies in 50,000 cellular genomes, Hiraoka et al. analysed RCR vector biodistribution in a mouse hepatic metastasis model using BALB/c mice and the syngeneic colon carcinoma cell line CT26 [60,61]. After locoregional delivery of 2x10e4 of RCR vector particles either expressing the eGFP or CD transgene, *via* intrasplenic injection followed by splenectomy, no detectable virus-related signals were observed in genomic DNA extracted from peritumoral normal liver tissue, bone marrow, lung, kidney, small intestine, and colon. As expected, proviral RCR signals were highly abundant in genomic DNA from RCR-transduced tumour tissues with 3,000 – 16,600 proviral copies per 50,000 cells [60,61]. The copy number was increased in DNA obtained from ACE-CD/PBS-treated control animals (11,000 – 16,600 copies/50,000 cells) compared to ACE-CD/5-FC-treated animals (8,000 – 11,000 copies/50,000 cells) [61]. Optical imaging analyses, flow cytometric analyses as well as immunohistochemistry using an anti-eGFP antibody consistently revealed strongly positive eGFP signals in the tumour masses but not in the other organs mentioned above [60].

Biodistribution of RCR vectors after intravenous injection into immune deficient as well as immune competent mice was analysed by Solly and colleagues [25]. Two weeks after RCR vector injection, a 4070Aenv-based quantitative real-time PCR revealed presence of proviral genomes in bone marrow and spleen of nude mice. On the contrary, no proviral genomes could be detected in any tissue from immunocompetent animals, which emphasizes the potency of anti-MLV specific immune responses [25]. In vivo biodistribution of wt-MLV and MMP-activatable RCR vectors and their ability to reach tumour tissue after systemic administration was analysed in CB17-SCID mice using an optimized PCR method detecting up to 50 copies of proviral DNA in 300 ng of genomic DNA [48]. After intravenous injection of RCR vectors corresponding to 60 U of RT activity into tumour-free mice, tissues were analysed at different time points after virus injection. A strong signal in spleen and weak signals in liver and bone marrow were obtained after administration of wt-MLV vector one day after infection. After two weeks, wt-MLV sequences were found in lung, spleen, liver, heart, bone marrow, and muscle, but not in brain. The increase in PCR signal intensity over time suggests continuous virus replication. This was further supported by the presence of infectious virus in the blood of these animals. On the contrary, no positive signals were detected in mice infected with the MMP-activatable RCR vectors [48]. A similar experiment was performed with U-87MG and HT-1080 *s.c.* tumour-bearing mice to quantify the virus load in the tumour tissue. Again, animals were injected intravenously with similar amounts of wt-MLV and MMP-activatable RCR vectors and genomic DNA was analysed 2 weeks later. For all viruses, tumour tissue revealed the highest virus load reaching 100 % of cells in case of the non-targeted wt-MLV and up to 30 % of cells for MMP-activatable RCR vectors [48]. In addition, wt-MLV infected on average 32 % of the cells in the bone marrow, 11 % of the cells in spleen, and 6 % of the cells in liver, whereas the MMP-activatable RCR vector infected only 0.02 % of cells in these organs [48]. Interestingly, the load of wt-MLV in bone marrow and the other extratumoral organs in tumour-bearing animals was generally lower compared to those obtained in tumour-free animals [48].

Recently, Ostertag et al. reported biodistribution of the clinical vector Toca 511 after intratumoral administration in an immunocompetent mouse model of brain cancer using aquantitative real-time PCR technique to detect integrated provirus sequences with high sensitivity (10-25 copies per μg of gDNA) [75]. Two animal models based on different mouse strains had been Involved; BALB/c mice permissive for virus infection, and poorly permissive C57BL/6 mice. In these animal models 10e5 and 10e6 RCR vector particles have been injected intracranially into the tumor mass. Quantitative DNA analyses were performed on samples from mice which survived for 90 days and 180 days for the CT26-BALB/c model and the Tu-2449-B6C3F1 model, respectively. In the CT26-BALB/c model, vector spread to other tissues, particularly to lymphoid organs (thymus, spleen, lymph node, blood) was detectable [75]. Up to 5x10e5 proviral copies/μg gDNA were detected in thymus, up to 1.5x10e5 proviral copies/μg gDNA in samples from salivary gland, oesophagus, lung, heart, spleen, lymph node, and blood, and less than 5x10e3 proviral copies/μg gDNA in samples from skin, ovary, intestine, liver, kidney, spinal cord, bone marrow, cerebellum and brain [75]. In the Tu-2449-B6C3F1 model vector spread was observed at low levels only. Less than 5x10e3 proviral copies/μg gDNA were detected and interestingly the oesophagus was the organ in which the proviral copy number was highest. The difference in viral distribution observed in both model systems could be explained by the presence of different APOBEC3 alleles in these mouse strains. BALB/c mice have been shown to carry an allele that does not restrict MLV, whereas B6C3F1 mice carry an active allele [82]. Both mouse strains produced antibodies against Toca 511 [75].

The issue of biodistribution of the vector to non-target sites, as well as the expression of the therapeutic gene in off-target cells could be addressed best by infection targeting of the vector or expression targeting of the therapeutic gene to cells of the tumour. This approach has already been applied using tumour- and tissue-specific regulatory sequences to drive virus replication and transgene expression, and by modifying the viral envelope protein to allow transduction in a tissue/tumour specific manner.

4. Conclusion

Very recently, RCR vectors have been employed as a novel gene transfer vehicle for the treatment of cancer. Due to their dense genome organisation and the need for presence of all virus genes to allow vector replication, an only limited capacity for the introduction of foreign sequences is available, rendering the design of such vectors rather challenging. Nevertheless, different vector designs in respect to transgene location and mode of transgene expression have been elaborated. Their analysis in in vitro and in vivo studies revealed that the vectors are genetically stable over several replication cycles and result in an efficient delivery of the therapeutic gene into solid tumours in various animal models. On the other hand, different risks are associated with the use of RCR vectors, such as the risk of insertional tumorigenesis of non-target cells or the risk of inadvertent vector spread resulting in severe side effects. Such risks need to be carefully examined in appropriate non-clinical studies. In case they can be adequately addressed and dispelled, RCR vectors will be a promising option for efficient tumour therapy in humans.

Author details

Matthias Renner[1] and Juraj Hlavaty[2,3]

1 Department of Medical Biotechnology, Paul-Ehrlich-Institut, Langen, Germany

2 Christian-Doppler Laboratory for Innovative Immunotherapy, University of Veterinary Medicine, Vienna, Austria

3 Institute of Virology, Department of Pathobiology, University of Veterinary Medicine, Vienna, Austria

References

[1] Cross D, Burmester JK. Gene therapy for cancer treatment: past, present and future. Clinical Medicine & Research 2006;4(3): 218–227.

[2] Touchefeu Y, Harrington KJ, Galmiche JP, Vassaux G. Review article: gene therapy, recent developments and future prospects in gastrointestinal oncology. Alimentary Pharmacology & Therapeutics 2010;32(8): 953–968.

[3] Bader AG, Brown D, Stoudemire J, Lammers P. Developing therapeutic microRNAs for cancer. Gene Therapy 2011;18(12): 1121–1126.

[4] Duarte S, Carle G, Faneca H, de Lima MCP, Pierrefite-Carle V. Suicide gene therapy in cancer: Where do we stand now. Cancer Letters 2012;324(2): 160–170.

[5] Shand N, Weber F, Mariani L, Bernstein M, Gianella-Borradori A, Long Z, Sorensen AG, Barbier N. A phase 1-2 clinical trial of gene therapy for recurrent glioblastoma multiforme by tumor transduction with the herpes simplex thymidine kinase gene followed by ganciclovir. GLI328 European-Canadian Study Group. Human Gene Therapy 1999;10(14): 2325–2335.

[6] Rainov NG, Ren H. Clinical trials with retrovirus mediated gene therapy--what have we learned. Journal of Neuro-Oncology 2003;65(3): 227–236.

[7] Smitt PS, Driesse M, Wolbers J, Kros M, Avezaat C. Treatment of relapsed malignant glioma with an adenoviral vector containing the herpes simplex thymidine kinase gene followed by ganciclovir. Molecular Therapy 2003;7(6): 851–858.

[8] Cavazzana-Calvo M, Hacein-Bey S, Saint Basile G de, Gross F, Yvon E, Nusbaum P, Selz F, Hue C, Certain S, Casanova JL, Bousso P, Deist FL, Fischer A. Gene therapy of human severe combined immunodeficiency (SCID)-X1 disease. Science 2000;288(5466): 669–672.

[9] Cavazzana-Calvo M, Lagresle C, Hacein-Bey-Abina S, Fischer A. Gene therapy for severe combined immunodeficiency. Annual Review of Medicine 2005;56: 585–602.

[10] Kang EM, Choi U, Theobald N, Linton G, Long Priel DA, Kuhns D, Malech HL. Retrovirus gene therapy for X-linked chronic granulomatous disease can achieve stable long-term correction of oxidase activity in peripheral blood neutrophils. Blood 2010;115(4): 783–791.

[11] Dalba C, Bellier B, Kasahara N, Klatzmann D. Replication-competent vectors and empty virus-like particles: new retroviral vector designs for cancer gene therapy or vaccines. Molecular Therapy 2007;15(3): 457–466.

[12] Tai CK, Kasahara N. Replication-competent retrovirus vectors for cancer gene therapy. Frontiers in Bioscience 2008;13: 3083–3095.

[13] Logg CR, Robbins JM, Jolly DJ, Gruber HE, Kasahara N. Retroviral replicating vectors in cancer. Methods in Enzymology 2012;507: 199–228.

[14] Suzuki Y, Craigie R. The road to chromatin - nuclear entry of retroviruses. Nature Reviews Microbiology 2007;5(3): 187–196.

[15] Bushman F, Lewinski M, Ciuffi A, Barr S, Leipzig J, Hannenhalli S, Hoffmann C. Genome-wide analysis of retroviral DNA integration. Nature Reviews Microbiology 2005;3(11): 848–858.

[16] Stuhlmann H, Jaenisch R, Mulligan RC. Construction and properties of replication-competent murine retroviral vectors encoding methotrexate resistance. Molecular and Cellular Biology 1989;9(1): 100–108.

[17] Stuhlmann H, Jaenisch R, Mulligan RC. Transfer of a mutant dihydrofolate reductase gene into pre- and postimplantation mouse embryos by a replication-competent retrovirus vector. Journal of Virology 1989;63(11): 4857–4865.

[18] Dillon PJ, Lenz J, Rosen CA. Construction of a replication-competent murine retrovirus vector expressing the human immunodeficiency virus type 1 tat transactivator protein. Journal of Virology 1991;65(8): 4490–4493.

[19] Jespersen T, Duch M, Carrasco ML, Warming S, Pedersen FS. Expression of heterologous genes from an IRES translational cassette in replication competent murine leukemia virus vectors. Gene 1999;239(2): 227–235.

[20] Bachrach E, Pelegrin M, Piechaczyk M, Pedersen FS, Duch M. Efficient gene transfer into spleen cells of newborn mice by a replication-competent retroviral vector. Virology 2002;293(2): 328–334.

[21] Logg CR, Logg A, Tai CK, Cannon PM, Kasahara N. Genomic stability of murine leukemia viruses containing insertions at the Env-3' untranslated region boundary. Journal of Virology 2001;75(15): 6989–6998.

[22] Logg CR, Tai CK, Logg A, Anderson WF, Kasahara N. A uniquely stable replication-competent retrovirus vector achieves efficient gene delivery in vitro and in solid tumors. Human Gene Therapy 2001;12(8): 921–932.

[23] Paar M, Schwab S, Rosenfellner D, Salmons B, Gunzburg WH, Renner M, Portsmouth D. Effects of viral strain, transgene position, and target cell type on replication kinetics, genomic stability, and transgene expression of replication-competent murine leukemia virus-based vectors. Journal of Virology 2007;81(13): 6973–6983.

[24] Paar M, Klein D, Salmons B, Gunzburg WH, Renner M, Portsmouth D. Influence of vector design and host cell on the mechanism of recombination and emergence of mutant subpopulations of replicating retroviral vectors. BMC Molecular Biology 2009;10: 8.

[25] Solly SK, Trajcevski S, Frisen C, Holzer GW, Nelson E, Clerc B, Abordo-Adesida E, Castro M, Lowenstein P, Klatzmann D. Replicative retroviral vectors for cancer gene therapy. Cancer Gene Therapy 2003;10(1): 30–39.

[26] Buchholz CJ, Peng KW, Morling FJ, Zhang J, Cosset FL, Russell SJ. In vivo selection of protease cleavage sites from retrovirus display libraries. Nature Biotechnology 1998;16(10): 951–954.

[27] Finger C, Sun Y, Sanz L, Alvarez-Vallina L, Buchholz CJ, Cichutek K. Replicating retroviral vectors mediating continuous production and secretion of therapeutic gene products from cancer cells. Cancer Gene Therapy 2005;12(5): 464–474.

[28] Erlwein O, Buchholz CJ, Schnierle BS. The proline-rich region of the ecotropic Moloney murine leukaemia virus envelope protein tolerates the insertion of the green fluorescent protein and allows the generation of replication-competent virus. Journal of General Virology 2003;84(2): 369–373.

[29] Sliva K, Erlwein O, Bittner A, Schnierle BS. Murine leukemia virus (MLV) replication monitored with fluorescent proteins. Virology Journal 2004;1: 14.

[30] Sliva K, Schnierle BS. Stable integration of a functional shRNA expression cassette into the murine leukemia virus genome. Virology 2006;351(1): 218–225.

[31] Vile RG, Diaz RM, Miller N, Mitchell S, Tuszyanski A, Russell SJ. Tissue-specific gene expression from Mo-MLV retroviral vectors with hybrid LTRs containing the murine tyrosinase enhancer/promoter. Virology 1995;214(1): 307–313.

[32] Diaz RM, Eisen T, Hart IR, Vile RG. Exchange of viral promoter/enhancer elements with heterologous regulatory sequences generates targeted hybrid long terminal repeat vectors for gene therapy of melanoma. Journal of Virology 1998;72(1): 789–795.

[33] Saller RM, Ozturk F, Salmons B, Gunzburg WH. Construction and characterization of a hybrid mouse mammary tumor virus/murine leukemia virus-based retroviral vector. Journal of Virology 1998;72(2): 1699–1703.

[34] Feuer G, Fan H. Substitution of murine transthyretin (prealbumin) regulatory sequences into the Moloney murine leukemia virus long terminal repeat yields infectious virus with altered biological properties. Journal of Virology 1990;64(12): 6130–6140.

[35] Logg CR, Logg A, Matusik RJ, Bochner BH, Kasahara N. Tissue-specific transcriptional targeting of a replication-competent retroviral vector. Journal of Virology 2002;76(24): 12783–12791.

[36] Metzl C, Mischek D, Salmons B, Gunzburg WH, Renner M, Portsmouth D. Tissue- and tumor-specific targeting of murine leukemia virus-based replication-competent retroviral vectors. Journal of Virology 2006;80(14): 7070–7078.

[37] Liu X, Xu W, Russ J, Eiden LE, Eiden MV. The host range of gammaretroviruses and gammaretroviral vectors includes post-mitotic neural cells. PloS One 2011;6(3): e18072.

[38] Miller AD, Garcia JV, Suhr N von, Lynch CM, Wilson C, Eiden MV. Construction and properties of retrovirus packaging cells based on gibbon ape leukemia virus. Journal of Virology 1991;65(5): 2220–2224.

[39] Laer D von, Thomsen S, Vogt B, Donath M, Kruppa J, Rein A, Ostertag W, Stocking C. Entry of amphotropic and 10A1 pseudotyped murine retroviruses is restricted in hematopoietic stem cell lines. Journal of Virology 1998;72(2): 1424–1430.

[40] Sandrin V, Russell SJ, Cosset FL. Targeting retroviral and lentiviral vectors. Current Topics in Microbiology and Immunology 2003;281: 137–178.

[41] van Zeijl M, Johann SV, Closs E, Cunningham J, Eddy R, Shows TB, O'Hara B. A human amphotropic retrovirus receptor is a second member of the gibbon ape leukemia virus receptor family. Proceedings of the National Academy of Sciences of the United States of America 1994;91(3): 1168–1172.

[42] Logg CR, Baranick BT, Lemp NA, Kasahara N. Adaptive evolution of a tagged chimeric gammaretrovirus. Journal of Molecular Biology 2007;369(5): 1214–1229.

[43] Roux P, Jeanteur P, Piechaczyk M. A versatile and potentially general approach to the targeting of specific cell types by retroviruses: application to the infection of human

cells by means of major histocompatibility complex class I and class II antigens by mouse ecotropic murine leukemia virus-derived viruses. Proceedings of the National Academy of Sciences of the United States of America 1989;86(23): 9079–9083.

[44] Russell SJ, Hawkins RE, Winter G. Retroviral vectors displaying functional antibody fragments. Nucleic Acids Research 1993;21(5): 1081–1085.

[45] Kasahara N, Dozy AM, Kan YW. Tissue-specific targeting of retroviral vectors through ligand-receptor interactions. Science 1994; 266 (5189): 1373–1376.

[46] Zhao Y, Zhu L, Lee S, Li L, Chang E, Soong NW, Douer D, Anderson WF. Identification of the block in targeted retroviral-mediated gene transfer. Proceedings of the National Academy of Sciences of the United States of America 1999;96(7): 4005–4010.

[47] Tai CK, Logg CR, Park JM, Anderson WF, Press MF, Kasahara N. Antibody-mediated targeting of replication-competent retroviral vectors. Human Gene Therapy 2003;14(8): 789–802.

[48] Duerner LJ, Schwantes A, Schneider IC, Cichutek K, Buchholz CJ. Cell entry targeting restricts biodistribution of replication-competent retroviruses to tumour tissue. Gene Therapy 2008;15(22): 1500–1510.

[49] Schneider RM, Medvedovska Y, Hartl I, Voelker B, Chadwick MP, Russell SJ, Cichutek K, Buchholz CJ. Directed evolution of retroviruses activatable by tumour-associated matrix metalloproteases. Gene Therapy 2003;10(16): 1370–1380.

[50] Hartl I, Schneider RM, Sun Y, Medvedovska J, Chadwick MP, Russell SJ, Cichutek K, Buchholz CJ. Library-based selection of retroviruses selectively spreading through matrix metalloprotease-positive cells. Gene Therapy 2005;12(11): 918–926.

[51] Soifer H, Higo C, Logg CR, Jih LJ, Shichinohe T, Harboe-Schmidt E, Mitani K, Kasahara N. A novel, helper-dependent, adenovirus-retrovirus hybrid vector: stable transduction by a two-stage mechanism. Molecular Therapy 2002;5(5): 599–608.

[52] Kubo S, Haga K, Tamamoto A, Palmer DJ, Ng P, Okamura H, Kasahara N. Adenovirus-retrovirus hybrid vectors achieve highly enhanced tumor transduction and antitumor efficacy in vivo. Molecular Therapy 2011;19(1): 76–82.

[53] Biermann V, Volpers C, Hussmann S, Stock A, Kewes H, Schiedner G, Herrmann A, Kochanek S. Targeting of high-capacity adenoviral vectors. Human Gene Therapy 2001;12(14): 1757–1769.

[54] Komarova S, Kawakami Y, Stoff-Khalili MA, Curiel DT, Pereboeva L. Mesenchymal progenitor cells as cellular vehicles for delivery of oncolytic adenoviruses. Molecular Cancer Therapeutics 2006;5(3): 755–766.

[55] Portsmouth D, Hlavaty J, Renner M. Suicide genes for cancer therapy. Molecular Aspects of Medicine 2007;28(1): 4–41.

[56] Wang WJ, Tai CK, Kasahara N, Chen TC. Highly efficient and tumor-restricted gene transfer to malignant gliomas by replication-competent retroviral vectors. Human Gene Therapy 2003;14(2): 117–127.

[57] Tai CK, Wang WJ, Chen TC, Kasahara N. Single-shot, multicycle suicide gene therapy by replication-competent retrovirus vectors achieves long-term survival benefit in experimental glioma. Molecular Therapy 2005;12(5): 842–851.

[58] Wang W, Tai CK, Kershaw AD, Solly SK, Klatzmann D, Kasahara N, Chen TC. Use of replication-competent retroviral vectors in an immunocompetent intracranial glioma model. Neurosurgery Focus 2006;20(4): E25.

[59] Hlavaty J, Jandl G, Liszt M, Petznek H, Konig-Schuster M, Sedlak J, Egerbacher M, Weissenberger J, Salmons B, Gunzburg WH, Renner M. Comparative evaluation of preclinical in vivo models for the assessment of replicating retroviral vectors for the treatment of glioblastoma. Journal of Neuro-Oncology 2011;102(1): 59–69.

[60] Hiraoka K, Kimura T, Logg CR, Kasahara N. Tumor-selective gene expression in a hepatic metastasis model after locoregional delivery of a replication-competent retrovirus vector. Clinical Cancer Research: 2006;12(23): 7108–7116.

[61] Hiraoka K, Kimura T, Logg CR, Tai CK, Haga K, Lawson GW, Kasahara N. Therapeutic efficacy of replication-competent retrovirus vector-mediated suicide gene therapy in a multifocal colorectal cancer metastasis model. Cancer Research 2007;67(11): 5345–5353.

[62] Kikuchi E, Menendez S, Ozu C, Ohori M, Cordon-Cardo C, Logg CR, Kasahara N, Bochner BH. Highly efficient gene delivery for bladder cancers by intravesically administered replication-competent retroviral vectors. Clinical Cancer Research 2007;13(15): 4511–4518.

[63] Kawasaki Y, Tamamoto A, Takagi-Kimura M, Maeyama Y, Yamaoka N, Terada N, Okamura H, Kasahara N, Kubo S. Replication-competent retrovirus vector-mediated prodrug activator gene therapy in experimental models of human malignant mesothelioma. Cancer Gene Therapy 2011;18(8): 571–578.

[64] Kikuchi E, Menendez S, Ozu C, Ohori M, Cordon-Cardo C, Logg CR, Kasahara N, Bochner BH. Delivery of replication-competent retrovirus expressing Escherichia coli purine nucleoside phosphorylase increases the metabolism of the prodrug, fludarabine phosphate and suppresses the growth of bladder tumor xenografts. Cancer Gene Therapy 2007;14(3): 279–286.

[65] Huber BE, Austin EA, Good SS, Knick VC, Tibbels S, Richards CA In vivo antitumor activity of 5-fluorocytosine on human colorectal carcinoma cells genetically modified to express cytosine deaminase. Cancer research 1993;53(19): 4619–4626.

[66] Parker WB, King SA, Allan PW, Bennett LL, Secrist JA, Montgomery JA, Gilbert KS, Waud WR, Wells AH, Gillespie GY, Sorscher EJ. In vivo gene therapy of cancer with E. coli purine nucleoside phosphorylase. Human Gene Therapy 1997;8(14): 1637–1644.

[67] Tai C, Wang W, Lai Y, Logg CR, Parker WB, Li Y, Hong JS, Sorscher EJ, Chen TC, Kasahara N. Enhanced efficiency of prodrug activation therapy by tumor-selective replicating retrovirus vectors armed with the Escherichia coli purine nucleoside phosphorylase gene. Cancer Gene Therapy 2010;17(9): 614–623.

[68] Perez OD, Logg CR, Hiraoka K, Diago O, Burnett R, Inagaki A, Jolson D, Amundson K, Buckley T, Lohse D, Lin A, Burrascano C, Ibanez C, Kasahara N, Gruber HE, Jolly DJ. Design and Selection of Toca 511 for Clinical Use: Modified Retroviral Replicating Vector With Improved Stability and Gene Expression. Molecular Therapy 2012;20(9): 1689-1698.

[69] Erbs P, Regulier E, Kintz J, Leroy P, Poitevin Y, Exinger F, Jund R, Mehtali M. In vivo cancer gene therapy by adenovirus-mediated transfer of a bifunctional yeast cytosine deaminase/uracil phosphoribosyltransferase fusion gene. Cancer Research 2000;60(14): 3813–3822.

[70] Bourbeau D, Lavoie G, Nalbantoglu J, Massie B Suicide gene therapy with an adenovirus expressing the fusion gene CD::UPRT in human glioblastomas: different sensitivities correlate with p53 status. The Journal of Gene Medicine 2004;6(12): 1320–1332.

[71] Suttle DP, Bugg BY, Winkler JK, Kanalas JJ. Molecular cloning and nucleotide sequence for the complete coding region of human UMP synthase. Proceedings of the National Academy of Sciences of the United States of America 1988;85(6): 1754–1758.

[72] Sakamoto E, Nagase H, Kobunai T, Oie S, Oka T, Fukushima M, Oka T. Orotate phosphoribosyltransferase expression level in tumors is a potential determinant of the efficacy of 5-fluorouracil. Biochemical and Biophysical Research Communications 2007;363(1): 216–222.

[73] Taomoto J, Yoshida K, Wada Y, Tanabe K, Konishi K, Tahara H, Fukushima M. Overexpression of the orotate phosphoribosyl-transferase gene enhances the effect of 5-fluorouracil on gastric cancer cell lines. Oncology 2006;70(6): 458–464.

[74] Johnson AJ, Ardiani A, Sanchez-Bonilla M, Black ME. Comparative analysis of enzyme and pathway engineering strategies for 5FC-mediated suicide gene therapy applications. Cancer Gene Therapy 2011;18(8): 533–542.

[75] Ostertag D, Amundson KK, Lopez Espinoza F, Martin B, Buckley T, Galvao da Silva AP, Lin AH, Valenta DT, Perez OD, Ibanez CE, Chen C, Pettersson PL, Burnett R, Daublebsky V, Hlavaty J, Gunzburg W, Kasahara N, Gruber HE, Jolly DJ, Robbins JM. Brain tumor eradication and prolonged survival from intratumoral conversion of 5-fluorocytosine to 5-fluorouracil using a nonlytic retroviral replicating vector. Neuro-Oncology 2012;14(2): 145–159.

[76] Sun Y, Finger C, Alvarez-Vallina L, Cichutek K, Buchholz CJ. Chronic gene delivery of interferon-inducible protein 10 through replication-competent retrovirus vectors suppresses tumor growth. Cancer Gene Therapy 2005;12(11): 900–912.

[77] Wang JM, Deng X, Gong W, Su S. Chemokines and their role in tumor growth and metastasis. Journal of Immunological Methods 1998;220(1-2): 1–17.

[78] Frederick MJ, Clayman GL. Chemokines in cancer. Expert Reviews in Molecular Medicine 2001;3(19): 1–18.

[79] Schaser T, Wrede C, Duerner L, Sliva K, Cichutek K, Schnierle B, Buchholz CJ. RNAi-mediated gene silencing in tumour tissue using replication-competent retroviral vectors. Gene Therapy 2011;18(10): 953–960.

[80] Ebeling SB, Simonetti ER, Borst HPE, Blok A, Schelen AM, Braakman E, Ederveen J, Hagenbeek A. Human primary T lymphocytes have a low capacity to amplify MLV-based amphotropic RCR and the virions produced are largely noninfectious. Gene Therapy 2003;10(21): 1800–1806.

[81] Powell SK, Artlip M, Kaloss M, Brazinski S, Lyons R, McGarrity GJ, Otto E. Efficacy of antiretroviral agents against murine replication-competent retrovirus infection in human cells. Journal of Virology 1999;73(10): 8813–8816.

[82] Takeda E, Tsuji-Kawahara S, Sakamoto M, Langlois M, Neuberger MS, Rada C, Miyazawa M. Mouse APOBEC3 restricts friend leukemia virus infection and pathogenesis in vivo. Journal of Virology 2008;82(22): 10998–11008.

Chapter 7

A Novel Therapy for Melanoma and Prostate Cancer Using a Non-Replicating Sendai Virus Particle (HVJ-E)

Toshihiro Nakajima, Toshimitsu Itai, Hiroshi Wada,
Toshie Yamauchi, Eiji Kiyohara and
Yasufumi Kaneda

Additional information is available at the end of the chapter

1. Introduction

The virotherapy approach to cancer therapy uses virus particles. It is based on the case reports since 1950s, which reported the regression of cancers including leukemia, Hodgkin's disease, and Burkitt's lymphoma after the infection of wild type viruses [1-11].

The earliest virotherapies involved injection of wild-type viruses and evaluation of their efficacies [1-3]. *Ex vivo* therapies using autologous irradiated tumors infected with oncolytic viruses were also investigated [12-18]. Deletion mutants of oncolytic viruses [19-24], and recombinant viruses carrying a therapeutic gene [25-32] that induce cancer apoptosis or cancer immunity have been developed and evaluated in the clinical setting.

Oncolytic viruses derived from adenovirus, poxvirus, reovirus, picornavirus, paramyxovirus, and herpes simplex virus are currently available and have been clinically evaluated [33-35]. In China, two adenovirus-based products (Gendicine and Ocorine) have been commercialized [36], while randomized phase III studies of two oncolytic viruses (reovirus and poxvirus) are ongoing in advanced countries [33-35]. Thus, virotherapy is expected to become available as a new approach for cancer treatment, and specific product approval is anticipated in the US, EU, and Japan [37].

The major drawback associated with virotherapy is safety since replicating viruses are used in this therapy. In order to reduce the toxicity to normal cells, oncolytic viruses with strict specificity for cancer cells were constructed [29, 38-42]. However, the use of these viruses is still considered to be high risk because it is theoretically possible that a virulent infection may occur after recombination with wild-type viruses [43].

An alternative option to avoid such a risk is to use a non-replicating oncolytic virus [44]. We found that a non-replicating oncolytic virus (HVJ-E: hemagglutinating virus of Japan-envelope) is able to induce cancer cell-specific apoptosis and immunity [45]. The induction of apoptosis and activation of dendritic cells *in vitro*, and anti-tumor activity *in vivo* are similar to the wild-type hemagglutinating virus of Japan (also known as Sendai virus, HVJ) [45].

The hemagglutinating virus of Japan was discovered in Sendai, Japan, in the 1950s [46]. It is a paramyxovirus with a minus-strand RNA genome. The virus has fusogenic activity [47, 48], and is used to prepare hybridoma cells for the production of monoclonal antibodies, and heterokaryons for chromosome analysis [49-51].

The hemagglutinating virus of Japan-envelope is an inactivated HVJ particle [52]. It is manufactured by a process similar to that used for whole virus particle vaccines. Good manufacturing practice (GMP)-regulated processes have been established in their production for use in preclinical and clinical studies [53].

We conducted dose-setting efficacy studies for HVJ-E in a murine cancer model in which dose-dependent anti-cancer activity was observed. We also conducted safety studies following good laboratory practices (GLP), including pharmacological safety studies and toxicokinetic (TK) studies in rats and monkeys, as part of an investigational new drug (IND) application.

Osaka University Hospital is currently conducting two investigational clinical studies with HVJ-E for the treatment of advanced melanoma and castration-resistant prostate cancer (CRPC) [54-56]. These clinical trials are the first human studies for HVJ-E and will reveal the safety and efficacy of the non-replicating virus (HVJ-E). Virotherapy with a non-replicating oncolytic virus is a new approach that is anticipated to provide a new strategy for cancer therapy.

2. A new strategy for cancer therapy

Most cancers are still incurable and new approaches are required to improve the efficacy of cancer treatments. However, conventional cancer therapies are problematic.

Chemotherapy with anti-cancer agents is useful in achieving tumor regression. However, the immune system, which is important in the removal of residual cancer cells, is also suppressed by these agents (Figure 1). Therefore, surviving cancer cells and cancer stem cells (CSC) eventually acquire drug resistance, resulting in tumor relapse (Figure 1) [57]. Thus, chemotherapy with cytotoxic drugs does not generally result in the necessary eradication of cancer cells required for long-term survival.

Immune therapies for cancer offer a new approach to cancer treatment, and several products, including sipuleucel-T, are currently approved in advanced countries [58, 59]. The aim of these therapies is the removal of cancers by the immune system. Numerous cancer immune therapies are currently under evaluation in clinical studies. However, these agents are not potent because of lack of cytotoxic effect on cancer cells (Figure 1).

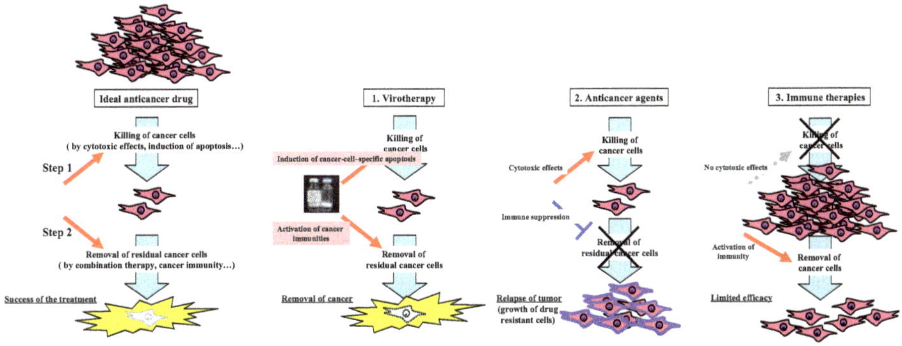

Figure 1. Problems with conventional therapies and a 2-step strategy for cancer treatment. Conventional anti-cancer therapies are problematic and a 2-step therapeutic strategy is proposed for effective cancer treatment. Virotherapy possesses ideal characteristics for such a 2-step therapy. Problems associated with conventional anti-cancer drugs and immune therapies, including cancer vaccines, are shown.

These observations suggest that a two-step strategy is necessary for the eradication of cancer cells (Figure 1).

During the first step, the direct killing of cancer cells is necessary for reduction of tumor volume. CSCs are usually resistant to conventional anti-cancer drugs and continue to proliferate during chemotherapy. Therefore, an agent that targets and kills CSCs is required for effective cancer treatment.

During the second step, the removal of residual cancer cells (and CSCs) from the body by a cancer-specific immune response is necessary to avoid relapse of the condition [57]. However, it is difficult for immune cells to recognize and remove CSCs because they exist as a minority population within the tumor, and possess a lower antigenicity than differentiated cancer cells [57]. Oncolytic viruses have the capability of both directly killing cancer cells and inducing cancer immunity.

It has been reported that several oncolytic viruses have the capability to kill CSCs [60-67]. The reovirus-based oncolytic virus [61], telomerase-specific oncolytic adenovirus [62], and herpes simplex virus-based oncolytic viruses (G47Delta and Delta 68H-6) [63, 64] reduced CSCs in murine models of breast cancer, esophageal cancer, and malignant glioma, respectively. Thus, a virotherapy approach in patients is expected to kill cancer cells and eradicate cancer cells including CSCs (Figure 1).

3. Non-replicating virus particles as anti-cancer agents

The use of non-replicating virus particles is a new approach in virotherapy.

A non-replicating virus particle, HVJ-E, is currently being developed as a potential new agent for the treatment of advanced melanoma and CRPC [44, 55, 56]. It is derived from HVJ, a member of the paramyxovirus family (Figure 2). The HVJ-E particle is prepared by inactivating the wild-type virus (HVJ) by treatment with an alkylating agent and UV irradiation [52, 53]. HVJ-E was originally developed as a drug delivery system (vector) for various biopharmaceuticals such as plasmid DNAs, siRNAs, decoy oligonucleotides, antibody proteins, and anti-cancer drugs [52, 68-75].

Kurooka and Kaneda discovered that the HVJ-E particle itself displayed anti-cancer effects in a murine model of colon cancer [45]. Similar to the live (replicating) virus, HVJ-E induced maturation and differentiation of human and murine dendritic cells (DCs). It also induced infiltration of immune cells into the tumor tissue followed by activation of cancer cell-specific cytotoxic T cells. Furthermore, HVJ-E suppressed the function of regulatory T cells (Treg), which have been reported to be negative regulators of cancer immunity. Thus, HVJ-E activates cancer immunity, and simultaneously suppresses Treg [45].

1. **Structure**
   a. **Spherical particle of diameter 200–300 nm**
   b. **Contains single strand RNA (ssRNA)**
   c. **Contains proteins+lipid for delivery (functions as a natural DDS for nucleic acid)**
2. **Mode of action**
   a. **The RNA in the particle acts as an RIG-I agonist and induces an induces cancer cell apoptosis**
   b. **Activates the RIG-I/MAVS pathway and also induces anticancer immune responses**
3. **Manufacture**
   a. **Process adapted to GMP guidelines, and pilot plant for clinical trial is available**
   b. **Freeze-dried formulation is stable for over 21 months in refrigerator.**

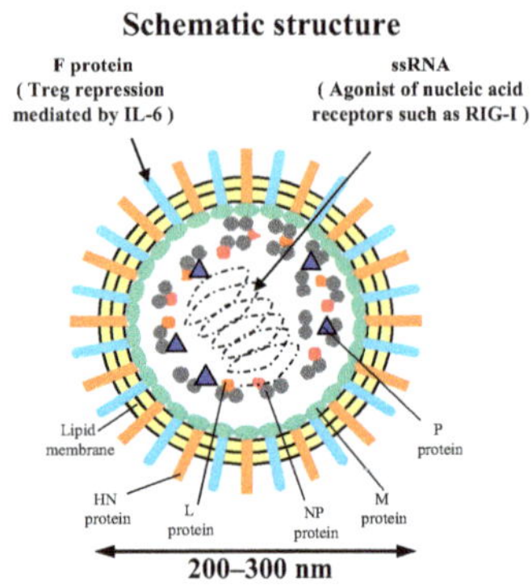

Figure 2. Characteristics and structure of HVJ-E/GEN0101. The characteristics of HVJ-E/GEN0101 are shown on the left. A schematic structure of the particle is shown on the right.

Fujiwara and Kaneda *et al.* reported that HVJ-E induced innate immunity [76]. Intratumoral injection of HVJ-E promoted infiltration and activation of natural killer (NK) cells by the induction of C-X-C motif chemokine 10 (CXCL10) and type I interferons. When HVJ-E was injected into the tumor of a murine model of renal cell carcinoma (RCC), NK cells exhibited cytotoxic activity against the RCC cell line *in vivo* [76]. The involvement of NK cells in the anti-tumor effect was also confirmed by showing the depletion of NK cells using an asialo-GM1 antibody [76]. Activated NK cells produced interferon-γ, which induces cancer-specific cytotoxic T cells [76]. These results indicated that HVJ-E is able to induce both innate and adaptive immunities.

In addition to the induction of cancer immunities, HVJ-E has the capability to induce cancer cell-specific apoptosis. Kawaguchi and Kaneda *et al.* reported that HVJ-E showed a dose-dependent, direct killing effect on human prostate cancer cell lines. In contrast, it showed no suppression of normal human prostate epithelium proliferation [77].

HVJ-E also induced apoptosis of prostate cancer cells *in vivo* because it showed an anti-tumor effect in severe combined immunodeficiency (SCID) mice that lack B lymphocyte- and T lymphocyte-mediated immunities [76, 77]. When NK cells were depleted from SCID mice by injection of the asialo-GM1 antibody, intratumoral injection of HVJ-E still showed an anti-tumor effect in a murine model of CRPC [77]. This result suggested that HVJ-E showed a direct killing activity *in vivo*. HVJ-E-mediated apoptosis of cancer cells was further confirmed in a murine model of prostate cancer using a NOD/SCID mouse, which lacks both innate (NK cell-mediated) and adaptive (antibody and CTL-mediated) immunities [54].

Numerous studies have revealed that the non-replicating HVJ-E particle shows anti-tumor effects in murine models of renal cell carcinoma, glioma, colon, bladder and CRPCs [45, 76-79].

In contrast, previous studies have reported that the non-replicating oncolytic Newcastle disease virus (NDV) failed to show an anti-tumor effect *in vivo* [80, 81]. These results are inconsistent with results obtained with HVJ-E [45, 76, 77, 79], and the putative reason is the difference between the number of particles used in the studies. In studies with NDV, 5×10^9 PFU of oncolytic virus were systemically or locally administrated [81], whereas the number of HVJ-E particles administered was estimated to be higher.

Another possibility is the difference in the capability of the virus to deliver its RNA fragments to target cancer cells. The Z strain-derived HVJ-E used in our studies has the highest level of membrane fusion activity [52]. Therefore, it is possible that HVJ-E has the ability to deliver more RNA component to the target cancer cells than the UV-inactivated NDV particle. The difference in process of inactivation may be responsible for the activity of non-replicating oncolytic viruses. The Newcastle disease virus was inactivated by UV irradiation, whereas HVJ-E was inactivated by a combination of treatment with an alkylating agent and UV irradiation [53]. Inactivation conditions affect the efficiency of delivery, and strictly regulated processes are necessary to obtain suitable performance [53].

4. Mode of actions

The major target cells of HVJ-E are cancer cells and dendritic cells (DCs) (Figure 3A) [44, 45, 76].

Treatment of cancer cells with HVJ-E enhanced the expression and activation (cleavage) of caspases 3, 8, and 9 (Figure 4A) [77], and induced dose-dependent apoptosis of melanoma, prostate, and other cancer cell lines *in vitro* (Figure 4B) [77]. Interestingly, no apoptotic effects were observed on normal epithelial cells derived from murine prostate [54, 77]. Thus, the apoptotic activity of HVJ-E is considered to be specific to cancer cells [54, 77].

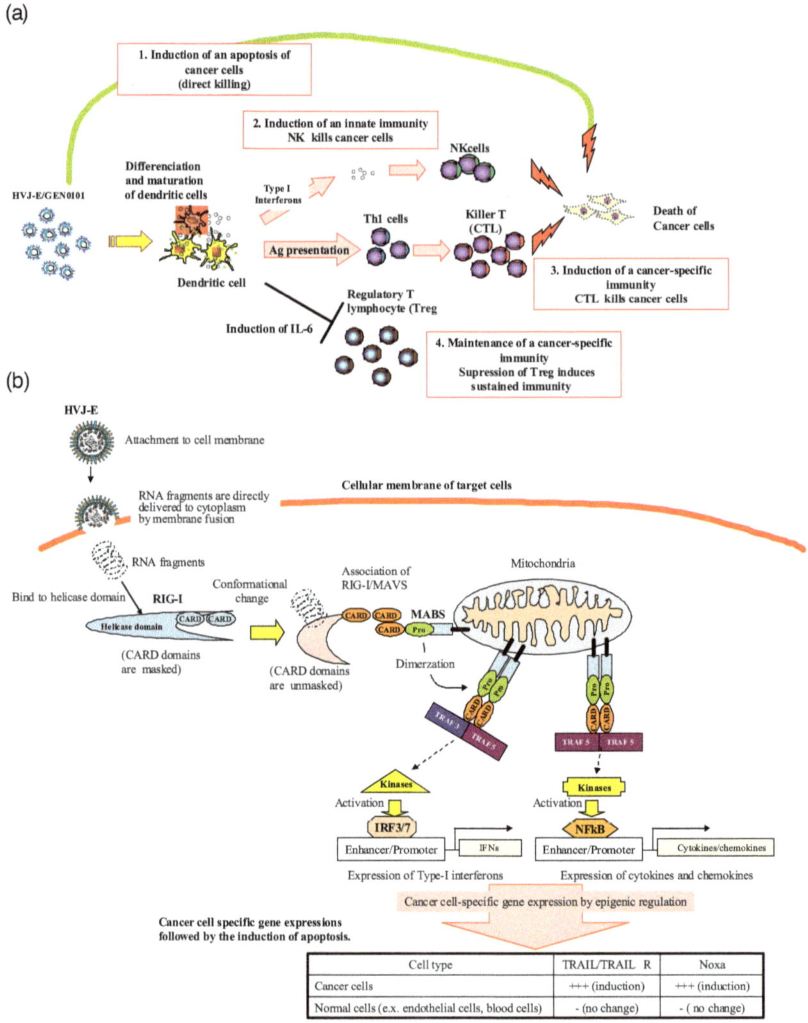

Figure 3. The mechanism of anti-cancer effects of HVJ-E/GEN0101. A novel type of virotherapy agent (HVJ-E/GEN0101) has a multi-mode of action that is ideal for 2-step cancer treatment. **(A)** Target cells and sequential anti-cancer effects of HVJ-E/GEN0101. **(B)** Signaling pathway induced by stimulation with HVJ-E/GEN0101. The RIG-I/MAVS pathway is the major pathway involved. RIG-I is a cytosolic receptor for nucleic acids: it usually functions as a sensor to recognize viral infection. The nucleic acids in the HVJ-E/GEN0101 particle act as an agonist for RIG-I and induce cancer cell-specific gene expression followed by the induction of apoptosis.

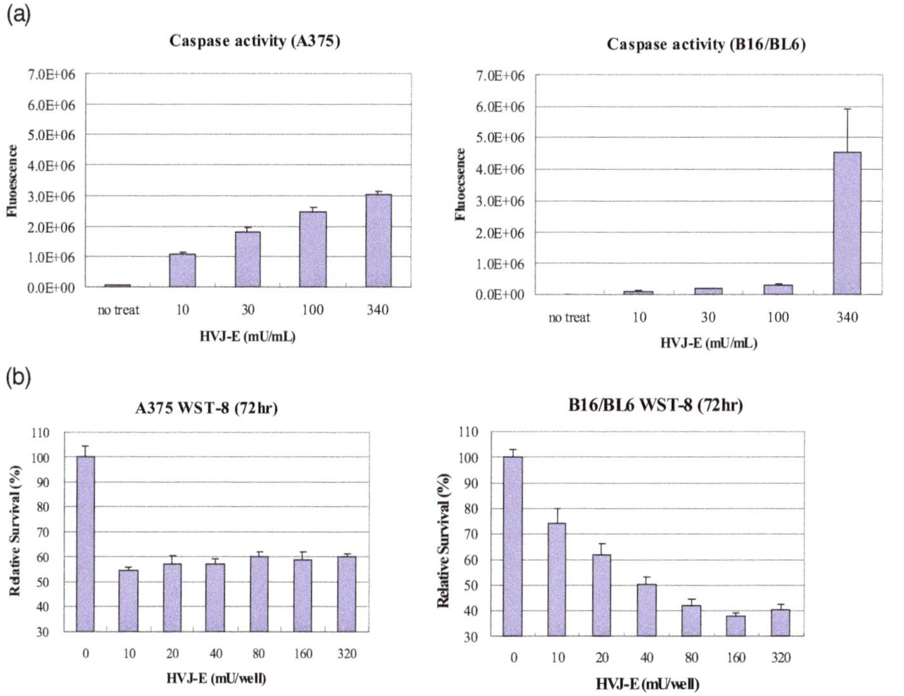

Figure 4. HVJ-E/GEN0101 induces apoptosis of human and murine melanoma cells. (A) Induction of caspase activity after treatment of melanoma cells with HVJ-E/GEN0101. Human (A375) and murine (B16/BL6) melanoma cells were treated with various amounts of HVJ-E/GEN0101, and caspase activities were measured 24 hours later. A dose-dependent activation was observed. **(B)** Survival of melanoma cells after treatment with various amounts of HVJ-E/GEN0101. Human (A375) and murine (B16/BL6) melanoma cells were treated with various amounts of HVJ-E/GEN0101 and cell survival was measured by WST-8 assay 72 hours later.

Matsushima and Kaneda *et al.* conducted an investigation to determine the active component for anti-cancer effects, and identified RNA fragments within the particle [54]. Moreover, Kaneda *et al.* analyzed the signaling pathway involved and revealed that retinoic acid inducible gene-I (RIG-I) is a key factor for signal transduction [44, 54, 77]. Retinoic acid inducible gene-I is a cytosolic nucleic acid receptor and was originally identified as a sensor that recognizes infection by single strand RNA viruses [82, 83]. Thus, RIG-I has been recognized as an inducer of immune response against infected viruses [82-84].

The RNA fragments delivered by HVJ-E bind the helicase domain of RIG-I in the cytoplasm and change the conformation to unmask the caspase activation and recruitment domain (CARD) (Figure 3B). After binding with the RNA fragments, RIG-I interacts with the mitochondrial antiviral signaling (MAVS) protein on the mitochondrial membrane (Figure 3B) [84]. The mitochondrial antiviral signaling protein forms a complex with an adaptor protein

(TRAF3/5), stimulates transcription factors (IRF3 and IRF7), and promotes the expression of interferon-α and β (Figure 3B) [85, 86]. It also stimulates kinases of regulator protein of transcription factor NK-κB, resulting in increased expression of cytokines, chemokines, and other genes (Figure 3B) [45, 54, 76, 77].

It has been reported that the RIG-I/MAVS pathway is activated after cancer cells are treated with HVJ-E [54]. Transfection of isolated RNA fragments from HVJ-E particle also induced apoptosis of cancer cells *in vitro* [54]. Thus, HVJ-E uses a natural oligonucleotide (RNA fragment from the inactivated virus genome) as an active ingredient, and a natural virus particle (envelope of HVJ) as a delivery system for a nucleic acid medicine (RNA fragments). The apoptosis induced by HVJ-E was cancer cell-specific because normal endothelial cells showed no apoptosis after the treatment with HVJ-E [54, 77].

Involvement of RIG-I in cancer cell-specific apoptosis has also been indicated in ovarian cancers and melanoma. Kübler and Barchet *et al.* reported that the RIG-I agonist (Poly(dAdT)) induced apoptosis and expression of MHC class I molecules in ovarian cancer cells [87, 88]. Van and Bell *et al.* also reported apoptosis of ovarian cancer cells after treatment with dsRNA [89]. Analysis by shRNA-mediated knockdown revealed that RIG-I and other receptors for dsRNA (TLR3 and MDA-5) were involved in the caspase 8/9-mediated apoptosis of cancer cells. Similar to sensitivity of HVJ-E, epithelial cells derived from ovarian surface was resistant to apoptosis mediated by RIG-I signal pathway. When combined with conventional chemotherapy (carboplatin/paclitaxel), treatment with dsRNA showed a synergistic suppression of ovarian cancer cell viability [89]. Besch *et al.* reported that stimulation of RIG-I and MDA-5 induced apoptosis of human melanoma cells [90]. The authors used pppRNA and poly(I:C) as ligands for RIG-I and MDA-5, and showed the involvement of caspase-9 and Apaf-1 during apoptosis. They also reported the reduction of lung metastasis by treatment with ligands for RIG-I and MDA-5 in the NOD/SCID mouse [90]. Details of the underlying pathways are currently being analyzed using siRNAs of apoptosis-related factors [54]. It has been suggested that differences in the expression of apoptotic genes such as Noxa, TRAIL, and TRAIL receptors in cancer cells and normal cells determine the specificity of apoptosis induced by HVJ-E (Figure 3B) [54].

HVJ-E also induced differentiation and maturation of murine and human DCs [45]. It induced the expression of surface markers on mature DCs, and the production of various cytokines and chemokines from DCs [45, 76, 77]. Activated DCs induce both innate (NK cell-mediated) and adaptive (cytotoxic T cell-mediated) immunities (Figure 3A) [45, 76]. It has been reported that an RIG-I agonist (Poly(dAdT)) induced the production of cytokines (IL-6 and TNF-α) and chemokines (CXCL1-and CCL5/RANTES) [87, 88] in human ovarian cancer cells.

5. Efficacy in preclinical studies

The efficacy of the non-replicating oncolytic virus (HVJ-E/GEN0101) was examined in murine models of melanoma and prostate cancer (Figure 5A). GEN0101 is the identification code for the agent. The data have indicated that the anti-tumor effect is dose-dependent similar to other non-viral anti-cancer agents (Figure 5B). This feature is important for the development of non-replicating oncolytic virus as a novel therapeutic agent; identification of the optimal dose for non-replicating oncolytic viruses is easier than determining the optimal dose for replicating oncolytic viruses as the latter are subject to change (increase) resulting from replication in target cancer cells. The effects of administration in a xenograft model of human CRPC were also examined (Figure 5A). Efficacy after subcutaneous administration was revealed (Figure 5C). It is known that the SCID mice lacks B lymphocyte- and T lymphocyte-mediated immunities such as antibody production, and induction of cytotoxic T cells but retains monocytes and NK cells important for innate immunity. Thus, the non-replicating virus (HVJ-E/GEN0101) is able to induce innate immunity, and show anti-cancer activity *in vivo* even in the absence of direct killing of cancer cells. Efficacy by subcutaneous administration is important for the development of a non-replicating virus because subcutaneous administration is more common than intratumoral administration. Intratumoral administration kills cancer cells directly and promotes the release of tumor antigens, which are recognized by immune cells. Subcutaneous administration is expected to enhance and sustain the immune response. Therefore, the combination of intratumoral and subcutaneous administration is suggested as a suitable regimen in the clinical setting.

In summary, the results of efficacy studies have indicated that the anti-cancer effect of the non-replicating oncolytic virus HVJ-E/GEN0101 is dose-dependent similar to conventional anti-cancer drugs, and subcutaneous administration may be the preferred administration route for the viral and non-replicating viral agents.

6. Safety studies

Safety of the non-replicating oncolytic virus (HVJ-E/GEN0101) has been confirmed in non-primate (rat) and primate (Cynomolgus monkey) animals. Lists of the studies that have been conducted are shown in Table 1A and B.

Results from single dose general toxicity studies revealed that no death or severe finding was observed even in the maximum dosage groups. Similar to the single dose studies, no severe finding was observed in repeated dose, general toxicity studies (Table 1A).

Results from immunological and genetic toxicity studies in rat and monkeys revealed that no abnormal symptoms related to the test agent were observed. The levels of IL-6 and IFN-γ in monkey serum were analyzed after subcutaneous injection of HVJ-E/GEN0101, and the levels of both cytokines were determined to be within the normal range (data not shown). A core battery of safety pharmaceutical studies was performed to determine the effects on major organs (central nervous, respiratory, and cardiovascular systems); no abnormal effect was observed with the exception of transient and non-severe pyrexia (Table 1B).

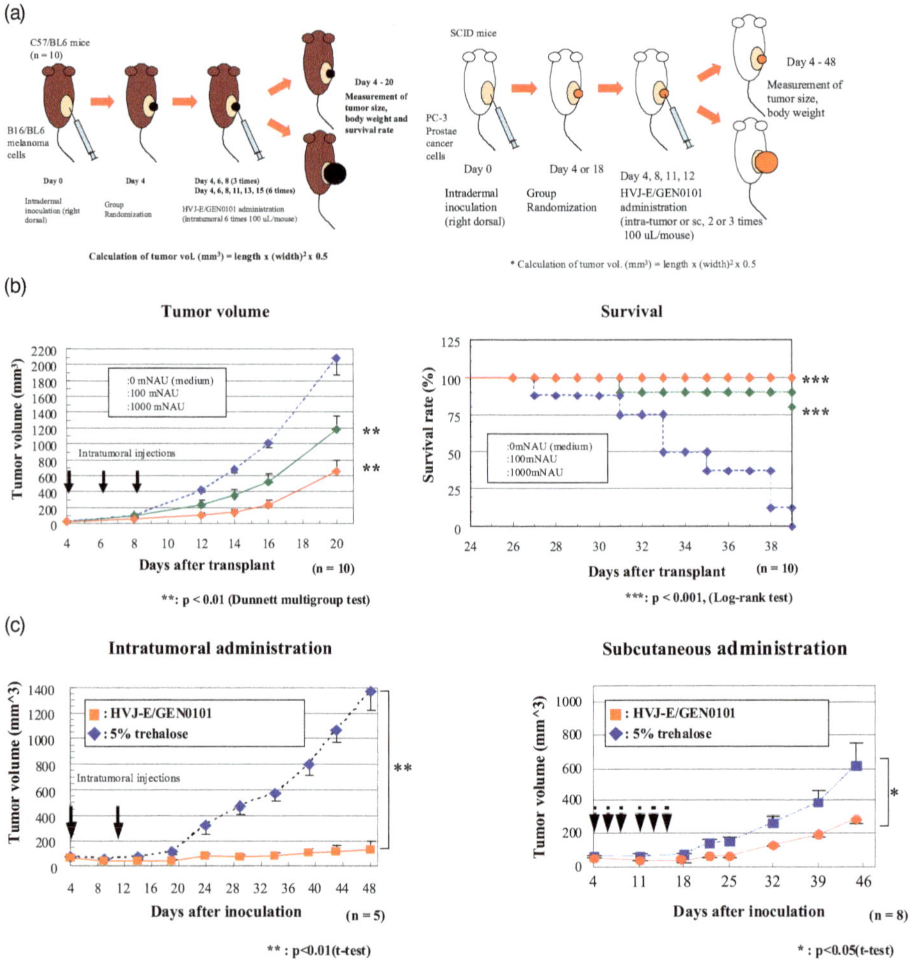

Figure 5. Efficacy studies of HVJ-E/GEN0101 in a murine model of melanoma and prostate cancer.(A) Protocols for the efficacy study using murine models of melanoma and prostate cancer. Left: C57/BL6 mice were transplanted with B16/BL6 cells and 3 intratumoral injections of HVJ-E/GEN0101 were administered after tumor formation (4 days after transplant). A time course study of change in tumor volume was performed, and the difference in tumor volume among the three groups was statistically analyzed at the end of the study. Significant differences were determined by Dunnett's multigroup test, and significant differences to the medium (control) group were observed ($p < 0.01$). The survival rate after the injection of HVJ-E/GEN0101 was also monitored in the melanoma model. A survival study was performed and the difference among the three groups was statistically analyzed at the end of the study. Significant differences were determined by log-rank analysis. Significant differences to the medium group were observed ($p < 0.001$). Right: Protocol for the efficacy study in a murine model of prostate cancer. Human CRPC (PC-3)-bearing mice were used for the study. A summary of the study protocol is shown. The anti-tumor effect of HVJ-E/GEN0101 for each administration route was examined. Severe combined immunodeficiency mice were transplanted with PC-3 cells. Two intratumoral injections or 6 subcutaneous injections of HVJ-E/GEN0101 were performed after tumor formation (4

days after transplant). A time course study of change in tumor volume was performed and differences in tumor volume between the two groups were statistically analyzed at the end of study. Significant differences were determined by t-test and significant differences to the medium were observed in both routes ($p < 0.01$ and $p < 0.05$). **(B)** Efficacy study in a murine model of melanoma. Dose-dependency of the anti-tumor effect of HVJ-E/GEN0101 was revealed. **(C)** Efficacy study in a murine model of prostate cancer. A time course study of change in tumor volume was performed and differences in tumor volume between the two groups were statistically analyzed at the end of the study. Significant differences were determined by t-test, and significant differences to the medium were observed for both administration routes ($p < 0.01$ and $p < 0.05$).

a) Toxicological study (1): General toxicity study

Dosing Regimen	Species	Route	Dose
Single Dose	Rat	iv	single
	Rat	sc	single
	Cynomolgus monkey	iv	single
	Cynomolgus monkey	sc	single
Repeated Dose	Rat	iv	7 days
	Rat	sc	6 times in 2 weeks
	Cynomolgus monkey	sc	6 times in 2 weeks

b) Toxicological study (2): Safety pharmacology and other studies

Study	Method	Species	Route	Dose
Safety pharmacology	Rat FOB	Rat	sc	single
	Respiratory	Rat	sc	single
	Cardiovascular	Cynomolgus monkey	sc	single
TK	Q-PCR	Rat	sc	6 times 2 weeks
Genetic toxicity	Micronucleus	Rat	sc	single
Antibody production	ELISA	Rat	sc	6 times 2 weeks

Table 1. Summary of toxicological studies

7. Clinical studies

Two clinical studies using the non-replicating oncolytic virus (HVJ-E/GEN0101) are currently being conducted in Osaka University Hospital. The target diseases are advanced melanoma (stage IIIC and stage IV) and CRPC [55, 56]. These proof-of-concept studies in melanoma and CRPC using the non-replicating oncolytic virus were initiated in July 2009 and July 2011, respectively [55, 56]. The respective summaries of both studies are shown in Table 2A and B. The primary endpoints of these studies were safety and tolerability based on the Common Terminology Criteria for Adverse Events (CTCAE) version 4.0, whereas the secondary endpoints were efficacy and confirmation of the mode of action. The major difference between the regimens for the melanoma and CRPC studies was the route of administration and number of administrations. A combination of intratumoral and subcutaneous routes of administration (one intratumoral and three subcutaneous injections) was adopted in the CRPC study. In addition, a new injection system developed by Okayama University was used in the CRPC study. This system permits stable refrigerated storage of the test article, and accurate injection into the prostate [91].

a) Advanced melanoma	
Study title	Phase I/II investigational clinical study of inactivated HVJ-E administration for advanced malignant melanoma patients
Condition	Malignant melanoma (AJCC stage IIIC or stage IV)
Study design	Masking: Open Label
	Allocation: Non-Randomized Primary endpoint: Safety and tolerability Secondary endpoint: Anti-tumor immunity and validity Target sample size: 6–12 patients Route: Intratumoral Dose: 6 times in 2 weeks/cycle, 2 cycles
Sponsor	Osaka University Graduate School of Medicine (Osaka University Hospital)
URL	https://upload.umin.ac.jp/cgi-open-bin/ctr/ctr.cgi?function=brows&action=brows&type=summary&recptno=R000002889&language=E
b) Castration-resistant prostate cancer	
Study title	Phase I/II investigational clinical study to assess safety and efficacy of intratumoral and subcutaneous injection of HVJ-E to castration-resistant prostate cancer patients
Condition	Castration resistant prostate cancer (CRPC)
Study design	Masking: Open Label
	Allocation: Non-Randomized Primary endpoint: Safety and tolerability Secondary endpoint: Anti-tumor immunity and validity Target sample size: 6–12 patients Route: Intratumoral × 1 then SC × 3 Dose: 4 times in 2 weeks/cycle, 2 cycles
Sponsor	Osaka University Graduate School of Medicine (Osaka University Hospital)
URL	https://upload.umin.ac.jp/cgi-open-bin/ctr/ctr.cgi?function=brows&action=brows&type=summary&recptno=R000007153&language=E

Table 2. Design of investigational clinical studies

8. Discussion and conclusion

The major disadvantages associated with oncolytic viruses are safety concerns because viral replication could theoretically cause the emergence of new pathogenic viruses [43]. The use of non-replicating oncolytic viruses is expected to resolve the safety issues associated with conventional oncolytic viruses because they are unable to replicate in target cells.

The modes of action underlying the anti-cancer effects of non-replicating virus on cancer cells and immune cells have been analyzed. One major signaling pathway is the RIG-I/MAVS pathway [54]. RIG-I is a cytosolic nucleic acid receptor that acts as a sensor that detects virus infection [82-84]. Similar to wild-type RNA viruses, the non-replicating virus (HVJ-E) is able to activate the RIG-I/MAVS pathway in DCs and induce both innate and adapted immunities. The non-replicating virus also activates the RIG-I/MAVS pathway in cancer cells and induces cancer cell-specific apoptosis. Genetic analyses suggest that differences in the expression of apoptosis-related genes define the sensitivity to the treatment with a non-replicating virus (HVJ-E) [54]. Furthermore, it is suggested that methylation of the respective enhancer/promoter regions underlies differences in transcription of apoptosis-related genes [54].

RIG-I, TLR3, and MDA-5 signaling pathways are involved in the apoptosis of ovarian cancers [87-89] and melanoma [90]. Thus, the RIG-I/MAVS pathway is likely to emerge as a new target for the development of drugs that induce cancer cell-specific apoptosis.

The non-replicating virus (HVJ-E) activates DCs to produce IL-6, which suppress the function of Treg [45]. This effect is expected to maintain the induced cancer immunity because Treg is known to be a negative regulator of immune responses [92-94]. It has been reported that cancer cells escape cancer immunity by the recruitment and activation of Treg. Therefore, it will be important to control the function of Treg for long-term effective induction and maintenance of cancer immunities. Suzuki and Kaneda *et al.* reported that the RIG-I/MAVS pathway was not required to induce the expression of IL-6 [95]. The attachment of the HVJ-E particle to the surface of DCs was sufficient for the production of IL-6, suggesting that the RNA fragments are unnecessary for the induction of this cytokine [95]. Detailed analyses identified that the F protein on the surface of HVJ-E is involved in the production of IL-6 [95]. Binding of the F protein to target cells requires expression of the HN protein [96]. Several gangliosides, such as GD1a and sialyl paragloboside, are implicated in the association of the HVJ-E particle and cancer cells because the HN protein binds the sialic acids of gangliosides. The receptor for the F protein remains unidentified to date. Taken together, the RIG-I/MAVS signal pathway, and a second pathway that induces the production of IL-6 may cooperate in the activation and sustainment of cancer immunity induced by the non-replicating virus (HVJ-E).

The development of a non-replicating oncolytic virus other than HVJ-E is possible because the manufacturing process for such a particle is similar to that of whole particle viral vaccines. In case of HVJ-E, the virus is inactivated by treatment with an alkylating agent and UV irradiation, a process used for the production of vaccines against viral diseases. Thus, the development of oncolytic viruses could be converted to the development of non-replicating oncolytic particles by similar manufacturing processes.

A disadvantage associated with non-replicating oncolytic viruses may be the defect in transmission ability. Therefore, it is possible that a greater amount of non-replicating oncolytic virus may be required for effective treatment compared with a live oncolytic virus. Alternatively, more frequent injections may be necessary for complete tumor eradication compared with the use of live oncolytic viruses. However, it is important to achieve a balance between the risks and benefits associated with the therapy. In our opinion, repeated administration of the non-replicating virus should be tolerable because no severe finding was observed during our safety studies.

In conclusion, non-replicating virus particles such as HVJ-E may resolve the safety issue of conventional virotherapy and provide a new strategy in cancer treatment.

9. Future perspectives

The first non-replicating oncolytic virus (HVJ-E) is currently under evaluation in clinical studies. Proof-of-concept data for non-replicating viruses in both clinical and non-clinical studies are necessary for further development of this approach. Osaka University Hospital is currently conducting two phase I/IIa studies: one for advanced melanoma and another for CRPC [55, 56]. The results of these studies will reveal the safety, efficacy, and optimal dosage regimen necessary for phase II study or randomized, double blind phase III study.

Combination treatment may be an effective approach to increase efficacy [97]. Indeed, an increase in therapeutic efficacy has been reported for virotherapies combined with photodynamic therapy [98, 99], radiotherapy [100], chemotherapy [101, 102], or gene therapy [103]. Kiyohara and Kaneda reported that combination of the non-replicating virus (HVJ-E) and gene therapy (IL-12) increased efficacy in a murine model of melanoma [104]. Furthermore, it was reported that a combination of non-replicating virus (HVJ-E) and chemotherapy [bleomycin or cis-diamminedichloroplatinum (CDDP)] increased efficacy in murine models of colon and bladder cancers [78, 105].

Technologies for systemic administration and targeting for HVJ-E are under development. The HN protein of HVJ-E has hemagglutinating activity and causes agglutination and lysis of erythrocytes *in vitro*. Currently, inactivation of the HN protein, decreased expression of the HN protein, and "masking" with platelets is being developed for intravenous injection of HVJ-E. Targeting after the intravenous injection is also important for systemic delivery. The addition of transferrin, a single chain antibody, or platelets have been suggested as suitable modifiers for HVJ-E.

The selection of viruses, or viral strains for the preparation of non-replicating oncolytic viruses is also important for obtaining higher efficacy because the level of immune response is dependent on the selection of virus strains [106]. A number of replicating oncolytic viruses are currently under clinical development [35, 97]. Therefore, it may be feasible to select a suitable virus for therapeutic application from the oncolytic viruses that have been developed [106, 107]. The tropism and complement resistance features of each virus should be considered for targeting and stabilization in serum.

HVJ-E is the only non-replicating oncolytic virus currently undergoing clinical investigation. These studies establish a new strategy for the virotherapy and gene therapy fields. The primary goal is to provide a novel approach for improving cancer therapy.

Summary

Conventional cancer therapies suffer from one paradox: although chemotherapeutic agents strongly kill cancer cells and decrease tumor volume, they simultaneously suppress the immune system. Chemotherapy frequently results in tumor relapse because residual cancer cells and cancer stem cells escape immune responses. In contrast, immune therapies including therapeutic cancer vaccines, effectively induce cancer immunity, but possess weak cytotoxic activity against cancer cells. Therefore, these treatments usually show weak efficacy. It has been reported that cancer is able to progress even after the activation and proliferation of cancer-specific cytotoxic T lymphocytes.

Virotherapy is predicted to become an alternative approach to obtain a model cancer therapy because it generally displays both oncolytic and immunostimulatory activities. However, the major drawback associated with current virotherapy is safety concerns. Virotherapy using a non-replicating virus is a new approach aimed at resolving safety issues. Thus, it is expected to become a novel concept for cancer therapy in the near future.

Acknowledgements

We appreciate T. Yamazaki for helpful discussions. We also appreciate H. Ueda and S. Ishikawa for their excellent administrative supports.

This study was supported by the advanced research for medical products Mining Program of the National Institute of Biomedical Innovation (NIBIO).

Author details

Toshihiro Nakajima[1], Toshimitsu Itai[1], Hiroshi Wada[1], Toshie Yamauchi[1], Eiji Kiyohara[2,3] and Yasufumi Kaneda[2]

1 GenomIdea, Inc., Midorigaoka, Ikeda, Osaka, Japan

2 Division of Gene Therapy Science, Department of Molecular Therapeutics, Graduate School of Medicine, Osaka University, Yamada-oka, Suita, Osaka, Japan

3 Department of Dermatology, Graduate School of Medicine, Osaka University, Yamada-oka, Suita, Osaka, Japan

T. Nakajima is a CEO of GenomIdea. T. Itai, H. Wada, and T. Yamauchi are employees of GenomIdea. The remaining authors have no conflicts of interest.

References

[1] Southam CM. and Moore AE., Clinical studies of viruses as antineoplastic agents with particular reference to Egypt 101 virus., Cancer 1952; 5:1025-1034.

[2] Bierman HR., Crike DM., Dod KS., Kelly KH., Petrakis NL., White LP. and Shimkin MD., Remissions in leukemia of childhood following acute infectious disease. Staphylococcus and Streptococcus, Varicella, and Feline Panleukopenia., Cancer 1953: 6:591-605.

[3] Newman W and Southam CM. Virus treatment in advanced cancer; a pathological study of fifty-seven cases., Cancer 1954; 7:106-118.

[4] Gallico E., The influence of viruses on the evolution of some malignant tumors., J. Natl. Med. Assoc. 1955 May; 47:158-161.

[5] Barley SL., Possible effect of measles on leukemia., Lancet 1971 January; 1(7690) :136

[6] Gross S., Measles and leukemia., Lancet 1971 February; 1(7695) :397–398.

[7] Zygiert Z., Hodgkin's disease: remissions after measles., Lancet. 1971 March;1(7699): 593.

[8] Bluming AZ, Ziegler JL., Regression of Burkitt's lymphoma in association with measles infection., Lancet 1971 July: 10;2(7715):105-106.

[9] Mota HC. Infantile Hodgkin's disease: remission after measles., Br Med J. 1973;2: 421.

[10] Ziegler JL., Spontaneous remission in Burkitt's lymphoma., Natl Cancer Inst Monogr. 1976;44: 61-65.

[11] Taqi AM., Abdurrahman MB., Yakubu AM. and Fleming AF., Regression of Hodgkin's disease after measles., Lancet. 1981 May 16;1(8229):1112.

[12] Schuepbach J. and Sauter C., Inverse correlation of antiviral antibody titers and the remission length in patients treated with viral oncolysate: a possible new prognostic sign in acute myelogenous leukemia., Cancer. 1981 Sep 15;48(6):1363-1367.

[13] Wallack MK., Bash JA., McNally KR. and Leftheriotis E., Serological evaluation of melanoma patients in a phase I/II trial of vaccinia melanoma oncolysate (VMO) immunotherapy., Cancer Detect Prev Suppl. 1987;1:351-359.

[14] Sauter C., Alberto P., Berchtold W., Fopp M., Gmür J., Gratwohl A., Imbach P., Maurice P., Obrecht P., Senn HJ., et al., Long-term results of two Swiss AML studies., Haematol Blood Transfus. 1987;30:38-44.

[15] Cassel WA. and Murray DR., Treatment of stage II malignant melanoma patients with a Newcastle disease virus oncolysate., Nat Immun Cell Growth Regul. 1988;7(5-6):351-352.

[16] Freedman RS, Bowen JM, Atkinson EN, Wallace S, Lotzová E, Silva E, Edwards CL, Delclos L, Scott W, Patenia B, et al., Randomized comparison of viral oncolysate plus radiation and radiation alone in uterine cervix carcinoma., Am J Clin Oncol. 1989 Jun;12(3):244-250.

[17] Wallack MK., Sivanandham M., Balch CM., Urist MM., Bland KI., Murray D., Robinson WA., Flaherty LE., Richards JM., Bartolucci AA., et al., A phase III randomized, double-blind multiinstitutional trial of vaccinia melanoma oncolysate-active specific immunotherapy for patients with stage II melanoma., Cancer. 1995 Jan 1;75(1):34-42.

[18] Batliwalla FM., Bateman BA., Serrano D., Murray D., Macphail S., Maino VC., Ansel JC., Gregersen PK. and Armstrong CA., A 15-year follow-up of AJCC stage III malignant melanoma patients treated postsurgically with Newcastle disease virus (NDV) oncolysate and determination of alterations in the CD8 T cell repertoire., Mol Med. 1998 Dec;4(12):783-794.

[19] DeWeese TL., van der Poel H., Li S, Mikhak B., Drew R., Goemann M., Hamper U., DeJong R., Detorie N., Rodriguez R., Haulk T., DeMarzo AM., Piantadosi S., Yu DC., Chen Y., Henderson DR., Carducci MA., Nelson WG. and Simons JW., A phase I trial of CV706, a replication-competent, PSA selective oncolytic adenovirus, for the treatment of locally recurrent prostate cancer following radiation therapy., Cancer Res. 2001 Oct 15;61(20):7464-7472.

[20] Kemeny N., Brown K., Covey A., Kim T., Bhargava A., Brody L., Guilfoyle B., Haag NP., Karrasch M., Glasschroeder B., Knoll A., Getrajdman G., Kowal KJ., Jarnagin WR. and Fong Y., Phase I, open-label, dose-escalating study of a genetically engineered herpes simplex virus, NV1020, in subjects with metastatic colorectal carcinoma to the liver., Hum Gene Ther. 2006 Dec;17(12):1214-1224.

[21] Nakao A., Takeda S., Shimoyama S., Kasuya H., Kimata H., Teshigahara O., Sawaki M., Kikumori T., Kodera Y., Nagasaka T., Goshima F., Nishiyama Y. and Imai T., Clinical experiment of mutant herpes simplex virus HF10 therapy for cancer., Curr Cancer Drug Targets. 2007 Mar;7(2):169-174.

[22] Fong Y., Kim T., Bhargava A., Schwartz L., Brown K., Brody L., Covey A., Karrasch M., Getrajdman G., Mescheder A., Jarnagin W. and Kemeny N., A herpes oncolytic virus can be delivered via the vasculature to produce biologic changes in human colorectal cancer., Mol Ther. 2009 Feb;17(2):389-394. Epub 2008 Nov 18.

[23] Geevarghese SK., Geller DA., de Haan HA., Hörer M., Knoll AE., Mescheder A., Nemunaitis J., Reid TR., Sze DY., Tanabe KK. and Tawfik H., Phase I/II study of oncolytic herpes simplex virus NV1020 in patients with extensively pretreated refractory colorectal cancer metastatic to the liver., Hum Gene Ther. 2010 Sep;21(9): 1119-1128.

[24] Nakao A., Kasuya H., Sahin TT., Nomura N., Kanzaki A., Misawa M., Shirota T., Yamada S., Fujii T., Sugimoto H., Shikano T., Nomoto S., Takeda S., Kodera Y. and Nishiyama Y., A phase I dose-escalation clinical trial of intraoperative direct intratu-

moral injection of HF10 oncolytic virus in non-resectable patients with advanced pancreatic cancer., Cancer Gene Ther. 2011 Mar;18(3):167-175. Epub 2010 Nov 19.

[25] Hu JC., Coffin RS., Davis CJ., Graham NJ., Groves N., Guest PJ., Harrington KJ., James ND., Love CA., McNeish I., Medley LC., Michael A., Nutting CM., Pandha HS., Shorrock CA., Simpson J., Steiner J., Steven NM., Wright D. and Coombes RC., A phase I study of OncoVEXGM-CSF, a second-generation oncolytic herpes simplex virus expressing granulocyte macrophage colony-stimulating factor., Clin Cancer Res. 2006 Nov 15;12(22):6737-6747.

[26] Park BH., Hwang T., Liu TC., Sze DY., Kim JS., Kwon HC., Oh SY., Han SY., Yoon JH., Hong SH., Moon A., Speth K., Park C., Ahn YJ., Daneshmand M., Rhee BG., Pinedo HM., Bell JC. and Kirn DH., Use of a targeted oncolytic poxvirus, JX-594, in patients with refractory primary or metastatic liver cancer: a phase I trial., Lancet Oncol. 2008 Jun;9(6):533-542. Epub 2008 May 19.

[27] Li JL., Liu HL., Zhang XR., Xu JP., Hu WK., Liang M., Chen SY., Hu F. and Chu DT., A phase I trial of intratumoral administration of recombinant oncolytic adenovirus overexpressing HSP70 in advanced solid tumor patients., Gene Ther. 2009 Mar;16(3): 376-382. Epub 2008 Dec 25.

[28] Kaufman HL., Kim DW., DeRaffele G., Mitcham J., Coffin RS. and Kim-Schulze S., Local and distant immunity induced by intralesional vaccination with an oncolytic herpes virus encoding GM-CSF in patients with stage IIIc and IV melanoma., Ann Surg Oncol. 2010 Mar;17(3):718-30.

[29] Nemunaitis J., Tong AW., Nemunaitis M., Senzer N., Phadke AP., Bedell C., Adams N., Zhang YA., Maples PB., Chen S., Pappen B., Burke J., Ichimaru D., Urata Y. and Fujiwara T., A phase I study of telomerase-specific replication competent oncolytic adenovirus (telomelysin) for various solid tumors., Mol Ther. 2010 Feb;18(2):429-434. Epub 2009 Nov 24.

[30] Galanis E., Hartmann LC., Cliby WA., Long HJ., Peethambaram PP., Barrette BA., Kaur JS., Haluska PJ Jr., Aderca I., Zollman PJ., Sloan JA., Keeney G., Atherton PJ., Podratz KC., Dowdy SC., Stanhope CR., Wilson TO., Federspiel MJ., Peng KW. and Russell SJ., Phase I trial of intraperitoneal administration of an oncolytic measles virus strain engineered to express carcinoembryonic antigen for recurrent ovarian cancer., Cancer Res. 2010 Feb 1;70(3):875-882. Epub 2010 Jan 26.

[31] Harrington KJ., Hingorani M., Tanay MA., Hickey J., Bhide SA., Clarke PM., Renouf LC., Thway K., Sibtain A., McNeish IA., Newbold KL., Goldsweig H., Coffin R. and Nutting CM., Phase I/II study of oncolytic HSV GM-CSF in combination with radiotherapy and cisplatin in untreated stage III/IV squamous cell cancer of the head and neck., Clin Cancer Res. 2010 Aug 1;16(15):4005-4015.

[32] Hwang TH., Moon A., Burke J., Ribas A., Stephenson J., Breitbach CJ., Daneshmand M., De Silva N., Parato K., Diallo JS., Lee YS., Liu TC., Bell JC. and Kirn DH., A mechanistic proof-of-concept clinical trial with JX-594, a targeted multi-mechanistic onco-

lytic poxvirus, in patients with metastatic melanoma., Mol Ther. 2011 Oct;19(10): 1913-1922. doi: 10.1038/mt.2011.132. Epub 2011 Jul 19.

[33] Hammill AM. and Conner J, Cripe TP., Oncolytic virotherapy reaches adolescence., Pediatr Blood Cancer. 2010 Dec 15;55(7):1253-1263. doi: 10.1002/pbc.22724. Epub 2010 Aug 23.

[34] Seymour LW. and Thrasher AJ., Gene therapy matures in the clinic., Nat Biotechnol. 2012 Jul 10;30(7):588-593. doi: 10.1038/nbt.2290.

[35] Russell SJ., Peng KW. and Bell JC., Oncolytic virotherapy., Nat Biotechnol. 2012 Jul 10;30(7):658-670.

[36] Shi J. and Zheng D., An update on gene therapy in China., Curr Opin Mol Ther. 2009 Oct;11(5):547-553.

[37] Bell J., Oncolytic viruses: an approved product on the horizon?, Mol Ther. 2010 Feb; 18(2):233-234.

[38] Vidal L., Pandha HS., Yap TA., White CL., Twigger K., Vile RG., Melcher A., Coffey M., Harrington KJ. and DeBono JS., A phase I study of intravenous oncolytic reovirus type 3 Dearing in patients with advanced cancer., Clin Cancer Res. 2008 Nov 1;14(21):7127-7137.

[39] Kimball KJ., Preuss MA., Barnes MN., Wang M., Siegal GP., Wan W., Kuo H., Saddekni S., Stockard CR., Grizzle WE., Harris RD., Aurigemma R., Curiel DT. and Alvarez RD., A phase I study of a tropism-modified conditionally replicative adenovirus for recurrent malignant gynecologic diseases., Clin Cancer Res. 2010 Nov 1;16(21): 5277-5287. Epub 2010 Oct 26.

[40] Rudin CM., Poirier JT., Senzer NN., Stephenson J Jr., Loesch D., Burroughs KD., Reddy PS., Hann CL. and Hallenbeck PL., Phase I clinical study of Seneca Valley Virus (SVV-001), a replication-competent picornavirus, in advanced solid tumors with neuroendocrine features., Clin Cancer Res. 2011 Feb 15;17(4):888-895. Epub 2011 Feb 8.

[41] Breitbach CJ., Burke J., Jonker D., Stephenson J., Haas AR., Chow LQ., Nieva J., Hwang TH., Moon A., Patt R., Pelusio A., Le Boeuf F., Burns J., Evgin L., De Silva N., Cvancic S., Robertson T., Je JE., Lee YS., Parato K., Diallo JS., Fenster A., Daneshmand M., Bell JC. and Kirn DH., Intravenous delivery of a multi-mechanistic cancer-targeted oncolytic poxvirus in humans., Nature. 2011 Aug 31;477(7362):99-102. doi: 10.1038/nature10358.

[42] Pesonen S., Diaconu I., Cerullo V., Escutenaire S., Raki M., Kangasniemi L., Nokisalmi P., Dotti G., Guse K., Laasonen L., Partanen K., Karli E., Haavisto E., Oksanen M., Karioja-Kallio A., Hannuksela P., Holm SL., Kauppinen S., Joensuu T., Kanerva A. and Hemminki A., Integrin targeted oncolytic adenoviruses Ad5 D24 RGD and Ad5 RGD-D24-GMCSF for treatment of patients with advanced chemotherapy refractory

solid tumors., Int J Cancer. 2012 Apr 15;130(8):1937-1947. doi: 10.1002/ijc.26216. Epub 2011 Aug 8.

[43] Peng KW., Ahmann GJ., Pham L., Greipp PR., Cattaneo R. and Russell SJ., Systemic therapy of myeloma xenografts by an attenuated measles virus., Blood. 2001 Oct 1;98(7):2002-7.

[44] Kaneda Y., A non-replicating oncolytic vector as a novel therapeutic tool against cancer., BMB Rep. 2010 Dec;43(12):773-780.

[45] Kurooka M. and Kaneda Y., Inactivated Sendai virus particles eradicate tumors by inducing immune responses through blocking regulatory T cells., Cancer Res. 2007 Jan 1;67(1):227-236.

[46] Kuroya M., Ishida N. and Shiratori T., Newborn virus pneumonitis (type Sendai). II. The isolation of a new virus., Tohoku J Exp Med. 1953 Jun;58(1):62.

[47] Okada Y. and Tadokoro J., The distribution of cell fusion capacity among several cell strains or cells caused by HVJ., Exp Cell Res. 1963 Dec;32:417-430.

[48] Okada Y., Yamada K. and Tadokoro J., Effect of antiserum on the cell fusion reaction caused by HVJ., Virology. 1964 Mar;22:397-409.

[49] Harris H. and Watkins JF., Hybrid cells derived from mouse and man: artificial heterokaryons of mammalian cells from different species., Nature. 1965 Feb 13;205:640-6..

[50] . Harris H., Watkins JF., Campbell GL., Evans EP. and Ford CE., Mitosis in hybrid cells derived from mouse and man., Nature. 1965 Aug 7;207(997):606-608.

[51] Köhler G. and Milstein C., Continuous cultures of fused cells secreting antibody of predefined specificity., Nature. 1975 Aug 7;256(5517):495-497.

[52] Kaneda Y., Nakajima T., Nishikawa T., Yamamoto S., Ikegami H., Suzuki N., Nakamura H., Morishita R. and Kotani H., Hemagglutinating virus of Japan (HVJ) envelope vector as a versatile gene delivery system., Mol Ther. 2002 Aug;6(2):219-226.

[53] Kaneda Y., Yamamoto S. and Nakajima T., Development of HVJ Envelope Vector and Its Application to Gene Therapy., Adv Genet. 2005;53PA:307-332.

[54] Matsushima-Miyagi T., Hatano K., Nomura M., Li-Wen L., Nishikawa T., Saga K., Shimbo T. and Kaneda Y., TRAIL and Noxa are selectively up-regulated in prostate cancer cells downstream of the RIG-I/MAVS signaling pathway by non-replicating Sendai virus particles., Clin Cancer Res. 2012 Oct 17. [Epub ahead of print].

[55] Phase I/II clinical trial of inactivated HVJ-E administration for advanced malignant melanoma patients., UMIN000002376 (2009/08/26), https://upload.umin.ac.jp/cgi-open-bin/ctr/ctr.cgi?function=brows&action=brows&type=summary&recptno=R000002889&language=E

[56] Phase I/II clinical trial to assess safety and efficacy of intratumoral and subcutaneous injection of HVJ-E to castration resistant prostate cancer patients. UMIN000006142(2011/09/01), https://upload.umin.ac.jp/cgi-open-bin/ctr/ctr.cgi?function=brows&action=brows&type=summary&recptno=R000007153&language=E

[57] Dey M., Ulasov IV., Tyler MA., Sonabend AM. and Lesniak MS., Cancer stem cells: the final frontier for glioma virotherapy., Stem Cell Rev. 2011 Mar;7(1):119-129.

[58] Drake CG., Prostate cancer as a model for tumour immunotherapy., Nat Rev Immunol. 2010 Aug;10(8):580-593.

[59] Sheikh NA., Petrylak D., Kantoff PW., Dela Rosa C., Stewart FP., Kuan LY., Whitmore JB., Trager JB., Poehlein CH., Frohlich MW. and Urdal DL., Sipuleucel-T immune parameters correlate with survival: an analysis of the randomized phase 3 clinical trials in men with castration-resistant prostate cancer., Cancer Immunol Immunother. 2012 Aug 3. doi 10.1007/s00262-012-1317-2

[60] Friedman GK., Cassady KA., Beierle EA., Markert JM. and Gillespie GY., Targeting pediatric cancer stem cells with oncolytic virotherapy., Pediatr Res. 2012 Apr;71(4 Pt 2):500-510. doi: 10.1038/pr.2011.58. Epub 2012 Feb 15.

[61] Marcato P., Dean CA., Giacomantonio CA. and Lee PW., Oncolytic reovirus effectively targets breast cancer stem cells., Mol Ther. 2009 Jun;17(6):972-979. Epub 2009 Mar 17.

[62] Zhang X., Komaki R., Wang L., Fang B. and Chang JY., Treatment of radioresistant stem-like esophageal cancer cells by an apoptotic gene-armed, telomerase-specific oncolytic adenovirus., Clin Cancer Res. 2008 May 1;14(9):2813-2823.

[63] Wakimoto H., Kesari S., Farrell CJ., Curry WT Jr., Zaupa C., Aghi M., Kuroda T., Stemmer-Rachamimov A., Shah K., Liu TC., Jeyaretna DS., Debasitis J., Pruszak J., Martuza RL. and Rabkin SD., Human glioblastoma-derived cancer stem cells: establishment of invasive glioma models and treatment with oncolytic herpes simplex virus vectors., Cancer Res. 2009 Apr 15;69(8):3472-3481. Epub 2009 Apr 7.

[64] Kanai R., Zaupa C., Sgubin D., Antoszczyk SJ., Martuza RL., Wakimoto H. and Rabkin SD., Effect of γ34.5 deletions on oncolytic herpes simplex virus activity in brain tumors., J Virol. 2012 Apr;86(8):4420-4431. Epub 2012 Feb 15.

[65] Alonso MM., Jiang H., Gomez-Manzano C. and Fueyo J., Targeting brain tumor stem cells with oncolytic adenoviruses., Methods Mol Biol. 2012;797:111-125.

[66] Bao S., Wu Q., Li Z., Sathornsumetee S., Wang H., McLendon RE., Hjelmeland AB. and Rich JN., Targeting cancer stem cells through L1CAM suppresses glioma growth., Cancer Res. 2008 Aug 1;68(15):6043-6048.

[67] Cheng L., Wu Q., Huang Z., Guryanova OA., Huang Q., Shou W., Rich JN. and Bao S., L1CAM regulates DNA damage checkpoint response of glioblastoma stem cells through NBS1., EMBO J. 2011 Mar 2;30(5):800-813. Epub 2011 Feb 4.

[68] Shimamura M., Morishita R., Endoh M., Oshima K., Aoki M., Waguri S., Uchiyama Y. and Kaneda Y., HVJ-envelope vector for gene transfer into central nervous system., Biochem Biophys Res Commun. 2003 Jan 10;300(2):464-471.

[69] Kaneda Y., New vector innovation for drug delivery: development of fusigenic non-viral particles., Curr Drug Targets. 2003 Nov;4(8):599-602.

[70] Kotani H., Nakajima T., Lai S., Morishita R. and Kaneda Y., The HVJ-envelope as an innovative vector system for cardiovascular disease., Curr Gene Ther. 2004 Jun;4(2): 183-194.

[71] Kaneda Y., Applications of Hemagglutinating Virus of Japan in therapeutic delivery systems., Expert Opin Drug Deliv. 2008 Feb;5(2):221-233.

[72] Kondo Y., Miyata K. and Kato F., Efficient delivery of antibody into living cells using hemagglutinating virus of Japan (HVJ) envelope., Curr Protoc Immunol. 2010 Apr;Chapter 2:Unit 2.16.1-12.

[73] Kondo Y., Miyata K. and Kato F., Use of the hemagglutinating virus of Japan (HVJ) envelope as a versatile delivery system for nucleic acids and proteins to leukocytes in vitro., Curr Protoc Immunol. 2010 Apr;Chapter 10:Unit 10.17D.1-9.

[74] Kaneda Y., HVJ liposomes and HVJ envelope vectors., Cold Spring Harb Protoc. 2011 Oct 1;2011(10):1281-1289. doi: 10.1101/pdb.prot065748.

[75] Kaneda Y., Development of liposomes and pseudovirions with fusion activity for efficient gene delivery., Curr Gene Ther. 2011 Dec;11(6):434-441.

[76] Fujihara A., Kurooka M., Miki T. and Kaneda Y., Intratumoral injection of inactivated Sendai virus particles elicits strong antitumor activity by enhancing local CXCL10 expression and systemic NK cell activation., Cancer Immunol Immunother. 2008 Jan; 57(1):73-84. Epub 2007 Jun 30.

[77] Kawaguchi Y., Miyamoto Y., Inoue T. and Kaneda Y., Efficient eradication of hormone-resistant human prostate cancers by inactivated Sendai virus particle., Int J Cancer. 2009 May 15;124(10):2478-2487.

[78] Kawano H., Komaba S., Yamasaki T., Maeda M., Kimura Y., Maeda A. and Kaneda Y., New potential therapy for orthotopic bladder carcinoma by combining HVJ envelope with doxorubicin., Cancer Chemother Pharmacol. 2008 May;61(6):973-978. Epub 2007 Jul 26.

[79] Tanaka M., Shimbo T., Kikuchi Y., Matsuda M. and Kaneda Y., Sterile alpha motif containing domain 9 is involved in death signaling of malignant glioma treated with inactivated Sendai virus particle (HVJ-E) or type I interferon., Int J Cancer. 2010 Apr 15;126(8):1982-1991.

[80] Lorence RM., Reichard KW., Katubig BB., Reyes HM., Phuangsab A., Mitchell BR., Cascino CJ., Walter RJ. and Peeples ME., Complete regression of human neuroblasto-

ma xenografts in athymic mice after local Newcastle disease virus therapy., J Natl Cancer Inst. 1994 Aug 17;86(16):1228-1233.

[81] Phuangsab A., Lorence RM., Reichard KW., Peeples ME. and Walter RJ., Newcastle disease virus therapy of human tumor xenografts: antitumor effects of local or systemic administration., Cancer Lett. 2001 Oct 22;172(1):27-36.

[82] Kawai T and Akira S., Innate immune recognition of viral infection., Nat Immunol. 2006 Feb;7(2):131-137.

[83] Takeuchi O. and Akira S., Innate immunity to virus infection., Immunol Rev. 2009 Jan;227(1):75-86.

[84] Seth RB., Sun L. and Chen ZJ., Antiviral innate immunity pathways., Cell Res. 2006 Feb;16(2):141-147.

[85] Saha SK. and Cheng G.., TRAF3: a new regulator of type I interferons., Cell Cycle. 2006 Apr;5(8):804-807. Epub 2006 Apr 17.

[86] Tang ED. and Wang CY., TRAF5 is a downstream target of MAVS in antiviral innate immune signaling., PLoS One. 2010 Feb 11;5(2):e9172.

[87] Kübler K., Gehrke N., Riemann S., Böhnert V., Zillinger T., Hartmann E., Pölcher M., Rudlowski C., Kuhn W., Hartmann G. and Barchet W., Targeted activation of RNA helicase retinoic acid-inducible gene-I induces proimmunogenic apoptosis of human ovarian cancer cells., Cancer Res. 2010 Jul 1;70(13):5293-5304. Epub 2010 Jun 15.

[88] Kübler K., tho Pesch C., Gehrke N., Riemann S., Dassler J., Coch C., Landsberg J., Wimmenauer V., Pölcher M., Rudlowski C., Tüting T., Kuhn W., Hartmann G. and Barchet W., Immunogenic cell death of human ovarian cancer cells induced by cytosolic poly(I:C) leads to myeloid cell maturation and activates NK cells., Eur J Immunol. 2011 Oct;41(10):3028-3039. doi: 10.1002/eji.201141555. Epub 2011 Aug 30.

[89] Van DN., Roberts CF., Marion JD., Lépine S., Harikumar KB., Schreiter J., Dumur CI., Fang X., Spiegel S. and Bell JK., Innate immune agonist, dsRNA, induces apoptosis in ovarian cancer cells and enhances the potency of cytotoxic chemotherapeutics., FASEB J. 2012 Aug;26(8):3188-3198. Epub 2012 Apr 24.

[90] Besch R., Poeck H., Hohenauer T., Senft D., Häcker G., Berking C., Hornung V., Endres S., Ruzicka T., Rothenfusser S. and Hartmann G., Proapoptotic signaling induced by RIG-I and MDA-5 results in type I interferon-independent apoptosis in human melanoma cells., J Clin Invest. 2009 Aug;119(8):2399-2411. doi: 10.1172/JCI37155. Epub 2009 Jul 20.

[91] Nasu Y., Saika T., Ebara S., Kusaka N., Kaku H., Abarzua F., Manabe D., Thompson TC. and Kumon H., Suicide gene therapy with adenoviral delivery of HSV-tK gene for patients with local recurrence of prostate cancer after hormonal therapy., Mol Ther. 2007 Apr;15(4):834-840. Epub 2007 Feb 27.

[92] Nishikawa H. and Sakaguchi S., Regulatory T cells in tumor immunity., Int J Cancer. 2010 Aug 15;127(4):759-767.

[93] Jacobs JF., Nierkens S., Figdor CG., de Vries IJ., Adema GJ., Regulatory T cells in melanoma: the final hurdle towards effective immunotherapy?, Lancet Oncol. 2012 Jan; 13(1):e32-42.

[94] Le DT. and Jaffee EM., Regulatory T-cell modulation using cyclophosphamide in vaccine approaches: a current perspective., Cancer Res. 2012 Jul 15;72(14):3439-3444. Epub 2012 Jul 3.

[95] Suzuki H., Kurooka M., Hiroaki Y., Fujiyoshi Y., Kaneda Y., Sendai virus F glycoprotein induces IL-6 production in dendritic cells in a fusion-independent manner., FEBS Lett. 2008 Apr 16;582(9):1325-1329. Epub 2008 Mar 20.

[96] Chang A. and Dutch RE., Paramyxovirus fusion and entry: multiple paths to a common end., Viruses. 2012 Apr;4(4):613-636. Epub 2012 Apr 19.

[97] Galanis E., Cancer: Tumour-fighting virus homes in., Nature. 2011 Aug 31;477(7362): 40-41. doi: 10.1038/477040a

[98] Fujii H., Matsuyama A., Komoda H., Sasai M., Suzuki M., Asano T., Doki Y., Kirihata M., Ono K., Tabata Y., Kaneda Y., Sawa Y. and Lee CM., Cationized gelatin-HVJ envelope with sodium borocaptate improved the BNCT efficacy for liver tumors in vivo., Radiat Oncol. 2011 Jan 20;6:8.

[99] Sakai M., Fujimoto N., Ishii K., Nakamura H., Kaneda Y. and Awazu K., In vitro investigation of efficient photodynamic therapy using a nonviral vector; hemagglutinating virus of Japan envelope., J Biomed Opt. 2012 Jul;17(7):078002.S

[100] Harrington KJ., Karapanagiotou EM., Roulstone V., Twigger KR., White CL., Vidal L., Beirne D., Prestwich R., Newbold K., Ahmed M., Thway K., Nutting CM., Coffey M., Harris D., Vile RG., Pandha HS., Debono JS. and Melcher AA., Two-stage phase I dose-escalation study of intratumoral reovirus type 3 dearing and palliative radiotherapy in patients with advanced cancers., Clin Cancer Res. 2010 Jun 1;16(11): 3067-3077. Epub 2010 May 18.

[101] Lolkema MP., Arkenau HT., Harrington K., Roxburgh P., Morrison R., Roulstone V., Twigger K., Coffey M., Mettinger K., Gill G., Evans TR. and de Bono JS., A phase I study of the combination of intravenous reovirus type 3 Dearing and gemcitabine in patients with advanced cancer., Clin Cancer Res. 2011 Feb 1;17(3):581-588. Epub 2010 Nov 24.

[102] Kanai R., Rabkin SD., Yip S., Sgubin D., Zaupa CM., Hirose Y., Louis DN., Wakimoto H. and Martuza RL., Oncolytic virus-mediated manipulation of DNA damage responses: synergy with chemotherapy in killing glioblastoma stem cells. J Natl Cancer Inst. 2012 Jan 4;104(1):42-55. Epub 2011 Dec 15.

[103] Hwang TH., Moon A., Burke J., Ribas A., Stephenson J., Breitbach CJ., Daneshmand M., De Silva N., Parato K., Diallo JS., Lee YS., Liu TC., Bell JC. and Kirn DH., A mechanistic proof-of-concept clinical trial with JX-594, a targeted multi-mechanistic oncolytic poxvirus, in patients with metastatic melanoma., Mol Ther. 2011 Oct;19(10): 1913-1922. doi: 10.1038/mt.2011.132. Epub 2011 Jul 19.

[104] Kaneda Y., Kiyohara E., Nakajima T. and Itai T., Gene Therapy of Melanoma Using Inactivated Sendai Virus Envelope Vector (HVJ-E) with Intrinsic Anti-Tumor Activities., Viral Gene Therapy, Ke Xu (Ed.), 2011, ISBN: 978-953-307-539-6 doi: 10.5772/17492, InTech, Available from: http://www.intechopen.com/books/viral-gene-therapy/gene-therapy-of-melanoma-using-inactivated-sendai-virus-envelope-vector-hvj-e-with-intrinsic-anti-tu

[105] Kawano H., Komaba S., Kanamori T. and Kaneda Y., A new therapy for highly effective tumor eradication using HVJ-E combined with chemotherapy., BMC Med. 2007 Sep 21;5:28.

[106] Apostolidis L., Schirrmacher V. and Fournier P., Host mediated anti-tumor effect of oncolytic Newcastle disease virus after locoregional application., Int J Oncol. 2007 Nov;31(5):1009-1019.

[107] Prestwich RJ., Ilett EJ., Errington F., Diaz RM., Steele LP., Kottke T., Thompson J., Galivo F., Harrington KJ., Pandha HS., Selby PJ., Vile RG.. and Melcher AA., Immune-mediated antitumor activity of reovirus is required for therapy and is independent of direct viral oncolysis and replication., Clin Cancer Res. 2009 Jul 1;15(13):4374-4381. Epub 2009 Jun 9.

Chapter 8

Development of Muscle-Directed Systemic Cancer Gene Therapy

Koichi Miyake and Takashi Shimada

Additional information is available at the end of the chapter

1. Introduction

In recent years, one of the main focuses of the effort to improve cancer treatment and patient prognosis has been gene therapy. Furthermore, the complex nature of cancer has meant that a variety of therapeutic strategies have been developed along two main avenues: local gene therapies and systemic gene therapies (Table 1). The strategies for local cancer gene therapy include suppression of an oncogene, activation of a tumor suppressor gene, and introduction of a suicide gene into cancer cells (McCormick 2001). Unfortunately, delivering a therapeutic gene to every individual cancer cell in a patient with metastatic cancer has so far proven to be an insurmountable task. It has not been possible to treat all cancerous lesions, which can include undetectable ones such as individual cancer cells and micrometastases. In addition, it is difficult to selectively target cancer cells without affecting normal cells. On the other hand, systemic cancer gene therapy such as immunotherapy appears more promising for both inhibiting tumor growth and preventing metastasis. This chapter will summarize the utility of viral vector-mediated systemic cancer gene therapy in the treatment of human malignancies, focusing on the powerful and promising approach of recombinant adeno-associated virus (AAV)-based systemic anti-angiogenic cancer gene therapy.

2. Muscle-directed systemic cancer gene therapy

2.1. Why gene therapy?

Because a neovasculature is essential for tumor growth and metastasis (Folkman 1971), inhibiting the development of the tumor vasculature using anti-angiogenic agents has emerged as an attractive new strategy for the treatment of cancer (Kerbel & Folkman 2002). For many types of cancer, targeted biological therapies that selectively interfere with tumor angiogenesis have the potential to improve survival among patients, and a number of angiogenesis inhibitors are currently being tested in clinical trials (Shojaei 2012). In addition, preclinical studies using purified anti-angiogenic factors have indicated the ability of anti-angiogenic compounds to minimize the size of established tumors. However, although they are capable of significantly inhibiting tumor cell growth in animal models, the clinical efficacy of administering purified anti-angiogenic factors would likely be limited by the peptides' short half-life. On the other hand, synthesis and secretion of anti-angiogenic factors following gene transfer may overcome that limitation. If so, gene therapy could play an important role in this field, as anti-angiogenic factors need to be delivered for long periods to control the progression of tumors.

Strategy		Target cells
1. Local gene therapy		
1) Suppression of oncogenes	RNAi, antisense etc.	Cancer cells
2) Activation of tumor suppressor genes	p53 etc.	Cancer cells
3) Suicide gene therapy	HSV-TK	Cancer cells
2. Systemic gene therapy		
1) Immuno gene therapy	Cytokine genes etc.	Lymphocytes, Cancer cells Antigen presenting cells,
2) Anti-angiogenic gene therapy	Endostatin etc.	All cells

Table 1. Strategy of cancer gene therapy

2.2. Why anti-angiogenic?

Anti-angiogenic gene therapy has several advantageous features (Table 2). As mentioned above, this strategy can potentially suppress both the main tumor and small metastatic tumors. Moreover, since angiogenesis is essential for the development of all tumors, this strategy could be applied to a wide variety of cancers. In contrast to genetic therapies targeting tumor cells directly, anti-angiogenic gene therapy does not require the targeting and transduction of cancer cells. Instead, systemic levels of anti-angiogenic factors may be achieved by targeting non-tumor cells, which provide a stable platform for transgene expression and subsequent secretion of the translated proteins. Finally, cancers do not develop resistance to anti-angiogenic therapy, and the patients experience no side effects or side effects that are much milder than those associated with conventional anti-cancer therapies.

1. Effective for almost all cancers
2. Inhibition of tumor growth and prevention of metastases
3. Targeting gene transfer is unnecessary
4. No resistance
5. No or mild side-effect

Table 2. Advantages of anti-angiogenic Cancer Gene Therapy

2.3. Why muscle directed?

To express therapeutic proteins, skeletal muscles are considered an attractive target for gene delivery because they are large, have a good capacity for protein synthesis and are easily accessible for intramuscular injection. In addition, muscle fibers are capable of expressing and secreting biologically active gene products that they do not normally synthesize (Arruda et al. 2001). Thus, direct injection of viral vectors into muscles has been widely used for both the treatment of muscular disorders and for expression of therapeutic proteins used for the treatment of metabolic disease, genetic bleeding disorders and malignant diseases (Liu et al. 2004; Noro et al. 2004; Yan et al. 2005).

2.4. Why an AAV vector?

The potential of anti-angiogenic gene therapy in cancer is currently being evaluated using viral and non-viral vectors. The development of an effective gene delivery system is absolutely critical to the effectiveness and safety of gene therapy. Among the several gene transfer strategies being considered at present, the AAV vector appears the most promising, in view of its lack of pathogenicity, wide tropisms and long-term transgene expression *in vivo*. Gene therapy studies using different serotypes of recombinant AAVs as delivery vehicles have demonstrated that AAVs are an effective modality for cancer gene therapy that meet the requirements necessary for anti-angiogenic therapy.

2.5. A concept of muscle-directed systemic cancer gene therapy

Figure 1 illustrates the concept of muscle-directed systemic cancer gene therapy. First, an AAV vector encoding anti-angiogenic agents is injected into a muscle. After a single injection, secreted anti-angiogenic agents are circulating throughout the entire body. These circulating factors suppress both the primary tumor and undetectable metastatic lesions through inhibition of tumor angiogenesis. If the gene therapy alone is not sufficient to suppress all the tumors, other therapies such as radiation, chemotherapy or immunotherapy can be added to enhance the effect.

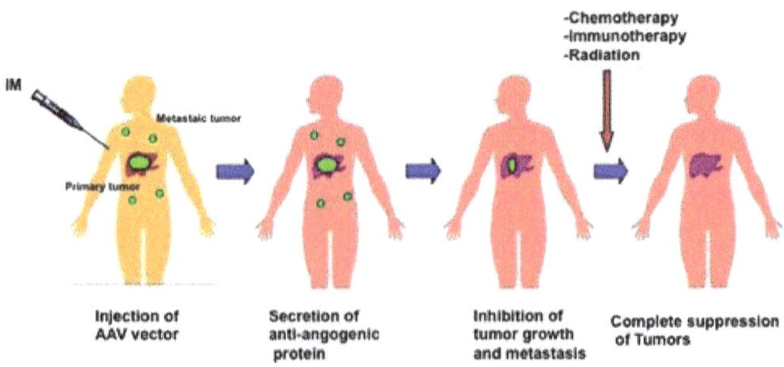

Figure 1. A concept of muscle-directed systemic cancer gene therapy

3. Applications of systemic cancer gene therapy

3.1. Systemic anti-angiogenic cancer gene therapy

To assess the feasibility of anti-angiogenic gene therapy using an AAV vector, we constructed an AAV vector encoding murine endostatin (AAV/mEnd) (Figure 2A), which is a tumor-derived angiogenesis inhibitor and is the first endogenous inhibitor of angiogenesis to be identified in a matrix protein (O'Reilly et al. 1997). We then attempted to use the vector to treat pancreatic cancer in an orthotopic model. When PGHAM-1 derived from chemically induced hamster pancreatic cancer cells is injected into the pancreas of hamsters, a ductal adenocarcinoma develops that closely resembles the human disease and, like its human counterpart, it frequently metastasizes to the liver (Matsushita et al. 2001; Yanagi et al. 2000). After AAV/mEnd ($5x10^{10}$ vector genomes) was intramuscularly injected into the left quadriceps, we assessed the ability of AAV-mediated systemic delivery of endostatin to suppress metastatic pancreatic cancer. We found that intramuscular injection of the AAV/mEnd vector increased serum endostatin levels, as compared to a control AAV vector encoding GFP (Figure 2B). In addition, the size of the primary pancreatic tumors and the sizes and number of liver metastases were all reduced in the treated animals (Figure 2C). This suggests that AAV-mediated systemic delivery of endostatin represents a potentially effective treatment for pancreatic cancer and liver metastases.

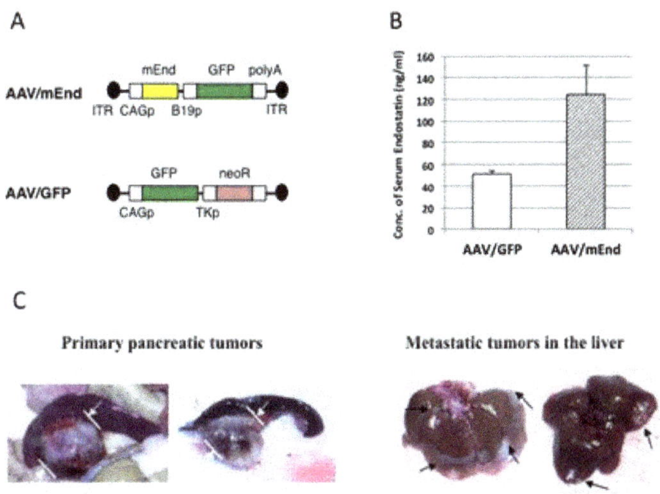

Figure 2. (A) Construction of recombinant AAV vector plasmids expressing murine endostatin (AAV/mEnd) and control GFP expressing vector (AAV/GFP). ITR: inverted terminal repeats, CAGp: CAG promoter, B19p: B19 promoter, TKp: thymidine kinase promoter, neoR: neomycin resistance gene (B) Serum levels of endostatin after intramuscular injection of AAV/End (42 days after vector injection). Intramuscular injection of AAV/End increased the serum endostatin level. (C) Effects of AAV-mediated endostatin expression on pancreatic tumor growth and liver metastasis.

To achieve the anti-angiogenic state in the model animals used in this experiment, we used classical AAV serotype 2 vectors (Noro et al. 2004). One problem with that vector is that it takes several weeks to reach the maximal level of transgene expression. Therefore, to evaluate the efficacy of cancer gene therapy in a transplantation model animal, the AAV vector must be injected before tumor inoculation. Recently, several different AAV serotypes have been characterized, and we investigated which AAV serotype would maximize the efficiency of the gene transfer into muscle.

3.2. The best AAV serotype

A number of novel AAV serotypes have been isolated from nonhuman primates (Gao et al. 2002), and we endeavored to determine which AAV vector most efficiently mediates muscle expression of anti-angiogenic proteins useful for treating cancer. Included among these were AAV serotypes 1, 7 and 8, which, when developed as vectors, mediate gene transfer into various tissues much more efficiently than those based on previously described serotypes. Therefore, to determine the AAV serotype that most efficiently mediates muscle expression of anti-angiogenic proteins, we injected 4 different AAV vector serotypes (AAV1, AAV2, AAV7 and AAV8) encoding mEnd together with GFP into a quadriceps muscle in C57BL/6 mice. The highest GFP expression and plasma mEnd levels were observed one week after injection in mice administered AAV8 (8>7>1>2) (Figure 3A). Moreover, expression of mEnd was sustained for at least 6 months. We then confirmed the transduction efficiency into the muscle using an AAV vector harboring the luciferase gene (AAV/Luc). *In vivo* imaging showed that the greatest expression occurred in mice administered AAV8 (Figure 3B). Taken together, these results clearly demonstrate that AAV8 is able to efficiently mediate gene transfer into muscle tissue, leading to prolonged expression and secretion of the gene product (Isotani et al. 2011).

3.3. Melanoma differentiation-associated gene-7/interleukin-24 (*mda-7/IL24*)

Another candidate gene for systemic cancer gene therapy is melanoma differentiation-associated gene-7/interleukin-24 (*mda-7/IL24*), which has anti-angiogenic properties (MDA-7/IL24 bioactivity was 20- to 50-fold greater than endostatin or angiostatin) as well as several other features useful for cancer gene therapy. *Mda-7/IL24* selectively induces apoptosis in cancer cells without harming normal cells, and it exerts both immunomodulatory effects and potent antitumor bystander effects. These multifunctional tumor-specific cytotoxic effects of MDA-7/IL24 make this molecule a promising gene-based therapeutic agent for the treatment of cancer. To assess the *in vivo* effects of AAV-mediated systemic delivery of MDA-7/IL24, we constructed an AAV vector encoding MDA-7/IL24 (AAV/IL24). A single intravenous injection of AAV/IL24 (2.0×10^{11} vector genomes) into a subcutaneous tumor induced by injecting Ehrlich ascites tumor cells into the dorsum of DDY mice significantly inhibited tumor growth and increased survival among the AAV/IL24-treated mice (Figure 4). In addition, TUNEL and immunohistochemical analyses showed significant induction of tumor cell-specific apoptosis and a reduction in microvessel formation within the tumors (Tahara et al. 2007). These results clearly demonstrate that continuous systemic delivery of MDA-7/IL24 can serve as an effective treatment for cancer.

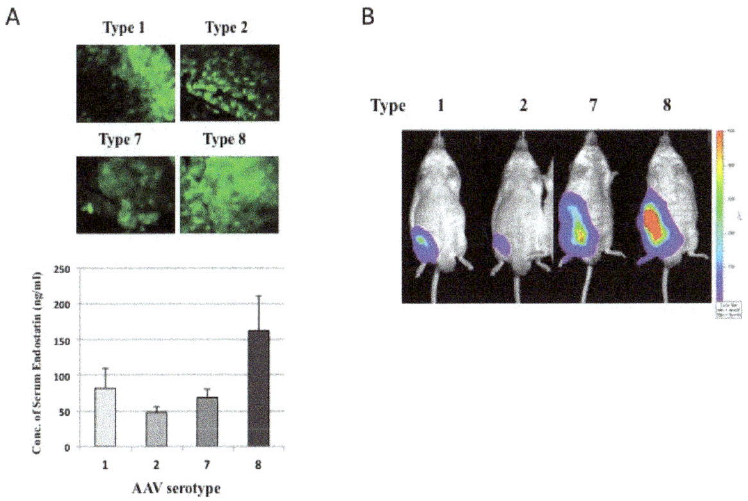

Figure 3. Expression of transgenes following intramuscular administration of AAVs. Following injection of the respective AAV serotypes of the AAV/mEnd vectors, which express murine endostatin together with GFP, into quadriceps muscles, expression of GFP and plasma concentrations of mEnd were analyzed (A). Four AAV serotypes of AAV/Luc, which express lucigerase, were injected into the quadriceps muscles of DDY mice. Four weeks after injection, these mice were analyzed by *in vivo* imaging system.

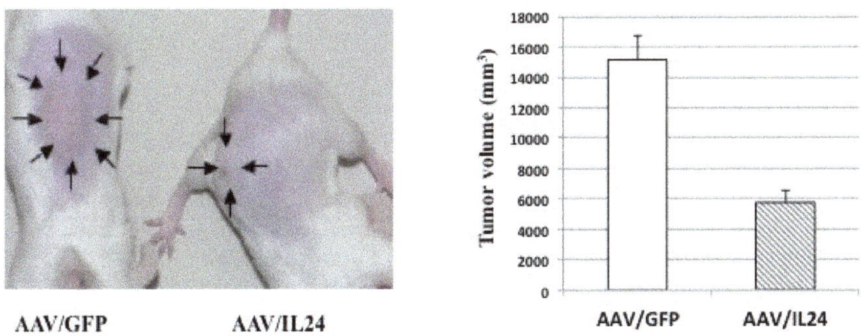

Figure 4. Inhibition of tumor growth after administration of AAV/IL24. One week after subcutaneous injection of Ehrlich ascites tumor cells, mice were treated with AAV/IL24 or control AAV/GFP. The mean tumor volumes 56 days after injection were significantly smaller in animals that received AAV/IL24 than in those that received AAV/GFP ($P < 0.001$).

To then assess the feasibility of AAV8-mediated muscle-directed cancer gene therapy using MDA-7/IL24, we established mixed-lineage leukemia (MLL)/AF4 transgenic (MLL/AF4 Tg) mice (Tamai et al. 2011). These mice developed pro-B cell ($CD45R/B220^{+}CD19^{+}CD43^{+}$) lymphoma as well as leukemia with high-level HOXA9 expression by 12 months of age, at which time lymphoma cells had infiltrated the liver, lung and spleen. In addition to multiple sites of tumor infiltration, a non-solid hematological malignancy, leukemia, was also present, making local gene therapy entirely impractical. This model is therefore well suited to analyze the utility of AAV-mediated systemic gene therapies. So far, we have observed that after a muscle-directed single AAV/IL24 injection, infiltration of tumor cells into all organs was suppressed (Tamai et al. 2012). Thus, AAV vector-mediated systemic delivery of MDA-7/IL24 represents a potentially important new approach to anticancer therapy.

4. Summary and future developments

Here we present evidence of the utility of AAV-mediated muscle-directed systemic cancer gene therapy using anti-angiogenic agents together with MDA-7/IL24. This new approach is safe and non-invasive, and could be used to treat primary tumors as well as undetectable metastatic tumors and hematological non-solid tumors without serious side effects. The potential utility of anti-angiogenic gene therapy in cancer is currently being evaluated in combination with radiation, chemotherapy or immunotherapy, which appear to provide a synergistic effect. Moreover, systemic cancer gene therapy may enable reduction of the dose of radiation, chemotherapy or immunotherapy needed to be effective, thereby reducing such side effects as bone marrow suppression. Thus, the combination of gene therapy with conventional anti-cancer therapy may overcome serious problems currently associated with cancer treatment.

Acknowledgements

We thank Dr. James Wilson at the University of Pennsylvania for providing AAV packaging plasmids (p5E18RXC1, p5E18-VD2/7 and p5E18-VD2/8). We also thank Takuya Noro, Ichiro Tahara, Noriko Miyake, Mayu Isotani and Hayato Tamai for helpful discussion and technical assistance. This work was supported in part by grants from the Ministry of Health and Welfare of Japan and the Ministry of Education, Science and Culture of Japan.

Author details

Koichi Miyake and Takashi Shimada

Department of Biochemistry and Molecular Biology, Division of Gene Therapy Research Center for Advanced Medical Technology, Nippon Medical School, Japan

References

[1] Arruda V. R., Hagstrom J. N., Deitch J., Heiman-Patterson T., Camire R. M., Chu K., Fields P. A., Herzog R. W., Couto L. B., Larson P. J. & High K. A. (2001). Posttranslational modifications of recombinant myotube-synthesized human factor IX. Blood 97,130-138.

[2] Folkman J. (1971). Tumor angiogenesis: therapeutic implications. The New England journal of medicine 285,1182-1186.

[3] Gao G. P., Alvira M. R., Wang L., Calcedo R., Johnston J. & Wilson J. M. (2002). Novel adeno-associated viruses from rhesus monkeys as vectors for human gene therapy. Proc Natl Acad Sci U S A 99,11854-11859.

[4] Isotani M., Miyake K., Miyake N., Hirai Y. & Shimada T. (2011). Direct comparison of four adeno-associated virus serotypes in mediating the production of antiangiogenic proteins in mouse muscle. Cancer investigation 29,353-359.

[5] Kerbel R. & Folkman J. (2002). Clinical translation of angiogenesis inhibitors. Nature reviews. Cancer 2,727-739.

[6] Liu Y. L., Mingozzi F., Rodriguez-Colon S. M., Joseph S., Dobrzynski E., Suzuki T., High K. A. & Herzog R. W. (2004). Therapeutic levels of factor IX expression using a muscle-specific promoter and adeno-associated virus serotype 1 vector. Hum Gene Ther 15,783-792.

[7] Matsushita A., Onda M., Uchida E., Maekawa R. & Yoshioka T. (2001). Antitumor effect of a new selective matrix metalloproteinase inhibitor, MMI-166, on experimental pancreatic cancer. International journal of cancer. Journal international du cancer 92,434-440.

[8] McCormick F. (2001). Cancer gene therapy: fringe or cutting edge? Nature reviews. Cancer 1,130-141.

[9] Noro T., Miyake K., Suzuki-Miyake N., Igarashi T., Uchida E., Misawa T., Yamazaki Y. & Shimada T. (2004). Adeno-associated viral vector-mediated expression of endostatin inhibits tumor growth and metastasis in an orthotropic pancreatic cancer model in hamsters. Cancer research 64,7486-7490.

[10] O'Reilly M. S., Boehm T., Shing Y., Fukai N., Vasios G., Lane W. S., Flynn E., Birkhead J. R., Olsen B. R. & Folkman J. (1997). Endostatin: an endogenous inhibitor of angiogenesis and tumor growth. Cell 88,277-285.

[11] Shojaei F. (2012). Anti-angiogenesis therapy in cancer: current challenges and future perspectives. Cancer letters 320,130-137.

[12] Tahara I., Miyake K., Hanawa H., Kurai T., Hirai Y., Ishizaki M., Uchida E., Tajiri T. & Shimada T. (2007). Systemic cancer gene therapy using adeno-associated virus type 1 vector expressing MDA-7/IL24. Molecular therapy : the journal of the American Society of Gene Therapy 15,1805-1811.

[13] Tamai H., Miyake K., Takatori M., Miyake N., Yamaguchi H., Dan K., Shimada T. & Inokuchi K. (2011). Activated K-Ras protein accelerates human MLL/AF4-induced leukemo-lymphomogenicity in a transgenic mouse model. Leukemia : official journal of the Leukemia Society of America, Leukemia Research Fund, U.K 25,888-891.

[14] Tamai H., Miyake K., Yamaguchi H., Takatori M., Dan K., Inokuchi K. & Shimada T. (2012). AAV8 vector expressing IL24 efficiently suppresses tumor growth mediated by specific mechanisms in MLL/AF4-positive ALL model mice. Blood 119,64-71.

[15] Yan H., Guo Y., Zhang P., Zu L., Dong X., Chen L., Tian J., Fan X., Wang N., Wu X. & Gao W. (2005). Superior neovascularization and muscle regeneration in ischemic skeletal muscles following VEGF gene transfer by rAAV1 pseudotyped vectors. Biochem Biophys Res Commun 336,287-298.

[16] Yanagi K., Onda M. & Uchida E. (2000). Effect of angiostatin on liver metastasis of pancreatic cancer in hamsters. Japanese journal of cancer research : Gann 91,723-730.

Chapter 9

Sendai Virus-Based Oncolytic Gene Therapy

Yosuke Morodomi, Makoto Inoue,
Mamoru Hasegawa, Tatsuro Okamoto,
Yoshihiko Maehara and Yoshikazu Yonemitsu

Additional information is available at the end of the chapter

1. Introduction

The first gene therapy that was used on humans was performed for adenosine deaminase (ADA) deficiency in 1990 [1]. In the early days of gene therapy, it was thought to be a breakthrough in the treatment of a number of human diseases including cancer, cardiovascular disease, genetic disease, and so on. However, two severe adverse events in gene therapy served as triggers for the rethinking of the safety of gene therapy. The use of adenoviral gene therapy in an 18-year-old with an inherited enzyme deficiency at the University of Pennsylvania's Institute for Human Gene Therapy resulted in the death of the patient 4 days after the injection of the vectors into the liver in 1999 [2]. The second accident involved derived carcinogenesis that was caused by gene therapy that was performed to treat severe combined immunodeficiency-X1 in 1999 [3]. On the other hand, nonviral vectors (e.g., plasmids, liposomes, polymers, and so on.) have been developed because of these safety concerns. However, the low effectiveness of nonviral vectors in gene transduction remains a serious problem.

The key to gene therapy is safety and effectiveness. Sendai virus (SeV) vectors are able to overcome many of these problems related to gene therapy. The advantages of SeV in terms of gene therapy are the following: 1) it is nonpathogenic to human, 2) it has a high efficiency of infection, and 3) it results in high levels of gene expression.

First, we would like to discuss the nonpathogenicity of SeV. The vector that is most used in gene therapy clinical trials is the Adenovirus, which is followed by the Retrovirus [4]. Adenovirus infections in humans cause pneumonia, bronchitis, croup, and so on. Retrovirus infections are one of the causes of human carcinogenesis or immunodeficiency. These vectors are pathogenic to human beings. Moreover, the infection of these vectors to human cells is associated with the risk of viral gene integration into the human genome, which contributes to gene mutations or structural changes to chromosomes. On the other hand, SeV was originally discovered as the cause of pneumonia in rodents. Because the SeV gene exists as RNA in the cell cytoplasm throughout the life cycle of the virus from infection of the target cells to viral budding, no genetic toxicities have been confirmed (Figure 1). For these reasons, the risk of pathogenicity to humans is surprisingly low, and its safety has already been assured when it is used as a gene therapy drug.

Second, we would like to discuss the features of SeV with respect to its high efficiency of infection. Hemagglutinin-neuraminidase (HN) proteins recognize sialic acid, which is expressed as a glycoprotein or glycolipid on the cell surface. Sialic acid is widely expressed in the cells of mammals or other species, and its expression enables a large variety of SeV infections, such as those in the airway epithelium [5], saphenous vein [6], or in a variety of tumors [7,8]. In contrast, adenoviruses require the coxsackievirus–adenovirus receptor (CAR) to attach to cells, and the CAR is selectively expressed among cells, which limits its infection. In addition, adenovirus-mediated gene transfer requires a relatively long exposure time to reach maximum gene transfer efficiency, and this is a common characteristic of other currently available vectors. In contrast, SeV can infect cells in a minute or less [6]. Moreover, SeV can infect dividing cells or nondividing cells.

The third feature of SeV is its high level of gene expression. SeV has a dramatically high gene transfer efficiency compared with adenovirus vectors [6,9]. Namely, SeV can efficiently load a therapeutic gene, and gene therapy using SeV is able to decrease the amount of administration vectors in the clinical setting, resulting in a lower risk of gene therapy.

We examined whether we can apply these outstanding characteristics of SeV to the gene therapy of cancer. In this chapter, we describe the history of the investigations of oncolytic gene therapy using SeV, the present developmental status of this therapy, and the future of this therapy.

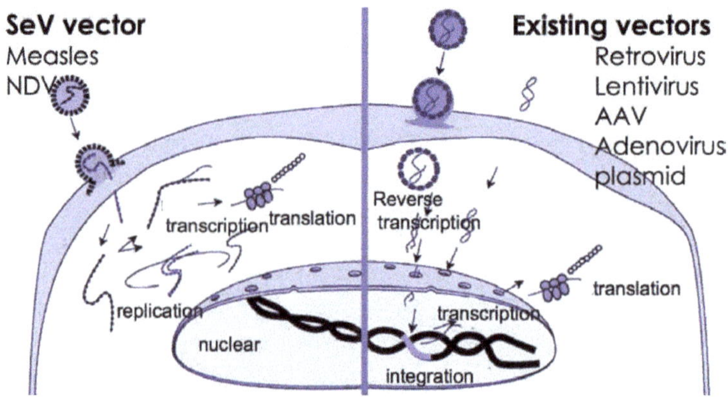

Figure 1. Redrawn with permission from Kinoh H et al., Front Biosci. 2008 Jan 1;13:2327-34. The life cycle of the Sendai Virus (SeV) and other vectors. SeV, Measles, and the Newcastle Disease Virus (NDV) do not result in chromosomal integration, whereas other existing vectors do. AAV, adeno-associated virus.

2. Structure of SeV

SeV is a negative-sense, single-stranded RNA virus of the Paramyxoviridae family. SeV genome consists of 15,384 base pairs and encodes the following 6 genes: nucleocapsid protein (N), which binds to RNA; phosphoprotein (P), which forms a small subunit of RNA polymerase; matrix protein (M), which lines the inside of viral particles; fusion protein (F), which is important for host cell penetration; HN, which is involved in the attachment to the host cells; and large protein (L), which forms a big subunit of RNA polymerase. The HN protein serves in the attachment to target cells by recognizing sialic acid on the cell surface. The F protein is cleaved through conformational change into F1 and F2, and this is triggered by local enzymatic activity, particularly that of trypsin. The cleaved F protein penetrates into the cellular membrane, which induces the membrane and the viral envelope to merge [10].

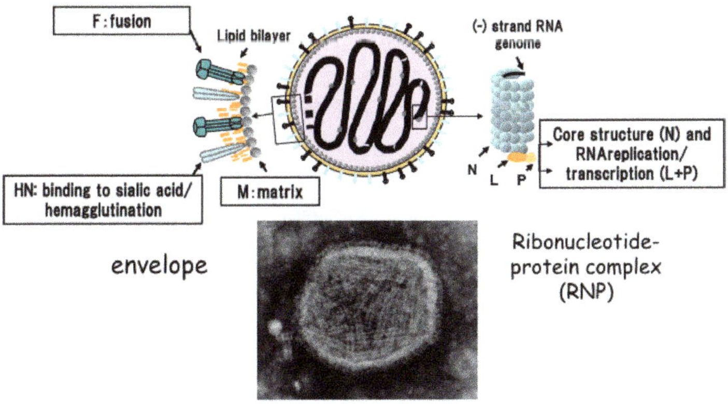

Figure 2. Schematic model and electron microscope photograph of SeV.

3. Fusogenic activity of SeV

Yoshio Okada discovered the phenomenon that SeV causes the fusion of Ehrlich's tumor cells [11]. Paramixoviridae family members including SeV have the property of cell-to-cell fusion. The fusion process, which occurs between the viral envelope and cells, may also occur between adjacent viral-infected cells when the Fusion protein is expressed on the cell surface, thus causing extensive membrane fusion and the formation of a syncytium. Cell-to-cell fusion induces apoptotic signals, resulting in cell death [12,13].

3.1. Oncolytic virotherapy with SeV

We have applied these fusogenic activity characteristics of SeV to cancer therapy. It is important in gene therapy for the treatment of cancer that 1) tumor-specific infections are enhanced and 2) secondary infection is prevented. In order to obtain these properties, we modified the SeV gene by altering the F gene and deleting the M gene.

First, we would like to describe the background of the tumor-specificity abilities of Bioknife™. We focused our attention on the urokinase-type plasminogen activator (uPA). uPA is a trypsin-like serine protease that is synthesized and secreted as pro-uPA, which has little or no proteolytic activity [14]. The urokinase-type plasminogen activator receptor (uPAR) is a 55–60-kD glycoprotein that is anchored on the cell surface by a glycosyl-phosphatidylinositol linkage [15,16]. uPA binds to uPAR with high affinity. uPAR anchors uPA to the cell membrane and converts pro-uPA to active uPA, thereby localizing the proteolytic activity around the cell surface [17]. Activated uPA plays an important role in extracellular matrix degradation and results in tumor invasion and metastasis [18]. A wide variety of cancers overexpress uPAR and are associated with poor prognosis [19-23]. However, uPAR is expressed less in normal tissue except for in unusual circumstances such as inflammation [21,22,24].

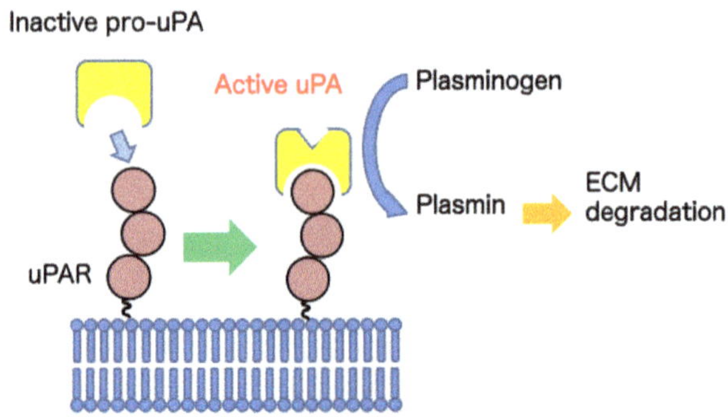

Figure 3. Schematic model of the urokinase activation system.

Bound and inactive pro-urokinase-type plasminogen activator (uPA) is converted to active uPA, inducing extracellular matrix (ECM) degradation. As a result, tumor invasion and metastasis are promoted.

Given that uPA activity is high around tumor cells and low around nontumor cells, we converted the F gene, which is specific to Trypsin in the wild type SeV, to a uPA-specific sequence (Figure 4). As a result, we succeeded in fusing infected cells to tumor cells only. Moreover, to optimize the fusion ability, the F gene was given an additional change, which truncated the cytoplasmic domain of the F protein (Figure 4). This genetic modification resulted in more efficient fusogenic abilities [8].

Second, we would like to describe the background of the deleting of the M gene (Figure 5). Deletion of the M gene resulted in avoidance of the budding of secondary viral particles because the M protein is indispensable for the budding of SeV. Consequently, the F proteins and HN proteins, which are expected to be the second particles in the viral spike, accumulate on the infected cell surface. If uPA is activated around the cell surface, the recombinant F

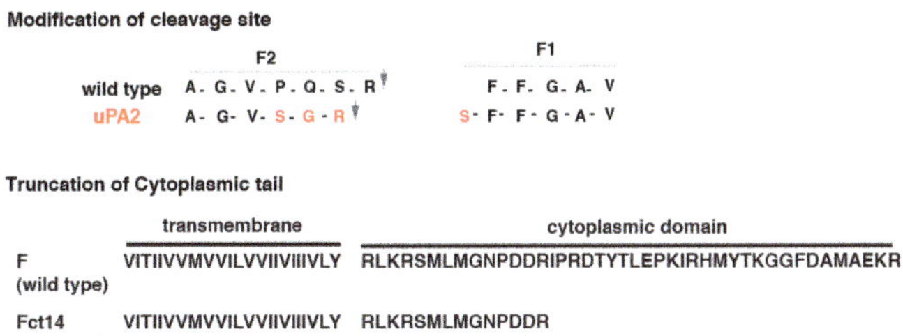

Figure 4. Modification of the cleavage site of the SeV-F protein, which is sensitive to the urokinase-type plasminogen activator, and truncation of the cytoplasmic tail resulted in optimization of the cell-fusion activity.

protein is cleaved, and the contiguous cells go into chain fusion reaction. These completely inhibited secondary viral particles served not only to promote fusion efficiency, but also to improve gene therapy safety.

I would like to emphasize that the oncolysis that is mediated by BioKnife™ is entirely different from conventional oncolysis. Oncolytic viruses, which is a term used to describe most viruses such as adenovirus or herpes simplex viruses, provoke the disruption of infected cells with a large number of secondary viral particles. However, the production of secondary viruses by these oncolytic viruses may limit gene therapy with respect to safety. Thus, a large number of viruses may evoke viremia and induce uncontrollable inflammatory reactions. In contrast, the oncolysis that is caused by BioKnife™ is cell death that is mediated by caspase-dependent apoptosis [13,25]. There is no need to worry about viremia, even if an explosive spread of infection is observed.

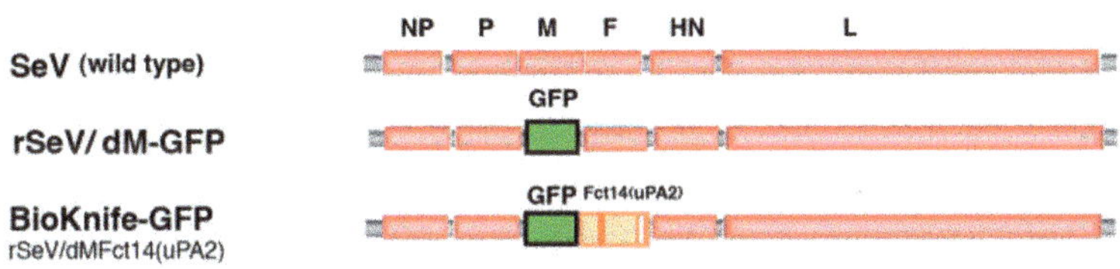

Figure 5. Gene structure of recombinant SeV. Wild type SeV is pictured at the top of the figure, which is followed by the M-gene deleted SeV with a substitutive load of the Green fluorescent protein (GFP) gene (rSeV/dM-GFP) in the middle. Finally, at the bottom, the F gene of rSeV/dM-GFP is transformed to a uPA-sensitive sequence (BioKnife™-GFP).

4. The potential of BioKnife™

To test the cytotoxicity of Bioknife™ against tumor cells, we conducted an *in vitro* infection experiment in many types of tumor cells. Cell fusion and cell death were observed in many tumor types, and this was dependent on the uPA activity of the tumor cells. As expected, nontumor cells were not injured [8]. Next, we tested the antitumor efficacy of BioKnife™ *in vivo*. Cells of the human prostate tumor cell line, PC3, were implanted into a nude mouse, and then BioKnife™ was injected into the tumor. BioKnife™-infected tumor presented GFP fluorescence from day 1 with the maximum GFP intensity on day 7. A microscopic examination of the subcutaneous tumor on day 16 showed that the tumor cells had been eradicated.

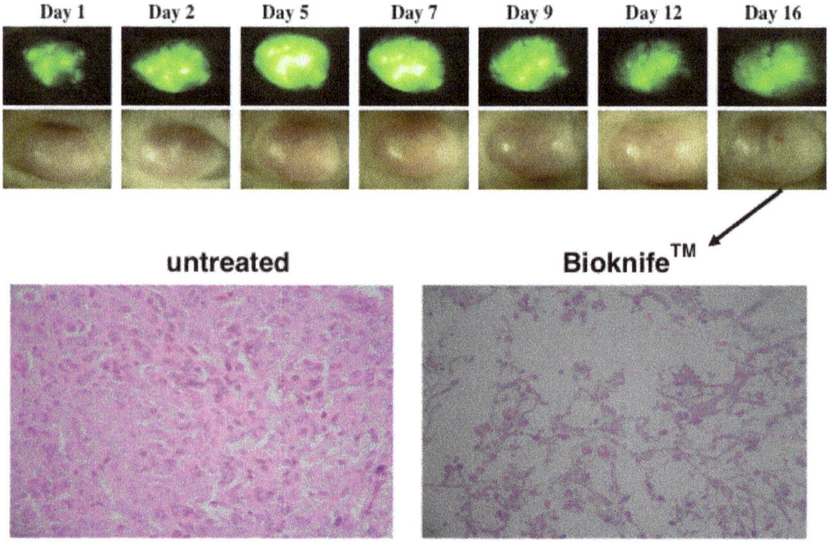

Figure 6. A time-course analysis of BioKnife™ infection of subcutaneously inoculated PC3 tumor cells in a nude mouse. Photomicrographs of tissue specimens on day 16 are presented in the bottom two panels.

5. BioKnife™ infections create a positive feedback loop of cell-to-cell fusion

The cell-to-cell fusion that is mediated by Bioknife™ provided another effect. We demonstrated that Bioknife™ infections induce simultaneous activation of the uPA expression. In addition, we found that the induction of uPA is mediated by the retinoic acid-inducible gene-1 (RIG-I), which is a viral RNA sensor that is activated by Bioknife™ infection and which activates the nuclear factor-kappa B (NF-κB) signaling pathway [25]. Activated RIG-I upregulates levels of uPA expression through the downstream protein, NFκB. Extracellularly secreted uPA binds uPAR on the tumor surface, which increases the activity of uPA. As a result, the F protein on BioKnife™-infected cells is activated and cleaved, resulting in cell fusion. It is possible that BioKnife™ results in self-induced fusion (Figure 7). This phenomenon suggests that uPAR is necessary for the cell fusion that is mediated by BioKnife™, even if uPA is not expressed in tumor cells, and BioKnife™ infection itself facilitates the fusion activity.

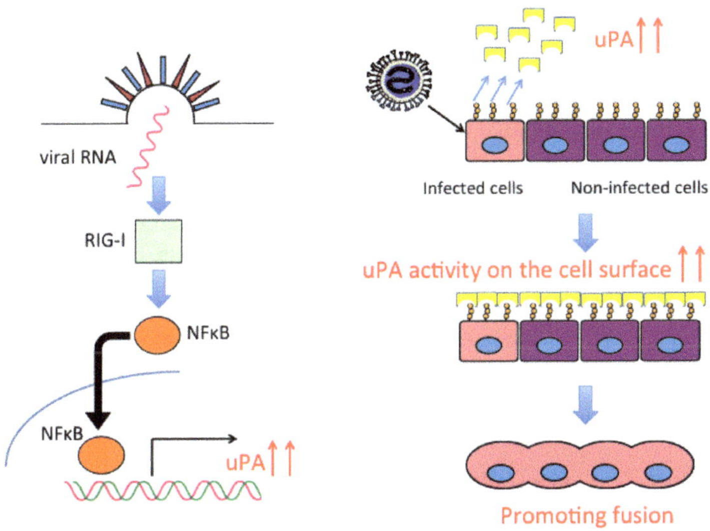

Figure 7. A schematic model of the induction of uPA expression through Bioknife™ infection. Retinoic acid-inducible gene-1 (RIG-I) activation promotes the fusion cascade.

In summary, we have demonstrated the potential and the mechanisms of Bioknife™ with numerous fundamental experiments. Admittedly, BioKnife™ has no ability to infect distant tumor lesions or metastatic lesions through intravascular routes because of its instability in the blood. However, the ability of local infections of the tumor cells and the killing power are outstanding. Next, we explored diseases in which gene therapy using BioKnife™ can be applied. We examined malignant mesothelioma (MPM) in particular.

MPM is a malignancy that arises from the pleural cavity. Because MPM has a long latency period after the inhalation of asbestos [26], the number of deaths by MPM is expected to increase in the next several decades, reflecting the past usage of asbestos [27]. MPM is highly malignant due to its intractableness to treatment. Although a large number of studies have examined approaches to MPM therapy, no marked progress has appeared to overcome this disease. The median overall survival rate is less than 30 months, even if it is treated with multimodality therapy [28,29]. Thus, novel therapeutics are highly desired. MPM spreads widely throughout the pleural cavity and rarely metastasizes to distant sites in the earlier stage. In addition, MPM expresses high levels of uPAR. These characteristics suggest favorable conditions for gene therapy with Bioknife™. Thus, we explored the possibility of treatment with Bioknife™ in this disease.

6. Antitumor effects of Bioknife™ in a MPM orthotopic murine model

To confirm the antitumor effects in MPM, we first established two independent human orthotopic murine models. The human MPM cell lines, MSTO-211H (biphasic subtype) and H226 (epithelioid subtype), were injected into the thoracic cavity of Balb/c nu/nu mice. The tumor cells spread and formed multiple nodules in the thoracic cavity, which is similar to the pathology observed during the clinical course of human MPM. Untreated mice eventually died due to MPM progression. We assessed the performance of Bioknife™ in these MPM murine models. MPM-bearing mice were treated with BioKnife™ at the following frequencies: once, three times, or six times. The result was that, in both murine models, BioKnife™-treated cohort exhibited a significantly prolonged survival compared with the control group. The greater the number of BioKnife™ injection times, the higher the survival rate. In the group receiving 6 injections of BioKnife™, long-term survivors were observed.

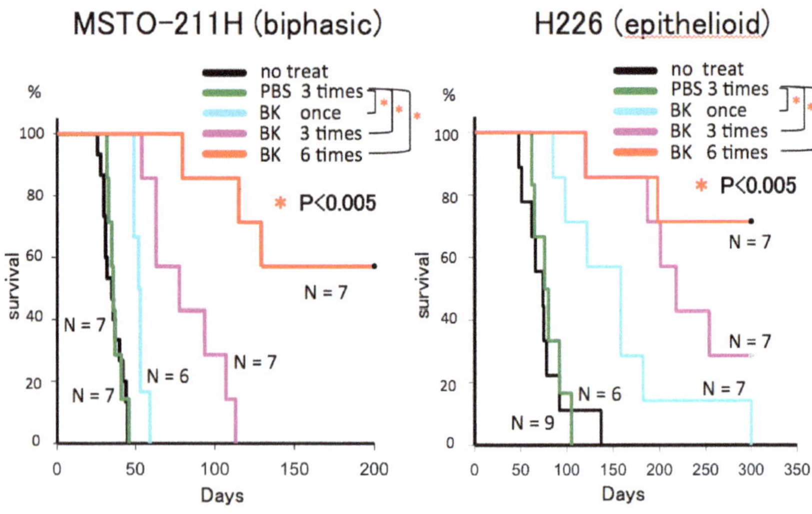

Figure 8. Kaplan–Meier survival plot of BALB/c nude mice bearing H226 or MSTO-211H tumors that were left untreated or treated with phosphate-buffered saline or BioKnife™ in multicycle treatments. No treat indicates no treatment, PBS indicates phosphate- buffered saline treatment, and BK indicates BioKnife™ treatment.

Considering these findings, MPM is a good target for BioKnife™ treatment because the biological characteristics of MPM match the characteristics of BioKnife™. MPM spreads in the thoracic cavity and rarely develops distant metastasis. BioKnife™ can spread to adjacent tumor cells, and local control is its primary advantage. Moreover, we would like to emphasize the accessibility of BioKnife™ in treatments of MPM. We suggest that video-assisted thoracoscopic surgery (VATS) and chest tubes are the best way to administer BioKnife™. MPM often forms nodular lesions on the pleural surface. For these targets, it is best to inject BioKnife™ intratumorally with VATS. In addition, because MPM frequently produces malignant pleural effusion [30], most cases need chest tubes. In these cases, it is convenient to administer BioKnife™ intrapleurally through the chest tube. This access route enables us to administer BioKnife™ repeatedly and safely because multiple cycles of the administration of BioKnife™ are more effective (Figure 8). Based on these results, we are planning a clinical trial using BioKnife™ to treat MPM.

7. BioKnife™ in the future

We described above the developmental history and the usefulness of BioKnife™. It should be noted that BioKnife™ has the ability to load other treatment genes, cytokines, tumor suppressing genes, or cancer antigens. Amazingly, the cytotoxicity of BioKnife™ depends solely on its fusion ability. In other words, there is still considerable room for improvements of this treatment modality. Moreover, there is room for further examination of the relationship between BioKnife™ and cancer immunity. Viral oncolysate is applied as a cancer vaccine in cancer immunotherapy. BioKnife™-lysed tumor cells make an extract of tumor cells. The extract contains both cancer cell proteins and virus proteins. This extract may facilitate the antigen presentation activity to dendritic cells or activate natural killer cells. Further studies are necessary to confirm this fact.

8. Conclusion

We developed BioKnife™, which is a uPA activity-dependent oncolytic SeV vector. This promising oncolytic vector, BioKnife™, may overcome the limitations of current gene therapy vectors. Further studies are needed to examine whether this new modality is effective in the clinical setting as a therapeutic alternative for this intractable disease.

Acknowledgements

We thank Chie Arimatsu, Aki Furuya, and Ryoko Nakamura for their assistance with the animal experiments, and Drs. Tagawa, Kanaya, Ban, and Hironaka for their excellent technical assistance in the vector construction and large-scale production. This work was supported in part by a grant from the Japanese Ministry of Education, Culture, Sports, Science, and Technology (to Y.M. and Y.Y.). Y.Y. is a member of the Scientific Advisory Board of DNAVEC Corporation. The other authors declare no conflicts of interest.

Author details

Yosuke Morodomi[1], Makoto Inoue[2], Mamoru Hasegawa[2], Tatsuro Okamoto[3], Yoshihiko Maehara[3] and Yoshikazu Yonemitsu[4]

1 Department of Thoracic Oncology, National Kyushu Cancer Center, Japan

2 DNAVEC Corporation, Japan

3 Department of Surgery and Science, Graduate School of Medicine, Kyushu University, Japan

4 R&D Laboratory for Innovative Biotherapeutics, Graduate School of Pharmaceutical Sciences, Kyushu University, Japan

References

[1] Blaese, R. M, Culver, K. W, Miller, A. D, Carter, C. S, Fleisher, T, Clerici, M, et al. T lymphocyte-directed gene therapy for ADA- SCID: initial trial results after 4 years. Science. (1995). Oct.;, 270(5235), 475-80.

[2] Lehrman, S. Virus treatment questioned after gene therapy death. Nature. (1999). Oct.;, 401(6753), 517-8.

[3] Hacein-bey-abina, S, Von Kalle, C, & Schmidt, M. Le Deist F, Wulffraat N, McIntyre E, et al. A serious adverse event after successful gene therapy for X-linked severe combined immunodeficiency. N. Engl. J. Med. (2003). Jan.;, 348(3), 255-6.

[4] Gene Therapy Clinical Trials Worldwide [cited (2012). JulAvailable from: http://www.wiley.com//legacy/wileychi/genmed/clinical/

[5] Yonemitsu, Y, Kitson, C, Ferrari, S, Farley, R, Griesenbach, U, Judd, D, et al. Efficient gene transfer to airway epithelium using recombinant Sendai virus. Nat. Biotechnol. (2000). Sep.;, 18(9), 970-3.

[6] Masaki, I. Recombinant Sendai virus-mediated gene transfer to vasculature: a new class of efficient gene transfer vector to the vascular system. The FASEB Journal. (2001). Mar. 28.

[7] Iwadate, Y. Recombinant Sendai Virus Vector Induces Complete Remission of Established Brain Tumors through Efficient Interleukin-2 Gene Transfer in Vaccinated Rats. Clin. Cancer Res. (2005). May 15;, 11(10), 3821-7.

[8] Kinoh, H, Inoue, M, Komaru, A, Ueda, Y, Hasegawa, M, & Yonemitsu, Y. Generation of optimized and urokinase-targeted oncolytic Sendai virus vectors applicable for various human malignancies. Gene Ther [Internet]. (2008). Nov. 27;Available from:

http://eutils.ncbi.nlm.nih.gov/entrez/eutils/elink.fcgi?
dbfrom=pubmed&id=19037241&retmode=ref&cmd=prlinks, 16(3), 392-403.

[9] Tokusumi, T, Iida, A, Hirata, T, Kato, A, Nagai, Y, & Hasegawa, M. Recombinant Sendai viruses expressing different levels of a foreign reporter gene. Virus Res. (2002). Jun.;86(1-2):33-8.

[10] Takimoto, T, Taylor, G. L, Connaris, H. C, Crennell, S. J, & Portner, A. Role of the hemagglutinin-neuraminidase protein in the mechanism of paramyxovirus-cell membrane fusion. J. Virol. (2002). Dec.;, 76(24), 13028-33.

[11] Okada, Y, & Tadokoro, J. Analysis of giant polynuclear cell formation caused by HVJ virus from Ehrlich's ascites tumor cells. II. Quantitative analysis of giant polynuclear cell formation. Exp. Cell Res. (1962). Feb.;, 26, 108-18.

[12] Scheller, C, & Jassoy, C. Syncytium Formation Amplifies Apoptotic Signals: A New View on Apoptosis in HIV Infection in Vitro. Virology. (2001). Mar. 30;, 282(1), 48-55.

[13] Villenave, R, Touzelet, O, Thavagnanam, S, Sarlang, S, Parker, J, Skibinski, G, et al. Cytopathogenesis of Sendai Virus in Well-Differentiated Primary Pediatric Bronchial Epithelial Cells. J. Virol. (2010). Oct. 25;, 84(22), 11718-28.

[14] Petersen, L. C, Lund, L. R, Nielsen, L. S, Danø, K, & Skriver, L. One-chain urokinase-type plasminogen activator from human sarcoma cells is a proenzyme with little or no intrinsic activity. J. Biol. Chem. (1988). Aug. 15;, 263(23), 11189-95.

[15] Nielsen, L. S, Kellerman, G. M, Behrendt, N, Picone, R, Danø, K, & Blasi, F. A. Mr receptor protein for urokinase-type plasminogen activator. Identification in human tumor cell lines and partial purification. J. Biol. Chem. (1988). Feb. 15;, 263(5), 2358-63.

[16] Ploug, M, Kjalke, M, Rønne, E, Weidle, U, Høyer-hansen, G, & Danø, K. Localization of the disulfide bonds in the NH2-terminal domain of the cellular receptor for human urokinase-type plasminogen activator. A domain structure belonging to a novel superfamily of glycolipid-anchored membrane proteins. J. Biol. Chem. (1993). Aug. 15;, 268(23), 17539-46.

[17] Vassalli, J. D, Baccino, D, & Belin, D. A cellular binding site for the Mr 55,000 form of the human plasminogen activator, urokinase. J. Cell Biol. (1985). Jan.;, 100(1), 86-92.

[18] Blasi, F, & Carmeliet, P. uPAR: a versatile signalling orchestrator. Nat. Rev. Mol. Cell Biol. (2002). Dec.;, 3(12), 932-43.

[19] AlpÃ zar-AlpÃ zar WNielsen BS, Sierra R, Illemann M, RamÃ rez JA, Arias A, et al. Urokinase plasminogen activator receptor is expressed in invasive cells in gastric carcinomas from high- and low-risk countries. Int. J. Cancer. (2010). Jan. 15;, 126(2), 405 15.

[20] Pedersen, H, Brünner, N, Francis, D, Osterlind, K, Rønne, E, Hansen, H. H, et al. Prognostic impact of urokinase, urokinase receptor, and type 1 plasminogen activa-

tor inhibitor in squamous and large cell lung cancer tissue. Cancer Res. (1994). Sep. 1;, 54(17), 4671-5.

[21] Bianchi, E, Cohen, R. L, & Thor, A. T. Todd RFIII, Mizukami IF, Lawrence DA, et al. The urokinase receptor is expressed in invasive breast cancer but not in normal breast tissue. Cancer Res. (1994). Feb.;, 54(4), 861-6.

[22] Li, Y, & Cozzi, P. J. Targeting uPA/uPAR in prostate cancer. Cancer Treat. Rev. (2007). Oct.;, 33(6), 521-7.

[23] De Bock, C. E, & Wang, Y. Clinical significance of urokinase-type plasminogen activator receptor (uPAR) expression in cancer. Med. Res. Rev. (2003). , 24(1), 13-39.

[24] Eddy, A. A. Serine proteases, inhibitors and receptors in renal fibrosis. Thromb. Haemost. (2009). Apr.;, 101(4), 656-64.

[25] Morodomi, Y, Yano, T, Kinoh, H, Harada, Y, Saito, S, Kyuragi, R, et al. BioKnife, a uPA activity-dependent oncolytic Sendai virus, eliminates pleural spread of malignant mesothelioma via simultaneous stimulation of uPA expression. Mol. Therapy. (2012). Apr.;, 20(4), 769-77.

[26] Marinaccio, A, Binazzi, A, Cauzillo, G, Cavone, D, Zotti, R. D, Ferrante, P, et al. Analysis of latency time and its determinants in asbestos related malignant mesothelioma cases of the Italian register. Eur. J. Cancer. (2007). Dec.;, 43(18), 2722-8.

[27] Murayama, T, Takahashi, K, Natori, Y, & Kurumatani, N. Estimation of future mortality from pleural malignant mesothelioma in Japan based on an age-cohort model. Am. J. Ind. Med. (2005). , 49(1), 1-7.

[28] Sugarbaker, D. J, Flores, R. M, Jaklitsch, M. T, Richards, W. G, Strauss, G. M, Corson, J. M, et al. Resection margins, extrapleural nodal status, and cell type determine postoperative long-term survival in trimodality therapy of malignant pleural mesothelioma: results in 183 patients. J. Thorac. Cardiovasc. Surg. (1999). Jan.;117(1):54-63-discussion, 63-5.

[29] Bölükbas, S, Manegold, C, Eberlein, M, Bergmann, T, Fisseler-eckhoff, A, & Schirren, J. Survival after trimodality therapy for malignant pleural mesothelioma: Radical Pleurectomy, chemotherapy with Cisplatin/Pemetrexed and radiotherapy. Lung Cancer. Elsevier Ireland Ltd; (2011). Jan. 1;, 71(1), 75-81.

[30] Kawashima, A, & Libshitz, H. I. Malignant pleural mesothelioma: CT manifestations in 50 cases. Am. J. Roentgenol. (1990). Nov.;, 155(5), 965-9.

Section 3

Gene Therapy for Cancer

Chapter 10

Cancer Gene Therapy: Targeted Genomedicines

Yadollah Omidi, Jaleh Barar and George Coukos

Additional information is available at the end of the chapter

1. Introduction

To date, traditional chemotherapy alone or in combination with immunotherapy and ionizing radiation modalities have been used to obliterate dividing aberrant cells in various tumors, while morbid statistics of cancer therapy show limited clinical successes.

Given the fact that malignant cells proliferate more rapidly than normal cells, damage to the cancer cells is anticipated to be markedly greater than normal cells. However, cancer cells generate chemoresistance mechanisms within the tumor microenvironment, while undesired toxicity may occur in the normal cells. For example, in colorectal cancer (CRC), there exist well-described sequences of mutational events that evince the shift of normal colon epithelium to premalignant adenoma and malignant adenocarcinoma. These events are 1) loss of the function of the adenomatous polyposis coli (APC) gene (encoding a protein involved in cell adhesion and transcription) in up to 85% of all cases of CRC, 2) mutation of KRAS (a GTP-ase that controls cell proliferation) in 50–60% of all cases of CRC, and 3) downregulated expression of the cell-adhesion transmembrane glycoprotein E-cadherin in almost 50–60% of all cases of CRC. Mutations in the mismatch-repair genes MLH1 and MSH2 contribute to genetic instability. Besides, there exist a number of genes alterations leading cells toward remodeling that include: 1) SMAD4 involved in the transforming growth factor signal transduction suppressing epithelial-cell growth, 2) INK4A involved in the retinoblastoma tumor-suppressor pathway, and 3) TP53 alterations increasing the resistance of cancer cells to apoptosis [1]. Similar molecular/cellular alterations occur in various solid tumors, highlighting the intricacy of biological events leading to initiation and progression of malignancies. Therefore, necessity for development and advancement of more effective modalities targeting such genetic changes is perceptible to achieve successful cancer treatment and cure. After decades of disappointment, targeted therapy of cancer has been advanced by integration of immunotherapy as well as gene and cell therapy. As proof-of-concept, recent clinical trials (e.g., anti-CTLA4 antibody, ipilimumab) have shown significant increase in survival for patients with metastatic melanoma, for which conventional therapies have failed [2].

Targeted therapy of cancer using mAbs has provided great outcomes [3], while cancer gene therapy has not been as productive as immunotherapy from translational stand point. Efficient gene transfer strategy, as a fundamental step, continues to be the major determining factor for clinical successes of the gene therapy. In fact, there exist some hurdles that make gene therapy a formidable task. There are problems with delivery of sufficient copies of a gene (e.g., short interfering RNA (siRNA), antisense) to all tumor cells, whose biology appear to be very complex and ideally all the cancer-related genes must be controlled. Another barrier is the lack of proper gene delivery systems (GDSs) since the nonspecificity of GDSs makes gene therapy strategy somewhat uncertain. Overall, the current gene therapy approaches are capable of introducing genes into cells in vivo without discrimination within target and non-target cells. However, such unselective approach can impact both normal and aberrant cells. Incorporation of a homing device (e.g., monoclonal antibodies (mAb), antibody (Ab) fragments, or target specific aptamers) with an appropriate delivery system may result in cell-specific targeting and greater clinical outcomes [4].

The main gist of this chapter is to concisely provide information upon the specific gene therapy strategies and gene targets. We will discuss impacts of oncogenes, tumor suppressor genes and apoptosis-inducing genes on cancer gene therapy strategies as well as methods that specifically reactivate pathways that render the mutated cells susceptible to antitumor agents and immunotherapy. We will also remark on the cancer therapy opportunities through exploiting targeted nanogenomedicines.

2. Trajectory of gene therapy

Of many cancer therapy endeavors, cancer gene therapy has granted great hopes even though it is in its developmental trajectory. So far, more than 65% of the gene therapy trials have been devoted to the cancer diseases using various vectors (retrovirus (20%), advenovirus (18%), adeno-associated virusade (5%), lipofection (6%)) and naked/plasmid DNA (18.5%). Despite conducting more than 1186 cancer gene therapy trials (out of 1843), 45 have reached to phase III and only 1 is in phase IV [5]. At this stage, there exist 9 clinical trials of gene therapy that have been conditionally approved [4]. Most of these trials are conducted as adjuvant therapies, which clearly highlight needs for more effective gene therapy systems.

The foremost basis of gene therapy is to fix the genomic defects; nonetheless the gene therapy concept is going to be revolutionized by illumination of epigenomics and targeted genomedicines. In tumor development, the origination of cancer is an intricate biological process, in which molecular changes at genomic/epigenomic levels play a central role. These molecular alterations can equip cancerous cells with unique molecular biostructures that play crucial roles in survival, progression and invasion of cancer cells. Such genomic/epigenomic alterations (e.g., changes in gene expression, mutations, gene deletion, DNA methylation/demethylation and histone acetylation/deacetylation) have directed scientists to devise genomedicines to fix the genomic defects. It should be evoked that, unlike treatment strategies for genetic defects that need permanent expression of the corrected genes, cancer gene therapy is based on temporary and locally limited stimulation/suppression effects on desired gene(s). Further, malignant cells display specific gene markers that are different in nature or magnitude compared to the normal cells. These characteristics of cancer cells are deemed to provide a robust platform for specific targeted gene therapy that provides major advantages over current chemotherapy and immunotherapy modalities [6, 7].

Up until now, some domains of cancer gene therapy have been devoted greater attention, including: a) suppression of cancer cells by introducing genes into tumor cells to lead cells toward apoptosis (e.g., herpes simplex virus thymidine kinase, cytosine deaminase); b) inhibition of growth of cancer cells; c) enhancement of cancer cells chemosensitivity (p53, Bax); d) specific stimulation of the host's immune response against the cancer cells (tumor antigen, DNA vaccines, cytokine genes) by introducing the relevant genes into tumor cells or dendritic cells. Although use of genomedicines (e.g., antisense RNA, siRNA, ribozymes, DNAzyme and aptamers) have shown positive outcomes, their combination with other cancer therapy modalities including chemotherapy and immunotherapy can open other avenues for cancer therapy [8-10].

In addition, immune gene therapies (e.g., targeted DNA vaccine) exploit the lymphocytes and dendritic cells potentials, activating the immune system defense mechanisms against cancer cells. DNA vaccines possess intrinsic ability to activate multiple pathways of innate immunity, that also provide a unique opportunity to guide defined antigens, accompanied by specific activator molecules, through a patient's compromised immune system [11]. Further, suicide gene therapy tackles to deliver genes to the cancer cells, upon which cancer cells convert nontoxic prodrugs into active chemotherapeuties. In this approach, cancerous cells containing suicide genes are solely targeted through a systemic administration of prodrug. The suicide gene therapy is deemed to provide maximal inhibitory effects in cancer cells, but minimal toxic effects in normal cells [12]. Other than these strategies, antisense oligodeoxynucleotides (AS-ODNs) as a new class of molecularly targeted agents are in transitional trajectory from the laboratory into the clinic. A number of very important transcriptomic elements (e.g., VEGF, Ang-1, MDM2, protein kinase C-a, c-myb, integrin subunit b3, PKA-I, H-ras, bcl-2, c-raf, R1/R2 subunits of ribonucleotide reductase) have successfully targeted by AS-ODNs [13].

In contrast to AS-ODNs technology, the mechanism of silencing an endogenous gene through a homologous double-stranded RNA (dsRNA), which is termed post-transcriptional gene silencing (PTGS) or RNA interference (RNAi), is a natural mechanism by which mammalian cells can regulate expansion of genes. Accordingly, short interfering RNA (siRNA) can be used for gene silencing. It is currently the fastest growing sector for target validation and therapeutic [14]. Further, considering cancer cells scape from immune system within the tumor microenvironment, immune targeted gene therapy appears to provide an effective tactic for activation of the immune systems in such intricate microenvironment, whereby targeted gene therapy of angiogenesis and lymphangiogenesis bestow robust treatment possibilities [15].

3. Gene silencing as gene therapy modality

It is clear that the tumorigenesis results from clusters of several genetic and/or epigenetic events. Therefore, identification of the involved genes provides new targets toward effective treatment of malignancies. Of various gene therapy approaches, it is deemed that the silencing of cancer-causing genes can control the biological consequences at its genetic root and thereby cure the disease. Hence, development of agents capable of gene silencing is now considered as a rational strategy for cancer therapy, which can be accomplished by genomedicines. We will review gene silencing technologies in the following sections.

3.1. Antisense oligodeoxynucleotides for suppression of mRNA

During the last decade, we have witnessed emergence of synthetic AS-ODNs. They are primarily designed to attach selectively to the target transcriptomes and to disrupt the expression of a target gene. It should be evoked that the overall utility of AS-ODN as therapeutic agent is dependent upon 1) the expression level of the target mRNA, 2) the optimal design of As-ODN, 3) the specificity of the AS-ODN to the target mRNA and 4) the availability of safe and highly efficient delivery systems. For example, we have shown that most of cationic polymers (CPs) and lipids used as GDSs to shuttle AS-ODNs specific to the epidermal growth factor receptor (EGFR) can also induce intrinsic cytotoxicity and toxicogenomics [16-22]. Previous studies have demonstrated that the viral vectors (e.g., adenovirus, adeno-associated virus (AAV), Epstein-Barr virus (EBV), herpes simplex virus type-1 (HSV-1), retrovirus, lentivirus, poxvirus, baculovirus) vectors can function as efficient vehicles for AS-ODN delivery. Of these, AAV vectors can be constructed to express short, distinct transcripts, a property that is useful for RNA - mediated inhibition of gene expression and successful delivery of the As-ODNs [23, 24]. Fig. 1 and Table 1 respectively represent the mechanism of action of AS-ODNs and their applications.

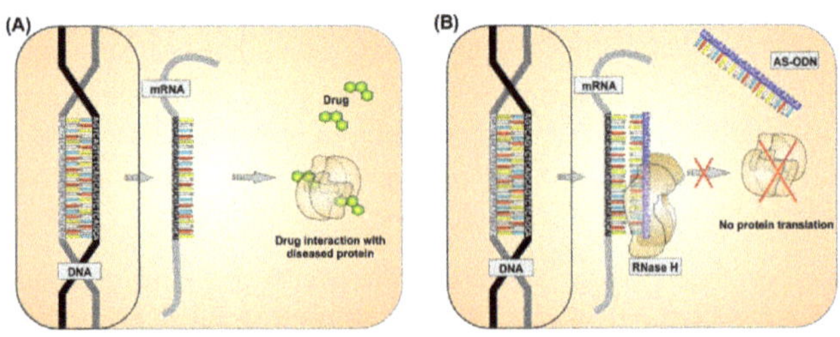

Figure 1. Mechanism of action of AS-ODN. A) Inhibition of proteins by small molecule drugs after translation. B) Suppression of mRNA by AS-ODN before translation in the presence of RNase H. This figure was adapted with permission from reference [4].

It is known that the oncogene E7 from high-risk human papillomavirus (HPV) strains has the potential to immortalize epithelial cells and increase cellular transformation in culture. Hence, to prevent the cervical cancer growth, the HPV16 E7 was inhibited by AS-ODN that was delivered by a recombinant AAV (rAAV). It was found that such genomedicines can inhibit cell proliferation, induce apoptosis, reduce cell migration, and restrain in vivo proliferation of the cervical cancer CaSki cells [24]. Table 1 shows selected oncogenes targeted by AS-ODNs.

Oncogene	Application	Ref
HER2 (c-erbB-2)	c-erbB-2 AS-ODN Inhibit serum-induced cell spreading of ovarian cancer cells	[27]
	Inhibitory effects of c-erbB-2 AS-ODN in uterine endometrial cancer Ishikawa cells	[28]
BCL-2	BCL-2 AS-ODN inhibits sensitize small cell lung cancer cells (in vitro and in vivo) to radiation	[29]
	Phase I/II study of G3139 (Bcl-2 AS-ODN) combined with doxorubicin and docetaxel in breast cancer	[30]
	Induction of apoptosis and increased chemosensitivity in human prostate cancer cells by Bcl-2 AS-ODN	[31]
c-RAF-1	Phase I study of the c-raf-1 AS-ODN (ISIS 5132) combined with carboplatin and paclitaxel in patients with advanced non-small cell lung cancer	[32]
	Phase I study of the c-raf-1 AS-ODN (ISIS 5132) in patients with advanced cancer	[33]
c-FOS	Tissue-targeted antisense c-fos retroviral vector inhibits established breast cancer xenografts in nude mice	[34]
	c-fos AS-ODN control prostaglandin E2-induced upregulation of vascular endothelial growth factor in human liver cancer cells	[35]
c-MYC	c-myc AS-ODN sensitize human colorectal cancer cells to chemotherapeutic drugs	[36]
	inhibition of c-MYC by antisense phosphorodiamidate morpholino oligomer in prostate cancer murine models and humans	[37]

Table 1. Selected oncogenes targeted by AS-ODNs.

The effectiveness of the AS-ODNs have so far been shown in both target cells/tissue as in vitro models and animal in vivo models in particular for cancer therapy [13]. The mechanisms of action of the AS-ODNs seem to vary in different systems. In the case of hybridization and intramolecular and/or intermolecular interactions, their degradation pattern appears to be different. Many investigations have shown the anti-oncogenic impacts of AS-ODNs through targeting specific oncogenes. We have used AS-ODNs specific to EGFR and showed substantial inhibition of EGFR in A431 cells [25] as well as A549 lung cancer cells [26] using non-viral vectors as delivery system. The inhibitory impacts of AS-ODNs have been assessed through alterations in growth rate, morphology and molecular analysis. Various oncogenes have been targeted by AS-ODNs.

3.2. Small interfering RNA

The siRNA (also called as short interfering RNA or silencing RNA) is double-stranded RNA (dsRNA) molecules of 20-25 nucleotides. The siRNA gene-silencing mechanism is induced by dsRNA and it is largely sequence-specific. RNA interference (RNAi) approach appears to be an extremely powerful tool for silencing gene expression in vitro [38]. Accordingly, huge researchers have been conducted to expand this technology toward in vivo applications [39]. Fig. 2 represents mechanism of siRNA in controlling the expression of a target mRNA.

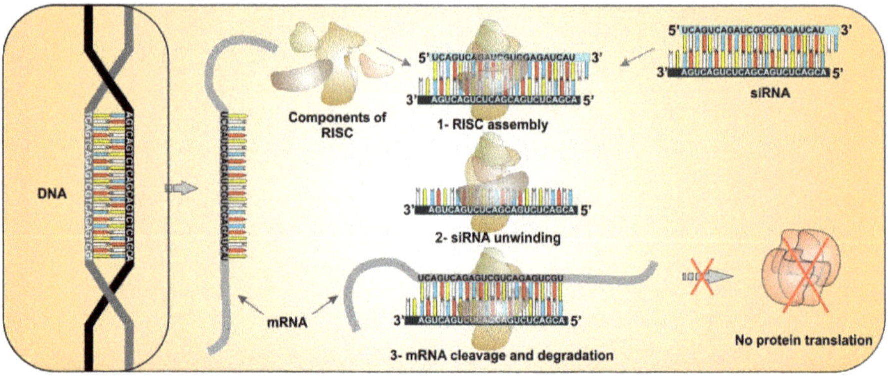

Figure 2. Cleavage and degradation of mRNA expression by siRNA. Short interfering RNAs (siRNAs) basically consist of two 21-25 single-stranded RNAs forming double stand RNA with overhangs at 3′ end. The antisense strand of the siRNA bound to RNA-induced silencing complex (RISC) can cleave the target mRNA. This figure was adapted with permission from reference [4].

Basically, investigation on RNAi has highlighted two distinct methodologies for gene silencing as: 1) cytoplasmic delivery of siRNA to target cells to imitate an endogenous RNAi mechanism and 2) nuclear delivery of gene expression cassettes expressing a short hairpin RNA (shRNA) that mimic the micro interfering RNA (miRNA) active intermediate of a different endogenous RNAi mechanism [40]. Both these approaches need safe delivery of gene materials into the target sites.

In fact, RNAi that was discovered initially in plants has been applied for various types of cancer as well as other diseases. Besides, RNAi technology seems to be the right tool for delineation of the functions and interactions of the thousands of human genes in high-throughput systems, which can also be harnessed in target validation technology. It is deemed that delivery of siRNAs as nanoformulations may resolve the inefficient delivery problem [41-43]. For example, a micelleplex system based on an amphiphilic and cationic triblock copolymer has been developed for delivery of siRNA specific to the acid ceramidase (AC) gene. In aqueous solution, the triblock copolymer (consisting of monomethoxy poly(ethylene glycol), poly(epsilon-caprolactone) and poly(2-aminoethyl ethylene phosphate)) can self assembles into positively charged (48 mV) micellar nanoparticles (MNPs) with an average diameter of 60 nm. Once exposed to siRNA, it can result in micelleplex that was shown to effectively internalize into the BT474 breast cancer cells and induce significant gene knockdown. Systemic delivery of micelleplex targeting AC gene was shown to significantly inhibit the tumor growth in a BT474 xenograft murine model without activation of the innate immune response [44].

Some chemotherapy agents are substrate of the efflux transporters (e.g., P-glycoprotein (P-gp), multidrug resistance proteins (MRPs)) that are often overexpressed on cancer cells developing resistance, while no safe inhibitor of P-gp is available. Simultaneous delivery of P-gp targeted siRNA and paclitaxel as poly(D,L-lactide-co-glycolide) (PLGA) nanoparticles (NPs) decorated with biotin has been shown to overcome tumor drug resistance in both in vitro and in vivo [42].

3.3. Ribozymes and DNAzyme

After being discovered in early 1980s, ribozymes as a class of RNA showing catalytic activity to cleave RNA molecules in a sequence specific manner have been used for cancer therapy. They have been shown to perform excellent catalytic reactions with great precision, which can be encoded and transcribed from DNA. It was a decade later that DNAzymes have entered the scene of nucleic acid-mediated catalysis [45]. They are special class of nucleic acid chains, which usually consist of both double and single stranded regions that fold into a specific three-dimensional structure performing catalytic functions. Various ribozyme formats (e.g., hammerhead, hairpin, axhead, group I intron, and RNAse P) can be used as trans-acting catalysts. Of these, the hammerhead and hairpin ribozymes seem to be the most commonly used. For example, the efficacy of an anti-KRAS hammerhead ribozyme targeting GUU-mutated codon 12 of the KRAS gene was evaluated in a cell-free system and also in cultured pancreatic carcinoma cells [46]. Fig. 3 schematically exemplifies a morphology and cleavage mechanisms of Ribozyme (A) and DNAzyme (B).

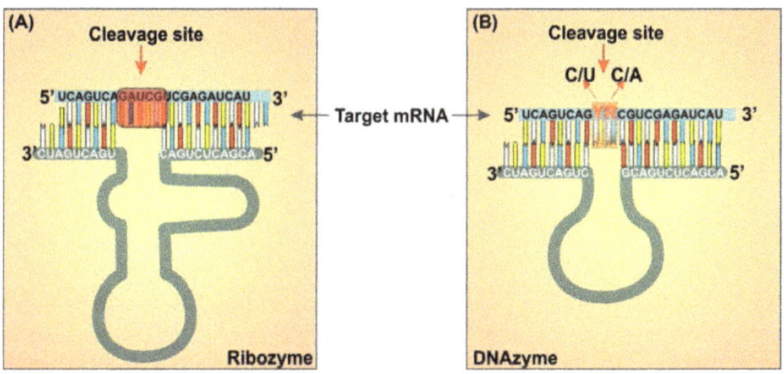

Figure 3. Schematic representation of morphology and cleavage mechanism of Ribozyme (A) and DNAzyme (B). This figure was adapted with permission from reference [4].

Tsuchida *et al.* showed that, in the cell-free system, the anti-KRAS ribozyme specifically cleaved KRAS RNA with GUU-mutation at codon 12. In the cell culture system, they showed that the anti-KRAS ribozyme significantly reduced KRAS mRNA level (GUU-mutated codon 12) in Capan-1 pancreatic carcinoma cells. Further, it has been proposed that trans-splicing ribozyme capable of specifically reprograming the human telomerase reverse transcriptase (hTERT) RNA can be harnessed as a useful tool for tumor-targeted gene therapy. Thus, a transcriptional targeting with the RNA replacement approach was implemented to target liver cancer cells through combining a liver-selective promoter with an hTERT-mediated cancer-specific ribozyme [47]. To this end, Song *et al.* validated it in vivo by constructing an adenovirus encoding the hTERT-targeting trans-splicing ribozyme under the control of a liver-selective phosphoenolpyruvate carboxy kinase promoter. They found that intratumoral injection of this virus produced selective and efficient regression of tumors in mice [47].

It should be emphasized that the catalytic ribozyme core is basically attached to the specific regions of the target transcript through flanking antisense sequences. They have been designed to effectively cleave the targets transcript resulting in suppressed gene expression. For inhibition of gene expression, it is deemed that ribozymes are more effective than AS-ODNs because they cleave the target transcripts catalytically.

The DNAzyme (the so called deoxyribozyme) molecules consist of the 10-23 nucleotides, which bind to mRNA in a highly sequence-specific manner and cleave the RNA independent from RNase with the relatively stable chemistries used in oligodeoxynucleotide-based antisense reagents. The major obstacle in the further development of these technologies is a phenomenon that requires substantial development efforts invested in drugs of various classes, the uphill battle to affect cellular delivery in a targeted manner. This challenge is being met with a multidisciplinary approach with the hope that a greater understanding of each step of this process will enhance DNAzyme pharmacodynamics [45].

Owing to DNA backbone, DNAzymes have the advantage of being highly stable and cost-effective in compassion with RNAzymes and proteins. DNAzymes, similar to aptamers, can be isolated through a combinatorial in vitro selection process. Hence, they can be literally manipulated to meet the requirements and applied for engineering of targeted genoceuticals. Such characteristics make them excellent choice for dynamic control of nanomaterials assembly [48].

4. Target antigens and oncogenes

Tumor epithelial and endothelial cells as well as tumor associated cells represent unique marker molecules that can be harnessed for targeted therapy of cancer. For example, tumor vasculature varies significantly from its normal counterpart, representing unique cancer marker molecules. This has been emphasized through recent technologies including: immunohistochemistry laser-capture microdissection (immuno-LCM), genome-wide high-throughput screening, and proteomics. It is deemed that the vast array of vascular bed-specific markers may provide an exceptional platform for discovery of new therapeutics that target tumor microvasculature in various malignancies [49]. It is the same for tumor epithelial cells and tumor associated cells (TACs). Regarding the epithelial cells, EGFRs are the most studied cancer marker molecules (CMMs), whose upregulation in cancer cells was shown to be substantially down regulated with gene based medicines such as siRNA and AS-ODN. Likewise, vascular EGF and EGF-receptors have been shown to be upregulated in tumor endothelial cells and they can also be suppressed by genomedicines [50].

Malignant brain tumors (high-grade glioma), pancreatic cancer and malignant melanoma are among the most aggressive tumors known. Despites these facts, necessary translational steps are needed to be fulfilled for their clinical applications. For example, Antisense Pharma has recently taken an AS-ODN medication (Trabedersen or AP 12009) in several clinical trials. Trabedersen is a DNA-oligonucleotide that inhibits the synthesis of the cytokine transforming growth factor beta 2 (TGF-ß2) through specific binding to mRNA of TGF-ß2 that is overexpressed in many highly aggressive tumors suppressing the immune system activity [51-53].

4.1. Tumor antigen–specific vaccines and DNA vaccines

Cancerous cells of different types of tumors often display expression of aberrant genes such as: 1) mutated genes (e.g., mutated P53, RAS, BCR-ABL), 2) unique genes resultant from viral oncogenes (e.g., HPV E6 or E7), 3) overexpressed cancer specific genes (e.g., Her2, TGF-ß2, carcinoembryonic antigen, mucin).

These aberrant genes could be recognized by the host immune system, resulting in elimination of the cancerous cells expressing such oncogenes. However, cancer cells can circumvent from the anticancer activity of immune system within the permissive tumor microenvironment. Accordingly, the basis of the tumor antigen-specific vaccines is boosting the immune system harnessing these aberrant antigens. Nevertheless, success of this approach depends on identification and appropriate use of tumor specific genes [54-56]. In fact, vaccination against tumors may provide a selective destruction of malignant cells by the host's immune system, which can be applied as integrated system containing target gene(s) in recombinant vectors. Of viral vectors use in cancer vaccination, the recombinant AAV vectors appear to grant better clinical responses because of their low intrinsic immunogenicity, hence they have been employed to generate immune responses against specific antigens. For example, the safety of cytotoxic T lymphocytes (CTLs) infusion by transfected dendritic cells (DCs) with rAAV carrying carcinoembryonic antigen (CEA) cDNA was investigated in advanced cancer patients. For example, a total of 27 cancer patients with tumor tissue and/or sera-elevated level of CEA were treated with the rAAV-DC immunovaccine, which was well-tolerated showing no severe side effects in patients [57].

As the most potent antigen-presenting cells, DCs originate from the bone marrow and play a key role in the generation of immune responses. Further, peptide-based vaccination in cancer patients using DCs have resulted in promising outcomes. For example, to control the relapse and succumb to progressive disease in patients with advanced ovarian cancer, an immunotherapy approach was applied using CDs loaded with Her2/neu, hTERT, and PADRE peptides in a randomized open-label phase I/II trial. Despite showing modest immune responses, these peptide-loaded DC vaccination showed promising survival rate [58]. Fig. 4 represents the radar pattern of DNA vaccines in each phase of clinical trials.

It appears that we need to develop much more rational consolidative strategies for treatment of solid tumor in advanced stages since the applied strategies exploiting DCs (e.g., peptide pulsing with tumor antigens, transfection with DNA/RNA and transduction with tumor antigens encoding viral vectors) have not substantially generated antitumor immune responses.

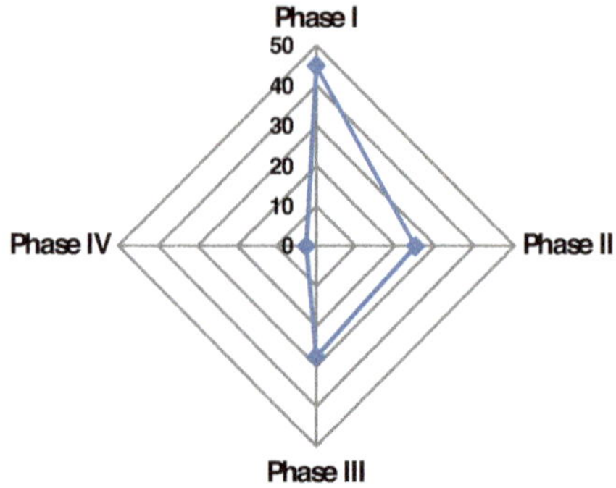

Figure 4. Selected DNA vaccines in clinical trials. Only 4 trials have reached to the phase IV trial, in which 3 of them are targeting human papillomavirus (HPV) and 1 targeting HPV and hepatitis B [59].

Ideally, for effective vaccination of any type of malignant disease, administered vaccine should activate both innate immunity and specific immune effector responses. Basically, the success of the vaccine therapy using immuno-stimulating genes depends on several parameters such as appropriateness of vector, suitable transgene design, inclusion/deletion of specific sequences, and optimization of necessary elements to induce secretion of the transgene product from the transduced cells. It also largely relies on the safe and efficient delivery of DNA into target cells. Development of the most current clinical trials has been based upon cytotoxic agents, immunotherapy and vaccination, while the mechanistic function of the DNA vaccines is different from these medicaments. They have several advantages over conventional vaccination modalities, including no risk of infection, antigen presentation by both MHC class I and class II molecules, polarizing T-cell helpers toward TH1/TH2 phenotypes, ease of preparation and cost-effectiveness [11, 60].

To date, over 730 DNA vaccines clinical trials have been undertaken. Of these, 156 are challenging different types of cancers [59]. A plasmid DNA encoding human tyrosinase (huTyr) has been approved by the US Department of Agriculture to treat canine melanoma [61]. The results supported the safety and efficacy of the huTyr DNA vaccine in dogs as adjunctive treatment for oral malignant melanoma. To date, no DNA vaccine has been approved by the U.S. Food and Drug Administration (FDA) for human, there exist more than 150 trials for different types of cancers. DNA-based vaccines have the advantage over conventional vaccines because they are able to induce both cell-mediated and humoral immunity, and to provide long-term responses with lower (in ng range) and fewer doses in a safer manner in comparison with conventional live vaccines. Further, they are cost-effective because of easier manufacturing process [56].

In 2010, sipuleucel-T (PROvenge®, Dendreon, USA) was approved by the FDA for treatment of asymptomatic/minimally symptomatic metastatic hormone-refractory prostate cancer (HRPC). PROvenge® is the first personalized medicine, which is a cellular immunotherapy agent and its administration demands 3 steps, as follow: 1) extraction of patient's antigen-presenting cells (APCs) through a leukapheresis procedure, 2) incubation with a fusion protein

PA2024 consisting of the antigen prostatic acid phosphatase (PAP) and an immune signaling factor granulocyte-macrophage colony stimulating factor (GM-CSF) that helps the APCs to mature, and 3) infusion of the activated blood product [62].

4.2. Tumor suppressor and apoptosis–inducing genes

It should be highlighted that the initiation of cancer is an intricate multi-cause process involving sequential activation of oncogenes and inactivation of tumor suppressor genes (TSGs) and apoptosis inducing genes (AIGs). Such genetic changes, subsequently, yield concomitant phenotypic alterations in the tumor cells resulting in cancer cells survival and progression. Thus, in addition to oncogenes, the tumor suppressor genes must be targeted by a designated genomedicine [63].

The pivotal roles of the TSGs and AIGs should be considered for cancer gene therapy, while little devotion has given to their biological impacts. The defects/mutated forms of these genes should be corrected through transfecting the normal forms which can be fulfilled through targeted systems; for more details on TSGs and AIGs, reader is directed to see reference [4].

4.3. Suicide gene therapy: A targeted genomedicine modality

Having harnessed suicide genes, a prodrug can be converted to a toxic metabolite. In fact, suicide gene therapy (SGT) is a unique approach that allows selective targeting through negative selection of malignant cells.

Using a designated prodrug, which can be activated only in aberrant cells producing the metabolizing enzyme, cancer cells can be specifically targeted by a nontoxic prodrug that metabolized into toxic metabolites. The herpes simplex virus thymidine kinase (HSV-TK) gene is the prototype gene, which can be transferred into tumor cells either by viral vectors or nonviral methods [64].

Suicide gene therapy using gene-directed enzyme/prodrug therapy (GEPT) was shown to improve the therapeutic efficacy of conventional cancer radiotherapy and chemotherapy without side-effects. Of the SGTs, the HSV- TK system gene therapy can sensitizes cells to the cytotoxic effects of designated drugs such as ganciclovir (GCV) and acyclovir (ACV). The HSV-TK-based SGT approach has resulted in promising outcomes in phase I/II study of glioblastoma, showing that brain injections of M11 retroviral vector-producing cells for glioblastoma HSV-1 TK gene therapy were well tolerated and associated with significant therapeutic responses [65]. Similar clinical outcomes have been reported for the treatment of melanoma [66]. In this study, although patients showed disease progression on long-term follow-up, retrovirus vector "M11"-mediated HSV-1 TK gene therapy was well tolerated over a wide dose range. Despite limited tumor response possibly due to poor gene transfer efficiency, necrosis following GCV administration in transduced tumors may indicate a potential for treatment efficacy. The HSV-TK based SGT has been reported as an effective system for treating experimental human pancreatic cancer [67].

In an interesting study, Aoi et al. capitalized on a physical method using ultrasound (US) and nano/microbubbles (NBs/MBs) to deliver exogenous genomedicines noninvasively into the target cancer cells. They successfully harnessed a low-intensity pulsed ultrasound (1 MHz; 1.3 W/cm^2) and NBs/MBs to transduce the HSV-TK system using an in vitro model. They showed that addition of GCV to the transduced cells can lead to HSV-TK/GCV-dependent apoptosis [68].

Other paradigms of this approach are cytosine deaminase/5-fluorocytosine (CD/5-FC) and carboxyl esterase/irinotecan (CE/CPT-11). Further, genetically engineered stem cells (GESTECs) have also been applied for GEPT [69]. While chemotherapy of brain tumors is often disrupted by the brain blood barrier (BBB) [70], GESTECs (consisting of neural stem cells (NSCs) expressing cytosine deaminase (CD) gene) have been employed as a novel cell therapy modality. The GESTECs were injected to xenograft mouse model of lung cancer metastasis to the brain produced through implanting the 549 lung cancer cells in the right hemisphere of the mouse brain. Two days after the injection of GESTECs, 5-fluorocytosine (5-FC) was administered via intraperitoneal injection. Histological analysis of extracted brain confirmed the therapeutic efficacy of GESTECs that converted the 5-FC into 5-fluorouracil resulting in the decreased density and aggressiveness of lung cancer cells [71].

Likewise, in a study, the GESTECs expressing either cytosine deaminase (CD) or carboxyl esterase (CE) showed profound inhibition of ovarian cancer cells SKOV-3 by converting prodrug 5-FC into 5-FU [72]. Table 2 represents the clinical trials for suicide gene therapy of cancer.

5. Immunogene therapy approaches for cancer

Cancer immunotherapy as an effective alternative treatment modality to chemotherapy arose from the notion that the immune system play a central role in prevention of the development/ progression of tumors, which is also called as immunosurveillance [73]. Perhaps the most compelling evidence for such tumor immunosurveillance is immune system activity in paraneoplastic diseases that are neurological disorders resultant from an anti-tumor immune response [74]. For progression, invasion and metastasis, a solid tumor must develop several critical abilities, including: 1) movement and migration potential, 2) capacity for degradation of extracellular matrix (ECM), 3) survival ability inside and outside of the tumor microenvironment escaping from immune system activity, and 4) propensity and quality of generation and progression in the new environment [75]. In fact, migrating malignant cells have capabilities to escape from immune system [76], invade and initiate a new life, perhaps through its pleiotrophic abilities activating a number of unique transcription factors, transporters and enzymes. Nevertheless, various solid tumors show some extend of immune system escape capabilities within the tumor microenvironment [76], where the anti-tumor immunity induced by T cells requires several mechanisms, including: a) recognition of an antigen by T cells receptors, b) co-stimulation by appropriate accessory molecules, and c) initiation of an inflammatory signal (the so called danger signal).

Inherently, based upon innate and adaptive responses of immune system, immunotherapy modalities are performed as "passive therapy" (using antibodies (Abs)/cytokines), "adaptive therapy" (in the form of the graft vs leukemia (GVL) reaction associated with the graft vs host

Clinical trial	US Trial ID	Malignancy	Intervention	Phase	Status
Randomized trial of suicide gene therapy and prostate cancer	NCT00583492	Prostate cancer	Biological: Ad5-yCD/ mutTKSR39rep-ADP; Radiation	II/III	Rg
Combining suicide gene therapy with chemoradiotherapy in the treatment of non-metastatic pancreatic adenocarcinoma	NCT00415454	Pancreatic cancer	Genetic: Ad5-yCD/ mutTKSR39rep-ADP	I	Td
Suicide gene therapy for donor lymphocytes infusion after allogeneic hematopoietic stem cell transplantation (ILD-TK01)	NCT01086735	Hematological malignancy	Biological: donor lymphocyte infusion	I/II	Rg
TK-based suicide gene therapy for hepatocellular carcinoma	NCT00844623	Carcinoma, hepatocellular	Genetic: TK99UN	I	Cd
An infectivity enhanced suicide gene expressing adenovirus for ovarian cancer in patients with recurrent ovarian and other selected gynecologic cancers	NCT00964756	Ovarian cancer	Genetic: Ad5.SSTR/ TK.RGD; Drug: GCV	I	Rg
CASPALLO: Allo-depleted T cells transduced with inducible caspase 9 suicide gene	NCT00710892	Lymphoblastic leukemia; lymphoma	Biological: Allodepleted T Cells	I	Active
Administration of donor T cells with the caspase-9 suicide gene	NCT01494103	Various types of leukemia; non-Hodgkin's lymphoma	Biological: Allodepleted T cells transduced with caspase 9; Drug: AP1903	I	Rg
Infusion of donor lymphocytes transduced with the suicide gene HSV-TK in patients with haematological malignancies	NCT00423124	Hematological malignancies	Genetic: HSV-TK	I/II	Active

Table 2. Clinical trials for suicide gene therapy of cancer. Ad5-yCD/mutTKSR39rep-ADP: Replication-competent adenovirus; Ad5: Adenovirus; yCD: Yeast cytosine deaminase; ADP: Adenovirus death protein; Td: terminated; Rg: recruiting; Cd: completed; IMRT: Intensity-modulated radiation therapy; TK99UN: An adenoviral vector containing herpes simplex virus's thymidine Kinase; GCV: Ganciclovir; AP1903: a lipid permeable, synthetic organic compound used exclusively in conjunction with a chemical inducers of dimerization (CID) therapy; HSV-TK: herpes simplex virus's thymidine Kinase. Data were adapted with permission from reference [4].

(GVH) reaction) or "active therapy" by stimulating the immune system [77]. Basically, autologous antigen-specific T cells can be expanded ex vivo and then re-infused into patients to boost T cells-based immune system activities. DCs, which play a central role in immune system activities due to their ability to control both immune tolerance and immunity, have been extensively used as a cell-based immunotherapy modality [74]. While tumor cells themselves are poor antigen-presenting cells (APCs), DCs are potent APCs. Fundamentally, the aim of DCs based immunotherapy is to elicit tumor-specific effector T cells ($CD4^+$ T cells, $CD8^+$ T cells and B cells) that can effectively reduce the tumor mass and can also induce immunological memory to control tumor relapse [74]. The first step of DCs-based vaccination is to provide DCs with tumor-specific antigens, which can be performed through ex vivo cultivation of the patients-derived DCs with an adjuvant for DC maturation and the tumor-specific antigen. The processed DCs can be then injected back into the patient. Alternatively, DCs can be induced to take up the tumor-specific antigen in vivo [74]. This approach has been harnessed as vaccination modality in various cancers. For example, phase I/II randomized trial of DCs-based vaccination with or without cyclophosphamide have recently been conducted for consolidation therapy of advanced ovarian cancer in first or second remission [58]. It was shown that the peptide-loaded DC vaccination induced modest immune responses, while the survival rate was promising [58].

In a study, Coukos' group has investigated the mechanism underlying cooperation between oncolytic HSV and host effector immune mechanisms in a syngeneic murine model of ovarian carcinoma. They showed that therapeutic administration of HSV-1716 (a replication-restricted mutant) can result in significant reduction of tumor growth and improved survival rate. Intratumoral injection of HSV-1716 elicited expression of some key elements (IFN-γ, MIG, and IP-10) and significant increase in the number of tumor-associated natural killer (NK) and CD8+ T cells. Ascites from HSV-1716-treated animals efficiently induced in vitro migration of NK and CD8+ T cells that was dependent upon the presence of MIG and IP-10, in which monocytes and DCs appeared to be responsible for the production of MIG and IP-10 [78]. This study clearly indicate that, in ovarian carcinoma, monocyte-derived DCs produced large amounts of IFN-gamma and upregulated MIG and IP-10 expression upon HSV-1716 infection, which may favor antitumor immune response upon oncolytic therapy.

Thus far, CDs-based vaccination has been harnessed in over 150 clinical trials [59]. Nevertheless, the overall results obtained from the human clinical trials capitalizing on DCs have shown promising clinical outcomes resulting in significant induction of clinically meaningful antitumor immunity even with no apparent side effects or toxicities. This modality is a perfect paradigm for personalized medicines.

6. Anti–angiogenesis gene therapy

Several critical steps are involved during angiogenesis, including: proliferation of the endothelial cells (ECs), migration of the ECs, degradation of the basement membrane, and formation of the new lumen organization. Such biological event is controlled by proangiogenesis and antiangiogenesis factors liberated by various cells (activated ECs, monocytes, smooth muscle cells, pericytes and platelets) into the blood circulation [79]. Tumors need angiogenesis for survival and growth, thus inhibition of angiogenesis can be an effective strategy for cancer therapy.

Administration of endogenous inhibitors of angiogenesis are associated with some hindrances (e.g., high dose requirements and some instability of the corresponding recombinant proteins), hence gene therapy of angiogenesis may be an effective approach to battle malignancies. It should be noted that tumors secrete a number of "angiogenesis" factors, whose encoding genes can be targeted.

Selected angiogenesis factors include: vascular endothelial growth factor (VEGF), thrombospondin-1 (THBS1), endostatin, tumstatin, arresten, canstatin, vastatin, restin, angiostatin, 16 kD human prolactin fragment (16K hPRL), platelet factor-4 (PF4), interferon-inducible protein-10 (IIP10), angiopoietins, interleukin-12 (IL-12), interleukin-18 (IL-18), interferons (IFNs), endothelial-monocyte activating polypeptide-II (EMAP-II), tissue Inhibitors of metalloproteinases (TIMPs), tumor necrosis factor-α (TNF-α, transforming growth factor (TGF), pleiotropin, fibroblast growth factor (FGF), placental growth factor (PGF), and platelet derived endothelial cell growth factor (PD-ECGF) [79]. Of these, VEGF is the most studied target. It carries out multifaceted functions in tumor development, in which several isoforms impose distinct biologic functions and clinical implications. Several strategies have been carried out to control VEGF with some successes. Coukos' group has successfully used DNA vector-based RNA interference (RNAi) by inserting RNAi sequences targeting murine VEGF isoforms in downstream of an RNA polymerase III (Pol III) promoter, which may have potential applications in isoform-specific "knock-down" of VEGF. They compared two Pol III promoters, U6 and H1, in their efficiency forsiRNA expression. Large molecular weight VEGF isoforms were specifically reduced in vitro in the presence of isoform-specific RNAi constructs. Additionally, H1 promoter may be superior to U6 promoter when used for vector-based RNAi of VEGF isoforms. They proposed this novel strategy as an effective tool to investigate the functionalities of various VEGF isoforms and also concluded that, to develop such novel RNAi strategy as a practical research tool and feasible cancer therapy approach, identifying the most efficient targeting sequence and developing an efficient delivery system are vital steps [80].

The effect of INF-β gene therapy on the growth of human prostate cancer was determined in nude mice bearing PC3MM2 cells. It was found that the intralesional delivery of adenoviaral vector encoding murine IFN-β was able to suppress the growth of tumor in a dose-dependent manner, perhaps through induction of INF-β and inducible nitric oxide synthase (iNOS) as well as reduction of basic FGF and TGF-β1 resulting in inhibition of angiogenesis [81].

In a study, rAAV vectors were constructed to express endostatin (rAAV-endostatin) or the antiangiogenic domain of thrombospondin-1 3TSR (rAAV-3TSR) and applied to a mouse angiogenesis model. The rAAV-mediated gene delivery resulted in inhibition of VEGF-induced angiogenesis, in which pretreatment of mice with i.m. or intrasplenic injection of rAAV-endostatin or rAAV-3TSR significantly inhibited tumor growth [82].

The rAAV vectors carrying IL-12 and angiostatin-like molecule (K1-3) were administered to a subcutaneous hepatoma model in mice (Hepa129 cells in C3H mice). It was found that injection of rAAV-K1-3 or rAAV-IL-12 into tumor nodules resulted in a significant dose-dependent reduction in tumor growth, while the survival rate was significantly improved in the IL-12 treated mice, but not in the K1-3 treated mice. Combined therapy of these genomedicines, however, did not further improve antitumor efficacy compared with the monotherapy [83]. Table 3 represents selected examples for angiogenic gene therapy trials.

Clinical trial	US Trial ID	Malignancy	Intervention	Phase	Status
Phase I - Pre-Radical Prostatectomy RTVP-1 Gene Therapy for Prostate Cancer	NCT00403221	Prostate Cancer	Genetic: RTVP-1 Gene	I	Cd
Trial of E10A in Head and Neck Cancer	NCT00634595	Head and neck squamous carcinoma; Nasopharyngeal carcinoma	Drug: E10A, Cisplatin, Paclitaxel	II	NA
Safety and Efficacy of Adenoviral Endostatin in the Treatment of Advanced Solid Tumor	NCT00262327	Advanced solid tumor	Drug: Antangiogenesis; Genetic: endostatin gene	I	NA
Gene Therapy in Treating Patients With Unresectable, Recurrent, or Refractory Head and Neck Cancer	NCT00004070	Head and neck cancer	Biological: interleukin-12 gene	I/II	NA
Interleukin-12 Gene Therapy in Treating Patients With Skin Metastases	NCT00028652	Metastatic cancers	Biological: interleukin-12 gene	I	Td
Interleukin-12 Gene and in Vivo Electroporation-Mediated Plasmid DNA Vaccine Therapy in Treating Patients With Merkel Cell Cancer	NCT01440816	Skin cancers	Biological: interleukin-12 gene; electroporation-mediated plasmid DNA vaccine therapy	II	Rg
Treatment of B-CLL With Autologous IL2 and CD40 Ligand-Expressing Tumor Cells + Lenalidomide	NCT01604031	Chronic lymphocytic leukemia	Biological: B-CLL Vaccine; Drug: Lenalidomide	I/II	NA

Table 3. Selected paradigms for angiogenic gene therapy trials. RTVP-1: related to testes-specific, vespid, and pathogenesis protein; Cd: completed; NA: not available; E10A: an adenovirus carrying human endostatin gene [84]; Td: terminated; Rg: recruiting. Data were adapted with permission from reference [4].

7. Targeted nanogenomedicines: Nanotechnology and gene therapy integration

Integration of nanotechnology with gene therapy has resulted in production of advanced nano-scaled genomedicines that can be armed with homing devices to deliver the gene-based cargos to the target sites through both passive and active targeting mechanisms. It should be highlighted that the lipids or polymers used for formulation should be positively charged to be able to condense the negatively charged nucleic acids. However, we have shown that both cationic lipids (CLs) and polymers may induce inadvertent intrinsic gene expression, masking/ stimulating some undesired gene activities [17, 19-21, 85, 86]. Fig. 5 represents schematic structure of the advanced nanoformulations for genomedicines.

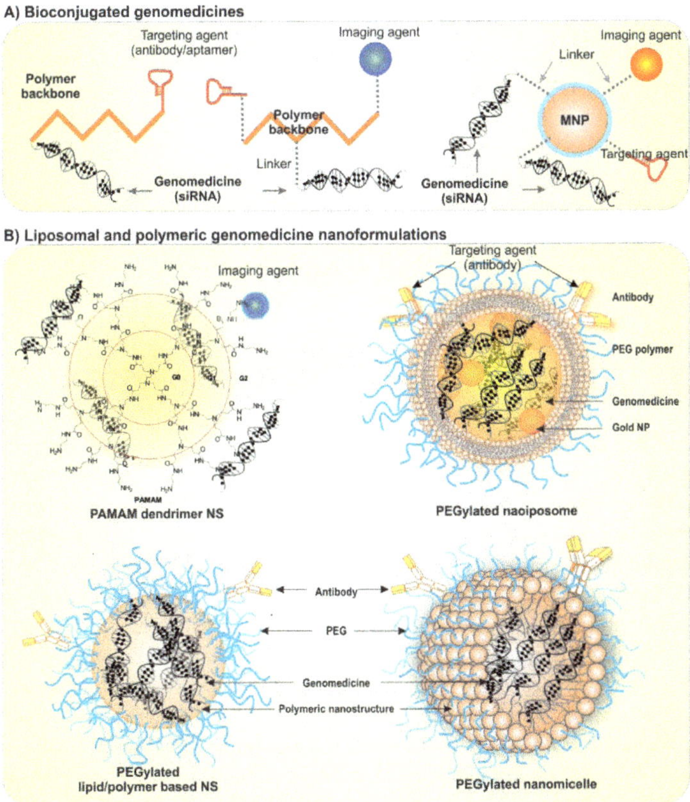

Figure 5. Schematic structures of advanced nanogenomedicines. A) Bioconjugations of genes with polymeric backbone and grafted homing and imaging moieties. B) Polymeric and liposomal gene containing nanoformulations. This figure was adapted with permission from reference [4].

7.1. Bioconjugation and PEGylation

Lipids and polymers, based upon their end groups, can be conjugated with different moieties such as imaging devices (fluorescent dyes, quantum dots) and homing devices (antibody, peptide, aptamer). Post-formulation conjugation of NPs are basically performed through chemical grafting using homobifunctional crosslinkers (*e.g.*, N-hydroxysuccinimide (NHS) esters, immidoesters, sulfhydryl-reactive crosslinkers, hydrazides) or heterobifunctional crosslinkers (*e.g.*, sulfhydryl-reactive and photoreactive crosslinkers like N-succinimidyl-3-(2-

pyridyldithio)propionate (SPDP), LC-SPDP, and Sulfo-LC-SPDP) [87]. Decoration with homing devices can arm them to target cancer cells and deliver the gene-based cargo directly to the tumor microenvironment and thereby cancer cells, but not normal cells/tissues. Antibodies can be modified via amine groups using 2-iminothiolane (Traut's reagent) and conjugated to NPs. They can also be activated with, N-succinimidyl S-acetylthioacetate (SATA) or SPDP, in which the active NHS ester end of SATA or SPDP can react with amino groups in proteins and other molecules to form a stable amide linkage. Further, conjugation of the NPs with PEG (the so called PEGylation) can favor the pharmacokinetics of these NPs prolonging the circulation period that grant a proper time frame for NPs' accumulation in the tumor microenvironment. Although attaching poly ethylene glycol (PEG) (i.e., PEGylation) is the most effective method to reduce protein immunogenicity and to avoid the RES system clearance, several other polymers have successfully been implemented as alternative to PEG, including poloxamer, polyvinyl alcohol, poly(amino acid)s, and polysaccharide. However, PEG is still the most widely used polymer to engineer stealth NPs [88]. For nanoliposomes, PEG-lipid (such as PEG-DSPE) is usually inserted into liposomes to form a hydrated layer on the liposome surface.

7.2. Bioimpacts of nanogenomedicines

Typically, tumor microvasculature display discontinuous fenestrated morphology characteristics with gaps and pores between endothelial cells, in which the pore sizes are at a range of 100 nm to 1000 nm [89]. For instance, subcutaneously grown tumors were reported to have profound fenestration, showing pore sizes at a range of 200 nm to 1200 nm [90]. Most tissues present tight junctions between cells with intercellular openings smaller than 2 nm and around 6 nm in post-capillary venules, and tissues with discontinuous fenestrated endothelium such as kidney glomerulus and sinusoidal endothelium of liver have larger junctions with pore sizes of 40-60 nm and 70-150 nm, respectively [91]. As a result, NPs with size ranging 150-250 nm can substantially extravasate showing significant enhanced permeation and retention (EPR) effects within the tumor microenvironment [92]. Since long circulation of NPs in blood is a pivotal requirement for their successful *in vivo* applications, they are basically grafted with PEG that provide greater hydrophilicity and longer circulation in blood resulting in greater accumulation within the tumor microenvironment [93]. The naked gene based medicines such as AS-ODN and siRNA can be simply degraded and destroyed by the nuclease enzymes within blood, thereby not being taken up by the target cells and even giving a rise to undesired harmful immune reactions. Thus, nano-scaled protected gene medicines will provide desired canonical outcomes. Recently, it was shown that the siRNA protected by cyclodextrin-containing polymers (the basis of the RONDEL platform) can literally get to the proposed target site and impose the intended impacts [94].

7.3. Liposomal NPs

Nanoliposomes are basically formulated using solvent evaporation method to make lipid film that is then subjected to hydration. In the presence of surfactant, the hydrated lipids form multilamellar vesicles (MLVs) and unilamellar vesicles (ULVs) with a diverse size, ranging from μm to nm, respectively. Sonication, homogenization and extrusion are the methods used for preparation of liposomes. In practice, based on end-point aims, different compositions of lipids can be used to engineer the intended liposomes. Mainly, lipophilic compounds (*e.g.*, phosphatidylcholine (PC), cholesterol (Chol), designated amounts of functionalized lipids and lipophilic drugs) are dissolved in a solvent (*e.g.*, chloroform or 3:1 ratio of chloroform: methanol). To form lipid film, the solvent is then evaporated using a rotary evaporator at 40-60 °C. The lipid film is rehydrated with stirring (~250 rpm) for 1 hr in the presence of surfactant such as Tween 20/Tween 80 under pulsed sonication (20 s ON, 10 s OFF intervals to avoid over-heating) for 10 min. As an alternative approach, the mixture can be homogenized by a high-speed homogenizer at 16,000 rpm for 5 min. To make uniform nanoliposomes, they can be extruded through polycarbonate filters with a designated pore size of (*e.g.*, 200 nm or 100 nm) for several times. The nanoliposomes can be then lyophilized for future use, reader is directed to see [95]. Mixture of polycationic lipids with plasmid DNAs can form self-assembled liposomal structures. To this end, several lipids have been exploited [96, 97], including: mixture of dioleoyl phosphatidylethanolamine (DOPE); 1,2-di-O-octadecenyl-3-trimethylammonium propane (DOTMA); N-(1-(2,3-dioleyloxy)propyl)-N-(2-(sperminecarboxamido)ethyl)-N,N-dimethy- lammonium trifluoroacetate (DOSPA); N,N-distearyl-N,N-dimethylammonium bromide (DDAB); dioctadecylamidoglycyl carboxyspermine (DOGS); N-(2,3-dioley-loxy)propyl)-N,N,N-trimethylammonium chloride (DOTAP); N-(1,2-dimyristyloxyprop-3-yl)-N,N-dimethyl-N-hydroxyethyl ammonium bromide (DMRIE); dioleyl-N,N-dimethylammonium chloride (DODAC); dipalmitoylphosphatidylcholine (DPPC); and 3β-(N-(N',N'-dimethylaminoethane)-carbamoyl)cholesterol (DC-Chol). However, most of these cationic lipids induce nonspecific gene expressions [17, 20, 85].

CLs are able to yield relatively high transfection efficiency in vitro and in vivo, and accordingly they have been progressed toward clinical trials. Precise advantages of this approach are 1) the simplicity of the DNA/liposome formulation as lipoplex, 2) the stability of the formulation and gene components protection, and 3) the robustness and applicability of the method for delivery to different types of solid tumors. For example, using cationic lipids, 16K hPRL was formulated as cationic liposomes and administered subcutaneously to a B16F10 mouse melanoma model. The results revealed that administration of the liposomal formulation of 16K hPRL gene can effectively maintain antiangiogenic activities in mice [98]. Table 4 represents selected gene therapy trials using liposomal formulations.

In another study, to monitor breast cancer processes, a unique liposomal formulation was applied as quantitative bioluminescence imaging (BLI) method. A breast cancer model was created by injection of 4T1 cells carrying a reporter system encoding a double fusion reporter gene consisting of firefly luciferase (Fluc) and green fluorescent protein (GFP) into BALB/c mice. Nanoliposomes loaded with a triple fusion gene containing HSV-TK and renilla luciferase (Rluc) and red fluorescent protein (RFP) were administered, and subsequently mice were treated with GCV. This approach resulted in monitoring of the tumor growth by BLI, while the treatment delivery of nanoliposomes was efficiently tracked by Rluc imaging [99]. Further, to avoid rapid clearance by RES after an intravenous injection, stealth PEGylated liposomes have resulted increased serum half-life and greater EPR. These stealth nanolipo-

Clinical trial	US Trial ID	Malignancy	Intervention	Phase	Status
Gene Therapy in Treating Patients With Advanced Head and Neck Cancer	NCT00009841	Advanced head and neck cancer	Liposomal formulation of EGFR antisense	I	NA
FUS1-nanoparticles and Erlotinib in Stage IV Lung Cancer	NCT01455389	Lung cancer	DOTAP:Chol-fus1; Erlotinib; Dexamethasone	I/II	Active
Study to Determine the Maximum Tolerated Dose of LErafAON in Patients With Advanced Solid Tumors	NCT00024661	Advanced solid tumors	LErafAON	I	Cd
EphA2 Gene Targeting Using Neutral Liposomal Small Interfering RNA Delivery	NCT01591356	Advanced solid tumors	siRNA-EphA2-DOPC liposomes	I	NA
C-VISA BikDD: Liposome in Advanced Pancreatic Cancer	NCT00968604	Advanced pancreatic cancer	BikDD Nanoparticles	I	Active

Table 4. Gene therapy clinical trials using liposomal formulations. EGFR: epidermal growth factor receptor; NA: not available; Cd: completed; LErafAON: liposomes carrying antisense oligonucleotide against the Raf-1 protein; siRNA: small interfering RNA; EphA2: ephrin type-A receptor 2; C-VISA BikDD: liposome consists of a pancreatic-cancer-specific expression vector "VISA" (VP16-GAL4-WPRE integrated systemic amplifier) and a pancreatic-cancer-specific promoter CCKAR (cholecystokinin type A receptor) (CCKAR-VISA or C-VISA) which drives expression of the gene BikDD, a mutant form of the potent proapoptotic gene Bik (Bcl-2 interacting killer). Data were adapted with permission from reference [4].

somes can be further decorated with homing devices (Ab, ligand) and imaging devices to develop targeted stealth nanoliposome for safe i.v. delivery of gene based medicines [100]. For example, transferrin (Trf) receptor-targeted liposomes (Trf-liposomes) encapsulating anti-BCR-ABL genomedicine (siRNA or AS-ODN) has resulted in significant delivery of cargo genes in chronic myeloid leukemia [101]. Folate receptor-targeted liposomes have also been used as cancer specific vectors [102]. For efficient delivery of siRNA to neuroblastoma (the most common solid tumor in early childhood), Adrian et al. engineered liposomal nanoformulation (190 to 240 nm) containing siRNA armed with anti-Disialoganglioside (GD2) Ab for selective interaction with neuroblastoma cells [103]. They showed a significant association of liposomes with neuroblastoma cells and effective delivery of siRNA with anti-GD2 Ab-armed liposomes.

7.4. Polymeric gene delivery nanosystems

To engineer polymeric NPs, various synthetic and biodegradable polymers have so far been exploited. Of these, biodegradable polymers provide better clinical outcomes. Among biodegradable polymers, poly(lactic-co-glycolic acid) (PLGA) as a copolymer approved by FDA is the most widely used polymer. For engineering PLGA NPs, depending on physicochemical property of drug and desired emulsion (single or double), solvent evaporation or solvent diffusion methods are mainly recruited [104]. We have developed folate receptor targeting PEGylated PLGA NPs for delivery of nucleic acids (Fig. 6).

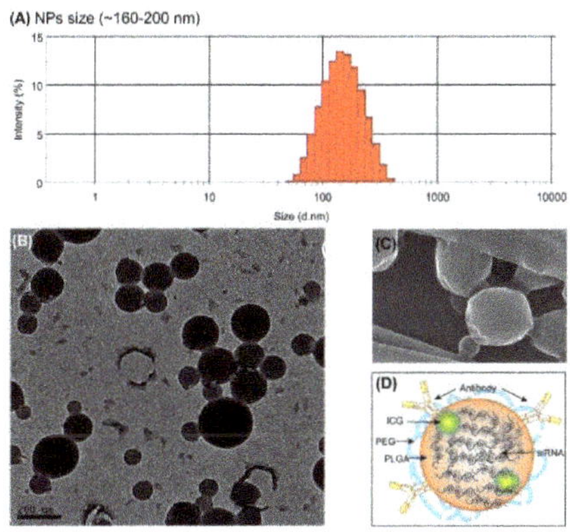

Figure 6. Size and morphology of PLGA nanoparticles. A) Dynamic light scattering (DLC) analysis of PEGylated PLGA NPs encapsulating siRNA. B) Transmission electron microscopy (TEM) micrograph of PLGA NPs. C) Scanning electron microscopy (SEM) micrograph of clusters of PLGA NPs. D) Schematic presentation of antibody armed PEGylated PLGA nanoparticle (our unpublished data).

Self-assembled micellar nanoformulations are another type of NPs that are widely used as gene delivery nanosystems, in which the positively charged polymers can interact with the negatively charged nucleic acids forming nanomicelles under sonication. Cationic polymers (e.g., linear and branched polyethyleneimine (l-PEI and b-PEI), poly(L-lysine), and polyamidoamine (PAMAM) dendrimers) can condense the nucleic acids forming polyplexes as either uni-molecular or multi-molecular complexes. Unfortunately, similar to CLs, cationic polymers can also induce intrinsic toxicogenomics [86] and cytotoxicity [16]. To achieve efficient target-specific gene transfer, these polymers can covalently be modified by conjugating targeting ligands. The ligand-armed systems can then target the cells that present the specific cellular receptors. Because of their nano-scaled size (100-200 nm in diameter), they can be taken up by cells through receptor-mediated endocytosis. For example, a Trf-modified cyclodextrin polymer-based gene delivery nanosystem has been developed. These Trf-armed PEGylated cyclodextrin show increased stability in biological fluids and active targeting potential via transferrin, retaining high binding affinity toward Trf receptor and profound transfection of the target leukemia cells (K562 cells) through both passive and active targeting [105]. Recently, Hatefi's group engineered a novel multi-domain biopolymer, consisting of: 1) repeating units of arginine and histidine to condense pDNA and lyse endosome membranes, 2) a HER2 affibody as targeting moety, 3) a pH responsive fusogenic peptide to destabilize endosome membranes and enhance endosomolytic activity of histidine residues, and 4) a nuclear localization signal to enhance translocation of pDNA towards the cell nucleus [106]. They showed that pDNA was condensed into biopolymeric Nps and protected from serum endonucleases, while targeting HER2 positive cancer cells, and metabolized by endogenous furin enzymes to reduce potential toxicity. Later on, synthesis of a targeted PEI polymer was reported, in which the PEI polymer was conjugated to angiogenic vessel-homing peptide Ala-Pro-Arg-Pro-Gly (APRPG) through PEG spacer [107]. The PEI-PEG-APRPG was shown to effectively condense siRNA into 20-50 nm NPs that can substantially impose inhibitory effects in vitro with profound EPR in vivo targeting tumor vasculature through VEGF.

8. Tissue specific gene therapy

In addition to targeted nanomedicine gene therapies, tissue specific gene therapy provides a robust targeted approach. We describe some of the cell/tissue specific applications in the following sections.

8.1. Cancer Stem Cells (CSCs)

Some of the transit-amplifying cells in the cancer population appear to remain immature within the differentiating cells. These classes of cells that act as cancer cells progenitor are called cancer stem cells, which are deemed to be one of the reasons for cancer relapse that are hardly responsive for treatment. The poor prognosis and responsiveness of patients with relapsed aggressive metastatic tumors necessitate the development of more effective tumor-selective therapies towards cells that cause such relapse, while the conventional therapy target the differentiated cancer cells. Therefore, to be maximally effective, gene therapy of cancer should target both the resting stem cells and the proliferating cells of the cancer [108]. To this end, several translational approaches have been undertaken to target CSCs, including use of oncolytic viruses that may offer an effective way to specifically target and eradicate CSCs. Of these, conditionally replicative adenoviruses (CRAd) are considered as promising virotherapy systems [109]. Considering the plasticity of CSCs, apoptosis-inducing strategy can be used to eliminate these cells by harnessing genes such as TRAIL, BCL-2 family and XIAP as targeted therapies [110].

8.2. Mesenchymal Stem Cells (MSCs) as a gene therapy carrier

To date, as a personalized medicine, cell-based therapy of cancer has been considered as a promising modality. Of these, MSCs seem to hold great potential as targeted-delivery vehicle in cancer gene therapy [111]. Their propagation in culture is simple, also shows contingency toward genetic modification in order to express therapeutic proteins. Above all, MSCs possess inherent tumor-tropic and migratory properties that allow them to serve as robust cell based carrier as targeted drug delivery systems for isolated tumors and metastatic diseases [112]. In a study, the migration ability of MSCs toward prostate cancer cells (in vitro and in vivo) and incorporating into the tumor mass was investigated. The infected cells with HSV-TK gene were shown to maintain their tumor tropism capabilities and significantly inhibited the growth of subcutaneous PC3 prostate cancer xenografts in nude mice in the presence of GCV [113]. Similar strategy was applied to evaluate the impact of the suicide gene therapy by MSCs in normal cells in brain using a rat model. It was found that the tumoricidal bystander effect in the HSV-TK gene therapy using MSCs and GCV does not injure normal brain tissues [114]. In another study, umbilical cord blood MSCs were used to deliver the transgenic LIGHT (TNFSF14) to the target tumor cells in vivo. The transfected MSCs with lentiviral vectors carrying LIGHT genes demonstrated a strong suppressive effect on tumor growth, in which pathological sections of the tumor tissues showed significant induction of apoptosis and occurrence of tumor necrosis in tumor cells [115]. The potential of genetically modified MSCs expressing IFN-β was assessed in an immuno-competent mouse model of prostate cancer lung metastasis. Significant reduction in tumor volume in lungs was seen following IFN- β expressing MSC therapy, perhaps through induction of apoptosis and increase in the natural kill cell activity [116]. The MSC-based gene therapy is still in its infancy era and need much more investigation prior to its clinical applications even though the MSCs themselves are under clinical trials [117].

8.3. Tissue–specific promoters and inducible promoters

Tissue-specific promoters (TSPs), a powerful tool for decreasing the toxicity of cancer gene therapy to normal tissues, have been used as targeted gene therapy approach. TSPs have been utilized for specific mutation compensation or delivery of prodrug-converting enzymes and also for controlling crucial viral replication regulators and consequent restriction of replication to tumor cells [118]. The safety and contingency of this approach has been shown in some initial clinical trials [119]. Of these, the cytomegalovirus (CMV) immediate-early promoter is often harnessed in gene therapy since it can express target genes at high levels in tumor cells. Lin et al. (2001) examined the effects of the involucrin (INV), keratin 14 (K14) and CMV promoters on the expression of the reporter gene beta-galactosidase. They introduce the plasmid DNA to BALB/c mice using a gene gun, and examined the skin biopsies. They found that the K14 and INV promoter constructs could induce the beta-galactosidase gene expression only in the epidermis, while the CMV promoter was able to elicit gene expression in both the dermis and epidermis [120]. To increase promoter strength while maintaining tissue specificity, Qiao et al. (2002) constructed a recombinant adenovirus encompassing a binary promoter system with a tumor-specific promoter carcinoembryonic antigen (CEA) driving a transcription transactivator with capability to express a HSV-TK. After successful application in vitro, they employed noninvasive nuclear imaging using a radioiodinated nucleoside (fraluridine (FIAU)) serving as a substrate for HSV-TK in BALB/C mice model. The results indicated the accumulated radioactivity only in the area of CEA-positive tumors after intratumoral injection, in which significantly less spread was observed to the adjacent liver tissue [121]. In another study, a vector with the human minimal tyrosinase promoter and two human enhancer elements (2hE-hTyrP) was compared with different hybrid promoter constructs containing tyrosinase regulatory sequences and the viral simian virus 40 (SV40) promoters. The hybrid SV40-based promoters were effective in vitro, and the in vivo tissue specificity of the 2hE-hTyrP vector was demonstrated in subcutaneous xenografted tumors model [122]. Another plausible approach to specifically target tumor cells for gene expression is to harness promoter elements that become activated in chemotherapy-resistant tumor cells [123]. In addition to TSPs, inducible promoters (IPs) can be exploited to minimize target gene expression in normal cells. Harnessing the IPs, the timing of the gene expression can be modulated and controlled. Of a large number of inducible systems developed, only a few were translated into clinical gene therapy trials, including radiation-inducible genes [124]. Using this cancer gene therapy modality, promoters of radiation-inducible genes are exploited to drive transcription of transgenes in response to radiation, resulting in increased responsiveness of cancer cells to radiotherapy. These constructs, delivered by adenoviral vectors, can activate a transgene encoding a cytotoxic protein in tumor cells, in which the tumoricidal effects can be then localized temporally and spatially by X-rays. Perhaps, TNFerade (GenVec, Inc) is the best paradigm, which is an adenoviral vector containing radiation-inducible elements of the early growth response-1 promoter upstream of a cDNA encoding human TNF-α [125]. It has been translated into several clinical applications, e.g., as the first-line treatment of locally advanced pancreatic cancer in combination with 5-FU and radiotherapy [126]. However, it has not been approved.

9. Translational hurdles

Over the last couple of decades, various gene-based medicines have been developed in vitro with great potential to be translated for in vivo uses in clinic. It has been evinced that the gene therapy approach by virtue carries a certain degree of risk, thus the design and development of such modality need to meet the entire scientific and regulatory requirements. Some of the risks are procedural hazards (e.g. for parenteral medicaments), while some others happen to be specific to the genomedicine per se (e.g., immunologic reaction of viral vectors or nonspecific impacts of the delivered genes). All scientific, ethical, legal and social implications of this novel modality to genetic disease are involved for its successful translation. Fig. 7 schematically epitomizes the complexity of the steps for development and translation of gene-medicine for immunogene therapy of ovarian cancer.

In immunogene therapy, for example, stimulation of the cellular immune system to recognize and obliterate the cancer cells with genes encoding a variety of cytokines (e.g., interleukin-2 (IL-2), granulocyte - macrophage colony-stimulating factor (GM-CSF), co-stimulatory molecules such as CD80 and CD86) can 1) increase the immunogenicity of the transfected autologous tumour cells, 2) increase the likelihood of generating a tumor-specific cytotoxic T-lymphocyte (CTL) response. In the ex vivo transfection of antigen-presenting cells (APCs), the cells are transfected with a gene encoding a tumor-specific antigen (e.g., carcinoembryonic antigen, CEA) that is presented by major histocompatibility complex (MHC) class I molecules to antigen-specific CTLs via the T-cell receptor (TCR). Stimulated CTLs can find and eradicate the residual CEA-expressing tumor cells, in which GM-CSF can increase the activation of APCs and their migration into the tumor microenvironment [1].

Further, some degree of knowledge of industrial drug development is critical for innovation in this new sector, while healthcare systems and industries need to undertake more translatable approaches to fasten the in terms of cancer gene therapy.

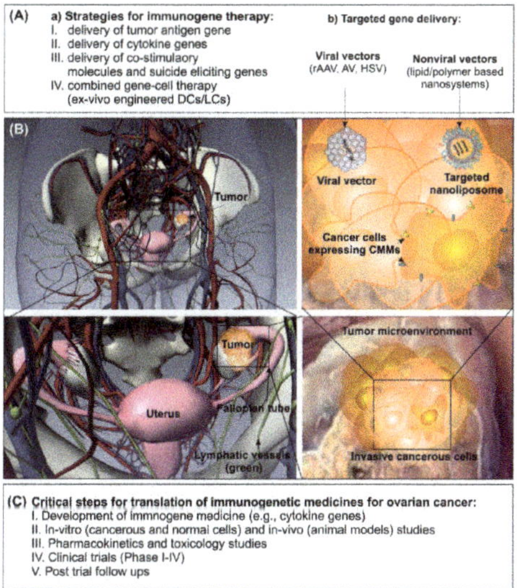

Figure 7. Schematic representation of translational approach for immunogene therapy of ovarian cancer. A) Design of the immunogene therapy based on a) different strategies of gene therapy and b) different gene delivery systems. B) Anatomical and cellular complexity of the ovarian cancer cells that need to be specifically targeted using advanced gene delivery systems and cancer marker molecules (CMMs). C) Various stages for translation of immunogenetic medicine.

10. Final remarks

Cancer gene therapy continues to grow even though clinical applications of this approach demand further investigations. Trajectory of gene therapy shows great impacts of genomedicines (i.e., As-ODNs, siRNA, Ribozymes, DNAzyme) both cell based and animal models, while tumor antigen-specific vaccines and DNA vaccines appear to be the most promising modalities. While suicide gene therapy, immunogene therapy and angiogenic gene therapy continue to become a mature modality, integration of nanotechnology toward development of multifunctional nanoparticles appear to provide a resilient, yet versatile, platform for targeted cancer gene therapy as "nano-genoceuticals". Rise of MSCs based cancer gene therapies may also open a new chapter as "cyto-genoceuticals". More than 65% of the gene therapy trials have been devoted to the cancer diseases; however, less than 3% of these trials have been progressed to the phase II/III stages and only few to the phase IV stage. The first approved cancer vaccination (Sipuleucel-T) has resulted in great clinical corollaries. Still many tumor suppressor and apoptosis-inducing genes can be evaluated for clinical applications. Attributable to intricate nature of malignant diseases, to achieve more effective gene therapy against cancer, genomedicines need to be advanced to be able to holistically target the most cancer causing genes. It is also essential to target both the tumor cells and other cancer associated players of the tumor microenvironment including: tumor microvasculature and tumor associated cells, stromal cells and CSCs.

Author details

Yadollah Omidi[1,2], Jaleh Barar[1,2] and George Coukos[1,3]

1 Ovarian Cancer Research Center, Perelman School of Medicine, University of Pennsylvania, Philadelphia, PA, USA

2 Research Center for Pharmaceutical Nanotechnology, Faculty of Pharmacy, Tabriz University of Medical Sciences, Tabriz, Iran

3 Ludwig Center for Cancer Research, University of Lausanne, Lausanne, Switzerland

References

[1] Kerr, D. Clinical development of gene therapy for colorectal cancer. Nat Rev Cancer. (2003)., 3(8), 615-22.

[2] Mellman, I, Coukos, G, & Dranoff, G. Cancer immunotherapy comes of age. Nature. (2011)., 480(7378), 480-9.

[3] Majidi, J, Barar, J, Baradaran, B, Abdolalizadeh, J, & Omidi, Y. Target therapy of cancer: implementation of monoclonal antibodies and nanobodies. Hum Antibodies. (2009)., 18(3), 81-100.

[4] Barar, J, & Omidi, Y. Translational Approaches toward Cancer Gene Therapy: Hurdles and Hopes. BioImpacts. (2012)., 2(3), 127-43.

[5] The Journal of Gene Medicine Clinical Trial siteJohn Wiley & Son (http://www.abedia.com/wiley/index.html),accessed on 12 Aug (2012).

[6] Weber, G. F. Molecular Mechanisms of Cancer. Dordrecht: Springer; (2007).

[7] King RJBRobins MW. Cancer Biology. 3rd ed. Harlow: Pearson Education Limited; (2006).

[8] Liu, X, Li, J, Tian, Y, Xu, P, Chen, X, Xie, K, et al. Enhanced pancreatic cancer gene therapy by combination of adenoviral vector expressing c-erb-B2 (Her-2/neu)-targeted immunotoxin with a replication-competent adenovirus or etoposide. Hum Gene Ther. (2010)., 21(2), 157-70.

[9] Candolfi, M, Kroeger, K. M, Muhammad, A. K, Yagiz, K, Farrokhi, C, Pechnick, R. N, et al. Gene therapy for brain cancer: combination therapies provide enhanced efficacy and safety. Curr Gene Ther. (2009)., 9(5), 409-21.

[10] Rachakatla, R. S, Pyle, M. M, Ayuzawa, R, Edwards, S. M, Marini, F. C, Weiss, M. L, et al. Combination treatment of human umbilical cord matrix stem cell-based inter-

feron-beta gene therapy and 5-fluorouracil significantly reduces growth of metastatic human breast cancer in SCID mouse lungs. Cancer Invest. (2008). , 26(7), 662-70.

[11] Stevenson, F. K, Ottensmeier, C. H, & Rice, J. DNA vaccines against cancer come of age. Curr Opin Immunol. (2010). , 22(2), 264-70.

[12] Vassaux, G, & Martin-duque, P. Use of suicide genes for cancer gene therapy: study of the different approaches. Expert Opin Biol Ther. (2004). , 4(4), 519-30.

[13] Wacheck, V, & Zangemeister-wittke, U. Antisense molecules for targeted cancer therapy. Crit Rev Oncol Hematol. (2006). , 59(1), 65-73.

[14] Devi, G. R. siRNA-based approaches in cancer therapy. Cancer Gene Ther. (2006). , 13(9), 819-29.

[15] Dougherty, G. J, & Dougherty, S. T. Exploiting the tumor microenvironment in the development of targeted cancer gene therapy. Cancer Gene Ther. (2009). , 16(3), 279-90.

[16] Kafil, V, & Omidi, Y. Cytotoxic impacts of linear and branched polyethylenimine nanostructures in A431 cells. BioImpacts. (2011). , 1(1), 23-30.

[17] Omidi, Y, Hollins, A. J, Benboubetra, M, Drayton, R, Benter, I. F, & Akhtar, S. Toxicogenomics of non-viral vectors for gene therapy: a microarray study of lipofectin- and oligofectamine-induced gene expression changes in human epithelial cells. J Drug Target. (2003). , 11(6), 311-23.

[18] Omidi, Y, Hollins, A. J, Drayton, R. M, & Akhtar, S. Polypropylenimine dendrimer-induced gene expression changes: the effect of complexation with DNA, dendrimer generation and cell type. J Drug Target. (2005). , 13(7), 431-43.

[19] Hollins, A. J, Omidi, Y, Benter, I. F, & Akhtar, S. Toxicogenomics of drug delivery systems: Exploiting delivery system-induced changes in target gene expression to enhance siRNA activity. J Drug Target. (2007). , 15(1), 83-8.

[20] Omidi, Y, Barar, J, Heidari, H. R, Ahmadian, S, Yazdi, H. A, & Akhtar, S. Microarray analysis of the toxicogenomics and the genotoxic potential of a cationic lipid-based gene delivery nanosystem in human alveolar epithelial a549 cells. Toxicol Mech Methods. (2008). , 18(4), 369-78.

[21] Barar, J, Hamzeiy, H, Mortazavi-tabatabaei, S. A, Hashemi-aghdam, S. E, & Omidi, Y. Genomic signature and toxicogenomics comparison of polycationic gene delivery nanosystems in human alveolar epithelial A549 cells. Daru. (2009). , 17(3), 139-47.

[22] Omidi, Y, & Barar, J. Induction of human alveolar epithelial cell growth factor receptors by dendrimeric nanostructures. Int J Toxicol. (2009). , 28(2), 113-22.

[23] Zhang, X, Chen, Z, Chen, Y, & Tong, T. Delivering antisense telomerase RNA by a hybrid adenovirus/ adeno-associated virus significantly suppresses the malignant

phenotype and enhances cell apoptosis of human breast cancer cells. Oncogene. (2003). , 22(16), 2405-16.

[24] Wu, S, Meng, L, Wang, S, Wang, W, Xi, L, Tian, X, et al. Reversal of the malignant phenotype of cervical cancer CaSki cells through adeno-associated virus-mediated delivery of HPV16 E7 antisense RNA. Clin Cancer Res. (2006). Pt 1) 2032-7.

[25] Hollins, A. J, Benboubetra, M, Omidi, Y, Zinselmeyer, B. H, Schatzlein, A. G, Uchegbu, I. F, et al. Evaluation of generation 2 and 3 poly(propylenimine) dendrimers for the potential cellular delivery of antisense oligonucleotides targeting the epidermal growth factor receptor. Pharm Res. (2004). , 21(3), 458-66.

[26] Nakhlband, A, Barar, J, Bidmeshkipour, A, Heidari, H. R, & Omidi, Y. Bioimpacts of anti epidermal growth factor receptor antisense complexed with polyamidoamine dendrimers in human lung epithelial adenocarcinoma cells. J Biomed Nanotechnol. (2010). , 6(4), 360-9.

[27] Wiechen, K. c-e. r. b. B. Antisense Oligonucleotides Inhibit Serum-Induced Cell Spreading of Ovarian Cancer Cells. Methods Mol Med. (2001).

[28] Zhao, F. J, Zhang, S. L, Ma, L, Gao, H, & Zong, Z. H. Inhibitory effects of c-erbB-2 antisense oligonucleotide transfection on uterine endometrial cancer Ishikawa cell lines. Eur J Gynaecol Oncol. (2009). , 30(1), 54-9.

[29] Loriot, Y, Mordant, P, Brown, B. D, Bourhis, J, Soria, J. C, & Deutsch, E. Inhibition of BCL-2 in small cell lung cancer cell lines with oblimersen, an antisense BCL-2 oligodeoxynucleotide (ODN): in vitro and in vivo enhancement of radiation response. Anticancer Res. (2010). , 30(10), 3869-78.

[30] Moulder, S. L, Symmans, W. F, Booser, D. J, Madden, T. L, Lipsanen, C, Yuan, L, et al. Phase I/II study of G3139 (Bcl-2 antisense oligonucleotide) in combination with doxorubicin and docetaxel in breast cancer. Clin Cancer Res. (2008). , 14(23), 7909-16.

[31] Yamanaka, K, Rocchi, P, Miyake, H, Fazli, L, So, A, Zangemeister-wittke, U, et al. Induction of apoptosis and enhancement of chemosensitivity in human prostate cancer LNCaP cells using bispecific antisense oligonucleotide targeting Bcl-2 and Bcl-xL genes. BJU Int. (2006). , 97(6), 1300-8.

[32] Fidias, P, Pennell, N. A, Boral, A. L, Shapiro, G. I, Skarin, A. T, Eder, J. P, et al. Phase I study of the c-raf-1 antisense oligonucleotide ISIS 5132 in combination with carboplatin and paclitaxel in patients with previously untreated, advanced non-small cell lung cancer. J Thorac Oncol. (2009). , 4(9), 1156-62.

[33] Rudin, C. M, Holmlund, J, Fleming, G. F, Mani, S, Stadler, W. M, Schumm, P, et al. Phase I Trial of ISIS 5132, an antisense oligonucleotide inhibitor of c-raf-1, administered by 24-hour weekly infusion to patients with advanced cancer. Clin Cancer Res. (2001). , 7(5), 1214-20.

[34] Arteaga, C. L, & Holt, J. T. Tissue-targeted antisense c-fos retroviral vector inhibits established breast cancer xenografts in nude mice. Cancer Res. (1996). , 56(5), 1098-103.

[35] Li, Y. Q, Tao, K. S, Ren, N, & Wang, Y. H. Effect of c-fos antisense probe on prostaglandin E2-induced upregulation of vascular endothelial growth factor mRNA in human liver cancer cells. World J Gastroenterol. (2005). , 11(28), 4427-30.

[36] Abaza, M. S, Al-saffar, A, & Al-sawan, S. Al-Attiyah R. c-myc antisense oligonucleotides sensitize human colorectal cancer cells to chemotherapeutic drugs. Tumour Biol. (2008). , 29(5), 287-303.

[37] Iversen, P. L, Arora, V, Acker, A. J, Mason, D. H, & Devi, G. R. Efficacy of antisense morpholino oligomer targeted to c-myc in prostate cancer xenograft murine model and a Phase I safety study in humans. Clin Cancer Res. (2003). , 9(7), 2510-9.

[38] Mcmanus, M. T, & Sharp, P. A. Gene silencing in mammals by small interfering RNAs. Nat Rev Genet. (2002). , 3(10), 737-47.

[39] Gondi, C. S, & Rao, J. S. Concepts in in vivo siRNA delivery for cancer therapy. J Cell Physiol. (2009). , 220(2), 285-91.

[40] Aigner, A. Cellular delivery in vivo of siRNA-based therapeutics. Curr Pharm Des. (2008). , 14(34), 3603-19.

[41] Taratula, O, Garbuzenko, O, Savla, R, Wang, Y. A, He, H, & Minko, T. Multifunctional nanomedicine platform for cancer specific delivery of siRNA by superparamagnetic iron oxide nanoparticles-dendrimer complexes. Curr Drug Deliv. (2011). , 8(1), 59-69.

[42] Patil, Y. B, Swaminathan, S. K, Sadhukha, T, Ma, L, & Panyam, J. The use of nanoparticle-mediated targeted gene silencing and drug delivery to overcome tumor drug resistance. Biomaterials. (2010). , 31(2), 358-65.

[43] Akita, H, Kogure, K, Moriguchi, R, Nakamura, Y, Higashi, T, Nakamura, T, et al. Nanoparticles for ex vivo siRNA delivery to dendritic cells for cancer vaccines: programmed endosomal escape and dissociation. J Control Release. (2010). , 143(3), 311-7.

[44] Mao, C. Q, Du, J. Z, Sun, T. M, Yao, Y. D, Zhang, P. Z, Song, E. W, et al. A biodegradable amphiphilic and cationic triblock copolymer for the delivery of siRNA targeting the acid ceramidase gene for cancer therapy. Biomaterials. (2011). , 32(11), 3124-33.

[45] Dass, C. R, Choong, P. F, & Khachigian, L. M. DNAzyme technology and cancer therapy: cleave and let die. Mol Cancer Ther. (2008). , 7(2), 243-51.

[46] Tsuchida, T, Kijima, H, Oshika, Y, Tokunaga, T, Abe, Y, Yamazaki, H, et al. Hammerhead ribozyme specifically inhibits mutant K-ras mRNA of human pancreatic cancer cells. Biochem Biophys Res Commun. (1998). , 253(2), 368-73.

[47] Song, M. S, Jeong, J. S, Ban, G, Lee, J. H, Won, Y. S, Cho, K. S, et al. Validation of tissue-specific promoter-driven tumor-targeting trans-splicing ribozyme system as a multifunctional cancer gene therapy device in vivo. Cancer Gene Ther. (2009). , 16(2), 113-25.

[48] Liu, J, & Lu, Y. Design of asymmetric DNAzymes for dynamic control of nanoparticle aggregation states in response to chemical stimuli. Org Biomol Chem. (2006). , 4(18), 3435-41.

[49] Li, C, Sasaroli, D, Chen, X, Hu, J, Sandaltzopoulos, R, Omidi, Y, et al. Tumor vascular biomarkers: new opportunities for cancer diagnostics. Cancer Biomark. (2010).

[50] Wang, F. Q, Barfield, E, Dutta, S, Pua, T, & Fishman, D. A. VEGFR-2 silencing by small interference RNA (siRNA) suppresses LPA-induced epithelial ovarian cancer (EOC) invasion. Gynecol Oncol. (2009). , 115(3), 414-23.

[51] Jaschinski, F, Rothhammer, T, Jachimczak, P, Seitz, C, Schneider, A, & Schlingensiepen, K. H. The antisense oligonucleotide trabedersen (AP 12009) for the targeted inhibition of TGF-beta2. Curr Pharm Biotechnol. (2011). , 12(12), 2203-13.

[52] Schlingensiepen, K. H, Jaschinski, F, Lang, S. A, Moser, C, Geissler, E. K, Schlitt, H. J, et al. Transforming growth factor-beta 2 gene silencing with trabedersen (AP 12009) in pancreatic cancer. Cancer Sci. (2011). , 102(6), 1193-200.

[53] Vallieres, L. Trabedersen, a TGFbeta2-specific antisense oligonucleotide for the treatment of malignant gliomas and other tumors overexpressing TGFbeta2. IDrugs. (2009). , 12(7), 445-53.

[54] Gomez, D. E, Vazquez, A. M, & Alonso, D. F. Cancer Antigen Prioritization: A Road Map to Work in Defining Vaccines Against Specific Targets. A Point of View. Front Oncol. (2012).

[55] Keilholz, U. Antigen-specific cancer vaccines. Recent Results Cancer Res. (2007).

[56] Bodles-brakhop, A. M, & Draghia-akli, R. DNA vaccination and gene therapy: optimization and delivery for cancer therapy. Expert Rev Vaccines. (2008). , 7(7), 1085-101.

[57] Di, L, Zhu, Y, Jia, J, Yu, J, Song, G, Zhang, J, et al. Clinical safety of induced CTL infusion through recombinant adeno-associated virus-transfected dendritic cell vaccination in Chinese cancer patients. Clin Transl Oncol. (2012).

[58] Chu, C. S, Boyer, J, Schullery, D. S, Gimotty, P. A, Gamerman, V, Bender, J, et al. Phase I/II randomized trial of dendritic cell vaccination with or without cyclophosphamide for consolidation therapy of advanced ovarian cancer in first or second remission. Cancer Immunol Immunother. (2012). , 61(5), 629-41.

[59] ClinicalTrials (http://wwwclinicaltrials.gov/), accessed on 12 Aug (2012).

[60] Lowe, D. B, Shearer, M. H, Jumper, C. A, & Kennedy, R. C. Towards progress on DNA vaccines for cancer. Cell Mol Life Sci. (2007). , 64(18), 2391-403.

[61] Grosenbaugh, D. A, Leard, A. T, Bergman, P. J, Klein, M. K, Meleo, K, Susaneck, S, et al. Safety and efficacy of a xenogeneic DNA vaccine encoding for human tyrosinase as adjunctive treatment for oral malignant melanoma in dogs following surgical excision of the primary tumor. Am J Vet Res. (2011). , 72(12), 1631-8.

[62] Huber, M. L, Haynes, L, Parker, C, & Iversen, P. Interdisciplinary critique of sipuleucel-T as immunotherapy in castration-resistant prostate cancer. J Natl Cancer Inst. (2012). , 104(4), 273-9.

[63] Vattemi, E, & Claudio, P. P. Tumor suppressor genes as cancer therapeutics. Drug News Perspect. (2007). , 20(8), 511-20.

[64] Singhal, S, & Kaiser, L. R. Cancer chemotherapy using suicide genes. Surg Oncol Clin N Am. (1998). , 7(3), 505-36.

[65] Klatzmann, D, Valery, C. A, Bensimon, G, Marro, B, Boyer, O, Mokhtari, K, et al. A phase I/II study of herpes simplex virus type 1 thymidine kinase "suicide" gene therapy for recurrent glioblastoma. Study Group on Gene Therapy for Glioblastoma. Hum Gene Ther. (1998). , 9(17), 2595-604.

[66] Klatzmann, D, Cherin, P, Bensimon, G, Boyer, O, Coutellier, A, Charlotte, F, et al. A phase I/II dose-escalation study of herpes simplex virus type 1 thymidine kinase "suicide" gene therapy for metastatic melanoma. Study Group on Gene Therapy of Metastatic Melanoma. Hum Gene Ther. (1998). , 9(17), 2585-94.

[67] Wang, J, Lu, X. X, Chen, D. Z, Li, S. F, & Zhang, L. S. Herpes simplex virus thymidine kinase and ganciclovir suicide gene therapy for human pancreatic cancer. World J Gastroenterol. (2004). , 10(3), 400-3.

[68] Aoi, A, Watanabe, Y, Mori, S, Takahashi, M, Vassaux, G, & Kodama, T. Herpes simplex virus thymidine kinase-mediated suicide gene therapy using nano/microbubbles and ultrasound. Ultrasound Med Biol. (2008). , 34(3), 425-34.

[69] Yi, B. R, Choi, K. J, Kim, S. U, & Choi, K. C. Therapeutic potential of stem cells expressing suicide genes that selectively target human breast cancer cells: Evidence that they exert tumoricidal effects via tumor tropism (Review). Int J Oncol. (2012). , 41(3), 798-804.

[70] Omidi, Y, & Barar, J. Impacts of Blood-Brain Barrier in Drug Delivery and Targeting of Brain Tumors. BioImpacts. (2012). , 2(1), 5-22.

[71] Yi, B. R, Kim, S. U, Kim, Y. B, Lee, H. J, Cho, M. H, & Choi, K. C. Antitumor effects of genetically engineered stem cells expressing yeast cytosine deaminase in lung cancer brain metastases via their tumor-tropic properties. Oncol Rep. (2012). , 27(6), 1823-8.

[72] Kim, K. Y, Kim, S. U, Leung, P. C, Jeung, E. B, & Choi, K. C. Influence of the prodrugs 5-fluorocytosine and CPT-11 on ovarian cancer cells using genetically engi-

neered stem cells: tumor-tropic potential and inhibition of ovarian cancer cell growth. Cancer Sci. (2010). , 101(4), 955-62.

[73] Ben-efraim, S. Cancer immunotherapy: hopes and pitfalls: a review. Anticancer Res. (1996). B) , 3235-40.

[74] Palucka, K, & Banchereau, J. Cancer immunotherapy via dendritic cells. Nat Rev Cancer. (2012). , 12(4), 265-77.

[75] Mbeunkui, F, & Johann, D. J. Jr. Cancer and the tumor microenvironment: a review of an essential relationship. Cancer Chemother Pharmacol. (2009). , 63(4), 571-82.

[76] Barar, J. Targeting Tumor Microenvironment: The Key Role of Immune System. Bio-Impacts. (2012). , 2(1), 1-3.

[77] Mathe, G. Passive, adoptive, and active immunotherapy: a review of clinical trials in cancer. Cancer Detect Prev Suppl. (1987).

[78] Benencia, F, Courreges, M. C, Conejo-garcia, J. R, Mohamed-hadley, A, Zhang, L, Buckanovich, R. J, et al. HSV oncolytic therapy upregulates interferon-inducible chemokines and recruits immune effector cells in ovarian cancer. Mol Ther. (2005). , 12(5), 789-802.

[79] Tandle, A, & Blazer, D. G. rd, Libutti SK. Antiangiogenic gene therapy of cancer: recent developments. J Transl Med. (2004).

[80] Zhang, L, Yang, N, Mohamed-hadley, A, Rubin, S. C, & Coukos, G. Vector-based RNAi, a novel tool for isoform-specific knock-down of VEGF and anti-angiogenesis gene therapy of cancer. Biochem Biophys Res Commun. (2003). , 303(4), 1169-78.

[81] Cao, G, Su, J, Lu, W, Zhang, F, Zhao, G, Marteralli, D, et al. Adenovirus-mediated interferon-beta gene therapy suppresses growth and metastasis of human prostate cancer in nude mice. Cancer Gene Ther. (2001). , 8(7), 497-505.

[82] Zhang, X, Xu, J, Lawler, J, Terwilliger, E, & Parangi, S. Adeno-associated virus-mediated antiangiogenic gene therapy with thrombospondin-1 type 1 repeats and endostatin. Clin Cancer Res. (2007). , 13(13), 3968-76.

[83] Schmitz, V, Tirado-ledo, L, Raskopf, E, Rabe, C, Wernert, N, Wang, L, et al. Effective antitumour mono- and combination therapy by gene delivery of angiostatin-like molecule and interleukin-12 in a murine hepatoma model. Int J Colorectal Dis. (2005). , 20(6), 494-501.

[84] Zhao, P, Luo, R, Wu, J, Xie, F, Li, H, Xiao, X, et al. E10A, an adenovirus carrying human endostatin gene, in combination with docetaxel treatment inhibits prostate cancer growth and metastases. J Cell Mol Med. (2008).

[85] Omidi, Y, Barar, J, & Akhtar, S. Toxicogenomics of cationic lipid-based vectors for gene therapy: impact of microarray technology. Curr Drug Deliv. (2005). , 2(4), 429-41.

[86] Omidi, Y, & Barar, J. Toxicogenomics of Nonviral Cationic Gene Delivery Nanosystems. In: Yuan X, (ed.). Non-viral Gene Therapy. Rijeka: InTech Open Access Publisher; (2011). , 547-576.

[87] Hermanson, G. T. Bioconjugate Techniques. 2nd ed. Amesterdam: Elsevier Inc. ; (2008).

[88] Guo, S, & Huang, L. Nanoparticles Escaping RES and Endosome: Challenges for siRNA Delivery for Cancer Therapy. J Nanomaterilas. (2011).

[89] Adiseshaiah, P. P, Hall, J. B, & Mcneil, S. E. Nanomaterial standards for efficacy and toxicity assessment. Wiley interdisciplinary reviews Nanomedicine and nanobiotechnology. (2010). , 2(1), 99-112.

[90] Hobbs, S. K, Monsky, W. L, Yuan, F, Roberts, W. G, Griffith, L, Torchilin, V. P, et al. Regulation of transport pathways in tumor vessels: role of tumor type and microenvironment. Proc Natl Acad Sci U S A. (1998). , 95(8), 4607-12.

[91] Seymour, L. W. Passive tumor targeting of soluble macromolecules and drug conjugates. Crit Rev Ther Drug Carrier Syst. (1992). , 9(2), 135-87.

[92] Li, Y, Wang, J, Wientjes, M. G, & Au, J. L. Delivery of nanomedicines to extracellular and intracellular compartments of a solid tumor. Adv Drug Deliv Rev. (2012). , 64(1), 29-39.

[93] Shan, X, Yuan, Y, Liu, C, Tao, X, Sheng, Y, & Xu, F. Influence of PEG chain on the complement activation suppression and longevity in vivo prolongation of the PCL biomedical nanoparticles. Biomed Microdevices. (2009). , 11(6), 1187-94.

[94] Heidel, J. D, & Schluep, T. Cyclodextrin-containing polymers: versatile platforms of drug delivery materials. J Drug Deliv. (2012).

[95] Mozafari, M. R. Nanoliposomes: preparation and analysis. Methods Mol Biol. (2010).

[96] Clark, P. R, & Hersh, E. M. Cationic lipid-mediated gene transfer: current concepts. Curr Opin Mol Ther. (1999). , 1(2), 158-76.

[97] Hirko, A, Tang, F, & Hughes, J. A. Cationic lipid vectors for plasmid DNA delivery. Curr Med Chem. (2003). , 10(14), 1185-93.

[98] Kinet, V, Nguyen, N. Q, Sabatel, C, Blacher, S, Noel, A, Martial, J. A, et al. Antiangiogenic liposomal gene therapy with 16K human prolactin efficiently reduces tumor growth. Cancer Lett. (2009). , 284(2), 222-8.

[99] Zhou, M, Wang, L, Su, W, Tong, L, Liu, Y, Fan, Y, et al. Assessment of therapeutic efficacy of liposomal nanoparticles mediated gene delivery by molecular imaging for cancer therapy. J Biomed Nanotechnol. (2012). , 8(5), 742-50.

[100] Sofou, S, & Sgouros, G. Antibody-targeted liposomes in cancer therapy and imaging. Expert Opin Drug Deliv. (2008). , 5(2), 189-204.

[101] Mendonca, L. S, Firmino, F, & Moreira, J. N. Pedroso de Lima MC, Simoes S. Transferrin receptor-targeted liposomes encapsulating anti-BCR-ABL siRNA or asODN for chronic myeloid leukemia treatment. Bioconjug Chem. (2010). , 21(1), 157-68.

[102] Shi, G, Guo, W, Stephenson, S. M, & Lee, R. J. Efficient intracellular drug and gene delivery using folate receptor-targeted pH-sensitive liposomes composed of cationic/ anionic lipid combinations. J Control Release. (2002).

[103] Adrian, J. E, Wolf, A, Steinbach, A, Rossler, J, & Suss, R. Targeted delivery to neuroblastoma of novel siRNA-anti-GD2-liposomes prepared by dual asymmetric centrifugation and sterol-based post-insertion method. Pharm Res. (2011). , 28(9), 2261-72.

[104] Omidi, Y, & Davaran, S. Impacts of Biodegradable Polymers: Towards Biomedical Applications. In: Sharma SK, Mudhoo A, Clark JH, (eds.). A Handbook of Applied Biopolymer Technology: Synthesis, Degradation and Applications. London: Royal Society of Chemistry; (2011). , 388-418.

[105] Bellocq, N. C, Pun, S. H, Jensen, G. S, & Davis, M. E. Transferrin-containing, cyclodextrin polymer-based particles for tumor-targeted gene delivery. Bioconjug Chem. (2003). , 14(6), 1122-32.

[106] Canine, B. F, Wang, Y, & Hatefi, A. Biosynthesis and characterization of a novel genetically engineered polymer for targeted gene transfer to cancer cells. J Control Release. (2009). , 138(3), 188-96.

[107] Lu, Z. X, Liu, L. T, & Qi, X. R. Development of small interfering RNA delivery system using PEI-PEG-APRPG polymer for antiangiogenic vascular endothelial growth factor tumor-targeted therapy. Int J Nanomedicine. (2011).

[108] Sell, S. Potential gene therapy strategies for cancer stem cells. Curr Gene Ther. (2006). , 6(5), 579-91.

[109] Short, J. J, & Curiel, D. T. Oncolytic adenoviruses targeted to cancer stem cells. Mol Cancer Ther. (2009). , 8(8), 2096-102.

[110] Kruyt, F. A, & Schuringa, J. J. Apoptosis and cancer stem cells: Implications for apoptosis targeted therapy. Biochem Pharmacol. (2010). , 80(4), 423-30.

[111] Hu, Y. L, Fu, Y. H, Tabata, Y, & Gao, J. Q. Mesenchymal stem cells: a promising targeted-delivery vehicle in cancer gene therapy. J Control Release. (2010). , 147(2), 154-62.

[112] Gao, Z, Zhang, L, Hu, J, & Sun, Y. Mesenchymal stem cells: a potential targeted-delivery vehicle for anti-cancer drug, loaded nanoparticles. Nanomedicine. (2012).

[113] Song, C, Xiang, J, Tang, J, Hirst, D. G, Zhou, J, Chan, K. M, et al. Thymidine kinase gene modified bone marrow mesenchymal stem cells as vehicles for antitumor therapy. Hum Gene Ther. (2011). , 22(4), 439-49.

[114] Amano, S, Gu, C, Koizumi, S, Tokuyama, T, & Namba, H. Tumoricidal bystander effect in the suicide gene therapy using mesenchymal stem cells does not injure normal brain tissues. Cancer Lett. (2011). , 306(1), 99-105.

[115] Zhu, X, Su, D, Xuan, S, Ma, G, Dai, Z, Liu, T, et al. Gene therapy of gastric cancer using LIGHT-secreting human umbilical cord blood-derived mesenchymal stem cells. Gastric Cancer. (2012).

[116] Ren, C, Kumar, S, Chanda, D, Kallman, L, Chen, J, Mountz, J. D, et al. Cancer gene therapy using mesenchymal stem cells expressing interferon-beta in a mouse prostate cancer lung metastasis model. Gene Ther. (2008). , 15(21), 1446-53.

[117] Rodriguez, R, Garcia-castro, J, & Trigueros, C. Garcia Arranz M, Menendez P. Multipotent mesenchymal stromal cells: clinical applications and cancer modeling. Adv Exp Med Biol. (2012).

[118] Saukkonen, K, & Hemminki, A. Tissue-specific promoters for cancer gene therapy. Expert Opin Biol Ther. (2004). , 4(5), 683-96.

[119] Shirakawa, T, Gotoh, A, Wada, Y, Kamidono, S, Ko, S. C, Kao, C, et al. Tissue-specific promoters in gene therapy for the treatment of prostate cancer. Mol Urol. (2000). , 4(2), 73-82.

[120] Lin, M. T, Wang, F, Uitto, J, & Yoon, K. Differential expression of tissue-specific promoters by gene gun. Br J Dermatol. (2001). , 144(1), 34-9.

[121] Qiao, J, Doubrovin, M, Sauter, B. V, Huang, Y, Guo, Z. S, Balatoni, J, et al. Tumor-specific transcriptional targeting of suicide gene therapy. Gene Ther. (2002). , 9(3), 168-75.

[122] Lillehammer, T, Tveito, S, Engesaeter, B. O, Fodstad, O, Maelandsmo, G. M, & Engebraaten, O. Melanoma-specific expression in first-generation adenoviral vectors in vitro and in vivo-- use of the human tyrosinase promoter with human enhancers. Cancer Gene Ther. (2005). , 12(11), 864-72.

[123] Yoon, T. K, Shichinohe, T, Laquerre, S, & Kasahara, N. Selectively replicating adenoviruses for oncolytic therapy. Curr Cancer Drug Targets. (2001). , 1(2), 85-107.

[124] Mezhir, J. J, Smith, K. D, Posner, M. C, Senzer, N, Yamini, B, Kufe, D. W, et al. Ionizing radiation: a genetic switch for cancer therapy. Cancer Gene Ther. (2006). , 13(1), 1-6.

[125] Mcloughlin, J. M, Mccarty, T. M, Cunningham, C, Clark, V, Senzer, N, Nemunaitis, J, et al. TNFerade, an adenovector carrying the transgene for human tumor necrosis factor alpha, for patients with advanced solid tumors: surgical experience and long-term follow-up. Ann Surg Oncol. (2005). , 12(10), 825-30.

[126] Hecht, J. R, Farrell, J. J, Senzer, N, Nemunaitis, J, Rosemurgy, A, Chung, T, et al. EUS or percutaneously guided intratumoral TNFerade biologic with 5-fluorouracil and radiotherapy for first-line treatment of locally advanced pancreatic cancer: a phase I/II study. Gastrointest Endosc. (2012). , 75(2), 332-8.

Chapter 11

Targeting Intercellular Communication in Cancer Gene Therapy

Mohamed Amessou and Mustapha Kandouz

Additional information is available at the end of the chapter

1. Introduction

Cells dedicate a considerable amount of energy and regulatory mechanisms to ensure cell-cell communication, for this biological process is an important aspect of their machinery of survival, behavior and fate within their immediate environment. For cells, communicating is vital not only because they are part of organs and tissues of which they contribute to maintaining the integrity and proper function [1-5], but also because many of their functions need to be coordinated, quantitatively fine-tuned and/or limited in space and time. Furthermore, cells make use of communication to minimize the energetic and signaling burden, whereas a single minimal signal could be amplified and propagated, as is for instance the case of gap junction-mediated transfer of pro-apoptotic signals [6-8]. Many types of intercellular communication have been studied, among which direct cell-cell interactions could be distinguished from cellular interactions via released growth factors and cytokines. Their studies have revealed a significant potential for use in cancer therapy. The importance of cell-cell communication is particularly well revealed when defects in this process result in serious diseases, as exemplified by mutations identified in many gap and tight junction proteins [9, 10].

The diversity of the types of intercellular communications (i.e. gap junctions (GJ), tight junctions (TJ), adherens junctions (AJ) and desmosomes), implicates a diversity of signaling pathways and biological functions at stake. It further emphasizes the need for cells to communicate in different ways and for different purposes: transfer of small molecules, reciprocal signaling, establishment of barriers and polarity, control of paracellular permeability and transmission of cytoskeleton-generated forces. All of these processes have been implicated in cancer development as reviewed previously for GJs [11-13], TJs [14, 15] and desmosomes [16].

In this chapter we will present an overview of how various types of direct cell-cell communication and different groups of intercellular-dependent protein interactions have been used in strategies of gene therapy of cancer. Important concepts and paradigms as well as successful approaches, limitations and possibilities for the future will be discussed.

2. Intercellular communication & gene therapy: The enzyme/prodrug strategy

Cancer gene therapy has since its beginnings faced a major hurdle, the inefficiency of the methods of gene delivery to target cells (i.e. transfection and infection). While attempts have later been made to identify promising alternatives, a key development was the discovery that gap junctions could provide an efficient method that, without directly reaching every cell, could transfer the cytotoxic signal originating from a limited number of target cells to their bystander neighboring cells, thus amplifying the therapeutic effect. This process has subsequently been called "bystander effect" (BE) [17]. Triggering apoptotic death process in target cells results in the transfer of the pro-apoptotic signaling molecules to other cells with which they interact via gap junction intercellular communications (GJICs), and ultimately in the demise of both cells. The BE thus plays an important role in the efficiency of cancer therapy [18]. It also impacts the therapeutic cytotoxic side effects: since high doses of drugs are not required to kill tumor cells, normal tissues may not be reached by the treatment.

3. Use of the bystander effect in the enzyme/prodrug cancer gene therapy

Gene therapy soon became the major therapeutic application of the BE in the so-called "suicide gene therapy" involving the use of Enzyme/Prodrug cytotoxic systems, whereby target cells express an enzyme that converts a prodrug into the cytotoxic active drug, which is then transferred via gap junctions to the interacting cells [19]. The general mechanism is that the active molecules are therefore transmitted to neighboring cells via GJIC and trigger their death [20]. GJIC and connexins are essential for the BE-based enzyme/prodrug therapy [21-26] (Figure 1). Different enzymes/prodrugs have been assayed among which cytosine deaminase (CD)/5-fluorocytosine (5-FC), carboxylesterase/Camptothecin, and Herpes Simplex Virus-thymidine kinase (HSV/tk)/Ganciclovir (GCV) are prominent [27]. The CD/5-FC combination is based on the conversion of the nontoxic prodrug 5-FC by bacterial or yeast enzyme cytosine deaminase into active 5-fluorouracil (5-FU) [28]. Similarly, GCV, a nontoxic purine analogue, is phosphorylated by the enzyme HSVtk and by endogenous kinases to GCV-triphosphate, which kills cells by inhibiting DNA synthesis [29] [30]. The carboxylesterase activates the prodrug irinotecan,7-ethyl-10-[4-(1-piperidino)-1-piperidino]carbonyloxycamptothecin (CPT-11) to the active metabolite SN-38. Another combination including the uracil phosphoribosyltransferase (UPRT) of E. coli and 5-fluorouracil (5-FU), has also been used in BE-based gene therapy, along with other less known systems. UPRT is an enzyme that catalyzes the synthesis of UMP from uracil and 5-phosphoribosyl-alpha-1-diphosphate [31].

The therapeutic potential of the HSVtk and nucleosides' combination has been assayed as early as the 70's and later extended to many types of cancers both *in vitro* and *in vivo* [32-41].

Originally tried using retroviral vectors, the same approach adapted to adenoviral vectors was later introduced and used successfully [42-44]. These and subsequent studies, all have in common the use of an efficient delivery system, mostly adenoviral, modified to improve the transduction efficiency or selectivity, in combination with an enzyme/prodrug system, most often the HSVtk/GCV, to achieve cancer cells' cytotoxicity. Virus-free delivery has also been attempted using liposomes for instance, with more or less good efficacy [45-47], but most of the studies have used viral delivery.

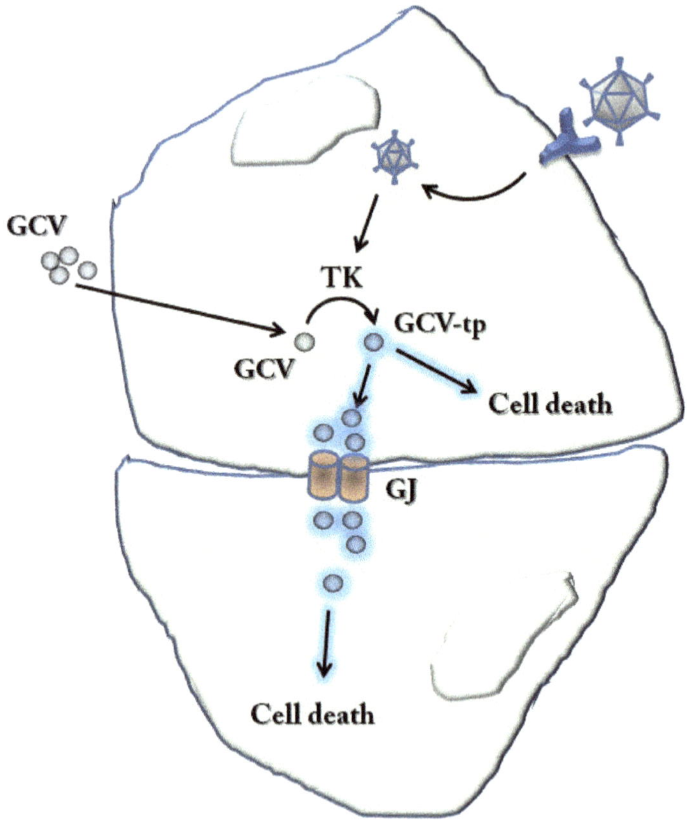

Figure 1. The enzyme/prodrug system and the bystander effect. Delivery via viral or non viral vectors of DNA sequences expressing an enzyme, here the herpes simplex virus thymidine kinase gene (TK) in the presence of the prodrug inactive substrate, here ganciclovir (GCV), results in the synthesis of the active metabolite, here GCV triphosphate (GCV-tp), which kills not only the target cell, but the neighboring bystander cell as well. This 'bystander effect' is mediated by a direct transfer of cytotoxic signals through gap junctions (GJ)-mediated intercellular communication.

3.1. Combination of oncolytic viruses and enzyme-prodrug gene therapy

Viruses are preferred vehicles for the transfer and delivery of engineered genes into host cells in gene therapy approaches. Recently, they have emerged as not only delivery vectors, but as *bona fide* therapeutic agents [74-77] (Figure 2). Oncolytic replication-competent viruses infect, replicate in and kill tumor cells. Examples abound of attempts to combine gene therapy and oncolytic virotherapy. Furthermore, the enzyme/prodrug systems have been used to improve the anti-tumor efficacy of oncolytic viruses. Early studies addressing the use of HSV vectors as oncolytic agents, showed that HSV-mediated oncolysis is enhanced by ganciclovir treatment through bystander effect [78]. A recombinant HSV (M012) was constructed to express the bacterial CD gene and was shown to enhance the prodrug-mediated anti-tumor effects after intracranial delivery in murine neuroblastoma and human glioma cells [79]. An oncolytic adenovirus modified to bear the human telomerase promoter (hTERT), was used to deliver the gene for the prodrug-activating enzyme carboxypeptidase G2 (CPG2) to tumors. The CPG2 metabolizes the prodrug ZD2767P into a cytotoxic drug and this strategy was shown to be effective in colorectal carcinomas via bystander effects and induction of apoptosis [80]. A recombinant Vesicular stomatitis virus (rVSV) encoding the CD/UPRT fusion gene was delivered intratumorally in the presence of the systemically administered 5-FU and significantly reduced growth of lymphoma and breast cancer cells *in vivo*. This effect involved three mechanisms: a strong bystander effect, the viral oncolytic activity as well as the activation of the immune system against the tumor [81]. Recombinant vesicular stomatitis virus (VSV) made to express CD/UPRT was delivered to breast cancer cells in combination with 5-fluorocytosine (5FC) [82]. An oncolytic adenovirus Ad5/3-Delta24FCU1 expressing the fusion suicide gene FCU1, which encodes a bifunctional fusion protein that metabolizes 5-FC, was found to exert significant anti-tumor activity *in vitro* and *in vivo* in a murine model of head and neck squamous cell carcinoma [83]. ONYX-015 (*dl*1520), a conditionally replicating adenovirus (CRAd) made of an E1B-55k-deleted oncolytic adenovirus and which has anti-tumor effects [84], has been combined with the CD/5-FC system and the enzyme/prodrug system involving *E. coli* nitroreductase (NTR) which can reduce nitro(hetero)aromatic compounds to hydroxylamines and amines, and both combinations showed enhanced efficacy *in vitro* and *in vivo* [85, 86]. Similarly, an oncolytic measles virus (MV) armed with the prodrug convertase, purine nucleoside phosphorylase (PNP) and the prodrug 6-methylpurine-2'-deoxyriboside (MeP-dR), was tested in a model of murine colon adenocarcinoma cells in syngeneic C57BL/6 mice and shown to have anti-tumorigenic effects after systemic delivery [87]. In spite of this available literature, many questions remain open. The factors defining the efficacy of this combinatorial therapy are not clearly identified and the strategy might not have any advantage in certain contexts. For instance, an oncolytic adenovirus, selective for the Rb/p16 pathway, killed ovarian cancer cells effectively by Tk/GCV-driven BE. However, while GCV improved the adenoviruses' antitumor efficacy over the replication-deficient virus counterpart, it did not further enhance its efficacy *in vivo*, suggesting that the prodrug strategy may not add antitumor activity to highly potent oncolysis [88].

3.2. Combined use of the enzyme/prodrug cancer gene therapy and gap junction communication restoration

Although since the beginning of the use of the enzyme/prodrug approach, it was found that the BE involves effects that do not depend on direct cell-cell interaction and are rather related to diffusible molecules released extracellularly and possibly to immune-related effects [48-51], the role of gap junctions-mediated intercellular communication (GJIC) and connexins was deemed essential [25, 26, 52-54] [55]. In light of the observed loss of connexins' expression in many cancers, the efficiency of the enzyme/prodrug approach could be limited by the ability of tumor cells to undergo GJICs between gene-transduced and bystander non-transduced cells. The levels of connexins and GJIC could modulate the impact of the bystander effect of the prodrug/enzyme systems, as shown for HSVtk/GCV *in vitro* and *in vivo* [56, 57]. This was suggested to be a reason behind the limited efficacy of the viral HSVtk/GCV delivery in many reports [58-60]. Nevertheless, many attempts have been made to bypass this limitation by restoring connexins' expression and the ability to undergo GJIC. This could be achieved either by the direct delivery of Cx-encoding vectors [61-64] or by pharmacological induction of Cx expression. The later approach involved for instance treating with DNA demethylating agents [65], histone deacetylases' inhibitors (HDACi) [66-68], ATP-sensitive potassium (KATP) channels' inhibitors [69], treatment with all-trans retinoic acid [70] or cyclic-AMP [71-73].

3.3. Applications of the enzyme/prodrug gene targeting of stem cells

Cellular vectors, including stem cells, have been used for effective gene delivery in cancer therapy. Stem and progenitor cells have been acknowledged as important for both normal and cancer homeostasis. In particular, according to the cancer stem cells' theory, tumors contain a very small sub-population of self-renewing and highly proliferating cells called cancer stem cells (CSCs), which are responsible for the tumorigenic activity [89]. Mesenchymal stem cells (MSCs), which have a strong tropism for tumor cells, are another type of stem cells of importance in cancer understanding and therapeutic targeting [90]. The use of allogeneic and hence escaping immune vigilance mesenchymal stromal cells (MSCs), sometimes called mesenchymal stem cells, as Trojan horses to deliver the enzyme/prodrug within the tumor mass is a relatively new development in gene therapy. MSCs are used as carriers of the enzyme via viral transduction, which subsequently activates the prodrug and kills not only the MSCs but their neighboring cancer cells (Figure 2). This strategy has been tested in many cancers, as illustrated by the following examples.

It has been shown that MSCs localize primarily to the perivascular environment in many organs and, when implanted or injected into animals, they show a tropism for primary tumors and metastases, and specifically for the perivascular niches within tumors [91, 92]. Based on this preferential migration, MSCs have been used as a vehicle in gene therapy strategies [93, 94]. The cytosine deaminase prodrug system has been partnered with the human MSCs and the combination increased the bystander effect and selective cytotoxicity on target tumor cells *in vitro* and *in vivo* [95-97]. Similarly, human neural stem cells (NSCs) have been successfully used to therapeutically target brain cancers. In fact, both MSCs and NSCs show high tropism for brain cancers and have been combined with the prodrug system to target brainstem gliomas, a form of childhood central nervous system tumors with poor prognosis or medulloblastomas [98-101], and even in disseminated brain metastases of non-neuronal origins such as melanoma and breast cancer [102-104]. The success of this approach now warrants clinical trials such as the one recently started to study the feasibility of intracerebral administration of NSCs in combination with oral 5-FC in patients with recurrent high-grade gliomas [105].

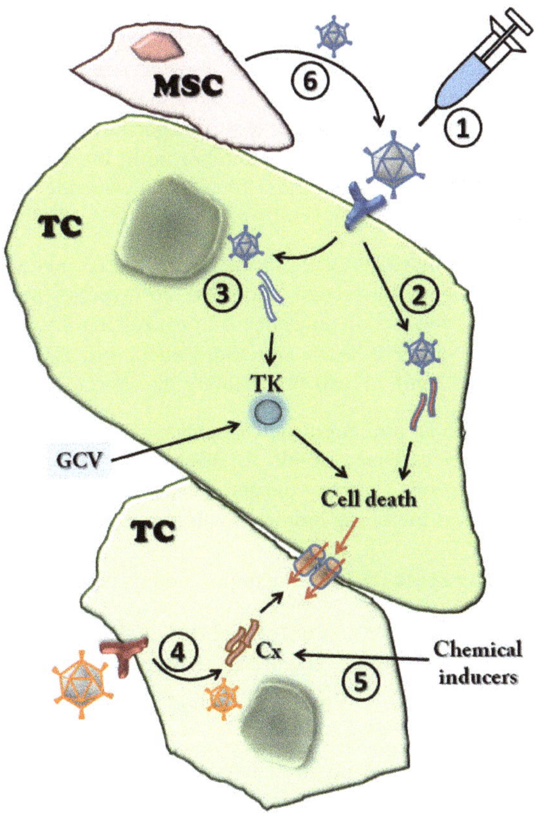

Figure 2. Different approaches of intercellular communication-based gene therapy. Tumor cells (TC) are targeted with oncolytic viruses which, in addition to their proper cytotoxic effects [1], could be combined with the bystander effect ensured by the enzyme/prodrug system, here for example the TK/GCV pair [3]. TCs are made sensitive to the bystander effect cytotoxic effects by inducing connexin (Cx) expression and the formation of gap junction intercellular communication. This is achieved by either 4) viral vectors, or 5) pharmacological inducers. Cellular delivery of the viral vectors for the enzyme/prodrug system could also be achieved using mesenchymal stem cells (MSCs) and other types of stem/progenitor cells [6].

Based on the tropism shown by neural stem cells (NSCs) for glioma cells, the herpes simplex virus-thymidine kinase (HSVtk)/GCV system has also been used in targeting gliomas [106-108]. However, for practical reasons related to the availability of cells, the use of MSCs might be more relevant clinically than the use of NSCs [109]. The system has also been tested for AT-MSCs [110] and bone marrow-derived tumor-infiltrating cells (BM-TICs) targeting of gliomas [111]. It was also proven to have a strong anti-tumor growth in medulloblastomas [112].

As discussed earlier, a major limitation to the efficacy of the therapeutic use of GJIC is the deficiency in the bystander effect due to low expression levels of connexins. Expectedly, this is also a challenge when using the prodrug/stem cells combined therapy. This can be bypassed by restoring connexin levels. For instance, GSCs showed more reduced GJIC and connexin levels than differentiated glioma cells [113]. Valproic acid (VPA) was able to upregulate Cx43 and Cx26 and to enhance the bystander effect of suicide gene therapy by human bone marrow MSCs expressing HSV-TK (MSCs-TK) [114]. In another study, the use of Bone marrow-derived stem cells (BMSCs) in combination with the (HSV-TK)/GCV suicide gene therapy of gliomas was improved by Cx43 overexpression *in vitro* and *in vivo* [115].

The MSC/Prodrug and Oncovirus/Prodrug strategies are often combined. For instance, MSCs transduced with an adenoviral vector modified to express integrin-binding motifs (Ad5lucRGD) for better transduction efficiency, and expressing thymidine kinase were able not only to kill ovarian cancer cells via bystander effect, but also support replication of adenoviruses which could result in further sustaining the effect [116].

MSCs can also act through an anti-angiogenic mechanism. They have been shown to target endothelial cells and inhibit capillary growth, establish Cx43-based GJIC with the target ECs, and to increase the production of reactive oxygen species (ROS). This effect culminates in the induction of apoptosis, thus inhibiting tumor growth in a model of melanomas [117].

3.4. The enzyme/prodrug approach in non-gap junctional communications

Curiously, unlike gap junctions, the number of studies delivering tight and adherens junctions or desmosomal proteins for cytotoxic gene therapy is limited. The adenoviral delivery of TK and E-cadherin genes improved TK/GCV cytotoxicity and antitumoral activity in pancreatic cancer cells [118].

Nevertheless, other cell-cell adhesion proteins, either or not with known links to these junctions, have been targeted in the enzyme/prodrug approach, as illustrated by the following examples. Carcinoembryonic antigen (CEA), a glycoprotein involved in cell-cell adhesion as well as cell-extracellular substrate adhesion, is a particularly prolific case. The expression of CEA in cancer cells with the exclusion of adult normal cells has been used in multiple ways to provide specificity to the Enzyme/Prodrug system. This directed enzyme/prodrug therapy, involves the generation of a recombinant plasmid, containing CEA promoter to specifically drive the expression of the enzyme/prodrug systems in CEA-expressing cancer cells [119-121]. The E. coli purine nucleoside phosphorylase (ePNP) under the control of CEA promoter sequences greatly improved the antitumor efficacy of the ePNP/MePdR killing system in pancreatic cancer cells [122]. The use of the double system including TK/GCV and CD/5-FC, in CEA-positive lung cancer cells, resulted in enhanced cytotoxicity [123]. A CEA promoter-regulated oncolytic adenovirus vector driving the Hsp70 gene expression in CEA-positive pancreatic cancer cells was also active *in vitro* and *in vivo* [124]. Similar results were obtained by targeting suicide gene CD expression to colon cancer cells [125]. An E1A, E1B double-restricted oncolytic adenovirus, AxdAdB-3, improved the therapeutic efficacy of the HSVtk/GCV system in gallbladder cancers when directed by the CEA promoter [126]. A modification of the approach done earlier, involved the addition of four tandem-linked NF-kappaB DNA-binding sites (kappaB4) and a kappaB4 enhancer upstream of the CEA promoter, thus sensitizing colon cancer cells to the thymidine phosphorylase (TP)/ 5-fluorouracil (5-FU) or 5'-deoxy-5-fluorouradine (5'-DFUR) combinations [127]. A different way of targeted delivery of adenoviral vectors involved the generation of a bispecific adapter protein (sCAR-MFE), consisting of a fusion of the ectodomain of the coxsackie/adenovirus receptor (sCAR) with a single-chain anti-CEA antibody (MFE-23) [128]. A specific CEA RNA-targeting ribozyme was developed and used for selective delivery of HSVtk/GCV cytotoxic activity, into CEA-expressing cancer cells [129].

A high affinity antibody for Neural cell adhesion molecule 2 (NCAM2), a cell-cell adhesion molecule, which is also capable of cell-extracellular matrix adhesion, was useful in increasing transduction efficiency of a fiber-modified adenoviral vector Adv-FZ33 in prostate and breast cancers, and restoring sensitivity to the UPRT/5-FU system in previously resistant cells [130]. An Adenoviral vector incorporating an IgG Fc-binding motif (Z33) from the Staphylococcus protein A (Ad-FZ33) combined with tumor-specific anti-EpCAM (epithelial cell adhesion molecule) antibodies improved the viral transduction and the growth suppression of biliary cancer xenografts in nude mice in response to the UPRT/FU combination in human biliary cancers [131]. A similar approach used the enzyme/prodrug system comprised of the enzyme carboxylesterase (CE) and its substrate the anticancer agent CPT-11 (irinotecan or 7-ethyl-10[4-(1-piperidino)-1-piperidino] carbonyloxycamptothecin). An adenoviral vector Ad.C28-sCE2 containing a fusion gene encoding a secreted form of human liver CE2 targeted to EpCAM was efficient in colon cancer spheroids [132]. As for CEA, the validation of the use of the EpCAM promoter to target the HSVtk/GCV therapy to cancer cells has been performed [133].

4. Gene therapy using bystander effect-independent intercellular communications

The prominence of BE-based gene therapy in the literature should not eclipse the importance of other intercellular communications which do not involve the BE as candidates for gene therapy. These include in addition to a GJIC-independent role of connexins, other types of cell-cell junctions as well as other types of protein-protein (ligand-receptor) interactions who depend on cell-cell interactions for their functions. Although to different extents, all these intercellular events have proven very amenable to gene therapy strategies.

4.1. GJIC-independent effects

The key players in the BE are connexins, the building blocks of gap junctional intercellular communication (GJIC) [23, 134, 135]. Even though the effectiveness of restoring Connexins' and GJIC's levels has traditionally been associated with the bystander effect in gene therapy, it has become clear that many functions of connexins, could be dissociated from both GJIC and the bystander effects [136-138] [139] [140] [141]. In this case, delivery of Cxs-encoding vectors could be used as a gene therapy approach, regardless of the use of enzyme/prodrug systems. However, future use of such application requires a better understanding of the non GJIC-related functions of these proteins, including their interacting partners and the mechanisms of their subcellular localization.

4.2. Desmosomes, adherens and tight junctions in gene therapy

Adherens junctions and their related desmosomes, as well as tight junctions are essential types of cell-cell adhesion in both normal homeostasis and tumor progression [142-148]. Claudins are key tight junction proteins whose expression is deregulated in many cancers [146, 149]. Claudins CLDN3 and CLDN4 function as receptors for the Clostridium perfringens enterotoxin (CPE) produced by the bacterial Clostridium type A strain, resulting in cell death. A gene therapy application based on CPE gene transfer-mediated cytoxicity has been achieved but, as expected, was limited to CLDN3- and CLDN4-overexpressing tumors [150]. SiRNA-mediated silencing of the expression of Epithelial Cell Adhesion Molecule (EpCAM or CD326), a cell-surface protein involved in tight junctions and metastasis in colon, breast and other epithelial carcinomas, was effective in decreasing the growth of breast cancer cells [151]. The same approach was used with an antibody against the carcinoembryonic antigen (CEA) in gastric cancer [152]. In fact, CEA has been extensively targeted in gene therapy approaches in different ways. A recombinant form of the oncolytic measles virus Edmonston strain (MV-Edm) changed to express CEA, demonstrated high cytotoxicity towards hepatocellular carcinoma cells *in vitro* and *in vivo* after either Intratumoral or intravenous delivery [153]. The cell adhesion molecule CECAM1, or carcinoembryonic antigen-related cell adhesion molecule 1, has served in an adenoviral gene therapy targeting prostate cancer cells and showed tumor suppressor activities *in vivo* [154].

It is noteworthy that even when targeting these cell-cell communications could not be directly performed or if it fails to affect tumor growth, there is no doubt about their impact on gene therapy applications. Cell-cell communications could indeed constitute a source of impediment to gene therapy, by constituting physical barriers to tumor targeting with oncolytic viruses *in vivo* [155] [156, 157]. This is particularly important in tissues such as the lung, intestine and reproductive system which show natural mechanisms of resistance to viral infection and might thus be less amenable to viral gene delivery. In fact, many junction proteins have been shown to be receptors for many viruses. The protein originally known as coxsackie-adenovirus receptor (hCAR), which was used in adenoviral-based gene therapy for cancer before realizing that it is a component of epithelial tight junctions [158, 159], affects the efficacy of the adenoviral gene therapy approach [160, 161]. Desmoglein-2 (DSG-2), a desmosomal adhesion glycoprotein, is a receptor used by adenoviruses

Ad3, Ad7, Ad11 and Ad14, which subsequently results in epithelial-to-mesenchymal transition-like changes and transient opening of intercellular junctions, a finding that could have an impact on the adenoviral gene delivery to normal or cancer cells [162, 163]. Adherens junction proteins Nectin-1 and -2 are entry receptors for the herpes simplex virus types 1 (HSV-1) and 2 (HSV-2) [164-166]. Increasing Nectin-1 expression resulted in increased susceptibility to HSV-1 infection and oncolytic activity and hence enhanced tumor regression *in vivo* [167]. Attenuated HSV-2 viral production in WB rat liver epithelial cells was found to depend on the viral protein co-localization with adherens junction proteins rather than by the status of gap junctions [168]. Taken together, these studies demonstrate the importance of junctional proteins in the infectivity of viruses and suggest that they might impact the efficacy of the viral oncolytic gene therapies. Compounds could thus be identified for example to improve viral gene transfer [169].

4.3. Intercellular communications-dependent protein-protein interactions

Many proteins, although not *bona fide* components of cell-cell junctions, are either affected by these interactions or are very important in the function of direct cell-cell interactions, whether junctional or not. Prototypes of these proteins are the ones involved in axon guidance, such as the Eph/Ephrin proteins. The Eph family is the largest family of receptor tyrosine kinases, and includes the A-type Eph (EphA1–10) and B-type Eph (EphB1–6) receptors as well as A-type Ephrin (EphrinA1-6) and B-type Ephrin (EphrinB1-3) ligands. A particularity of this family is that, with few exceptions, the receptor-ligand interactions depend on direct cell-cell contacts, as both Ephs and Ephrins are anchored in interacting cellular membranes and in fact their role in cell-cell repulsion/attraction and cell sorting is one of their main features. Study of Ephs/Ephrins' role in cancer has dramatically boomed in the last decade [170] and attempts are currently underway to target them in cancer therapy. Targeting of Ephs and Ephrins for gene therapy has been very timid so far. EphA2 is probably one of the most sought after receptors of this family, as its expression is increased in many cancers and it has shown pro-oncogenic functions. A human adenoviral type 5 (HAd) vector expressing a secreted fusion protein constituted of the extracellular domain of EphrinA1, an EphA2 ligand, fused to the Fc portion of IgG1, was used to infect mammary epithelial cells and was found to activate and induce the degradation of EphA2, thus showing anti-tumor effects. After intratumoral inoculation, the HAd-EphrinA1-Fc vector significantly inhibited tumor growth *in vivo* [171, 172]. On the other hand, taking advantage of the high expression levels of EphA2 in cancer cells, an EphA2-binding peptide has been added to an Adenoviral vector (Ad) to target pancreatic cancer cells and bypass the limitation of low Ad transduction due to low levels of the major Ad receptor called Coxsackie and Ad receptor (CAR) [173]. Recently, EphA2 has been shown to be an essential receptor for the Kaposi's sarcoma–associated herpesvirus, a major oncogenic virus in endothelial cells [174, 175]. EphrinB2 and EphrinB3, other family members, have also been identified as entry receptors for the Hendra virus and Nipah virus [176-178]. These data suggest that interfering with Ephs and Ephrins could be an interesting strategy in gene therapy applications by improving the transduction of viral vectors.

5. Concluding remarks & perspectives

Over the years, it has become clear that various systems of cell-cell communication play critical roles not only in the normal development, architecture, remodeling and function of various tissues and organs, but in the onset of diseases as well. Cells are social entities and need to interact with each other in a way that ensures a favorable response to input from their immediate micro-environment (growth, survival, cytotoxicity) and a flexible adaptation to various roles and stress conditions. They also need to communicate during their death and demise. These communication processes are subject to various regulatory mechanisms which, when going awry, could result in various pathologies. One such instance where cell-cell communication has a particularly dramatic role is cancer progression, metastasis and response to therapeutic interventions. This reliance of cancer cells on cell-cell communication provides a therapeutic opportunity that will be fully exploited only if the mechanisms of its normal and aberrant functions are elucidated. This is for instance obvious when attempting to restore GJIC to render cancer cells sensitive to enzyme/prodrug therapies.

Also, cancer cells share their microenvironment with many other cell types who are not just neutral bystanders. In particular, invasive cancer cells have very unstable intercellular contacts, as they keep migrating, constantly adhering to and detaching from cells on their way and thus changing the nature of their cell-cell communications. This might be a challenging fact when thinking of gene therapy strategies, and in fact any other type of therapy. Thus understanding these dynamics of change during the course of tumor progression is of utmost importance.

As progress continues in developing strategies for a more efficient and selective viral delivery of gene therapeutics, the role of different junctions in the resistance of cancer epithelial cells to viral infections, needs to be balanced by the advantageous use of these proteins to render this approach more cancer-specific. In this respect, the enzyme/prodrug strategies need to be reconsidered in the light of the new findings that involve both gap junctions and other types of intercellular communications in the bystander effect. Examining the links between the different types of cell-cell communication will be critical for future applications.

Finally, the impact of protein-protein interactions which are not necessarily engaged in cell junctions but are involved in direct cell-cell interactions, and the therapeutic opportunities they provide, will constitute a way for the future.

Author details

Mohamed Amessou[1] and Mustapha Kandouz[1,2]

1 Department of Pathology, Wayne State University School of Medicine, Detroit, Michigan, USA

2 Karmanos Cancer Institute, Wayne State University, Detroit, MI, USA

References

[1] Nakahama K. Cellular communications in bone homeostasis and repair. Cell Mol Life Sci 2010;67:4001-9.

[2] Brooke MA, Nitoiu D, Kelsell DP. Cell-cell connectivity: desmosomes and disease. J Pathol 2012;226:158-71.

[3] Chanson M, Derouette JP, Roth I, Foglia B, Scerri I, Dudez T, et al. Gap junctional communication in tissue inflammation and repair. Biochim Biophys Acta 2005;1711:197-207.

[4] Bruzzone R, Dermietzel R. Structure and function of gap junctions in the developing brain. Cell Tissue Res 2006;326:239-48.

[5] Bosco D, Haefliger JA, Meda P. Connexins: key mediators of endocrine function. Physiol Rev 2011;91:1393-445.

[6] Decrock E, Vinken M, De VE, Krysko DV, D'Herde K, Vanhaecke T, et al. Connexin-related signaling in cell death: to live or let die? Cell Death Differ 2009;16:524-36.

[7] Krysko DV, Leybaert L, Vandenabeele P, D'Herde K. Gap junctions and the propagation of cell survival and cell death signals. Apoptosis 2005;10:459-69.

[8] Vinken M, Vanhaecke T, Papeleu P, Snykers S, Henkens T, Rogiers V. Connexins and their channels in cell growth and cell death. Cell Signal 2006;18:592-600.

[9] Zoidl G, Dermietzel R. Gap junctions in inherited human disease. Pflugers Arch 2010;460:451-66.

[10] Lai-Cheong JE, Arita K, McGrath JA. Genetic diseases of junctions. J Invest Dermatol 2007;127:2713-25.

[11] Carystinos GD, Bier A, Batist G. The role of connexin-mediated cell-cell communication in breast cancer metastasis. J Mammary Gland Biol Neoplasia 2001;6:431-40.

[12] Cronier L, Crespin S, Strale PO, Defamie N, Mesnil M. Gap junctions and cancer: new functions for an old story. Antioxid Redox Signal 2009;11:323-38.

[13] Mesnil M, Crespin S, Avanzo JL, Zaidan-Dagli ML. Defective gap junctional intercellular communication in the carcinogenic process. Biochim Biophys Acta 2005;1719:125-45.

[14] Martin TA, Mason MD, Jiang WG. Tight junctions in cancer metastasis. Front Biosci 2011;16:898-936.

[15] Feigin ME, Muthuswamy SK. Polarity proteins regulate mammalian cell-cell junctions and cancer pathogenesis. Curr Opin Cell Biol 2009;21:694-700.

[16] Dusek RL, Attardi LD. Desmosomes: new perpetrators in tumour suppression. Nat Rev Cancer 2011;11:317-23.

[17] van D, I, Mulder NH, Vaalburg W, de Vries EF, Hospers GA. Influence of the bystander effect on HSV-tk/GCV gene therapy. A review. Curr Gene Ther 2002;2:307-22.

[18] Mothersill C, Seymour CB. Radiation-induced bystander effects--implications for cancer. Nat Rev Cancer 2004;4:158-64.

[19] Altaner C. Prodrug cancer gene therapy. Cancer Lett 2008;270:191-201.

[20] Hamel W, Magnelli L, Chiarugi VP, Israel MA. Herpes simplex virus thymidine kinase/ganciclovir-mediated apoptotic death of bystander cells. Cancer Res 1996;56:2697-702.

[21] Dilber MS, Abedi MR, Christensson B, Bjorkstrand B, Kidder GM, Naus CC, et al. Gap junctions promote the bystander effect of herpes simplex virus thymidine kinase *in vivo*. Cancer Res 1997;57:1523-8.

[22] Vrionis FD, Wu JK, Qi P, Waltzman M, Cherington V, Spray DC. The bystander effect exerted by tumor cells expressing the herpes simplex virus thymidine kinase (HSVtk) gene is dependent on connexin expression and cell communication via gap junctions. Gene Ther 1997;4:577-85.

[23] Elshami AA, Saavedra A, Zhang H, Kucharczuk JC, Spray DC, Fishman GI, et al. Gap junctions play a role in the 'bystander effect' of the herpes simplex virus thymidine kinase/ganciclovir system in vitro. Gene Ther 1996;3:85-92.

[24] Fick J, Barker FG, Dazin P, Westphale EM, Beyer EC, Israel MA. The extent of heterocellular communication mediated by gap junctions is predictive of bystander tumor cytotoxicity in vitro. Proc Natl Acad Sci U S A 1995;92:11071-5.

[25] Mesnil M, Piccoli C, Tiraby G, Willecke K, Yamasaki H. Bystander killing of cancer cells by herpes simplex virus thymidine kinase gene is mediated by connexins. Proc Natl Acad Sci U S A 1996;93:1831-5.

[26] Mesnil M, Yamasaki H. Bystander effect in herpes simplex virus-thymidine kinase/ganciclovir cancer gene therapy: role of gap-junctional intercellular communication. Cancer Res 2000;60:3989-99.

[27] Xu G, McLeod HL. Strategies for enzyme/prodrug cancer therapy. Clin Cancer Res 2001;7:3314-24.

[28] Mullen CA, Kilstrup M, Blaese RM. Transfer of the bacterial gene for cytosine deaminase to mammalian cells confers lethal sensitivity to 5-fluorocytosine: a negative selection system. Proc Natl Acad Sci U S A 1992;89:33-7.

[29] Chen SH, Shine HD, Goodman JC, Grossman RG, Woo SL. Gene therapy for brain tumors: regression of experimental gliomas by adenovirus-mediated gene transfer *in vivo*. Proc Natl Acad Sci U S A 1994;91:3054-7.

[30] Thompson TC. In situ gene therapy for prostate cancer. Oncol Res 1999;11:1-8.

[31] Kanai F, Kawakami T, Hamada H, Sadata A, Yoshida Y, Tanaka T, et al. Adenovirus-mediated transduction of Escherichia coli uracil phosphoribosyltransferase gene

sensitizes cancer cells to low concentrations of 5-fluorouracil. Cancer Res 1998;58:1946-51.

[32] Elion GB, Furman PA, Fyfe JA, de MP, Beauchamp L, Schaeffer HJ. Selectivity of action of an antiherpetic agent, 9-(2-hydroxyethoxymethyl) guanine. Proc Natl Acad Sci U S A 1977;74:5716-20.

[33] Nishiyama Y, Rapp F. Anticellular effects of 9-(2-hydroxyethoxymethyl) guanine against herpes simplex virus-transformed cells. J Gen Virol 1979;45:227-30.

[34] Furman PA, McGuirt PV, Keller PM, Fyfe JA, Elion GB. Inhibition by acyclovir of cell growth and DNA synthesis of cells biochemically transformed with herpesvirus genetic information. Virology 1980;102:420-30.

[35] Davidson RL, Kaufman ER, Crumpacker CS, Schnipper LE. Inhibition of herpes simplex virus transformed and nontransformed cells by acycloguanosine: mechanisms of uptake and toxicity. Virology 1981;113:9-19.

[36] Moolten FL. Tumor chemosensitivity conferred by inserted herpes thymidine kinase genes: paradigm for a prospective cancer control strategy. Cancer Res 1986;46:5276-81.

[37] Moolten FL, Wells JM. Curability of tumors bearing herpes thymidine kinase genes transferred by retroviral vectors. J Natl Cancer Inst 1990;82:297-300.

[38] Culver KW, Ram Z, Wallbridge S, Ishii H, Oldfield EH, Blaese RM. *In vivo* gene transfer with retroviral vector-producer cells for treatment of experimental brain tumors. Science 1992;256:1550-2.

[39] Ezzeddine ZD, Martuza RL, Platika D, Short MP, Malick A, Choi B, et al. Selective killing of glioma cells in culture and *in vivo* by retrovirus transfer of the herpes simplex virus thymidine kinase gene. New Biol 1991;3:608-14.

[40] Caruso M, Panis Y, Gagandeep S, Houssin D, Salzmann JL, Klatzmann D. Regression of established macroscopic liver metastases after in situ transduction of a suicide gene. Proc Natl Acad Sci U S A 1993;90:7024-8.

[41] Vile RG, Hart IR. Use of tissue-specific expression of the herpes simplex virus thymidine kinase gene to inhibit growth of established murine melanomas following direct intratumoral injection of DNA. Cancer Res 1993;53:3860-4.

[42] Smythe WR, Hwang HC, Amin KM, Eck SL, Davidson BL, Wilson JM, et al. Use of recombinant adenovirus to transfer the herpes simplex virus thymidine kinase (HSVtk) gene to thoracic neoplasms: an effective in vitro drug sensitization system. Cancer Res 1994;54:2055-9.

[43] Bonnekoh B, Greenhalgh DA, Bundman DS, Eckhardt JN, Longley MA, Chen SH, et al. Inhibition of melanoma growth by adenoviral-mediated HSV thymidine kinase gene transfer *in vivo*. J Invest Dermatol 1995;104:313-7.

[44] Rosenfeld ME, Feng M, Michael SI, Siegal GP, Alvarez RD, Curiel DT. Adenoviral-mediated delivery of the herpes simplex virus thymidine kinase gene selectively

sensitizes human ovarian carcinoma cells to ganciclovir. Clin Cancer Res 1995;1:1571-80.

[45] Calvez V, Rixe O, Wang P, Mouawad R, Soubrane C, Ghoumari A, et al. Virus-free transfer of the herpes simplex virus thymidine kinase gene followed by ganciclovir treatment induces tumor cell death. Clin Cancer Res 1996;2:47-51.

[46] Vile RG, Nelson JA, Castleden S, Chong H, Hart IR. Systemic gene therapy of murine melanoma using tissue specific expression of the HSVtk gene involves an immune component. Cancer Res 1994;54:6228-34.

[47] Nagamachi Y, Tani M, Shimizu K, Yoshida T, Yokota J. Suicidal gene therapy for pleural metastasis of lung cancer by liposome-mediated transfer of herpes simplex virus thymidine kinase gene. Cancer Gene Ther 1999;6:546-53.

[48] Dong Y, Wen P, Manome Y, Parr M, Hirshowitz A, Chen L, et al. *In vivo* replication-deficient adenovirus vector-mediated transduction of the cytosine deaminase gene sensitizes glioma cells to 5-fluorocytosine. Hum Gene Ther 1996;7:713-20.

[49] Hirschowitz EA, Ohwada A, Pascal WR, Russi TJ, Crystal RG. *In vivo* adenovirus-mediated gene transfer of the Escherichia coli cytosine deaminase gene to human colon carcinoma-derived tumors induces chemosensitivity to 5-fluorocytosine. Hum Gene Ther 1995;6:1055-63.

[50] Princen F, Robe P, Lechanteur C, Mesnil M, Rigo JM, Gielen J, et al. A cell type-specific and gap junction-independent mechanism for the herpes simplex virus-1 thymidine kinase gene/ganciclovir-mediated bystander effect. Clin Cancer Res 1999;5:3639-44.

[51] Bi W, Kim YG, Feliciano ES, Pavelic L, Wilson KM, Pavelic ZP, et al. An HSVtk-mediated local and distant antitumor bystander effect in tumors of head and neck origin in athymic mice. Cancer Gene Ther 1997;4:246-52.

[52] Pitts JD. Cancer gene therapy: a bystander effect using the gap junctional pathway. Mol Carcinog 1994;11:127-30.

[53] Denning C, Pitts JD. Bystander effects of different enzyme-prodrug systems for cancer gene therapy depend on different pathways for intercellular transfer of toxic metabolites, a factor that will govern clinical choice of appropriate regimes. Hum Gene Ther 1997;8:1825-35.

[54] Yang L, Chiang Y, Lenz HJ, Danenberg KD, Spears CP, Gordon EM, et al. Intercellular communication mediates the bystander effect during herpes simplex thymidine kinase/ganciclovir-based gene therapy of human gastrointestinal tumor cells. Hum Gene Ther 1998;9:719-28.

[55] Kawamura K, Bahar R, Namba H, Seimiya M, Takenaga K, Hamada H, et al. Bystander effect in uracil phosphoribosyltransferase/5-fluorouracil-mediated suicide gene therapy is correlated with the level of intercellular communication. Int J Oncol 2001;18:117-20.

[56] Dilber MS, Abedi MR, Christensson B, Bjorkstrand B, Kidder GM, Naus CC, et al. Gap junctions promote the bystander effect of herpes simplex virus thymidine kinase *in vivo*. Cancer Res 1997;57:1523-8.

[57] Vrionis FD, Wu JK, Qi P, Waltzman M, Cherington V, Spray DC. The bystander effect exerted by tumor cells expressing the herpes simplex virus thymidine kinase (HSVtk) gene is dependent on connexin expression and cell communication via gap junctions. Gene Ther 1997;4:577-85.

[58] Sacco MG, Benedetti S, Duflot-Dancer A, Mesnil M, Bagnasco L, Strina D, et al. Partial regression, yet incomplete eradication of mammary tumors in transgenic mice by retrovirally mediated HSVtk transfer '*in vivo*'. Gene Ther 1996;3:1151-6.

[59] Shinoura N, Chen L, Wani MA, Kim YG, Larson JJ, Warnick RE, et al. Protein and messenger RNA expression of connexin43 in astrocytomas: implications in brain tumor gene therapy. J Neurosurg 1996;84:839-45.

[60] Rosolen A, Frascella E, di FC, Todesco A, Petrone M, Mehtali M, et al. *In vitro* and *in vivo* antitumor effects of retrovirus-mediated herpes simplex thymidine kinase gene-transfer in human medulloblastoma. Gene Ther 1998;5:113-20.

[61] Cirenei N, Colombo BM, Mesnil M, Benedetti S, Yamasaki H, Finocchiaro G. *In vitro* and *in vivo* effects of retrovirus-mediated transfer of the connexin 43 gene in malignant gliomas: consequences for HSVtk/GCV anticancer gene therapy. Gene Ther 1998;5:1221-6.

[62] Ghoumari AM, Mouawad R, Zerrouqi A, Nizard C, Provost N, Khayat D, et al. Actions of HSVtk and connexin43 gene delivery on gap junctional communication and drug sensitization in hepatocellular carcinoma. Gene Ther 1998;5:1114-21.

[63] Marconi P, Tamura M, Moriuchi S, Krisky DM, Niranjan A, Goins WF, et al. Connexin 43-enhanced suicide gene therapy using herpesviral vectors. Mol Ther 2000;1:71-81.

[64] Tanaka M, Fraizer GC, De La CJ, Cristiano RJ, Liebert M, Grossman HB. Connexin 26 enhances the bystander effect in HSVtk/GCV gene therapy for human bladder cancer by adenovirus/PLL/DNA gene delivery. Gene Ther 2001;8:139-48.

[65] Hagiwara H, Sato H, Ohde Y, Takano Y, Seki T, Ariga T, et al. 5-Aza-2'-deoxycytidine suppresses human renal carcinoma cell growth in a xenograft model via up-regulation of the connexin 32 gene. Br J Pharmacol 2008;153:1373-81.

[66] Ammerpohl O, Thormeyer D, Khan Z, Appelskog IB, Gojkovic Z, Almqvist PM, et al. HDACi phenylbutyrate increases bystander killing of HSV-tk transfected glioma cells. Biochem Biophys Res Commun 2004;324:8-14.

[67] Ammerpohl O, Trauzold A, Schniewind B, Griep U, Pilarsky C, Grutzmann R, et al. Complementary effects of HDAC inhibitor 4-PB on gap junction communication and cellular export mechanisms support restoration of chemosensitivity of PDAC cells. Br J Cancer 2007;96:73-81.

[68] Hernandez M, Shao Q, Yang XJ, Luh SP, Kandouz M, Batist G, et al. A histone deacetylation-dependent mechanism for transcriptional repression of the gap junction gene cx43 in prostate cancer cells. Prostate 2006;66:1151-61.

[69] Paino T, Gangoso E, Medina JM, Tabernero A. Inhibition of ATP-sensitive potassium channels increases HSV-tk/GCV bystander effect in U373 human glioma cells by enhancing gap junctional intercellular communication. Neuropharmacology 2010;59:480-91.

[70] Park JY, Elshami AA, Amin K, Rizk N, Kaiser LR, Albelda SM. Retinoids augment the bystander effect *in vitro* and *in vivo* in herpes simplex virus thymidine kinase/ganciclovir-mediated gene therapy. Gene Ther 1997;4:909-17.

[71] Carystinos GD, Katabi MM, Laird DW, Galipeau J, Chan H, Alaoui-Jamali MA, et al. Cyclic-AMP induction of gap junctional intercellular communication increases bystander effect in suicide gene therapy. Clin Cancer Res 1999;5:61-8.

[72] Kunishige I, Samejima Y, Moriyama A, Saji F, Murata Y. cAMP stimulates the bystander effect in suicide gene therapy of human choriocarcinoma. Anticancer Res 1998;18:3411-9.

[73] Robe PA, Princen F, Martin D, Malgrange B, Stevenaert A, Moonen G, et al. Pharmacological modulation of the bystander effect in the herpes simplex virus thymidine kinase/ganciclovir gene therapy system: effects of dibutyryl adenosine 3',5'-cyclic monophosphate, alpha-glycyrrhetinic acid, and cytosine arabinoside. Biochem Pharmacol 2000;60:241-9.

[74] Bourke MG, Salwa S, Harrington KJ, Kucharczyk MJ, Forde PF, de KM, et al. The emerging role of viruses in the treatment of solid tumours. Cancer Treat Rev 2011;37:618-32.

[75] de VJ, Willemsen RA, Lindholm L, Hoeben RC, Bangma CH, Barber C, et al. Adenovirus-derived vectors for prostate cancer gene therapy. Hum Gene Ther 2010;21:795-805.

[76] Wollmann G, Ozduman K, van den Pol AN. Oncolytic virus therapy for glioblastoma multiforme: concepts and candidates. Cancer J 2012;18:69-81.

[77] Russell SJ, Peng KW, Bell JC. Oncolytic virotherapy. Nat Biotechnol 2012;30:658-70.

[78] Carroll NM, Chase M, Chiocca EA, Tanabe KK. The effect of ganciclovir on herpes simplex virus-mediated oncolysis. J Surg Res 1997;69:413-7.

[79] Guffey MB, Parker JN, Luckett WS, Jr., Gillespie GY, Meleth S, Whitley RJ, et al. Engineered herpes simplex virus expressing bacterial cytosine deaminase for experimental therapy of brain tumors. Cancer Gene Ther 2007;14:45-56.

[80] Schepelmann S, Ogilvie LM, Hedley D, Friedlos F, Martin J, Scanlon I, et al. Suicide gene therapy of human colon carcinoma xenografts using an armed oncolytic adenovirus expressing carboxypeptidase G2. Cancer Res 2007;67:4949-55.

[81] Porosnicu M, Mian A, Barber GN. The oncolytic effect of recombinant vesicular stomatitis virus is enhanced by expression of the fusion cytosine deaminase/uracil phosphoribosyltransferase suicide gene. Cancer Res 2003;63:8366-76.

[82] Leveille S, Samuel S, Goulet ML, Hiscott J. Enhancing VSV oncolytic activity with an improved cytosine deaminase suicide gene strategy. Cancer Gene Ther 2011;18:435-43.

[83] Dias JD, Liikanen I, Guse K, Foloppe J, Sloniecka M, Diaconu I, et al. Targeted chemotherapy for head and neck cancer with a chimeric oncolytic adenovirus coding for bifunctional suicide protein FCU1. Clin Cancer Res 2010;16:2540-9.

[84] Johnson L, Shen A, Boyle L, Kunich J, Pandey K, Lemmon M, et al. Selectively replicating adenoviruses targeting deregulated E2F activity are potent, systemic antitumor agents. Cancer Cell 2002;1:325-37.

[85] Zhan J, Gao Y, Wang W, Shen A, Aspelund A, Young M, et al. Tumor-specific intravenous gene delivery using oncolytic adenoviruses. Cancer Gene Ther 2005;12:19-25.

[86] Singleton DC, Li D, Bai SY, Syddall SP, Smaill JB, Shen Y, et al. The nitroreductase prodrug SN 28343 enhances the potency of systemically administered armed oncolytic adenovirus ONYX-411(NTR). Cancer Gene Ther 2007;14:953-67.

[87] Ungerechts G, Springfeld C, Frenzke ME, Lampe J, Parker WB, Sorscher EJ, et al. An immunocompetent murine model for oncolysis with an armed and targeted measles virus. Mol Ther 2007;15:1991-7.

[88] Raki M, Hakkarainen T, Bauerschmitz GJ, Sarkioja M, Desmond RA, Kanerva A, et al. Utility of TK/GCV in the context of highly effective oncolysis mediated by a serotype 3 receptor targeted oncolytic adenovirus. Gene Ther 2007;14:1380-8.

[89] Reya T, Morrison SJ, Clarke MF, Weissman IL. Stem cells, cancer, and cancer stem cells. Nature 2001;414:105-11.

[90] Houthuijzen JM, Daenen LG, Roodhart JM, Voest EE. The role of mesenchymal stem cells in anti-cancer drug resistance and tumour progression. Br J Cancer 2012;106:1901-6.

[91] Crisan M, Yap S, Casteilla L, Chen CW, Corselli M, Park TS, et al. A perivascular origin for mesenchymal stem cells in multiple human organs. Cell Stem Cell 2008;3:301-13.

[92] Bexell D, Scheding S, Bengzon J. Toward brain tumor gene therapy using multipotent mesenchymal stromal cell vectors. Mol Ther 2010;18:1067-75.

[93] Okada T, Ozawa K. Vector-producing tumor-tracking multipotent mesenchymal stromal cells for suicide cancer gene therapy. Front Biosci 2008;13:1887-91.

[94] Dwyer RM, Khan S, Barry FP, O'Brien T, Kerin MJ. Advances in mesenchymal stem cell-mediated gene therapy for cancer. Stem Cell Res Ther 2010;1:25.

[95] Kucerova L, Altanerova V, Matuskova M, Tyciakova S, Altaner C. Adipose tissue-derived human mesenchymal stem cells mediated prodrug cancer gene therapy. Cancer Res 2007;67:6304-13.

[96] Cavarretta IT, Altanerova V, Matuskova M, Kucerova L, Culig Z, Altaner C. Adipose tissue-derived mesenchymal stem cells expressing prodrug-converting enzyme inhibit human prostate tumor growth. Mol Ther 2010;18:223-31.

[97] Chang DY, Yoo SW, Hong Y, Kim S, Kim SJ, Yoon SH, et al. The growth of brain tumors can be suppressed by multiple transplantation of mesenchymal stem cells expressing cytosine deaminase. Int J Cancer 2010;127:1975-83.

[98] Lee DH, Ahn Y, Kim SU, Wang KC, Cho BK, Phi JH, et al. Targeting rat brainstem glioma using human neural stem cells and human mesenchymal stem cells. Clin Cancer Res 2009;15:4925-34.

[99] Aboody KS, Brown A, Rainov NG, Bower KA, Liu S, Yang W, et al. Neural stem cells display extensive tropism for pathology in adult brain: evidence from intracranial gliomas. Proc Natl Acad Sci U S A 2000;97:12846-51.

[100] Nakamizo A, Marini F, Amano T, Khan A, Studeny M, Gumin J, et al. Human bone marrow-derived mesenchymal stem cells in the treatment of gliomas. Cancer Res 2005;65:3307-18.

[101] Kim SK, Kim SU, Park IH, Bang JH, Aboody KS, Wang KC, et al. Human neural stem cells target experimental intracranial medulloblastoma and deliver a therapeutic gene leading to tumor regression. Clin Cancer Res 2006;12:5550-6.

[102] Aboody KS, Najbauer J, Schmidt NO, Yang W, Wu JK, Zhuge Y, et al. Targeting of melanoma brain metastases using engineered neural stem/progenitor cells. Neuro Oncol 2006;8:119-26.

[103] Brown AB, Yang W, Schmidt NO, Carroll R, Leishear KK, Rainov NG, et al. Intravascular delivery of neural stem cell lines to target intracranial and extracranial tumors of neural and non-neural origin. Hum Gene Ther 2003;14:1777-85.

[104] Joo KM, Park IH, Shin JY, Jin J, Kang BG, Kim MH, et al. Human neural stem cells can target and deliver therapeutic genes to breast cancer brain metastases. Mol Ther 2009;17:570-5.

[105] http://clinicaltrials.gov/ identifier#NCT01172964)

[106] Li S, Tokuyama T, Yamamoto J, Koide M, Yokota N, Namba H. Bystander effect-mediated gene therapy of gliomas using genetically engineered neural stem cells. Cancer Gene Ther 2005;12:600-7.

[107] Rath P, Shi H, Maruniak JA, Litofsky NS, Maria BL, Kirk MD. Stem cells as vectors to deliver HSV/tk gene therapy for malignant gliomas. Curr Stem Cell Res Ther 2009;4:44-9.

[108] Li S, Gao Y, Tokuyama T, Yamamoto J, Yokota N, Yamamoto S, et al. Genetically engineered neural stem cells migrate and suppress glioma cell growth at distant intracranial sites. Cancer Lett 2007;251:220-7.

[109] Amano S, Li S, Gu C, Gao Y, Koizumi S, Yamamoto S, et al. Use of genetically engineered bone marrow-derived mesenchymal stem cells for glioma gene therapy. Int J Oncol 2009;35:1265-70.

[110] Matuskova M, Hlubinova K, Pastorakova A, Hunakova L, Altanerova V, Altaner C, et al. HSV-tk expressing mesenchymal stem cells exert bystander effect on human glioblastoma cells. Cancer Lett 2010;290:58-67.

[111] Miletic H, Fischer Y, Litwak S, Giroglou T, Waerzeggers Y, Winkeler A, et al. Bystander killing of malignant glioma by bone marrow-derived tumor-infiltrating progenitor cells expressing a suicide gene. Mol Ther 2007;15:1373-81.

[112] Pu K, Li SY, Gao Y, Ma L, Ma W, Liu Y. Bystander effect in suicide gene therapy using immortalized neural stem cells transduced with herpes simplex virus thymidine kinase gene on medulloblastoma regression. Brain Res 2011;1369:245-52.

[113] Yu SC, Xiao HL, Jiang XF, Wang QL, Li Y, Yang XJ, et al. Connexin 43 reverses malignant phenotypes of glioma stem cells by modulating E-cadherin. Stem Cells 2012;30:108-20.

[114] Ryu CH, Park KY, Kim SM, Jeong CH, Woo JS, Hou Y, et al. Valproic acid enhances anti-tumor effect of mesenchymal stem cell mediated HSV-TK gene therapy in intracranial glioma. Biochem Biophys Res Commun 2012;421:585-90.

[115] Huang Q, Liu XZ, Kang CS, Wang GX, Zhong Y, Pu PY. The anti-glioma effect of suicide gene therapy using BMSC expressing HSV/TK combined with overexpression of Cx43 in glioma cells. Cancer Gene Ther 2010;17:192-202.

[116] Pereboeva L, Komarova S, Mikheeva G, Krasnykh V, Curiel DT. Approaches to utilize mesenchymal progenitor cells as cellular vehicles. Stem Cells 2003;21:389-404.

[117] Otsu K, Das S, Houser SD, Quadri SK, Bhattacharya S, Bhattacharya J. Concentration-dependent inhibition of angiogenesis by mesenchymal stem cells. Blood 2009;113:4197-205.

[118] Garcia-Rodriguez L, bate-Daga D, Rojas A, Gonzalez JR, Fillat C. E-cadherin contributes to the bystander effect of TK/GCV suicide therapy and enhances its antitumoral activity in pancreatic cancer models. Gene Ther 2011;18:73-81.

[119] DiMaio JM, Clary BM, Via DF, Coveney E, Pappas TN, Lyerly HK. Directed enzyme pro-drug gene therapy for pancreatic cancer *in vivo*. Surgery 1994;116:205-13.

[120] Osaki T, Tanio Y, Tachibana I, Hosoe S, Kumagai T, Kawase I, et al. Gene therapy for carcinoembryonic antigen-producing human lung cancer cells by cell type-specific expression of herpes simplex virus thymidine kinase gene. Cancer Res 1994;54:5258-61.

[121] Richards CA, Austin EA, Huber BE. Transcriptional regulatory sequences of carcinoembryonic antigen: identification and use with cytosine deaminase for tumor-specific gene therapy. Hum Gene Ther 1995;6:881-93.

[122] Deharvengt S, Wack S, Aprahamian M, Hajri A. Transcriptional tumor-selective promoter targeting of E. coli purine nucleoside phosphorylase for pancreatic cancer suicide gene therapy. J Gene Med 2005;7:672-80.

[123] Qiu Y, Peng GL, Liu QC, Li FL, Zou XS, He JX. Selective killing of lung cancer cells using carcinoembryonic antigen promoter and double suicide genes, thymidine kinase and cytosine deaminase (pCEA-TK/CD). Cancer Lett 2012;316:31-8.

[124] Xu C, Sun Y, Wang Y, Yan Y, Shi Z, Chen L, et al. CEA promoter-regulated oncolytic adenovirus-mediated Hsp70 expression in immune gene therapy for pancreatic cancer. Cancer Lett 2012;319:154-63.

[125] Zhang G, Liu T, Chen YH, Chen Y, Xu M, Peng J, et al. Tissue specific cytotoxicity of colon cancer cells mediated by nanoparticle-delivered suicide gene *in vitro* and *in vivo*. Clin Cancer Res 2009;15:201-7.

[126] Fukuda K, Abei M, Ugai H, Kawashima R, Seo E, Wakayama M, et al. E1A, E1B double-restricted replicative adenovirus at low dose greatly augments tumor-specific suicide gene therapy for gallbladder cancer. Cancer Gene Ther 2009;16:126-36.

[127] Guo X, Evans TR, Somanath S, Armesilla AL, Darling JL, Schatzlein A, et al. In vitro evaluation of cancer-specific NF-kappaB-CEA enhancer-promoter system for 5-fluorouracil prodrug gene therapy in colon cancer cell lines. Br J Cancer 2007;97:745-54.

[128] Li HJ, Everts M, Pereboeva L, Komarova S, Idan A, Curiel DT, et al. Adenovirus tumor targeting and hepatic untargeting by a coxsackie/adenovirus receptor ectodomain anti-carcinoembryonic antigen bispecific adapter. Cancer Res 2007;67:5354-61.

[129] Jung HS, Lee SW. Ribozyme-mediated selective killing of cancer cells expressing carcinoembryonic antigen RNA by targeted trans-splicing. Biochem Biophys Res Commun 2006;349:556-63.

[130] Takahashi S, Kato K, Nakamura K, Nakano R, Kubota K, Hamada H. Neural cell adhesion molecule 2 as a target molecule for prostate and breast cancer gene therapy. Cancer Sci 2011;102:808-14.

[131] Kawashima R, Abei M, Fukuda K, Nakamura K, Murata T, Wakayama M, et al. EpCAM- and EGFR-targeted selective gene therapy for biliary cancers using Z33-fiber-modified adenovirus. Int J Cancer 2011;129:1244-53.

[132] Oosterhoff D, Overmeer RM, de GM, van der Meulen IH, Giaccone G, van Beusechem VW, et al. Adenoviral vector-mediated expression of a gene encoding secreted, EpCAM-targeted carboxylesterase-2 sensitises colon cancer spheroids to CPT-11. Br J Cancer 2005;92:882-7.

[133] Gires O, Pockl S, Chapman RD, Munz M. Targeted gene expression using a 1.1 kilobase promoter fragment of the tumour-associated antigen EpCAM. Anticancer Res 2004;24:3715-21.

[134] Asklund T, Appelskog IB, Ammerpohl O, Langmoen IA, Dilber MS, Aints A, et al. Gap junction-mediated bystander effect in primary cultures of human malignant gliomas with recombinant expression of the HSVtk gene. Exp Cell Res 2003;284:185-95.

[135] Yamasaki H, Katoh F. Novel method for selective killing of transformed rodent cells through intercellular communication, with possible therapeutic applications. Cancer Res 1988;48:3203-7.

[136] Li Z, Zhou Z, Welch DR, Donahue HJ. Expressing connexin 43 in breast cancer cells reduces their metastasis to lungs. Clin Exp Metastasis 2008;25:893-901.

[137] Kalra J, Shao Q, Qin H, Thomas T, aoui-Jamali MA, Laird DW. Cx26 inhibits breast MDA-MB-435 cell tumorigenic properties by a gap junctional intercellular communication-independent mechanism. Carcinogenesis 2006;27:2528-37.

[138] Qin H, Shao Q, Thomas T, Kalra J, aoui-Jamali MA, Laird DW. Connexin26 regulates the expression of angiogenesis-related genes in human breast tumor cells by both GJIC-dependent and -independent mechanisms. Cell Commun Adhes 2003;10:387-93.

[139] McLachlan E, Shao Q, Wang HL, Langlois S, Laird DW. Connexins act as tumor suppressors in three-dimensional mammary cell organoids by regulating differentiation and angiogenesis. Cancer Res 2006;66:9886-94.

[140] Sato H, Iwata H, Takano Y, Yamada R, Okuzawa H, Nagashima Y, et al. Enhanced effect of connexin 43 on cisplatin-induced cytotoxicity in mesothelioma cells. J Pharmacol Sci 2009;110:466-75.

[141] Sato H, Hagiwara H, Ohde Y, Senba H, Virgona N, Yano T. Regulation of renal cell carcinoma cell proliferation, invasion and metastasis by connexin 32 gene. J Membr Biol 2007;216:17-21.

[142] Dusek RL, Attardi LD. Desmosomes: new perpetrators in tumour suppression. Nat Rev Cancer 2011;11:317-23.

[143] Brooke MA, Nitoiu D, Kelsell DP. Cell-cell connectivity: desmosomes and disease. J Pathol 2012;226:158-71.

[144] Chidgey M, Dawson C. Desmosomes: a role in cancer? Br J Cancer 2007;96:1783-7.

[145] Baum B, Georgiou M. Dynamics of adherens junctions in epithelial establishment, maintenance, and remodeling. J Cell Biol 2011;192:907-17.

[146] Turksen K, Troy TC. Junctions gone bad: claudins and loss of the barrier in cancer. Biochim Biophys Acta 2011;1816:73-9.

[147] Martin TA, Mason MD, Jiang WG. Tight junctions in cancer metastasis. Front Biosci 2011;16:898-936.

[148] Feigin ME, Muthuswamy SK. Polarity proteins regulate mammalian cell-cell junctions and cancer pathogenesis. Curr Opin Cell Biol 2009;21:694-700.

[149] Escudero-Esparza A, Jiang WG, Martin TA. The Claudin family and its role in cancer and metastasis. Front Biosci 2011;16:1069-83.

[150] Walther W, Petkov S, Kuvardina ON, Aumann J, Kobelt D, Fichtner I, et al. Novel Clostridium perfringens enterotoxin suicide gene therapy for selective treatment of claudin-3- and -4-overexpressing tumors. Gene Ther 2012;19:494-503.

[151] Osta WA, Chen Y, Mikhitarian K, Mitas M, Salem M, Hannun YA, et al. EpCAM is overexpressed in breast cancer and is a potential target for breast cancer gene therapy. Cancer Res 2004;64:5818-24.

[152] Tanaka T, Huang J, Hirai S, Kuroki M, Kuroki M, Watanabe N, et al. Carcinoembryonic antigen-targeted selective gene therapy for gastric cancer through FZ33 fiber-modified adenovirus vectors. Clin Cancer Res 2006;12:3803-13.

[153] Blechacz B, Splinter PL, Greiner S, Myers R, Peng KW, Federspiel MJ, et al. Engineered measles virus as a novel oncolytic viral therapy system for hepatocellular carcinoma. Hepatology 2006;44:1465-77.

[154] Kleinerman DI, Zhang WW, Lin SH, Nguyen TV, von Eschenbach AC, Hsieh JT. Application of a tumor suppressor (C-CAM1)-expressing recombinant adenovirus in androgen-independent human prostate cancer therapy: a preclinical study. Cancer Res 1995;55:2831-6.

[155] Strauss R, Lieber A. Anatomical and physical barriers to tumor targeting with oncolytic adenoviruses *in vivo*. Curr Opin Mol Ther 2009;11:513-22.

[156] Strauss R, Sova P, Liu Y, Li ZY, Tuve S, Pritchard D, et al. Epithelial phenotype confers resistance of ovarian cancer cells to oncolytic adenoviruses. Cancer Res 2009;69:5115-25.

[157] Bals R, Xiao W, Sang N, Weiner DJ, Meegalla RL, Wilson JM. Transduction of well-differentiated airway epithelium by recombinant adeno-associated virus is limited by vector entry. J Virol 1999;73:6085-8.

[158] Reimer D, Steppan I, Wiedemair A, Concin N, Hofstetter G, Marth C, et al. Soluble isoforms but not the transmembrane form of coxsackie-adenovirus receptor are of clinical relevance in epithelial ovarian cancer. Int J Cancer 2007;120:2568-75.

[159] Cohen CJ, Shieh JT, Pickles RJ, Okegawa T, Hsieh JT, Bergelson JM. The coxsackievirus and adenovirus receptor is a transmembrane component of the tight junction. Proc Natl Acad Sci U S A 2001;98:15191-6.

[160] Li Y, Pong RC, Bergelson JM, Hall MC, Sagalowsky AI, Tseng CP, et al. Loss of adenoviral receptor expression in human bladder cancer cells: a potential impact on the efficacy of gene therapy. Cancer Res 1999;59:325-30.

[161] Okegawa T, Li Y, Pong RC, Bergelson JM, Zhou J, Hsieh JT. The dual impact of coxsackie and adenovirus receptor expression on human prostate cancer gene therapy. Cancer Res 2000;60:5031-6.

[162] Wang H, Li ZY, Liu Y, Persson J, Beyer I, Moller T, et al. Desmoglein 2 is a receptor for adenovirus serotypes 3, 7, 11 and 14. Nat Med 2011;17:96-104.

[163] Wang H, Li Z, Yumul R, Lara S, Hemminki A, Fender P, et al. Multimerization of adenovirus serotype 3 fiber knob domains is required for efficient binding of virus to desmoglein 2 and subsequent opening of epithelial junctions. J Virol 2011;85:6390-402.

[164] Krummenacher C, Nicola AV, Whitbeck JC, Lou H, Hou W, Lambris JD, et al. Herpes simplex virus glycoprotein D can bind to poliovirus receptor-related protein 1 or herpesvirus entry mediator, two structurally unrelated mediators of virus entry. J Virol 1998;72:7064-74.

[165] Linehan MM, Richman S, Krummenacher C, Eisenberg RJ, Cohen GH, Iwasaki A. *In vivo* role of nectin-1 in entry of herpes simplex virus type 1 (HSV-1) and HSV-2 through the vaginal mucosa. J Virol 2004;78:2530-6.

[166] Warner MS, Geraghty RJ, Martinez WM, Montgomery RI, Whitbeck JC, Xu R, et al. A cell surface protein with herpesvirus entry activity (HveB) confers susceptibility to infection by mutants of herpes simplex virus type 1, herpes simplex virus type 2, and pseudorabies virus. Virology 1998;246:179-89.

[167] Yu Z, Li S, Huang YY, Fong Y, Wong RJ. Calcium depletion enhances nectin-1 expression and herpes oncolytic therapy of squamous cell carcinoma. Cancer Gene Ther 2007;14:738-47.

[168] Miezeiewski B, McShane-Kay K, Woodruff RI, Mbuy GK, Knabb MT. Role of Adherens Junction Proteins in Differential Herpes Simplex Virus Type 2 Infectivity in Communication-Competent and -Deficient Cell Lines. Intervirology 2012.

[169] Sorscher EJ, Harris J, Alexander M, Rottgers A, Hardy K, Ponnazhagan S, et al. Activators of viral gene expression in polarized epithelial monolayers identified by rapid-throughput drug screening. Gene Ther 2006;13:781-8.

[170] Kandouz M. The Eph/Ephrin family in cancer metastasis: communication at the service of invasion. Cancer Metastasis Rev 2012;31:353-73.

[171] Noblitt LW, Bangari DS, Shukla S, Knapp DW, Mohammed S, Kinch MS, et al. Decreased tumorigenic potential of EphA2-overexpressing breast cancer cells following treatment with adenoviral vectors that express EphrinA1. Cancer Gene Ther 2004;11:757-66.

[172] Noblitt LW, Bangari DS, Shukla S, Mohammed S, Mittal SK. Immunocompetent mouse model of breast cancer for preclinical testing of EphA2-targeted therapy. Cancer Gene Ther 2005;12:46-53.

[173] Van Geer MA, Brevoord D, Kuhlmann KF, Bakker CT, Mizuguchi H, Wesseling JG, et al. A fiber modified adenovirus vector that targets to the EphrinA2 receptor reveals enhanced gene transfer to ex vivo pancreatic cancer. Int J Oncol 2010;36:233-44.

[174] Hahn AS, Kaufmann JK, Wies E, Naschberger E, Panteleev-Ivlev J, Schmidt K, et al. The ephrin receptor tyrosine kinase A2 is a cellular receptor for Kaposi's sarcoma-associated herpesvirus. Nat Med 2012;18:961-6.

[175] Chakraborty S, Veettil MV, Bottero V, Chandran B. Kaposi's sarcoma-associated herpesvirus interacts with EphrinA2 receptor to amplify signaling essential for productive infection. Proc Natl Acad Sci U S A 2012;109:E1163-E1172.

[176] Bonaparte MI, Dimitrov AS, Bossart KN, Crameri G, Mungall BA, Bishop KA, et al. Ephrin-B2 ligand is a functional receptor for Hendra virus and Nipah virus. Proc Natl Acad Sci U S A 2005;102:10652-7.

[177] Negrete OA, Levroney EL, Aguilar HC, Bertolotti-Ciarlet A, Nazarian R, Tajyar S, et al. EphrinB2 is the entry receptor for Nipah virus, an emergent deadly paramyxovirus. Nature 2005;436:401-5.

[178] Xu K, Broder CC, Nikolov DB. Ephrin-B2 and ephrin-B3 as functional henipavirus receptors. Semin Cell Dev Biol 2012;23:116-23.

Chapter 12

Identification and Validation of Targets for Cancer Immunotherapy: From the Bench-to-Bedside

Ghazala Khan, Suzanne E. Brooks, Frances Denniss, Dagmar Sigurdardottir and Barbara-ann Guinn

Additional information is available at the end of the chapter

1. Introduction

The link between immune responses and cancer is evident from findings such as, a compromised immune system resulting in an increased tumour incidence [1] and cancer patient sera evidencing recognition of autologous cancer antigens [2]. The identification of tumour associated antigens (TAAs) plays a central role in our understanding of how cancer cells can inhibit the immune system and how we can overcome this tumour immune suppression to break tolerance and achieve cancer destruction [3]. Antibodies reacting with TAAs on the surface of cancer cells provoke an extremely effective immune response [4] which can be exquisitely specific to the tumour cells present in the body. However not many surface proteins are present on tumour cells and limited otherwise in expression to healthy non-essential tissues.

TAAs are most often proteins which have acquired mutations or have elevated expression levels which are expressed at the sub-cellular level. The ideal immunotherapy targets should also play a role in tumour progression [5]. For example p53 [6] is one of the most desirable targets for immunotherapy – targeting p53 can kill both the evolving tumour cell population and any cancer "stem" cell which harbours this as an early tumourigenesis aberration and supports further tumour growth. In addition, a number of tumour antigens have been shown to be useful biomarkers for cancer diagnosis [7] and survival [8].

In this chapter, we will examine how tumour antigens are identified and characterised to demonstrate their potential as immunotherapy targets and examine their role as biomarkers for treatment response and patient survival, and targets for personalised therapies.

2. Which tumour antigens?

Many of the tumour antigens identified by serological identification of antigens by recombinant expression cloning (SEREX) can be classified into one or more categories which are: cancer-testis, mutational, differentiation, amplified/overexpressed, splice variant and viral antigens [9]. Cancer-testis (CT) antigens [10] have been found to be highly expressed in tumours but not in normal tissues with the exception of immunologically protected sites (those tissues which lack major histocompatibility complex (MHC) class I and therefore do not present self-antigens). CT antigens make attractive targets as due to their limited expression, they should therefore induce specific anti-tumour immune responses and less toxicity to healthy tissue [11]. However some debate remains as to the definition of a CT antigen [12] with some suggestion of differential levels of expression and others suggesting no expression in normal tissues expect those in immunologically protected sites (such as ovary, placenta and testis). TAAs that are frequently found in tumours and provide excellent targets for immunotherapy include Wilms tumour 1 [13] and PRAME [14].

3. Identification of tumour antigens

Strategies are required to help identify potential targets which can be used for cancer immunotherapy. Some of the most commonly used and successful techniques are described as follows:-

3.1. Reverse-Transcription-Polymerase Chain Reaction (RT-PCR) and real-time PCR (RQ-PCR)

Reverse-transcription-polymerase chain reaction (RT-PCR) and real-time PCR (RQ-PCR) has been used to examine known TAA expression in a range of solid and haematological malignancies [15-19]. Although this has provided important expression information and a good starting point to identify potential antigenic targets in a range of cancers, these studies are entirely limited to tumour antigens which had already been discovered.

3.2. Representational difference analysis

Representational difference analysis was developed by Thierry Boon's group and used to discover a number of CT antigens [20, 21] including the MAGE family of antigens, typically from melanoma with one exception, RAGE, from renal cancer. Briefly, total RNA was extracted from normal tissue (driver) and a tumour sample (tester) and used to construct double-stranded cDNA. Both cDNA samples were digested with the restriction enzymes DpnII and ligated to adapters which contained primer binding sites. The fragments were amplified by PCR, the adapters removed and new adapters for unrelated primers ligated to the tester. The tester and driver were then mixed and hybridized leading to three combinations of product: driver-driver (no amplification), tester-driver (linear amplification) and tester-tester (exponential amplification). A further two hybridization and amplification steps generate greater variation in the products which are subsequently cloned and sequenced.

3.3. Serological identification of antigens by recombinant expression cloning (SEREX)

Serological identification of antigens by recombinant expression cloning (SEREX) provided a much needed boost to the area of antigen identification at a time when few cancer antigen identification options existed [2]. SEREX was not limited to immunogenic cancers such as melanoma and has now been used to identify more than 2,000 antigens [22-23] in a large range of different solid [24-26] and haematological malignancies [27-30]. cDNA libraries are created from tumour samples, cell lines or healthy normal donor cells (such as testes). RNA from these cells were reverse transcribed and inserted as cDNA into phage vectors and expressed as recombinant proteins on the capsid surface of phage which survived on permissive E.coli. Expressed proteins were transferred to nitrocellulose membranes and following the removal of excess E.coli waste, phage plaques were immunoscreened using pre-cleared patient sera. Any positive plaques were isolated, eluted and used for secondary confirmatory screening, prior to cDNA sequencing of phagemid inserts [31].

3.4. Serological proteome analysis (SERPA)

Serological proteome analysis (SERPA) was first described by Klade *et al* in 2001 [32]. Proteins were extracted from primary tumours or cell lines, separated concurrently on two 2D gels and transferred to nitrocellulose membranes. A third gel is stained with Coomassie Blue as a preparative gel. The membranes are incubated with cancer patient's sera and normal control. The two gels are directly compared and any bright spots on the cancer sera membrane were cut from the preparative gel and indentified using mass spectrometry [33, 34].

3.5. CDNA microarrays

The differential expression of tumour antigens and/or protein biomarkers between cell and disease subtypes have been directly compared on cDNA microarrays and has allowed our improved understanding of lymphomas [35] and aided our development of personalised therapies [36]. Microarray technology is able to distinguish between different subtypes of a particular cancer as well as identify the expression of novel antigens [37]. Minimal residual disease is a very important tool in the detection of impending relapse in patients who have had some form of treatment. Markers for minimal residual disease in acute lymphocytic leukaemia were identified by gene profiling [38]. cDNA microarray has been used to identify the frequency of elevated tumour antigen expression in acute myeloid leukaemia [28] and also associations between specific cytogenetic abnormalities and relative levels of tumour antigen expression [39]. Micorarray has also been used to elucidate the possible function of tumour antigens such as Synovial Sarcoma X breakpoint 2 Interacting Protein (SSX2IP) in the subversion of cells harbouring cytogenetic abnormalities (t(8;21) associated with mitotic spindle failure and the association between the elevated expression of some tumour antigens (SSX2IP, RHAMM and SURVIVIN) at disease presentation and patient survival [8] in acute myeloid leukaemia.

3.6. Mass Spectroscopy (MS)

Mass Spectroscopy (MS) involves the analysis of peptides eluted from the MHC of antigen presenting cells [40-42] or proteins in serum [43]. This area is reviewed more completely in the following reviews [44,45]. By using mass spectrometry, it has been demonstrated that as many as 10,000 different peptide species are presented by individual class I MHC alleles [46]. The technique, its strengths and limitations are extensively reviewed [47].

3.7. Protein microarrays

Protein microarrays involve the immunoscreening of protein arrays (approximately 9,000 full length proteins and functional domains) which may be purchased from companies such as Invitrogen, Functional Genomics or Cambridge Protein Arrays. Antibodies in sera from patients [33,48,49] can be detected using generic secondary antibodies (fluorescently conjugated anti-human IgG) and visualised on microarray scanners.

4. Validation of the expression of tumour antigens in tumour cells

Once TAAs have been identified their expression in tumour cells needs to be confirmed. There are a number of assays which can be used to validate the expression of antigens in tumour cells. Many of the most frequently used rely on an available antibody which has been validated [50,51]. Techniques frequently used include:-

4.1. Reverse Transcription (RT-PCR)/Real-time PCR

Total RNA is extracted from cells and used to make cDNA using reverse transcriptase. The cDNA product is amplified by PCR and run on an agarose gel to identify the presence of the transcribed gene in the cell [52]. This technique is sensitive and real-time PCR can provide relative quantitation, however both techniques only indicate the presence/level of gene expression and not protein translation, which can vary greatly between antigens.

4.2. Enzyme-Linked Immunosorbent Assay (ELISA)

Enzyme-Linked Immunosorbent Assay (ELISA) is a straightforward procedure which can be used to detect an antigen using an antibody [53]. The antigen is attached to the bottom of a 96-well plate, or bound by a capture antibody on the bottom of a plate (in the case of a sandwich ELISA). The protein of interest is then incubated with a chemically labelled detection antibody. In most experiments the chemical label is an enzyme and a substrate is added which will produce a colour change detectable by a microplate reader. The technique is sensitive and quantitative when used in conjunction with appropriate protein concentration controls but is better fitted to the analysis of protein in urine and blood, rather than in tissues.

4.3. Immunoblotting

Other systems which use antigen-antibody interactions are techniques such as Western blot. Extracted proteins from tumours or cells are separated by 2-dimensional electrophoretic gels and then blotted onto nitrocellulose membranes. The membranes are incubated with primary and then secondary antibody. The secondary antibody is covalently labelled with an enzyme which reacts with a substrate solution generating colour, which then can be measured [54].

4.4. Immunoprecipitation

The protein of interest can be purified by incubating lysed cell extracts with its specific antibody in solution. Once the antibody has bonded with the protein, the resulting complex can be precipitated using agarose or G Sepharose beads which remove the required protein. The complex can be separated using sodium dodecyl sulphate-polyacrylamide gel electrophoresis [55]. The sample can then be used to determine how much protein is present relative to other cells or other treatment conditions but denaturation is often required and details about sub-cellular localisation are not possible.

4.5. Immunocytochemistry/histochemistry

The antigen of interest can be detected in cells (cytochemistry) or in tissues (histochemistry). The cells or tissue sections are fixed onto slides using a fixative such as paraformaldehyde to immobilise them. They are incubated with the primary antibody and then the secondary which is labelled with a detection molecule. The technique is qualitative informing the user about the sub-cellular localisation of the antigen in tissue and which cell types express it (Figure 1). However quantitation is often lacking and like most methods this requires optimised reagents.

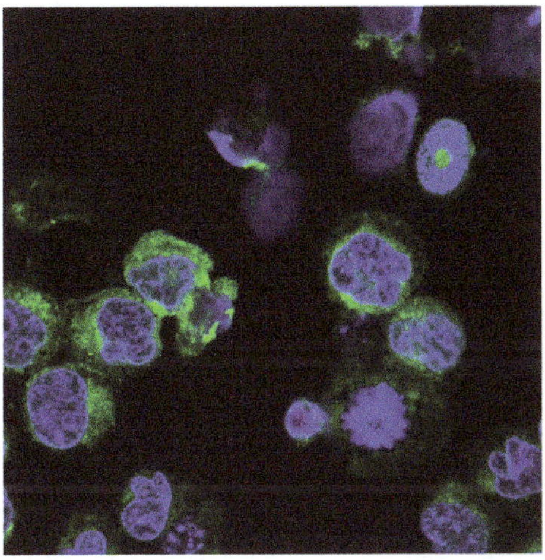

Figure 1. Demonstration of the sub-cellular localisation of the tumour antigen SSX2IP in K562 cells using immunofluoresence microscopy. Cells were air dried for 4-18hours onto glass microscope slides and stored at -20°C wrapped in saranwrap. Cells were defrosted and stained with antigen specific primary and fluorescently labelled secondary antibodies. Using confocal microscopy we detected SSX2IP expression (observed as a green colour by virtue of anti-SSX2IP-fluorescein isothiocyanate) was detectable on the surface of the K562 cells. Cell nuclei were stained blue using 4,6'-diamino-2-phenylindole (DAPI).

The advent of multiple tissue arrays from collaborators or commercial sources provides a screening opportunity once the cancer(s) of interest for the antigen has been defined.

4.6. Flow cytometry

This technique allows the analyses of cells with a variety of parameters such as extracellular or intracellular markers, granularity, size and shape. Cancer cells are labelled with fluorescent antibodies for the required antigen. The cells are passed in a stream and intersected with a laser beam. The intensity of the fluorescence is measured and plotted in the form of dot plots and histograms. This technique is sensitive and informative to allow specific cell types to be "gated" by virtue of size, granularity and detectable protein expression. Machines can measure up to 19 parameters in the most sophisticated machines allowing multiple proteins and cell types to be analysed simultaneously [56]. However the technique requires validated antibodies that have been shown to be appropriate for fluorescence activated cell sorting analysis and enough tumour cells in suspension for analysis.

5. Identification of HLA-binding epitopes — *in vitro* assays

Immune responses in the body can ensure that any foreign matter is eliminated effectively. Class I and II major histocompatability complexes (MHC) are present on the surface of nucleated cells and present processed peptides from proteins inside the cell to T cells. T cells can destroy infected cells if peptides in the context of "danger" are detected [57]. MHC in humans is known as the human leukocyte antigen (HLA) system. MHC class I HLA molecules are highly polymorphic and generally the best defence against infections.

5.1. MHC Peptide binding assay

Peptide antigens are stripped from the HLA class I molecules by mild acid treatment, cells are then incubated with a fluorescent reference peptide together with different concentrations of the peptide of interest. The efficiency with which the required peptide competes for binding to the HLA class I molecules is examined by measuring the amount of HLA-bound reference peptide with fluorescence activated cell sorting analysis [58].

5.2. T2 *in vitro* HLA-A2 binding assay

T2 *in vitro* HLA-A2 binding assay is more frequently used to determine the strength of peptide binding to the most common HLA molecule in Caucasian populations. The HLA-A2 expressing, TAP-1 deficient human T-cell line T2 is used as an assay of HLA-A2 peptide binding efficiency. T2 cells are washed and resuspended in serum-free RPMI media and plated in 96-well microtitre plates. Human β2-microglobulin and often nonamers (nine amino acids long peptides) are added and the cells are incubated overnight at 37°C/5% CO_2. The cells are washed and probed with a HLA-A2-specific monoclonal antibody and appropriate secondary antibody prior to flow cytometry. Only HLA-A2 molecules bound to peptide are stabilised and detectable on the cell surface. Results are reported as a relative mean fluorescence index (MFI), calculated as the MFI of peptide-pulsed T2 cells compared with the MFI of unpulsed T2 cells [59]. Time course assays may be used to indicate how long the peptide remains on the HLA-

A2, indicating how long T cells will have to interact with peptide bound HLA-A2 before the complex falls apart.

6. *In silico* identification of epitopes

There are a number of databases which can be mined to find epitopes which have already been shown to bind to HLA molecules. These have been used to identify established epitopes that may be used in immunotherapy strategies.

6.1. The SYFPEITHI

The SYFPEITHI database allows the prediction of MHC class I and II binding ligands for different mammalian species. When a search is carried out using a protein sequence, a prediction is made based on the amino acids in the anchor and auxiliary anchor positions and other frequent amino acids which can bind to MHC molecules. A score is then calculated which follows certain rules which are: a numerical value of 10 is given to amino acids that regularly arise in anchor positions, the value 8 is set for amino acids occurring in a significant number of ligands, six is for unusual anchors such as auxiliary anchors and less frequent residues of the same set have a value of four. Preferred amino acids have coefficients between 1–4 depending on the signal strength in pool sequencing or the occurrence of individual sequences. Amino acids that are considered as having an adverse effect on binding have a coefficient of –1 to –3 [60]. SYFPEITHI database gets updated regularly and has been used to identify various ligands; p28 peptide as an epitope for the CT antigen PLAC1 in breast cancer [61], p101-111 is the first CTA-derived peptide which induces CD4(+), CD8(+), and B-cell responses *in vitro* [62], p43-57 epitope stimulates T cells in HCA587-derived tumours [63] and PASD1(1) – PASD1(5) [51].

6.2. Bioinformatics and Molecular Analysis Section (BIMAS)

Bioinformatics and Molecular Analysis Section (BIMAS) develops computational processes to analyse data generated from molecular biology and genetics research; and provides bioinformatics guidance, support and resources for the collection, management, and display of biological sequence and genomic information for scientists involved in genomics and genetic analysis [64]. Other online software which can be used to identify epitopes includes EpiJen, Rankpep, nHLApred, NetCTL and Multipred [65].

7. Cell based assays — *In vitro* demonstration of T cell reactivity

There are a number of assays which can be used to determine if T cells are activated in response to antigen.

7.1. Carboxyfluorescein diacetate Succinimidyl Ester (CFSE)

Carboxyfluorescein diacetate succinimidyl ester (CFSE) is a cytoplasmic dye which is absorbed by all cell types. Once the CFSE labelled cells divide, the dye is shared amongst the daughter cells equally therefore the fluorescence is halved after each round of the cell cycle. This difference in fluorescence can be measured. The more cells proliferate, the greater the decrease in the fluorescent signal. The fluorescence peaks can be measured by flow cytometry [66]. CFSE labelling is increasingly used to measure target tumour cell killing [67], superseding radiation based assays, as well as T cell proliferation in response to tumour cells *in vivo* [68]. CFSE labelling can also be performed *in vivo* where the dye is injected into the host animal's spleen or lymph nodes, however the labelling is not uniform and it is sometimes difficult to obtain individual peaks once lymphocyte cell division has occurred [66].

7.2. Lymphocyte proliferation assays

Lymphocyte proliferation assays can be used to determine activation of T cells. Peripheral blood mononuclear cells are isolated and cultured in microtitre plates. The specific antigen is incubated with the cells, which causes the T cells to divide and grow. The MTT colorimetric assay is based upon (3-(4,5-Dimethylthiazol-2-yl)-2,5-diphenyltetrazolium bromide, a yellow tetrazolium salt which gets cleaved by enzymes in the mitochondria to produce blue formazan. Viable, dividing cells will create more formazan which can be quantified using a plate reader. MTT assay is very convenient, however some considerations need to be assessed to avoid false positives such as cell densities, correct culture medium, filtration of media to remove precipitate, optimisation of MTT concentrations and incubation times [69].

7.3. [^{3}H]-Thymidine incorporation assay

[^{3}H]-Thymidine incorporation assay is based on the use of [^{3}H]-thymidine a radioactive molecule which can be incorporated into DNA during the S-phase of cell division. As new DNA is synthesised, occasional thymidine bases are replaced by [^{3}H]-thymidine and subsequently the incorporated radioactivity is measured, following washes to remove unincorporated radioactivity, using a Scintillation Counter [70]. As [^{3}H]-thymidine is radioactive an analogue called bromodeoxyuridine (BrdU) was developed to replace it in assays. BrdU integrates into DNA strands and can be measured using immunohistochemistry and flow cytometry protocols using fluorescent conjugates and can be observed over a longer duration. BrdU is also used to look at the number of cells in each part of the cell cycle by flow cytometry [71]. However BrdU has been found to be more toxic than [^{3}H]-thymidine, possibly because it is structurally very different to the original DNA nucleotides. It also adversely affects cell division, the pattern of cell migration, final position of migrating cells and the fate of labelled cells [72].

7.4. Peptide-MHC (pMHCs)

Peptide-MHC (pMHCs) based assays circumvent issues caused by measuring T cell proliferation. T cell proliferation assays can provide information on whether an immune response has been generated but won't determine which T cells, if they are indeed T cells, have been activated. pMHCs, often referred to as tetramers, can be used to identify antigen specific T cells. They are produced through the refolding of β2-microglobulin and heavy chains in MHC molecules with the appropriate epitope of interest. The pMHC is then labelled with biotin using BirA enzyme. A streptavidin molecule conjugated to a fluorescent detector binds to four (tetramers) pMHCs or can used to create multimers (for example dimers, pentamers, dextramers) of these constructed MHC molecules courtesy of the biotin-avidin interaction [73]. T cell populations are added to this mixture and T cells with the specific receptor for the epitope of interest will bind and be measurable by flow cytometry [74]. Shen *et al* [74] have found that cross-reactive T cells i.e. T cells which recognise two different antigens can be identified providing an extra tool in vaccine development. In some cases antigen specific T cells may not bind tetramers due to being undifferentiated and unable to accumulate T cell receptor (TCR) molecules close to the antigen. Another reason could be low affinity between TCR and MHC [75]. Other techniques based on the use of pMHCs include pMHC arrays [76] (Section 7.5), NACS [77] and the combinatorial approach [78,79]. These techniques all provide high throughput analysis of multiple T cell populations with a variety of pros and cons to each technique including issues with background, specificity/binding capacity of individual pMHC complexes, activated induced cell death of pMHC bound T cells, internalisation of pMHCs following T cell binding [80], cost and labour intensity. Sequencing of TCRs (2-3 million every 2-3 days) by companies such as TRON gGmbH (Johannes Gutenberg University Mainz, Germany) and Adaptive Biotechnologies (Seattle, USA) will provide a new way of analysing T cell populations which will be informative with regards to which TCRs are present but not necessarily whether they are present on mature, anergic, activated or functional T cells nor which sub-group of T cells are harbouring them (helper T cells, cytotoxic T cells, Th17 cells or indeed regulatory T cells (Tregs)). This technology allows the first opportunity to examine an extremely large number of TCRs in a very short time and will revolutionise how we examine T cell responses in patients in the future.

7.5. pMHC arrays

pMHC or tetramer arrays [76,81] (Figure 2) provides a strategy to determine which specific $CD8^+$ T cell populations are present in the peripheral blood of patients. Antigens identified by the techniques described already can be used to help expand the pMHC array for future studies. In addition, the pMHC array provides a means to investigate epitope spreading and changes in T cell specificities with disease progression. The technique benefits from the low number of purified $CD8^+$ T cells required for each array ($0.5\text{-}2 \times 10^6$), which can be purified from 20ml of patient peripheral blood using StemCell $CD8^+$ negative isolation beads providing "untouched" T cells (Bonney, Guinn *et al*, in preparation). The purified $CD8^+$ T cells are then lipophyllically dyed with DiD (Molecular Probes), washed and incubated with the pMHC array. The pMHC array has a detection limit of 0.02% matching the sensitivity we can reproducibly achieve with flow cytometry when analysing patient samples. Where sample availability permits, pMHC array data should be validated by flow cytometry [82] using the same pMHC tetramers as in the pMHC array. The pMHC array has the added advantage that it can be used for the initial screening of a relatively small number of CD8+ T cells against a large number of pMHCs on the array, and a short-list of T cell populations which are shown to exist on the pMHC array can then be quantitated by flow cytometry (limiting the amount of sample required in subsequent studies). The pMHC array can be used to analyse patient samples at a number of disease time-points (presentation, post-treatment (surgery and/or radiotherapy) and with disease progression) to examine how T cell responses to tumour antigens change with treatment, to examine epitope spreading and to correlate changing immune responses with clinical responses.

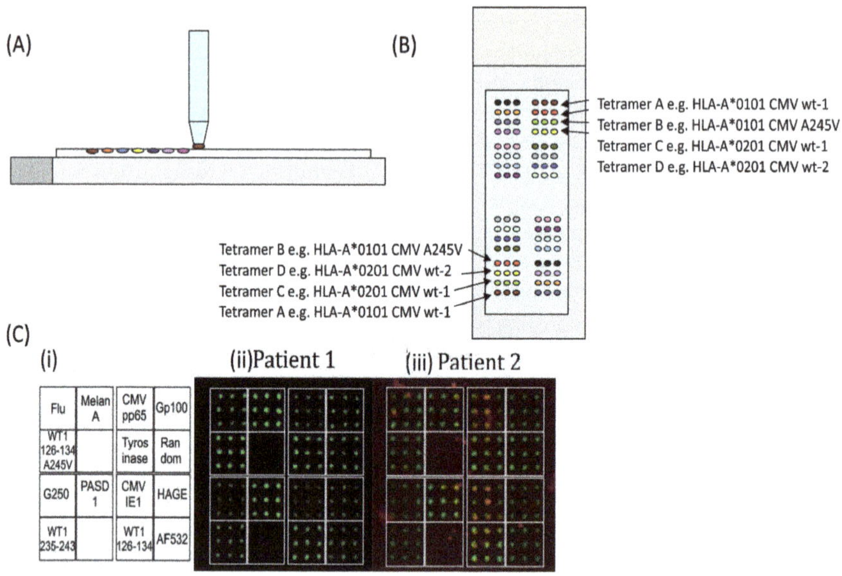

Figure 2. pMHC arrays for the simultaneous detection of T cell populations in patient peripheral blood. (A) Using a QArray^2 printer and HPLF 0.3mm solid tip pins (Genetix) we printed multiplexed AF532-conjugated pMHCs at a concentration of 0.5mg/ml so that 1ng was placed in each spot (shown as coloured ovals). Each spot is 400uM wide with a 700uM inter-spot distance. (B) At least six spots per pMHC are applied in each of two independent sites. Each hydrogel slide can hold up to 1,000 spots of tetramer in total. (C) We applied 0.8-1.5 x 10^6 lipophillically-dyed CD8+ T cells/slide (seen in red). pMHCs included a range of HLA restrictions and had already been shown to work in flow cytometry studies,(i) pMHCs are spotted across the gel, (seen as green spots) (ii) even some HLA-A2 positive patients show no reactivity with any pMHCs (iii) while others show the presence of multiple T cell populations which recognise tumour antigens. Based on figure in [144].

7.6. Intracellular cytokine staining assay

Intracellular cytokine staining assay detects particular cytokines released by immune cells which can provide a useful insight into the responding T cell populations. Such cytokines could include interferon-gamma (IFNγ), interleukin-2 (IL-2), IL-4 and tumour necrosis factor-α. Cells are plated and incubated with the antigen to stimulate cytokine production. To prevent the cytokine from exiting the cell a transport inhibitor is added e.g. brefeldin A. The cells are then fixed in paraformaldehyde and permeabilized to allow the anti-cytokine antibody to bind. The results are analysed by flow cytometry. The use of intracellular cytokine staining assay to detect the cytokine IFNγ shows high reproducibility and linearity with little background [83]. Duration of culture prior to antigen stimulation, as well as the cytokine accumulation period, are critical parameters of these methods. In both murine and cattle models, following 2-6 hours in culture, T cells produced a mixture of cytokines IFNγ, IL-2 and tumour necrosis factor-α, however following 6-16 hours of culture only IFN-γ cytokine was found [84].

Using multiple peptides from distinct TAAs to stimulate immune cells may prove the most effective for peptide vaccines. A cocktail of four multiple myeloma antigen peptides were used to stimulate T lymphocytes from HLA-A2 positive people to induce IFNγ production, cell proliferation and cytotoxicity against HLA-A2 positive multiple myeloma patients' cells [85]. Indeed long peptides may offer the advantage of allowing the immune system to choose the epitope(s) it can best process and present from a peptide sequence and induce an effective cytotoxic T cell response in the presence of longer CD4$^+$ helper motifs [86]. Conversely sometimes longer proteins can inhibit CD8$^+$ T cells responses [87] but this may vary depending on the constituents of individual protein sequences.

8. Cell based assays — *In vivo* assays

There are a number of approaches that can be taken when using mouse models to detect T cell immune responses. Animals can be used in transplantable tumour (xenografts) models or genetically engineered tumour models. In xenograft models human tumour cells are taken and injected into immunodeficient mice so that complex immune responses involving multiple cell types can be investigated. In contrast, in genetically engineered models, genes known to cause cancer are activated or tumour suppressor genes are "switched off" to allow their effects on tumour growth to be examined. In addition transgenic mice can be used to examine T cell responses to epitopes presented on MHC molecules as described in this section.

8.1. Immunodeficient mice

Immunodeficient mice such as athymic nude mice, severely compromised immunodeficient (SCID) mice and non-obese diabetic severe combined immunodeficiency mice will accept xenografts of human cells [88]. Depending upon the number of cells injected, or the size of the tumour transplanted, the tumour can develop over weeks to months and the response to appropriate therapeutic agents studied *in vivo* [89]. Indeed such models have been used to examine the effectiveness of various immunotherapeutic strategies including whole cell vaccines [90], dendritic cell (DC) vaccines [91], peptide vaccines [92] and DNA vaccines [67,87,93].

8.2. Genetically modified mice

Genetically modified mice may have genes which are overexpressed or deleted and the effects of these genes on tumour development can be studied. Examples include p53 null and heterogenous mice [94,95] demonstrated that these genes can act as oncogenes and lead to tumour development. Possible therapies for these oncogenes/tumour suppressor genes are tested for their response in an *in vivo*, full organism context [89] and examples include Ad-p53, AAV-HGFK1 [96].

HLA-A2 transgenic mice have genes inserted into the DNA so they will express the HLA molecules known in mice as H-2. In order to prevent the presentation of murine H-2-restricted cytotoxic T lymphocyte (CTL) epitopes in HLA-A2 (AAD) transgenic mice, HLA-A2.1 transgenic/H-2 class I knockout mice (HHD mice) were created [97]. In HHD mice, the H-2 class I gene is knocked out, and a chimeric HLA-A2.1 monochain (HHD) is produced by linking the C terminal of the human β2-microglobulin (unit of the class 1 MHC) covalently to the N-terminus of the chimeric HLA-A2 heavy chain (which contain the α1&2 domains of HLA-A2.1 and the α3 domain of H-2Db) by means of a peptide bond. This guarantees the sole expression of the HHD molecule on the cell surface, making sure that any identified CTL epitopes are HLA-A2 restricted [98]. HHD mice allow epitopes which are presented on human HLA-A2 to be examined for their ability to induce T cell responses in a variety of studies; for example STEAP, a prostate tumour antigen has been shown to be targeted by anti-tumour T cells [99] and DNA vaccines encoding Wilms tumour antigen 1 induce cytotoxic responses in mice [100] using this model system.

9. Modes of immunotherapy

One of the biggest debates in cancer immunotherapy remains which mode will be the most effective. The National Cancer Institute have suggested that immunotherapy studies should focus on a limited number of antigenic targets to maximise the chances of success [101]. However for some cancers effective immunotherapy targets have yet to be discovered (i.e. ovarian cancer, adult acute lymphocytic leukaemia) and better targets may yet be determined.

When T cells were found to be able to identify cancer cells [102] it was thought that T cell therapies would be the most effective with the aim being to stimulate $CD8^{+}$/CTL cells to kill tumour cells. This can be achieved by a number of ways such as through the use of DCs [103], peptide vaccines [85], DNA vaccines [104] and natural killer cells [105]. In recent years monoclonal antibodies (mAb) have become standard treatments for cancer. Ultimately if there is an antibody and it recognises a surface antigen solely on cancer and non-essential cells then this will likely be the most effective way to cause tumour destruction. mAbs are derived by vaccinating an animal with the target antigen and testing to see if the B cells are producing antibodies against it. Then the B cells are extracted from its spleen and infused with myeloma cells to produce hybridomas. Hybridomas divide perpetually and produce the mAb to the antigen in large amounts [106].

Rosenberg *et al* [107] showed that only 2.6% of immunotherapy clinical trials had worked and therefore an overhaul was needed in the practice of immunotherapy. Subsequently the same group showed that adoptive T cell therapy could be very promising with cell numbers being returned to the patient [108] and their status – activated but not mature [109] and cell numbers being the main issues. It is also likely that the best strategy may include a combination of conventional and immunotherapy techniques [110] or even a combination of immunotherapy techniques as demonstrated in increasing numbers of mouse models [111] and clinical trials [112].

DCs are antigen presenting cells therefore they have received some attention for possible use in cancer immunotherapy. DCs pulsed by peptide and injected into the skin showed a response rate of 28%. This percentage increased to 35.7% when immature DCs are injected straight into the tumour and even higher to 40% for advanced pancreatic cancer [113].

Tumour-infiltrating T cells (TIL) therapy has been used in stage IV melanoma patients. TILs are obtained from the blood, lymph nodes or from a tumour tissue biopsy. TILs are isolated, activated and expanded using IL-2 *in vitro*. The patient undergoes lympho-depleting chemotherapy prior to the T cells being injected back in to the blood [114].

When a tumour antigen is secreted into the circulation in high levels immune tolerance can be induced in the thymus. CD8α^-Sirpα^+, a subset of DCs, are able to capture tumour antigens in the blood, which can induce tolerance through Tregs or negative selection. Tregs are cells which are part of the tolerance system which prevents autoimmunity [115, 116]. Simultaneous Treg depletions (using anti-CD25 antibodies for instance) may aid the effectiveness of immunotherapy in some cancer types where Treg infiltration into the tumour is rife [117,118].

There are a number of reviews in this area of research which aim to look into effective immunotherapy strategies for the future. These include cellular immunotherapy [119], whole call vaccines [120], multidrug resistance [121] and DCs [122]. Targeted therapeutic strategies along with ever improving designs in clinical trials pave the way for further success [123].

10. Clinical trials

Clinical trials are undertaken after a large amount of data has been obtained on the antigen of interest in the lab. This data is required to ensure treatment safety and efficacy as far as is possible. It remains imperative in most countries that treatments have been tested on live animals prior to first-in-man clinical trials and that favourable results are apparent in order for treatments to be taken into clinical trials. People, often patients, are recruited as compensated or full volunteers. The drug is given to participants initially to show that it is safe and then that it is effective. Dose escalation is also important so that an effective and safe dosage in humans is used.

Clinical trials have four phases, very basically as follows: I – evaluation of safety, II – safety and efficacy (with Phase I/II often including dose escalation), III – efficacy in a large cohort of patients and IV – post-approval studies. Phase I trials look at the safety and the best dose of the drug to administer. Such trials often involve 13 patients or less, and these patients are often have late stage cancer and are refractory to all other treatments with little chance of recovery. Phase II trials start to look at the efficacy of the medicine and often involve 20 patients with late stage disease. Phase I and II trials have to be completed successfully in order for testing to proceed to Phase III. Current "best practise" treatment is compared to the new drug being tested in phase III trials. Only if the new drug offers an improvement over best practise does the new medicine have a chance of becoming the standard treatment. At this time the drug will need to be licensed and approved by the authoritative body e.g. the US Food and Drug Administration, and once licensed, phase IV trials investigate the long term benefits and unexpected side effects. In some cases the drug may go through one of the phases more than once before moving forward and even then may get rejected [124].

It is very important that trials follow certain rules for the results to be considered legitimate. Phase III trials need to be randomised i.e. a computer randomly puts people into one of two groups. These can also be double-blind trials so that neither the patient nor the investigator knows which treatment is being given, thus avoiding any bias. In some cases there may not be any treatment to compare a new therapy against, in which case a placebo (inactive treatment) is given to one group [125]. In the UK the Medicines and Healthcare products Regulatory Agency is responsible for the regulation of medicines and medical devices and equipment used in healthcare, and the investigation of harmful incidents as well as overseeing the use of blood and blood products [126].

Cohen *et al* [127] have created an online website called BreastCancerTrials.org which matches patients to current trials taking place depending on the information they provide. This provides a valuable source for cancer patients who may want initial guidance on which clinical trials may be beneficial to them.

11. Assays to demonstrate efficacy of the response

Assays tend to reflect the immunotherapy strategy employed with the efficacy of antibody therapies being measured by tumour destruction, ertumaxomab destroys tumour cells expressing HER2/neu [128], bispecific antibodies represent a new class of anticancer therapeutics [129] and antibody-targeted delivery of a vaccine can improve tumour cell killing [130].

11.1. Enzyme-Linked Immunosorbent Spot (ELISPOT) assay

Enzyme-Linked Immunosorbent Spot (ELISPOT) assay was developed by Cecil Czerkinskdy in 1983 [131] and shows most similarity to the ELISA technique. It is based on the use of a 96 well plate with a polyvinyl-difluoride membrane to which antigen specific monoclonal "capture" antibodies are attached. The cells are grown in media on the capture antibody coated membrane usually for several hours to overnight and secreted protein (often cytokines such as IFNγ) bind to the capture antibody. A second "detection" antibody specific to the protein is used. This is often conjugated to an enzyme allowing a chemical reaction to occur. Black spots form on the membrane wherever protein is present and these can be counted by an ELISPOT reader [131]. ELISPOT assays are one of the most sensitive *ex vivo* detection methods available with low detection thresholds in peripheral blood. ELISPOT is also able to identify patients with allergies through the detection of drug-specific T cells in their blood [132].

11.2. Cultured ELISPOT

Cultured ELISPOT measures memory T cells. Cells are stimulated and plated on a 24-well plate. After an incubation period half of the cell culture supernatant is removed and replaced with Lymphocult (an IL-2 containing growth factor supplement). Fresh Lymphocult is added again on day 7. On day 9, the cells are incubated overnight. On day 10, around $2.5x10^4$ of the originally plated cells are plated for a standard ELISPOT assay. Cultured ELISPOT assays revealed the existence of longer-lasting T cell memory responses [133].

12. Conclusions

This chapter has focussed predominantly on the identification of epitopes within tumour antigens and their validation as they enter clinical trials. Focus on clinical trials using antibody therapies, DCs, natural killer cells, and adoptive therapy among many other options are the focus of other excellent reviews in the field [134-136].

Cancer immunotherapy is a vital area of research that continues to progress at a pace. Our understanding of the immune response and its potential to recognise and kill tumour cells with mans guidance offers hope to the patients for whom few other treatment options exist. Many tumour antigens have been identified, but some cancers still lack antigen targets that are expressed in the majority of the cancer cells by the majority of cancer patients. New techniques to extend antigen discovery will allow the improvement of immunotherapy strategies while the identification of new biomarkers will assist in the development of personalised therapies. Personalised therapies will decrease the cost (quantitative and qualitative) of treatment on patients who are unlikely to respond to it, allowing patients to avoid unpleasant and harmful side effects while maximising patient quality of life.

Target antigen	Mode of immunotherapy	Patient group	Phase of clinical trial	Outcome	Reference
CD22	Monoclonal antibody conjugated to calecheamicin	Refractory and relapsed acute lymphocytic leukaemia	Phase 2	18% patients had complete response, 39% had marrow complete response, 39% had resistant disease, and 4% died within 4 weeks of starting treatment	[137]
TG4010 targeting MUC1 & IL-2	Poxvirus (modified vaccinia virus Ankara) in combination with first-line chemotherapy	Advanced non-small-cell lung cancer	Phase 2B	6-month progression-free survival was 43·2% in the TG4010 plus chemotherapy group, and 35·1% in the chemotherapy alone group	[138]
LY6K and TTK	peptide vaccines in combination with CpG-7909	Metastatic oesophageal squamous cell carcinoma	Phase 1	Vaccination with peptides in combination with CpG-7909 increased and activated pDC populations and NK cell populations	[139]
CTLA-4	Monoclonal antibody with glycoprotein 100 (gp100) peptide vaccine	Previously treated metastatic melanoma	Phase 3	The median overall survival was 10.0 months among patients receiving ipilimumab plus gp100, as compared with 6.4 months among patients receiving gp100 alone	[140]
Prostate-specific antigen	Poxviral vaccines	Prostate cancer	Phase 2	The primary end point was progression-free survival which was similar in the two groups (treated, controls). However, at 3 years post study, treated patients had a overall survival rate of 30% compared to 17% of controls	[141]
CD20	Monoclonal antibody	Relapsed or refractory follicular lymphoma	Phase 1/2	Treatment caused immediate and profound B-cell depletion, and 65% of patients reverted to negative BCL2 status.	[142]
CA-125	Abagovomab, an anti-idiotype antibody	Ovarian Cancer	Phase 1	Improved CA125-specific cellular cytotoxicity might indicate that longer vaccination (nine injections) would be preferred to short (six injections)	[143]

Table 1. Examples of completed clinical trials showing the cancer antigen targets. Representation of the various modes of immunotherapy employed to date, cancer patients treated and the outcome of the trials.

Abbreviations

BIMAS: Bioinformatics and Molecular Analysis Section; BrdU: bromodeoxyuridine; CFSE: Carboxyfluorescein diacetate succinimidyl ester; CTL: Cytotoxic T lymphocyte; CT: cancer-testis; DC: dendritic cell; ELISA: Enzyme-linked immunosorbent assay; ELISPOT: Enzyme-linked immunosorbence assay; HLA: human leukocyte antigen; IFNγ: interferon-gamma; IL: interleukin; mAb: monoclonal antibodies; MFI: mean fluorescence index; MHC: major histocompatibility complex; PCR: polymerise chain reaction; pMHC: peptide and major histocompatibility complex; SEREX: Serological identification of antigens by recombinant expression cloning; SSX2IP: Synovial Sarcoma X breakpoint 2 Interacting Protein; TAA: tumour associated antigens; TCR: T cell receptor; TIL: Tumour-infiltrating T cells; Tregs: regulatory T cells.

Acknowledgements

SEB was funded by Cancer Research U.K. Research by our group has been supported by Leukaemia and Lymphoma Research, Wessex Cancer Trust and a Wessex Medical Research Innovations grant.

Author details

Ghazala Khan[1], Suzanne E. Brooks[2], Frances Denniss[3], Dagmar Sigurdardottir[4] and Barbara-ann Guinn[1,2,3*]

*Address all correspondence to: barbara.guinn@beds.ac.uk

1 Division of Science, University of Bedfordshire, Park Square, Luton, UK

2 Cancer Sciences Division (MP824), Southampton University Hospitals, University of Southampton, Southampton, UK

3 Department of Haematological Medicine, King's College London School of Medicine, The Rayne Institute, London, UK

4 Department of Immunology, Institute for Cell Biology, University of Tübingen, Tübingen, Germany

References

[1] Penn, C.G. Halgrimson, T.E. Starzl, De novo malignant tumors in organ transplant recipients, Transplant. Proc. 1 (1971) 773-778.

[2] U. Sahin, O. Tureci, H. Schmitt, B. Cochlovius, T. Johannes, R. Schmits, F. Stenner, G. Luo, I. Schobert, M. Pfreundschuh, Human neoplasms elicit multiple specific immune responses in the autologous host, Proc. Natl. Acad. Sci. U. S. A. 25 (1995) 11810-11813.

[3] L.T. Nguyen, A.R. Elford, K. Murakami, K.M. Garza, S.P. Schoenberger, B. Odermatt, D.E. Speiser, P.S. Ohashi, Tumor growth enhances cross-presentation leading to limited T cell activation without tolerance, J. Exp. Med. 4 (2002) 423-435.

[4] E.M. Tan, Autoantibodies as reporters identifying aberrant cellular mechanisms in tumorigenesis, J. Clin. Invest. 10 (2001) 1411-1415.

[5] J.Y. Zhang, K.S. Looi, E.M. Tan, Identification of tumor-associated antigens as diagnostic and predictive biomarkers in cancer, Methods Mol. Biol. (2009) 1-10.

[6] T. Soussi, p53 Antibodies in the sera of patients with various types of cancer: a review, Cancer Res. 7 (2000) 1777-1788.

[7] E. Haralambieva, K.A. Pulford, L. Lamant, S. Pileri, G. Roncador, K.C. Gatter, G. Delsol, D.Y. Mason, Anaplastic large-cell lymphomas of B-cell phenotype are anaplastic lymphoma kinase (ALK) negative and belong to the spectrum of diffuse large B-cell lymphomas, Br. J. Haematol. 3 (2000) 584-591.

[8] B. Guinn, J. Greiner, M. Schmitt, K.I. Mills, Elevated expression of the leukemia-associated antigen SSX2IP predicts survival in acute myeloid leukemia patients who lack detectable cytogenetic rearrangements, Blood. 113 (2009) 1203-1204.

[9] Y.T. Chen, Identification of human tumor antigens by serological expression cloning: an online review on SEREX, *Cancer Immun.* (2004) http://www.cancerimmunity.org/serex

[10] M. Kalejs, J. Erenpreisa, Cancer/testis antigens and gametogenesis: a review and "brainstorming" session, Cancer. Cell. Int. 1 (2005) 4.

[11] S.H. Lim, Y. Zhang, J. Zhang, Cancer-testis antigens: the current status on antigen regulation and potential clinical use, Am. J. Blood Res. 1 (2012) 29-35.

[12] M.J. Scanlan, C.M. Gordon, B. Williamson, S.Y. Lee, Y.T. Chen, E. Stockert, A. Jungbluth, G. Ritter, D. Jager, E. Jager, A. Knuth, L.J. Old, Identification of cancer/testis genes by database mining and mRNA expression analysis, Int. J. Cancer. 4 (2002) 485-492

[13] Van Driessche, Z.N. Berneman, V.F. Van Tendeloo, Active specific immunotherapy targeting the Wilms' tumor protein 1 (WT1) for patients with hematological malignancies and solid tumors: lessons from early clinical trials, Oncologist. 2 (2012) 250-259.

[14] F. Wadelin, J. Fulton, P.A. McEwan, K.A. Spriggs, J. Emsley, D.M. Heery, Leucine-rich repeat protein PRAME: expression, potential functions and clinical implications for leukaemia, Mol. Cancer. (2010) 226.

[15] A.M. Krackhardt, M. Witzens, S. Harig, F.S. Hodi, A.J. Zauls, M. Chessia, P. Barrett, J.G. Gribben, Identification of tumor-associated antigens in chronic lymphocytic leukemia by SEREX, Blood. 6 (2002) 2123-2131.

[16] M. Forgber, U. Trefzer, W. Sterry, P. Walden, Proteome serological determination of tumor-associated antigens in melanoma, PLoS One. 4 (2009) e5199.

[17] K. Wang, X. Xu, Y. Nie, L. Dai, P. Wang, J. Zhang, Identification of tumor-associated antigens by using SEREX in hepatocellular carcinoma, Cancer Lett. 2 (2009) 144-150.

[18] J. Qian, J. Xie, S. Hong, J. Yang, L. Zhang, X. Han, M. Wang, F. Zhan, J.D. Shaughnessy Jr, J. Epstein, L.W. Kwak, Q. Yi, Dickkopf-1 (DKK1) is a widely expressed and potent tumor-associated antigen in multiple myeloma, Blood. 5 (2007) 1587-1594.

[19] S.P. Adams, S.S. Sahota, A. Mijovic, B. Czepulkowski, R.A. Padua, G.J. Mufti, B.A. Guinn, Frequent expression of HAGE in presentation chronic myeloid leukaemias, Leukemia. 16 (2002) 2238-2242.

[20] V. Martelange, C. De Smet, E. De Plaen, C. Lurquin, T. Boon, Identification on a human sarcoma of two new genes with tumor-specific expression, Cancer Res. 14 (2000) 3848-3855.

[21] K.L. Tyson, P.L. Weissberg, C.M. Shanahan, Heterogeneity of gene expression in human atheroma unmasked using cDNA representational difference analysis, Physiol. Genomics. 2 (2002) 121-130.

[22] http://www.licr.org/D_programs/d4a1i_SEREX.php

[23] S. Zhou, T Yi, B Zhang, F Huang, H Huang, J Tang, X Zhao. Mapping the high throughput SEREX technology screening for novel tumor antigens, Comb Chem High Throughput Screen. 15 (2012) 202-15.

[24] D. Jäger, Potential target antigens for immunotherapy identified by serological expression cloning (SEREX), Methods Mol Biol. 360 (2007) 319-26.

[25] M.J. Edelman, L. Hodgson, P.Y. Rosenblatt, R.H. Christenson, E.E. Vokes, X. Wang, R. Kratzke, CYFRA 21-1 as a prognostic and predictive marker in advanced non-small-cell lung cancer in a prospective trial: CALGB 150304, J. Thorac. Oncol. 4 (2012) 649-654.

[26] K. Imai, S. Hirata, A. Irie, S. Senju, Y. Ikuta, K. Yokomine, M. Harao, M. Inoue, Y. Tomita, T. Tsunoda, H. Nakagawa, Y. Nakamura, H. Baba, Y. Nishimura, Identification of HLA-A2-restricted CTL epitopes of a novel tumour-associated antigen, KIF20A, overexpressed in pancreatic cancer, Br. J. Cancer. 2 (2011) 300-307.

[27] A.P. Liggins, B.A. Guinn, C.S. Hatton, K. Pulford, A.H. Banham, Serologic detection of diffuse large B-cell lymphoma-associated antigens, Int. J. Cancer. 110 (2004) 563-569.

[28] B.A. Guinn, E.A. Bland, U. Lodi, A.P. Liggins, K. Tobal, S. Petters, J.W. Wells, A.H. Banham, G.J. Mufti, Humoral detection of leukaemia-associated antigens in presentation acute myeloid leukaemia, Biochem. Biophys. Res. Commun. 335 (2005) 1293-1304.

[29] S. Patel, H. Chen, L. Monti, E. Gould, E. Haralambieva, J. Schmid, D. Toomey, W. Woessmann, G. Roncador, C.S. Hatton, A.P. Liggins, R. Taramelli, A.H. Banham, F. Acquati, D. Murphy, K. Pulford, RNASET2 - An autoantigen in anaplastic large cell lymphoma identified by protein array analysis, J Proteomics. 75 (2012) 5279-5292.

[30] S. Tschiedel, C. Gentilini, T. Lange, C. Wolfel, T. Wolfel, V. Lennerz, S. Stevanovic, H.G. Rammensee, C. Huber, M. Cross, D. Niederwieser, Identification of NM23-H2 as a tumour-associated antigen in chronic myeloid leukaemia, Leukemia. 8 (2008) 1542-1550.

[31] Y. Wang, Q. Gu, B. Liu, Z. Zhu, Perspectives of SEREX-defined antigens in diagnosis and immunotherapy for gastric cancer, Cancer. Biol. Ther. 9 (2004) 806-811.

[32] C.S. Klade, T. Voss, E. Krystek, H. Ahorn, K. Zatloukal, K. Pummer, G.R. Adolf, Identification of tumor antigens in renal cell carcinoma by serological proteome analysis, Proteomics. 7 (2001) 890-898.

[33] C.G. Gunawardana, E.P. Diamandis, High throughput proteomic strategies for identifying tumour-associated antigens, Cancer Lett. 249 (2007) 110-119.

[34] C.A. Casiano, M. Mediavilla-Varela, E.M. Tan, Tumor-associated antigen arrays for the serological diagnosis of cancer, Mol. Cell. Proteomics. 5 (2006) 1745-1759.

[35] M. Nishiu, R. Yanagawa, S. Nakatsuka, M. Yao, T. Tsunoda, Y. Nakamura, K. Aozasa, Microarray analysis of gene-expression profiles in diffuse large B-cell lymphoma: identification of genes related to disease progression, Jpn. J. Cancer Res. 8 (2002) 894-901.

[36] D.J. Brennan, C. Kelly, E. Rexhepaj, P.A. Dervan, M.J. Duffy, W.M. Gallagher, Contribution of DNA and tissue microarray technology to the identification and validation of biomarkers and personalised medicine in breast cancer, Cancer Genomics Proteomics. 3 (2007) 121-134.

[37] C. De Pitta, L. Tombolan, M. Campo Dell'Orto, B. Accordi, G. te Kronnie, C. Romualdi, N. Vitulo, G. Basso, G. Lanfranchi, A leukemia-enriched cDNA microarray platform identifies new transcripts with relevance to the biology of pediatric acute lymphoblastic leukemia, Haematologica. 7 (2005) 890-898.

[38] J.S. Chen, E. Coustan-Smith, T. Suzuki, G.A. Neale, K. Mihara, C.H. Pui, D. Campana, Identification of novel markers for monitoring minimal residual disease in acute lymphoblastic leukemia, Blood. 7 (2001) 2115-2120.

[39] B.A. Guinn, L. Bullinger, N.S. Thomas, K.I. Mills, J. Greiner, SSX2IP expression in acute myeloid leukaemia: an association with mitotic spindle failure in t(8;21), and cell cycle in t(15;17) patients, Br. J. Haematol. 140 (2008) 250-251.

[40] V. Dutoit, C. Herold-Mende, N. Hilf, O. Schoor, P. Beckhove, J. Bucher, K. Dorsch, S. Flohr, J. Fritsche, P. Lewandrowski, J. Lohr, H.G. Rammensee, S. Stevanovic, C. Trautwein, V. Vass, S. Walter, P.R. Walker, T. Weinschenk, H. Singh-Jasuja, P.Y. Dietrich, Exploiting the glioblastoma peptidome to discover novel tumour-associated antigens for immunotherapy, Brain. 135 (2012) 1042-1054.

[41] J.S. Stickel, A.O. Weinzierl, N. Hillen, O. Drews, M.M. Schuler, J. Hennenlotter, D. Wernet, C.A. Muller, A. Stenzl, H.G. Rammensee, S. Stevanovic, HLA ligand profiles

of primary renal cell carcinoma maintained in metastases, Cancer Immunol. Immunother. 9 (2009) 1407-1417.

[42] A.J. Knights, A.O. Weinzierl, T. Flad, B.A. Guinn, L. Mueller, G.J. Mufti, S. Stevanovic, G. Pawelec, A novel MHC-associated proteinase 3 peptide isolated from primary chronic myeloid leukaemia cells further supports the significance of this antigen for the immunotherapy of myeloid leukaemias, Leukemia. 20 (2006) 1067-1072.

[43] Mohamedali, B.A. Guinn, S. Sahu, N.S. Thomas, G.J. Mufti, Serum profiling reveals distinctive proteomic markers in chronic myeloid leukaemia patients, Br. J. Haematol. 144 (2009) 263-265.

[44] N. Hillen, S. Stevanovic S. Contribution of mass spectrometry-based proteomics to immunology. Expert Rev Proteomics. 3 (2006) 653-64.

[45] L.J. Stern, Characterizing MHC-associated peptides by mass spectrometry, J. Immunol. 5 (2007) 2667-2668.

[46] A.L. Zarling, S.B. Ficarro, F.M. White, J. Shabanowitz, D.F. Hunt, V.H. Engelhard, Phosphorylated peptides are naturally processed and presented by major histocompatibility complex class I molecules *in vivo*, J. Exp. Med. 12 (2000) 1755-1762.

[47] J.R. Yates, C.I. Ruse, A. Nakorchevsky, Proteomics by mass spectrometry: approaches, advances, and applications, Annu. Rev. Biomed. Eng. (2009) 49-79.

[48] R. Chen, M. Snyder, Yeast proteomics and protein microarrays, J. Proteomics. 11 (2010) 2147-2157.

[49] Anonymous ProtoArray® Human Protein Microarrays | Life Technologies http://www.invitrogen.com/site/us/en/home/Products-and-Services/Applications/Protein-Expression-and-Analysis/Biomarker-Discovery/ProtoArray.html?CID=fl-protoarray.

[50] C.D. Cooper, A.P. Liggins, K. Ait-Tahar, G. Roncador, A.H. Banham, K. Pulford, PASD1, a DLBCL-associated cancer testis antigen and candidate for lymphoma immunotherapy, Leukemia. 12 (2006) 2172-2174.

[51] K. Ait-Tahar, A.P. Liggins, G.P. Collins, A. Campbell, M. Barnardo, C. Lawrie, D. Moir, C. Hatton, A.H. Banham, K. Pulford, Cytolytic T-cell response to the PASD1 cancer testis antigen in patients with diffuse large B-cell lymphoma, Br. J. Haematol. 4 (2009) 396-407.

[52] W.L. Chen, K.T. Kuo, T.Y. Chou, C.L. Chen, C.H. Wang, Y.H. Wei, L.S. Wang, The role of cytochrome c oxidase subunit Va in non-small cell lung carcinoma cells: association with migration, invasion and prediction of distant metastasis, BMC Cancer. 12 (2012) 273.

[53] http://www.piercenet.com/browse.cfm?fldID=F88ADEC9-1B43-4585-922E-836FE09D8403#detectionmethods

[54] B. Magi, S. Liberatori, Immunoblotting techniques, Methods Mol. Biol. (2005) 227-254.

[55] L.A. Goff, J. Davila, M.R. Swerdel, J.C. Moore, R.I. Cohen, H. Wu, Y.E. Sun, R.P. Hart, Ago2 immunoprecipitation identifies predicted microRNAs in human embryonic stem cells and neural precursors, PLoS One. 9 (2009) e7192.

[56] S.P. Perfetto, P.K. Chattopadhyay, M. Roederer. Seventeen-colour flow cytometry: unravelling the immune system. Nature Reviews Immunol. 4 (2004) 648-655.

[57] P. Matzinger, The danger model: a renewed sense of self, Science. 296 (2002) 301-305.

[58] J.H. Kessler, W.E. Benckhuijsen, T. Mutis, C.J. Melief, S.H. van der Burg, J.W. Drijfhout, Competition-based cellular peptide binding assay for HLA class I, Curr. Protoc. Immunol. (2004) Unit 18.12.

[59] B.M. Olson, T.P. Frye, L.E. Johnson, L. Fong, K.L. Knutson, M.L. Disis, D.G. McNeel, HLA-A2-restricted T-cell epitopes specific for prostatic acid phosphatase, Cancer Immunol. Immunother. 6 (2010) 943-953.

[60] H. Rammensee, J. Bachmann, N.P. Emmerich, O.A. Bachor, S. Stevanovic, SYFPEITHI: database for MHC ligands and peptide motifs, Immunogenetics. 3-4 (1999) 213-219.

[61] W. Liu, M. Zhai, Z. Wu, Y. Qi, Y. Wu, C. Dai, M. Sun, L. Li, Y. Gao, Identification of a novel HLA-A2-restricted cytotoxic T lymphocyte epitope from cancer-testis antigen PLAC1 in breast cancer, Amino Acids. 6 (2012) 2257-2265.

[62] F. Neumann, B. Kubuschok, K. Ertan, C. Schormann, S. Stevanovic, K.D. Preuss, W. Schmidt, M. Pfreundschuh, A peptide epitope derived from the cancer testis antigen HOM-MEL-40/SSX2 capable of inducing CD4(+) and CD8(+) T-cell as well as B-cell responses, Cancer Immunol. Immunother. 9 (2011) 1333-1346.

[63] W. Wen, L. Zhang, J. Peng, J. Chen, J. Hao, X. Li, X. Qian, P. Zeng, Y. Zhang, Y. Yin, Identification of promiscuous HLA-DR-restricted CD4(+) T-cell epitopes on the cancer-testis antigen HCA587, Cancer. Sci. 8 (2011) 1455-1461.

[64] K.C. Parker, M.A. Bednarek, J.E Coligan, Scheme for ranking potential HLA-A2 binding peptides based on independent binding of individual peptide side-chains, J Immunol 152 (1994) 163–175

[65] N. Seyed, F. Zahedifard, S. Safaiyan, E. Gholami, F. Doustdari, K. Azadmanesh, M. Mirzaei, N. Saeedi Eslami, A. Khadem Sadegh, A. Eslami Far, I. Sharifi, S. Rafati, *In silico* analysis of six known Leishmania major antigens and *in vitro* evaluation of specific epitopes eliciting HLA-A2 restricted CD8 T cell response, PLoS Negl Trop. Dis. 9 (2011) e1295.

[66] B. Asquith, C. Debacq, A. Florins, N. Gillet, T. Sanchez-Alcaraz, A. Mosley, L. Willems, Quantifying lymphocyte kinetics *in vivo* using carboxyfluorescein diacetate succinimidyl ester (CFSE), Proc. Biol. Sci. 1590 (2006) 1165-1171.

[67] J.N. Radcliffe, J.S. Roddick, F.K. Stevenson, S.M. Thirdborough, Prolonged antigen expression following DNA vaccination impairs effector CD8+ T cell function and memory development, J. Immunol. 12 (2007) 8313-8321.

[68] D. Bagnara, M.S. Kaufman, C. Calissano, S. Marsilio, P.E. Patten, R. Simone, P. Chum, X.J. Yan, S.L. Allen, J.E. Kolitz, S. Baskar, C. Rader, H. Mellstedt, H. Rabbani, A. Lee, P.K. Gregersen, K.R. Rai, N. Chiorazzi, A novel adoptive transfer model of chronic lymphocytic leukemia suggests a key role for T lymphocytes in the disease, Blood. 20 (2011) 5463-5472.

[69] P.W. Sylvester, Optimization of the tetrazolium dye (MTT) colorimetric assay for cellular growth and viability, Methods Mol. Biol. (2011) 157-168.

[70] R.K. Paul, A. Ramamoorthy, J. Scheers, R.P. Wersto, L. Toll, L. Jimenez, M. Bernier, I.W. Wainer, Cannabinoid receptor activation correlates with the pro-apoptotic action of the beta2-adrenergic agonist, (R,R')-4-methoxy-1-naphthylfenoterol, in HepG2 hepatocarcinoma cells, J. Pharmacol. Exp. Ther. 343 (2012) 157-166.

[71] B. Piovesan, N. Pennell, N.L. Berinstein, Human lymphoblastoid cell lines expressing mutant p53 exhibit decreased sensitivity to cisplatin-induced cytotoxicity, Oncogene. 18 (1998) 2339-2350.

[72] Duque, P. Rakic, Different effects of bromodeoxyuridine and [3H]thymidine incorporation into DNA on cell proliferation, position, and fate, J. Neurosci. 42 (2011) 15205-15217.

[73] S. Sims, C. Willberg, P. Klenerman, MHC-peptide tetramers for the analysis of antigen-specific T cells, Expert Rev. Vaccines. 7 (2010) 765-774.

[74] Z.T. Shen, M.A. Brehm, K.A. Daniels, A.B. Sigalov, L.K. Selin, R.M. Welsh, L.J. Stern, Bi-specific MHC heterodimers for characterization of cross-reactive T cells, J. Biol. Chem. 43 (2010) 33144-33153.

[75] N. Khan, M. Cobbold, J. Cummerson, P.A. Moss, Persistent viral infection in humans can drive high frequency low-affinity T-cell expansions, Immunology. 4 (2010) 537-548.

[76] D.S. Chen, Y. Soen, T.B. Stuge, P.P. Lee, J.S. Weber, P.O. Brown, M.M. Davis, Marked differences in human melanoma antigen-specific T cell responsiveness after vaccination using a functional microarray, PLoS Med. 10 (2005) e265.

[77] G.A. Kwong, C.G. Radu, K. Hwang, C.J. Shu, C. Ma, R.C. Koya, B. Comin-Anduix, S.R. Hadrup, R.C. Bailey, O.N. Witte, T.N. Schumacher, A. Ribas, J.R. Heath, Modular nucleic acid assembled p/MHC microarrays for multiplexed sorting of antigen-specific T cells, J. Am. Chem. Soc. 28 (2009) 9695-9703.

[78] S.R. Hadrup, T.N. Schumacher, MHC-based detection of antigen-specific CD8+ T cell responses, Cancer Immunol. Immunother. 9 (2010) 1425-1433.

[79] E.W. Newell, L.O. Klein, W. Yu, M.M. Davis, Simultaneous detection of many T-cell specificities using combinatorial tetramer staining, Nat. Methods. 7 (2009) 497-499.

[80] J.A. Whelan, P.R. Dunbar, D.A. Price, M.A. Purbhoo, F. Lechner, G.S. Ogg, G. Griffiths, R.E. Phillips, V. Cerundolo, A.K. Sewell, Specificity of CTL interactions with peptide-

MHC class I tetrameric complexes is temperature dependent, J. Immunol. 8 (1999) 4342-4348.

[81] Y. Soen, D.S. Chen, D.L. Kraft, M.M. Davis, P.O. Brown, Detection and characterization of cellular immune responses using peptide-MHC microarrays, PLoS Biol. 3 (2003) E65.

[82] J. Dittmann, K. Keller-Matschke, T. Weinschenk, T. Kratt, T. Heck, H.D. Becker, S. Stevanovic, H.G. Rammensee, C. Gouttefangeas, CD8+ T-cell response against MUC1-derived peptides in gastrointestinal cancer survivors, Cancer Immunol. Immunother. 8 (2005) 750-758.

[83] I.E. Flesch, N.A. Hollett, Y.C. Wong, D.C. Tscharke, Linear fidelity in quantification of anti-viral CD8(+) T cells, PLoS One. 6 (2012) e39533.

[84] D.A. Kaveh, A.O. Whelan, P.J. Hogarth, The duration of antigen-stimulation significantly alters the diversity of multifunctional CD4 T cells measured by intracellular cytokine staining, PLoS One. 6 (2012) e38926.

[85] J. Bae, R. Smith, J.F. Daley, N. Mimura, Y.T. Tai, K.C. Anderson, N.C. Munshi, Myeloma-specific multiple peptides able to generate cytotoxic T lymphocytes: A potential therapeutic application in multiple myeloma and other plasma cell disorders, Clin. Cancer Res. 18 (2012) 4850-4860.

[86] S. Zwaveling, S.C. Ferreira Mota, J. Nouta, M. Johnson, G.B. Lipford, R. Offringa, S.H. van der Burg, C.J. Melief, Established human papillomavirus type 16-expressing tumors are effectively eradicated following vaccination with long peptides, J. Immunol. 1 (2002) 350-358.

[87] J. Rice, S. Buchan, F.K. Stevenson, Critical components of a DNA fusion vaccine able to induce protective cytotoxic T cells against a single epitope of a tumor antigen. J Immunol. 169 (2002) 3908-13.

[88] C.L. Morton, P.J. Houghton, Establishment of human tumor xenografts in immunodeficient mice, Nat. Protoc. 2 (2007) 247-250.

[89] Richmond, Y. Su, Mouse xenograft models vs GEM models for human cancer therapeutics, Dis. Model. Mech. 2-3 (2008) 78-82.

[90] B.A. Guinn, M.A. DeBenedette, T.H. Watts, N.L. Berinstein, 4-1BBL cooperates with B7-1 and B7-2 in converting a B cell lymphoma cell line into a long-lasting antitumor vaccine, J. Immunol. 162 (1999) 5003-5010.

[91] S. Spranger, B. Frankenberger, D.J. Schendel, NOD/scid IL-2Rg(null) mice: a preclinical model system to evaluate human dendritic cell-based vaccine strategies *in vivo*, J. Transl. Med. (2012) 30.

[92] Y. Motomura, Y. Ikuta, T. Kuronuma, H. Komori, M. Ito, M. Tsuchihara, Y. Tsunoda, H. Shirakawa, H. Baba, Y. Nishimura, T. Kinoshita, T. Nakatsura, HLA-A2 and -A24-restricted glypican-3-derived peptide vaccine induces specific CTLs: preclinical study using mice, Int. J. Oncol. 5 (2008) 985-990.

[93] B.B. Williams, M. Wall, R.Y. Miao, B. Williams, I. Bertoncello, M.H. Kershaw, T. Mantamadiotis, M. Haber, M.D. Norris, A. Gautam, P.K. Darcy, R.G. Ramsay, Induction of T cell-mediated immunity using a c-Myb DNA vaccine in a mouse model of colon cancer, Cancer Immunol. Immunother. 11 (2008) 1635-1645.

[94] L.D. Attardi, S.W. Lowe, J. Brugarolas, T. Jacks, Transcriptional activation by p53, but not induction of the p21 gene, is essential for oncogene-mediated apoptosis, EMBO J. 14 (1996) 3693-3701.

[95] E.L. Volk, L. Fan, K. Schuster, J.E. Rehg, L.C. Harris, The MDM2-a splice variant of MDM2 alters transformation *in vitro* and the tumor spectrum in both Arf- and p53-null models of tumorigenesis, Mol. Cancer. Res. 6 (2009) 863-869.

[96] B. Nie, Z. Shen, J.B. Wen, O.G. Wong, W.D. Hsueh, L.F. Huo, H.F. Kung, B. Jiang, M.C. Lin, AAV-HGFK1 and Ad-p53 cocktail therapy prolongs survival of mice with colon cancer, Mol. Cancer. Ther. 9 (2008) 2855-2865.

[97] S. Pascolo, N. Bervas, J.M. Ure, A.G. Smith, F.A. Lemonnier, B. Perarnau, HLA-A2.1-restricted education and cytolytic activity of CD8(+) T lymphocytes from beta2 microglobulin (beta2m) HLA-A2.1 monochain transgenic H-2Db beta2m double knockout mice, J. Exp. Med. 12 (1997) 2043-2051.

[98] S. Peng, C. Trimble, L. He, Y.C. Tsai, C.T. Lin, D.A. Boyd, D. Pardoll, C.F. Hung, T.C. Wu, Characterization of HLA-A2-restricted HPV-16 E7-specific CD8(+) T-cell immune responses induced by DNA vaccines in HLA-A2 transgenic mice, Gene Ther. 1 (2006) 67-77.

[99] P.M. Alves, O. Faure, S. Graff-Dubois, S. Cornet, I. Bolonakis, D.A. Gross, I. Miconnet, S. Chouaib, K. Fizazi, J.C. Soria, F.A. Lemonnier, K. Kosmatopoulos, STEAP, a prostate tumor antigen, is a target of human CD8+ T cells, Cancer Immunol. Immunother. 12 (2006) 1515-1523.

[100] C. Chaise, S.L. Buchan, J. Rice, J. Marquet, H. Rouard, M. Kuentz, G.E. Vittes, V. Molinier-Frenkel, J.P. Farcet, H.J. Stauss, M.H. Delfau-Larue, F.K. Stevenson, DNA vaccination induces WT1-specific T-cell responses with potential clinical relevance, Blood. 7 (2008) 2956-2964.

[101] M.A. Cheever, J.P. Allison, A.S. Ferris, O.J. Finn, B.M. Hastings, T.T. Hecht, I. Mellman, S.A. Prindiville, J.L. Viner, L.M. Weiner, L.M. Matrisian, The prioritization of cancer antigens: a national cancer institute pilot project for the acceleration of translational research, Clin. Cancer Res. 17 (2009) 5323-5337.

[102] T. Wolfel, E. Klehmann, C. Muller, K.H. Schutt, K.H. Meyer zum Buschenfelde, A. Knuth, Lysis of human melanoma cells by autologous cytolytic T cell clones. Identification of human histocompatibility leukocyte antigen A2 as a restriction element for three different antigens, J. Exp. Med. 3 (1989) 797-810.

[103] I.G. Zizzari, F. Veglia, F. Taurino, H. Rahimi, E. Quaglino, F. Belleudi, F. Riccardo, M. Antonilli, C. Napoletano, F. Bellati, P. Benedetti-Panici, M.R. Torrisi, L. Frati, M. Nuti,

A. Rughetti, HER2-based recombinant immunogen to target DCs through FcgammaRs for cancer immunotherapy, J. Mol. Med. (Berl). 12 (2011) 1231-1240.

[104] T. Nguyen-Hoai, G. Baldenhofer, M.S. Ahmed, M. Pham-Duc, M. Gries, M. Lipp, B. Dorken, A. Pezzutto, J. Westermann, CCL19 (ELC) improves TH1-polarized immune responses and protective immunity in a murine Her2/neu DNA vaccination model, J. Gene Med. 2 (2012) 128-137.

[105] M.W. Anderson, S. Zhao, A.G. Freud, D.K. Czerwinski, H. Kohrt, A.A. Alizadeh, R. Houot, D. Azambuja, I. Biasoli, J.C. Morais, N. Spector, H.F. Molina-Kirsch, R.A. Warnke, R. Levy, Y. Natkunam, CD137 Is Expressed in Follicular Dendritic Cell Tumors and in Classical Hodgkin and T-Cell Lymphomas: Diagnostic and Therapeutic Implications, Am. J. Pathol. 3 (2012) 795-803.

[106] Tazi, H. Nafil, L. Mahmal, Monoclonal antibodies in hematological malignancies: past, present and future, J. Cancer. Res. Ther. 4 (2011) 399-407.

[107] S.A. Rosenberg, J.C. Yang, N.P. Restifo, Cancer immunotherapy: moving beyond current vaccines, Nat. Med. 9 (2004) 909-915.

[108] L. Gattinoni, S.E. Finkelstein, C.A. Klebanoff, P.A. Antony, D.C. Palmer, P.J. Spiess, L.N. Hwang, Z. Yu, C. Wrzesinski, D.M. Heimann, C.D. Surh, S.A. Rosenberg, N.P. Restifo, Removal of homeostatic cytokine sinks by lymphodepletion enhances the efficacy of adoptively transferred tumor-specific CD8+ T cells, J. Exp. Med. 7 (2005) 907-912.

[109] C.A. Klebanoff, L. Gattinoni, D.C. Palmer, P. Muranski, Y. Ji, C.S. Hinrichs, Z.A. Borman, S.P. Kerkar, C.D. Scott, S.E. Finkelstein, S.A. Rosenberg, N.P. Restifo, Determinants of successful CD8+ T-cell adoptive immunotherapy for large established tumors in mice, Clin. Cancer Res. 16 (2011) 5343-5352.

[110] Z. Peng, Current status of gendicine in China: recombinant human Ad-p53 agent for treatment of cancers, Hum. Gene Ther. 9 (2005) 1016-1027.

[111] Bose, D.B. Lowe, A. Rao, W.J. Storkus, Combined vaccine+axitinib therapy yields superior antitumor efficacy in a murine melanoma model, Melanoma Res. 3 (2012) 236-243.

[112] D. Karan, P. Van Veldhuizen, Combination immunotherapy with prostate GVAX and ipilimumab: safety and toxicity, Immunotherapy. 6 (2012) 577-580.

[113] Nakamura, M. Kanazawa, Y. Sato, A. Irisawa, T. Takagi, T. Ogata, S. Kashimura, A. Kenjo, H. Suzuki, M. Shibata, T. Shimura, H. Ohira, M. Goto, S. Takenoshita, H. Ohto, Clinical evaluation of dendritic cells vaccination for advanced cancer patients at Fukushima Medical University, Fukushima J. Med. Sci. 1 (2012) 40-48.

[114] P. Kvistborg, C.J. Shu, B. Heemskerk, M. Fankhauser, C.A. Thrue, M. Toebes, N. van Rooij, C. Linnemann, M.M. van Buuren, J.H. Urbanus, J.B. Beltman, P. thor Straten, Y.F. Li, P.F. Robbins, M.J. Besser, J. Schachter, G.G. Kenter, M.E. Dudley, S.A. Rosenberg,

J.B. Haanen, S.R. Hadrup, T.N. Schumacher, TIL therapy broadens the tumor-reactive CD8+ T cell compartment in melanoma patients, Oncoimmunology. 4 (2012) 409-418.

[115] R. Pacholczyk, J. Kern, The T-cell receptor repertoire of regulatory T cells, Immunology. 4 (2008) 450-458.

[116] T. Baba, S. Badr Mel, U. Tomaru, A. Ishizu, N. Mukaida, Novel Process of Intrathymic Tumor-Immune Tolerance through CCR2-Mediated Recruitment of Sirpalpha(+) Dendritic Cells: A Murine Model, PLoS One. 7 (2012) e41154.

[117] W. Jing, X. Yan, W.H. Hallett, J.A. Gershan, B.D. Johnson, Depletion of CD25(+) T cells from hematopoietic stem cell grafts increases posttransplantation vaccine-induced immunity to neuroblastoma, Blood. 25 (2011) 6952-6962.

[118] Baba, S. Watanabe, Y. Saida, T. Tanaka, T. Miyabayashi, J. Koshio, K. Ichikawa, K. Nozaki, T. Koya, K. Deguchi, C. Tan, S. Miura, H. Tanaka, J. Tanaka, H. Kagamu, H. Yoshizawa, K. Nakata, I. Narita, Depletion of radio-resistant regulatory T cells enhances antitumor immunity during recovery from lymphopenia, Blood. 120 (2012) 2417-27.

[119] E.L. Smits, C. Lee, N. Hardwick, S. Brooks, V.F. Van Tendeloo, K. Orchard, B.A. Guinn, Clinical evaluation of cellular immunotherapy in acute myeloid leukaemia, Cancer Immunol. Immunother. 60 (2011) 757-769.

[120] B.P. Keenan, E.M. Jaffee, Whole cell vaccines--past progress and future strategies, Semin. Oncol. 3 (2012) 276-286.

[121] T.J. Curiel, Immunotherapy: a useful strategy to help combat multidrug resistance, Drug Resist Updat. 1-2 (2012) 106-113.

[122] Palucka, J. Banchereau, Cancer immunotherapy via dendritic cells, Nat. Rev. Cancer. 4 (2012) 265-277.

[123] Mellman, G. Coukos, G. Dranoff, Cancer immunotherapy comes of age, Nature. 7378 (2011) 480-489.

[124] http://cancerhelp.cancerresearchuk.org/trials/types-of-trials/phase-1-2-3-and-4-trials

[125] http://www.macmillan.org.uk/Cancerinformation/Cancertreatment/Clinicaltrials/Understandingtrials/Trialdesign.aspx

[126] http://www.mhra.gov.uk/#page=DynamicListMedicines

[127] E. Cohen, J. Belkora, J. Tyler, J. Schreiner, M.J. Deering, L. Grama, B. Duggan, J. Illi, J. Pederson, A. Anand, A. Teng, E. McCreary, D. Moore, D. Tripathy, M. Hogarth, M. Lieberman, J. Park, L. Esserman, Adoption, acceptability, and accuracy of an online clinical trial matching website for breast cancer, J. Med. Internet Res. 4 (2012) e97.

[128] Jager, A. Schoberth, P. Ruf, J. Hess, H. Lindhofer, The trifunctional antibody ertumaxomab destroys tumor cells that express low levels of human epidermal growth factor receptor 2, Cancer Res. 10 (2009) 4270-4276.

[129] E.A. Rossi, D.M. Goldenberg, T.M. Cardillo, R. Stein, C.H. Chang, Hexavalent bispecific antibodies represent a new class of anticancer therapeutics: 1. Properties of anti-CD20/ CD22 antibodies in lymphoma, Blood. 24 (2009) 6161-6171.

[130] A.J. Marks, M.S. Cooper, R.J. Anderson, K.H. Orchard, G. Hale, J.M. North, K. Ganeshaguru, A.J. Steele, A.B. Mehta, M.W. Lowdell, R.G. Wickremasinghe, Selective apoptotic killing of malignant hemopoietic cells by antibody-targeted delivery of an amphipathic peptide, Cancer Res. 6 (2005) 2373-2377.

[131] C.C. Czerkinsky, L.A. Nilsson, H. Nygren, O. Ouchterlony, A. Tarkowski, A solid-phase enzyme-linked immunospot (ELISPOT) assay for enumeration of specific antibody-secreting cells, J. Immunol. Methods. 1-2 (1983) 109-121.

[132] D.G. Ebo, J. Leysen, C. Mayorga, A. Rozieres, E.F. Knol, I. Terreehorst, The *in vitro* diagnosis of drug allergy: status and perspectives, Allergy. 10 (2011) 1275-1286.

[133] J.M. Vuola, S. Keating, D.P. Webster, T. Berthoud, S. Dunachie, S.C. Gilbert, A.V. Hill, Differential immunogenicity of various heterologous prime-boost vaccine regimens using DNA and viral vectors in healthy volunteers, J. Immunol. 1 (2005) 449-455.

[134] A.M. Scott, J.D. Wolchok, L.J. Old, Antibody therapy of cancer, Nat. Rev. Cancer. 4 (2012) 278-287.

[135] J.E. Boudreau, A. Bonehill, K. Thielemans, Y. Wan, Engineering dendritic cells to enhance cancer immunotherapy, Mol. Ther. 5 (2011) 841-853.

[136] J. Copier, M. Bodman-Smith, A. Dalgleish, Current status and future applications of cellular therapies for cancer, Immunotherapy. 4 (2011) 507-516.

[137] H. Kantarjian, D. Thomas, J. Jorgensen, E. Jabbour, P. Kebriaei, M. Rytting, S. York, F. Ravandi, M. Kwari, S. Faderl, M.B. Rios, J. Cortes, L. Fayad, R. Tarnai, S.A. Wang, R. Champlin, A. Advani, S. O'Brien, Inotuzumab ozogamicin, an anti-CD22-calecheamicin conjugate, for refractory and relapsed acute lymphocytic leukaemia: a phase 2 study, Lancet Oncol. 4 (2012) 403-411.

[138] E. Quoix, R. Ramlau, V. Westeel, Z. Papai, A. Madroszyk, A. Riviere, P. Koralewski, J.L. Breton, E. Stoelben, D. Braun, D. Debieuvre, H. Lena, M. Buyse, M.P. Chenard, B. Acres, G. Lacoste, B. Bastien, A. Tavernaro, N. Bizouarne, J.Y. Bonnefoy, J.M. Limacher, Therapeutic vaccination with TG4010 and first-line chemotherapy in advanced non-small-cell lung cancer: a controlled phase 2B trial, Lancet Oncol. 12 (2011) 1125-1133.

[139] Iwahashi, M. Katsuda, M. Nakamori, M. Nakamura, T. Naka, T. Ojima, T. Iida, H. Yamaue, Vaccination with peptides derived from cancer-testis antigens in combination with CpG-7909 elicits strong specific CD8+ T cell response in patients with metastatic esophageal squamous cell carcinoma, Cancer. Sci. 12 (2010) 2510-2517.

[140] F.S. Hodi, S.J. O'Day, D.F. McDermott, R.W. Weber, J.A. Sosman, J.B. Haanen, R. Gonzalez, C. Robert, D. Schadendorf, J.C. Hassel, W. Akerley, A.J. van den Eertwegh, J. Lutzky, P. Lorigan, J.M. Vaubel, G.P. Linette, D. Hogg, C.H. Ottensmeier, C. Lebbe,

C. Peschel, I. Quirt, J.I. Clark, J.D. Wolchok, J.S. Weber, J. Tian, M.J. Yellin, G.M. Nichol, A. Hoos, W.J. Urba, Improved survival with ipilimumab in patients with metastatic melanoma, N. Engl. J. Med. 8 (2010) 711-723.

[141] P.W. Kantoff, T.J. Schuetz, B.A. Blumenstein, L.M. Glode, D.L. Bilhartz, M. Wyand, K. Manson, D.L. Panicali, R. Laus, J. Schlom, W.L. Dahut, P.M. Arlen, J.L. Gulley, W.R. Godfrey, Overall survival analysis of a phase II randomized controlled trial of a Poxviral-based PSA-targeted immunotherapy in metastatic castration-resistant prostate cancer, J. Clin. Oncol. 7 (2010) 1099-1105.

[142] Hagenbeek, O. Gadeberg, P. Johnson, L.M. Pedersen, J. Walewski, A. Hellmann, B.K. Link, T. Robak, M. Wojtukiewicz, M. Pfreundschuh, M. Kneba, A. Engert, P. Sonneveld, M. Flensburg, J. Petersen, N. Losic, J. Radford, First clinical use of ofatumumab, a novel fully human anti-CD20 monoclonal antibody in relapsed or refractory follicular lymphoma: results of a phase 1/2 trial, Blood. 12 (2008) 5486-5495.

[143] J. Pfisterer, A. du Bois, J. Sehouli, S. Loibl, S. Reinartz, A. Reuss, U. Canzler, A. Belau, C. Jackisch, R. Kimmig, K. Wollschlaeger, V. Heilmann, F. Hilpert, The anti-idiotypic antibody abagovomab in patients with recurrent ovarian cancer. A phase I trial of the AGO-OVAR, Ann. Oncol. 10 (2006) 1568-1577.

[144] B.A. Guinn, A. Mohamedali, N.S. Thomas, K.I. Mills, Immunotherapy of myeloid leukaemia, Cancer Immunol. Immunother. 7 (2007) 943-957.

Chapter 13

Challenges in Advancing the Field of Cancer Gene Therapy: An Overview of the Multi-Functional Nanocarriers

Azam Bolhassani and Tayebeh Saleh

Additional information is available at the end of the chapter

1. Introduction

Recent developments in molecular biology and cell biology have led to the discovery of novel genes and proteins having therapeutic potentials for various diseases including cancers. Based on these findings, novel categories of therapeutic biomacromolecules including genes, small interfering RNA (siRNAs), antisense oligonucleic acids, bioactive proteins and peptides have been developed. These macromolecules can be more advantageous than small-molecular-weight therapeutic agents in terms of their specificity and high potency to the target molecules [Nakase et al., 2010]. Gene therapy is the newest therapeutic strategy for treating human diseases. The basic idea of gene therapy is a gene or gene product that can be selectively delivered to a specific cell/tissue with minimal toxicity. This product can inhibit the expression of a specific defective gene or express a normal gene. Efficient and safe delivery is one of the key issues for the clinical application of nucleic acids as therapeutic agents [Du et al., 2010]. The goal of the Pharmaceutical Industry is to have a gene therapy medical product that can be delivered systemically. *In vivo* gene therapies have focused on viral vectors for gene delivery and have had marginal clinical successes. Major disadvantage of these delivery systems is the integration of some viral vectors into human chromosomes of normal tissue. There are four issues to be solved before cancer gene therapy will be successful: 1) Identification of key target genes critical for the disease pathology and progression; 2) Determination of the correct therapeutic gene to inhibit disease progression; 3) Optimal trans-gene expression for suppressing the target gene; and 4) Delivery of therapeutic product to the target tissue at an efficient dose [Scanlon, 2004].

Delivery is one of the most difficult challenges facing the gene therapy field. It is needed to use an efficient transfer system that can stabilize, transduce and express a transgene in the target tissue. Recently, non-viral technologies have been widely used as a significant alternative for gene delivery. The non-viral delivery systems have reduced adverse immune responses, are easier to manufacture and can be produced for the pharmaceutical industry in large quantities. The current progresses of gene therapy are further focused on synthesized nano-particle technologies. Some of these new chemical compositions are cationic molecules such as polymers, lipids and peptides [Scanlon, 2004; Gao et al., 2007].

However, for successful clinical trial, ideal non-viral vectors should be degradable into low molecular weight components, in response to biological stimuli, for lowered cytotoxicity and effective systemic clearance. They should also be efficient in overcoming extracellular and intracellular barriers, tissue/cell-targeted for specific accumulations and multi-functional for synergistic therapeutic and diagnostic outcomes. Recently, a broad range of different stimuli-responsive strategies (virus-mimicking gene delivery systems) has been employed to develop non-viral nucleic acid carriers that efficiently enhance multiple extracellular and intracellular gene delivery pathways by altering their physico-chemical properties in response to a variety of extra- and intra-cellular stimuli (e.g., pH, redox potential, and enzyme), as well as external triggers (e.g., light) [Zhu and Torchilin, 2012].

Therefore, numerous challenges remain to be overcome before gene therapy becomes available as a safe and effective treatment option. For instance, the cationic molecules (e.g., polymers, lipids and peptides) have the potential to be systemically delivered but selectivity for the target tissue needs to be validated. The best method for delivering genes will depend on the type of tissue targeted [Scanlon, 2004]. Recently, the development of virus-mimicking, multi-functional gene delivery systems is considered to be a potent strategy in the future, in particular for intravenous administration. This chapter summarizes the challenges for cancer gene therapy as well as addressing the advances in the multi-functional nano-carriers as a potent non-viral delivery system.

2. Gene therapy

Medicine has a long history of treating patients with cell therapies (i.e., blood transfusions) and protein therapies (i.e., growth factors and cytokines). Gene therapies are the newest therapeutic strategy for treating human diseases especially cancer [Scanlon, 2004]. This technology has been used to develop new strategies for killing cells selectively or inhibiting their growth. The field of cancer gene therapy comprises a range of technologies from direct attack on tumor cells to inducing the immune response to tumor antigens [McCormick, 2001]. However, there are serious doubts about gene therapy; for example, short-lived nature of gene therapy, immune response to a foreign object, problems with viral vectors and insertional mutagenesis inducing a tumor [Korthof, 1999].

2.1. History

In 1972, Friedmann and Roblin published a paper in Science entitled as "Gene therapy for human genetic disease" [Friedmann and Roblin, 1972; Rogers, 1970]. The first approved gene therapy case in the United States took place in 1990, at the National Institute of Health. It was performed on a four year old girl with a genetic defect associated to an immune system deficiency. The effects were only temporary, but successful [Blaese et al., 1995]. In addition, sickle cell disease was successfully treated in mice [Fisher, 1995]. At the same time, the researchers were able to create tiny liposomes 25 nanometers (nm) that can carry therapeutic DNA through pores in the nuclear membrane [www. newscientist.com, 2002]. In 1992, Claudio Bordignon performed the first procedure of gene therapy using hematopoietic stem cells as vectors to deliver genes aimed to correct hereditary diseases [Abbott, 1992]. In 2002, this work led to the publication of the first successful gene therapy treatment for adenosine deaminase-deficiency (SCID) [Cavazzana-Calvo et al., 2004]. In 2003, a Los Angeles research team inserted genes into the brain using liposomes coated in a polymer called polyethylene glycol (PEG). The transfer of genes into the brain is a significant achievement because viral vectors are too big to get across the blood–brain barrier. This method had potential for treating Parkinson's disease. At the same time, RNA interference or gene silencing was considered as a new way to treat Huntington's disease [www. newscientist.com, 2003]. In 2006, scientists at the National Institutes of Health have successfully treated metastatic melanoma in two patients using killer T cells genetically retargeted to attack the cancer cells. For the first time, this study demonstrated that gene therapy can be effective in treating cancer. In November 2006, Preston Nix reported on VRX496, a gene-based immunotherapy for the treatment of human immunodeficiency virus (HIV) that uses a lentiviral vector for delivery of an antisense gene against the HIV envelope [Levine et al., 2006; www.eurekalert.org, 2009].

Leber's congenital amaurosis is an inherited blinding disease caused by mutations in the RPE65 gene. In 2007-2008, the world's first gene therapy trial was announced for inherited retinal disease. They determined the safety of the sub-retinal delivery of recombinant adeno-associated virus (AAV) carrying RPE65 gene and found the positive results in vision and without the apparent side-effects [www. news.bbc.co.uk, 2007]. In 2009, the researchers were succeeded at arresting a fatal brain disease, adrenoleukodystrophy, using a vector derived from HIV to deliver the gene for the missing enzyme [Kaiser, 2009]. A paper published in 2010, deals with gene therapy for a form of achromatopsia in dogs. Achromatopsia, or complete color blindness, is presented as an ideal model to develop gene therapy directed to cone photoreceptors [Komáromy et al., 2010]. In 2011, a study carried out using genetically modified T cells to fight the chronic lymphocytic leukemia (CLL) disease. Moreover, Human HGF plasmid DNA therapy of cardiomyocytes was examined as a potential treatment for coronary artery disease as well as myocardial infarction [www. nature.com, 2011; Yang et al., 2008; Hahn et al., 2011]. However, most of the approved European and United States gene therapy protocols are for cancer (~ 66%), in contrast to monogenetic diseases (~ 11%) and cardiovascular diseases (~ 8%). The focus of cancer gene therapy has been on melanoma, prostate and ovarian cancer and leukemia [Scanlon, 2004].

2.2. The challenges of gene therapy

Recently, the use of gene therapy in medicine using plasmid DNA (pDNA), oligodeoxynucleotide (ODN) or small interfering RNA (siRNA) represents a promising new approach for treating a variety of genetic and acquired diseases (e.g., cancer). To date, more than 1000 different gene-therapy clinical trials for the treatment of many different diseases are in progress worldwide, but, the success with gene therapy has been limited. This lack of success can be assigned to difficulties related to the effective delivery of nucleic acids into target cells [Mastrobattista et al., 2006]. Naked DNA is unable to efficiently cross cellular barriers by passive diffusion because of its large size, strong negative charge, hydrophilicity and susceptibility to nuclease attack. Hence, the major challenge for *in vitro* DNA delivery is designing suitable vectors which can protect DNA and efficiently deliver it to the targeted sites in the cell. Successful application of such therapeutic vector-DNA formulations *in vivo* requires them to be stable during circulation in blood, resistant against rapid metabolic clearance and efficiently targeted to the appropriate tissue/cell [Mann et al., 2008].

3. Delivery systems in gene therapy

3.1. Viral delivery

Delivery is one of the most difficult challenges facing the gene therapy field. An efficient transfer system has not yet been found to stabilize, transduce and express a transgene in the target tissue. Limitations of the present vector technologies have slowed the progress of clinical gene therapy [Scanlon, 2004]. Various viruses, such as *influenza* viruses and *adenoviruses,* can efficiently deliver genes into the nucleus via sophisticated mechanisms. Despite the potent immunogenicity of viral vectors, their developed cell entry mechanism and high transfection efficiency in both dividing and non-dividing cells is desirable [Wagner, 2011; Mastrobattista et al., 2006]. All the viral gene strategies used to date have significant delivery limitations. The best method for delivering genes may depend on the type of targeted tissue. There are some promising delivery technologies for viral therapies, including the use of replication competent viruses. *Adenoviruses, herpes simplex virus* and *Newcastle disease virus* have all been modified for replication competent properties in human tumor cells. This has been one of the most popular areas in gene therapy and offers promises for treating cancer, especially when combined with chemotherapy [Scanlon, 2004]. Recently, the viral vectors have been developed into gene vectors and have provided convincing successes in gene therapy. Viruses have developed mechanisms to survive in the extracellular environment, attach to cells, cross cellular membranes, steal intracellular transport systems and subsequently deliver their genomes into the appropriate sub-cellular compartment (e.g., cytosol or nucleus) [Wagner, 2011; Sasaki et al., 2008]. For example, *influenza viruses* infect cells in a multi-step process: a) the virus binds to a receptor on the cell surface mediated by hemagglutinin (HA) protein; b) the virus invades via receptor-mediated endocytosis; c) the internalized virus is trafficked to a late endosome; d) the acidic endosomal environment induces membrane fusion between the virus and endosome, which is brought about by a conformational change of HA and the ribonucleoprotein complex core is released into cytoplasmic space; e) the core is transferred to the nucleus and viral gene expression progresses. Due to this very efficient cell-entry mechanism, the transfection efficiencies of viral vectors remain uniqe [Sasaki et al., 2008].

However, there are several problems to overcome before this therapy can be successful in clinical settings such as a) Enhanced lytic properties of these viruses; b) Improved yields with better manufacturing procedures of production for clinical studies; c) Systemic delivery; d) limited DNA-carrying capacity; e) lack of target-cell specificity; f) immunogenicity and h) for some viral vectors, insertional mutagenesis [Scanlon, 2004; Mastrobattista et al., 2006].

3.2. Non-viral delivery

There are some non-viral technologies that offer several advantages over the viral methodologies. Non-viral delivery systems have reduced adverse immune responses (relatively safe), are easier to manufacture, can be produced for the pharmaceutical industry in large quantities and modified by the incorporation of ligands for targeting to specific cell types [Scanlon, 2004; Mastrobattista et al., 2006]. Chemically synthesized nanoparticles constitute a new technology and offer several new strategies for successful systemic gene therapy delivery. Synthetic gene-delivery systems consist of a self-assembling complex of DNA with positively charged molecules (for example, polymers, peptides, lipids or their combinations). These complexes are small in size (40-150 nm) and usually have a net positive surface charge, which enables adsorption-mediated cell binding and internalization [Mastrobattista et al., 2006]. Some of these new chemical compositions are polymers containing either DNA/stearyl polylysine-coated lipids or peptoids (DNA coated with glycine oligomers) or cationic molecules (DNA/combined with positively charged B-cyclodextrin/adamantane and PEG). These molecules have been shown to be effective in cancer-related angiogenesis. These new agents have the potential to be systemically delivered, but their selectivity for the target tissue needs to be validated [Scanlon, 2004]. However, the levels of gene expression and the transfection efficiency mediated by synthetic vectors are low compared to viral vectors [Mastrobattista et al., 2006].

3.3. Cell delivery

One of the opportunities for gene therapy is to combine therapeutic genes with a cell to overcome the delivery to target tissues. The advantages of cell delivery of therapeutic products include minimal immune response; tissue directed therapy; selectivity and improved potency of the product. However, there are several problems to be solved: a) Determining optimal transduction of cells; b) Gene-transformed cells will require a selective growth advantage over defective cells to re-populate the host; c) DNA repair genes action (minimized mutations in the gene-transformed cells); d) Genomic stability (for optimal gene expression); e) Determining cell type for therapy (e.g., embryonic stem cells or activated, differentiated cells); f) Incorporation of a safety mechanism (*i.e.* a suicide gene) to destroy the gene-transformed cells if a problem arises. In addition, other cell therapies are currently being developed using bacteria, such as modified *Salmonella*, for gene delivery in cancer patients. These modified bacterial cells are already in Phase I clinical studies [Scanlon, 2004].

4. The challenges of nucleic acid delivery

There are many biological barriers for efficient gene delivery that need to be overcome [Mastrobattista et al., 2006]. This inefficiency of gene delivery is primarily a result of the inability of these vectors to overcome the numerous barriers encountered between the site of administration and localization in the cell nucleus. This series of barriers to efficient non-viral gene delivery is thought to include: a) the physical and chemical stability of DNA and its delivery vehicle in the extracellular space, b) cellular uptake by endocytosis, c) escape from the endosomal compartments prior to trafficking to lysosomes, d) cytosolic transport and e) nuclear localization of the plasmid for transcription. In addition to these physical and chemical obstacles, biological barriers, such as immunogenic responses to the vector itself as well as immune stimulation by certain DNA sequences containing a central un-methylated CpG motif, are present. The studies have shown that it is possible to minimize biological barriers by optimizing the plasmid sequence, thus physical and chemical barriers appear to be the negative factors to successful non-viral gene delivery [Wiethoff and Middaugh, 2003]. These barriers are briefly described as following:

4.1. Stability in extracellular compartments

The stability of non-viral delivery systems in the extracellular milieu, such as intercellular or intravascular spaces, is related to the chemical stability of the DNA as well as the physical stability of the delivery system [Wiethoff and Middaugh, 2003]. In extracellular environment, the carrier is exposed to blood components such as nucleases. This can result in premature destabilization with simultaneous release and degradation of the plasmid DNA. The half-life of naked plasmid DNA in blood is on the order of minutes. Therefore, carrier-mediated protection during transport through the blood circulation is a prerequisite to make the DNA inaccessible to degradative enzymes [Mastrobattista et al., 2006]. Condensing the DNA with a variety of polycations or by complexing with polymers that bind to DNA protects it from degradation [Wiethoff and Middaugh, 2003].

4.2. Cellular association of DNA

Irrespective of the injection route, the gene carriers should be able to bind to cells for allowing cellular uptake [Mastrobattista et al., 2006]. Association of DNA with the cell surface is typically very low in the absence of any delivery agent as an immediate consequence of the relatively high negative charge density of both the DNA and the cell surface. Polycations have been shown to substantially increase the cellular association of DNA by neutralization of the DNA negative charge, with the charge ratio of the complex modulating the extent of this contact. The degree of cellular association has also been shown to be related to the colloidal stability of these delivery systems, with those that aggregate often manifesting a greater degree of cellular association *in vitro*. The association of non-viral gene delivery systems containing either cationic lipids or polymers is thought to be mediated by interactions with cell surface heparin sulfate proteoglycans (HSPGs). These proteoglycans are ubiquitous to the surface of all cells and are involved in a variety of cellular processes, including differentiation, adhesion and migration. More recently they have been found to mediate the binding and internalization of several viruses, including HIV-1, HSV-2, AAV-2, and *adenovirus*. The composition of heparin sulfate proteoglycans (HSPGs) includes a protein core with one or more attached glycosaminoglycans [Wiethoff and Middaugh, 2003].

In general, binding of nano-carrier to the cell surfaces is not, a problem if the gene carriers have a net positive surface charge, which readily induces adsorption onto negatively charged cell membranes. However, this form of binding is random and does not allow restricted delivery to target cells (e.g., tumor cells) [Mastrobattista et al., 2006]. Several additional strategies have been attempted to increase the specificity of DNA binding to cells and induce targeting to particular cell types [Wiethoff and Middaugh, 2003]. Active targeting can be achieved by the functionalization of NPs with ligands such as antibodies, peptides, nucleic acids (aptamers), carbohydrates and small molecules [Gu et al., 2007].

4.3. Intracellular trafficking of non-viral gene delivery systems

Since many chemotherapeutic drugs and particularly gene therapeutics, would benefit from intracellular targeting, nano-carrier systems can be designed for receptor-mediated cell uptake, intracellular drug protection and intracellular target delivery [van Vlerken et al., 2007]. Once inside the cell, several intracellular barriers need to be crossed before the foreign DNA can be transcribed and translated [Mastrobattista et al., 2006]. These barriers contain endosomal escape, cytosolic transport of DNA and nuclear localization of plasmid DNA that described briefly in below:

4.3.1. Endosomal escape

The endocytic pathway is one of the uptake mechanisms of cells. In general, non-viral nano vectors have been developed to mimic the receptor-mediated cell entry mechanism of viruses and the main mechanism of internalization was confirmed to be endocytosis. This pathway is composed of vesicles known as endosomes with an internal pH around 5 that mature in a unidirectional manner from early endosomes to late endosomes before fusing with intracellular organelles called lysosomes which contain certain digestive enzymes. Thus, particles entering the cells via the endocytic pathway become entrapped in endosomes and eventually end up in the lysosome, where active enzymatic degradation processes take place [Varkouhi et al., 2011]. The entrapment of internalized DNA carriers in endocytic compartments prevents further intracellular transport towards the nucleus and will often result in degradation of the carrier and its associated DNA in the endosomal/lysosomal compartments [Mastrobattista et al., 2006]. While many viruses have evolved quite efficient systems for endosomal release, the situation is different for non-viral vectors, where in many cases the lack of endosomal escape is a major obstacle for efficient biological delivery, implying that more efficient methods for endosomal release would lead to improvements in designing synthetic transfection systems. In contrast to synthetic vectors, viral vectors are known to be efficient both for *in vitro* and *in vivo* applications [Varkouhi et al., 2011].

4.3.2. Cytosolic transport of DNA

After endosomal escape, DNA must traverse the cytosol to access the nucleus. Those DNA carriers that manage to escape the endosomal compartments are then challenged by the complex environment of the cytosol, which contains many filamentous structures that hinder the free diffusion of large particles such as DNA carriers. Dissociation of the carrier at this stage might be required to allow further transport of the plasmid DNA molecules. However, several studies have found evidence that plasmid DNA is largely immobile in the cytosol and is rapidly degraded by cytosolic nucleases [Mastrobattista et al., 2006]. Diffusion of DNA in the cytoplasm has been found to be substantially less than that observed in dilute solution. For DNA >2000 base pairs in length, the diffusion co-efficient in the cytosol is <1% of that in water, suggesting a substantial diffusional barrier. This decreased mobility has been ascribed to molecular crowding of the plasmid, but may also reflect an increased viscosity of the cytoplasm. As expected, the diffusion coefficient of DNA in the cytoplasm is inversely related to the size of the plasmid, suggesting smaller plasmids may be more desirable. No evidence for active transport of DNA in the cytoplasm has been reported. In addition to the considerable diffusional barrier for DNA in the cytosol, the presence of calcium-sensitive cytosolic nucleases pose a significant metabolic barrier. Micro-injection of DNA into the cytoplasm results in significant degradation of the DNA with a half-life of 50-90 min [Wiethoff and Middaugh, 2003].

4.3.3. Nuclear localization of plasmid DNA

Ultimately, delivery of DNA to the nucleus must occur for transcription of the transgene to take place. The mechanism of DNA nuclear translocation and whether the DNA is still associated with the delivery system are not fully understood but appear to depend on the type of delivery vehicle employed. At least three possible routes exist for DNA transport to the nucleus. The DNA can pass into the nucleus through nuclear pores, it can become physically associated with chromatin during mitosis when the nuclear envelope breaks down or it could traverse the nuclear envelope. Of these three possibilities, the latter seems impossible and without experimental support. Nuclear pores are embedded in the nuclear envelope at fairly high surface densities (3000-4000/nucleus) and exist in at least two conformational states. The closed state permits the passive diffusion of molecules of < 9 nm in diameter, whereas the open state facilitates transport of particles < 26 nm. This latter state could certainly assist the "threading" of supercoiled plasmid through the nuclear pore but not passage of typical non-viral gene delivery complexes [Wiethoff and Middaugh, 2003]. Small molecules (< 40 kDa) can diffuse freely through the pores of the nuclear pore complexes (NPC), whereas larger molecules and particles (up to 40 nm in size) can only be imported through the NPC by an active transport mechanism [Mastrobattista et al., 2006]. In a few cases, collapsed particles of < 30 nm have been produced, which could presumably enter the nucleus by this mechanism. The second and perhaps quite widespread mechanism by which DNA is thought to gain access to the nucleus is by association with nuclear material on breakdown of the nuclear envelope during mitosis [Wiethoff and Middaugh, 2003]. In this case, the nuclear barrier breaks down, which explains the increased levels of transfection in dividing cells as compared to their growth-arrested counterparts. However, as most cells do not divide or divide only slowly, an active transport mechanism is needed to carry the DNA from the cytosol into the nucleus [Mastrobattista et al., 2006].

4.4. Toxicity of non-viral delivery system

An important obstacle to effective non-viral gene delivery is the cytotoxicity of the delivery vectors [Wiethoff and Middaugh, 2003]. Inside the nucleus, the transgene encoded on the plasmid vector should be expressed to establish therapeutic levels of recombinant proteins within the affected cell. This requires gene transcription regulatory elements such as promoters and enhancers, to drive the expression of the transgene in mammalian cells. Viral promoters are often used because of their strong transcriptional activation. However, their constitutive nature does not allow control over the level of transgene expression. For the expression of proteins with a narrow therapeutic window, tight control over the level of transgene expression is essential. In addition, the introduction of foreign DNA into mammalian cells can induce a profound immune response, presumably triggered by differences in the degree of methylation of the foreign DNA compared with the mammalian genome [Mastrobattista et al., 2006]. Induction of innate immune responses by un-methylated CpG sequences in plasmid DNA is perhaps a more serious concern because these species have been demonstrated to greatly reduce the efficiency of non-viral gene delivery. This immunotoxicity is thought to be related to the efficient transfection of immune cells because polycation/DNA complexes evoke a considerably greater immune response than DNA or cationic vector alone. Initial observations suggest that delivery systems that are phagocytosed, due to their large size, may promote a greater immune response. Removal of CpG motifs from DNA containing the transgene has proven a successful means of improving gene expression. The methods involved in producing vectors without these motifs are not insignificant, and currently present a major limitation to their widespread usage. It has therefore been proposed that avoidance of transfection of immune cells either by specific targeting to particular cell types or by manipulation of the physicochemical properties of the delivery systems is necessary for significant improvements in non-viral gene delivery [Wiethoff and Middaugh, 2003].

5. Multi-functional nanocarriers

Currently used pharmaceutical nanocarriers, such as liposomes, micelles, nanoemulsions, polymeric nano-particles and many others demonstrate a broad variety of useful properties including: a) longevity in the blood allowing for their accumulation in pathological areas; b) specific targeting to certain disease sites due to various targeting ligands attached to the surface of the nanocarriers; c) enhanced intracellular penetration with the help of surface-attached cell-penetrating molecules; d) contrast properties due to the carrier loading with various contrast materials allowing for direct carrier visualization *in vivo*; e) stimuli-sensitivity allowing for drug release from the carriers under certain physiological conditions and etc. Some of those pharmaceutical carriers have already made their way into clinic, while others are still under preclinical development. However, the combination of pharmaceutical nanocarriers with several mentioned abilities, are rare. For example, long-circulating immunoliposomes capable of prolonged residence in the blood and specific target recognition represent one of few examples of this kind. At the same time, the engineering of multi-functional pharmaceutical nanocarriers combinig several useful properties in one particle can significantly enhance the efficacy of many therapeutic and diagnostic protocols [Torchilin, 2006].

The use of cationic lipids and cationic polymers as transfection vectors for efficient intracellular delivery of DNA was suggested in 1987. Complexes between cationic lipids (such as Lipofectin®, an equimolar mixture of N-[1-(2,3-dioleyloxy) propyl]-N,N,N-trimethylammonium chloride–DOTMA and dioleoyl phosphatidylethanolamine –DOPE) and DNA (lipoplexes) and complexes between cationic polymers, such as PEI and DNA (polyplexes) are formed because of strong electrostatic interactions between the positively charged carrier and negatively charged DNA. A slight net positive charge of formed lipoplexes and polyplexes is believed to facilitate their interaction with negatively charged cells and improve transfection efficiency. Endocytosis (including the receptor mediated endocytosis) was repeatedly confirmed as the main mechanism of lipoplex/polyplex internalization by cells [Torchilin, 2006]. Of special importance is the fact that despite of endocytosis-mediated uptake lipolexes and polyplexes, DNA does not end in lysosomes but releases in the cytoplasm due to the destabilization of the endosomal membrane provoked by lipid or polymeric component of the complexes. In particular, lipoplexes fuse with the endosomal membrane when they contain a fusogenic lipid, dioleylphosphatidylethanolamine (DOPE), which easily undergoes the transition from bilayer to hexagonal phase facilitating the fusion. In case of polyplexes, which cannot directly destabilize the endosomal membrane, the mechanism of DNA escape from endosomes, is associated with the ability of polymers, strongly protonate under the acidic pH inside endosome and create a charge gradient ultimately provoking a water influx and endosomal swelling and disintegration. In both cases, DNA-containing complexes when released into the cytosol, dissociate allowing for nuclear entry of free DNA. Nuclear translocation of the plasmid DNA is relatively inefficient because of the barrier function of the nuclear membrane and small size of nuclear pores (25 nm), as well as DNA degrades fast under the action of cytoplasmic nucleases. It was estimated that only 0.1% of plasmids undergo nuclear translocation from the cytosol. The attachment of nuclear localization sequences to plasmid DNA may significantly enhance its nuclear translocation and transfection efficiency. New approaches in using multifunctional carriers for DNA delivery include the application of bimetallic nano-rods that can simultaneously bind compacted DNA plasmid and targeting ligands in a spatially defined manner [Torchilin, 2006].

DNA–lipid amphiphiles self-assemble into novel "DNAsomes"-liposome-like core-shell structures with subunits composed of branched DNA-lipid hybrid molecules. These DNAsomes can be precisely modified over a wide range in terms of both size and surface charge. More importantly, DNAsome is a natural carrier of small interfering RNA (siRNA) due to DNA-RNA base-pairing, enabling efficient co-delivery of drugs and siRNA. The DNAsome represents a universal multi-functional drug vector for simultaneous delivery of drugs, tracer dyes, or antibodies, along with genes, siRNA or antisense nucleic acids [Roh et al., 2011].

6. Different types of nanocarrier systems

Over the last eight years, a laboratory at Northeastern University has developed an array of multi-functional nanocarriers for the delivery of genes, drugs and imaging modalities. These flexible platforms consist of polymeric and lipid systems that combine different modalities and stimuli-responsive release properties [Jabr-Milane et al., 2008].

The diagnostic and/or therapeutic objectives of a multi-functional nanocarrier system determine the design of the formulation. A review of the literature shows that there are many different types of nanocarrier formulations for the diagnosis, imaging and treatment of a wide spectrum of diseases. These multi-functional carriers share three main design components: platform (core) material, encapsulated payload/biologically active agents and targeting/surface properties. Nanocarrier platforms can be categorized as organic-based, inorganic-based or a hybrid combination. Organic nano-platforms include polymeric nanocarriers, lipid-based nanocarriers (e.g., liposomes and nanoemulsions), dendrimers and carbon-based nanocarriers (e.g., fullerenes and carbon nanotubes) [Jabr-Milane et al., 2008]. Inorganic nano-platforms include metallic nanostructures, silica nanoparticles and quantum dots. An example of a hybrid platform is colloidal gold encapsulated in liposomes or superparamagnetic iron oxide particles encapsulated in polymeric nanoparticles. Selection of the core material is highly dependent on the properties of the biologically active agents. Inherent and dynamic properties of the agents such as therapeutic index, lipophilicity, charge and size should be considered. When combining therapeutic agents with each other, with an imaging/diagnostic modality, or with energy delivery, the interaction of system components (i.e., synergy, quenching, enhanced toxicity) and release kinetics should also be considered. Surface properties are the third design component of multi-functional nanocarriers. A common surface modification technique that decreases reticuloendothelial system (RES) clearance is the physical or covalent attachment of PEG chains to the nanocarrier platform. Since tumor microvasculature is known to be highly fenestrated, colloidal particles can accumulate by the enhanced permeability and retention (EPR) effect. PEG surface modification increases circulatory residence time, which increases the probability of accumulation at the target. Block co-polymers of poly (ethylene oxide) (PEO) and poly (propylene oxide) (PPO) (e.g., Pluronics®) have also been used as surface conjugates to enhance circulation and achieve passive targeted delivery [Jabr-Milane et al., 2008].

Recently, nanoparticulate systems have been also developed for therapeutic gene delivery. Some researchers have developed glutathione-responsive nanoparticles for the delivery of plasmid DNA. The nanocarrier platform consisted of thiolated gelatin which was synthesized using 2-iminothiolane to covalently modify type B gelatin (pI ~ 4.5). The release profiles of cross-linked and non-cross-linked thiolated gelatin nanoparticles and gelatin nanoparticles (control) loaded with fluorescein isothiocyanate-conjugated dextran (FITC-dextran) were assessed in the presence of different glutathione concentrations (from 0.1 mM to 5 mM). A higher percentage of FITC–dextran was released from non-crosslinked nanoparticles compared to the cross-linked nanoparticles. The rate of FITC–dextran release from thiolated gelatin nanoparticles enhanced with increasing concentrations of glutathione. Glutathione in the media enhanced the release of FITC-dextran from thiolated gelatin nanoparticles by about 40%, while only a 20% enhancement was seen with gelatin nanoparticles [Jabr-Milane et al., 2008]. After establishing the rapid, stimuli-responsive release profile of these particles, the thiolated gelatin nanoparticles were loaded with plasmid DNA expressing green fluorescent protein (GFP). Upon incubation of the formulations with murine fibroblast cells, fluorescence imaging revealed transfection and protein expression after 6 h continuing as long as 96 h. Flow cytometry indicated that the cross-linked thiolated gelatin nanoparticles had the highest transfection efficiency. These nanocarriers are capable of rapid DNA delivery in response to intracellular glutathione. This nanocarrier platform was further modified to develop an anti-angiogenic gene therapy for the treatment of cancer. This platform consisted of PEG-modified thiolated gelatin nanoparticles loaded with plasmid DNA encoding the soluble form of the extracellular domain of vascular endothelial growth factor (VEGF) receptor-1 (sFlt-1). VEGF receptor over-expression in cancer is associated with neo-vascularization; sFlt-1 was selected as it blocks the VEGF receptor and the associated signal cascade [Jabr-Milane et al., 2008]. The PEG modified thiolated gelatin nanoparticles showed superior *in vitro* transfection in human breast adenocarcinoma cells when compared to plain gelatin nanoparticles, PEG-modified gelatin nanoparticles, thiolated gelatin nanoparticles, Lipofectin–plasmid DNA complexes and naked plasmid. *In vivo* evaluation of the formulation in *nu/nu* mice bearing orthotopic human breast adenocarcinoma (MDA-MB-435) xenografts established transfection and expression of sFlt-1 as assessed by ELISA, western blot analysis, tumor volume, microvessel density and immunostaining. PEG-modified thiolated gelatin nanoparticles were effective in transfection with sFlt-1 expressing plasmid DNA *in vivo* and showed significant suppression of tumor growth in MDAMB-435 tumor-bearing mice. The expressed sFlt-1 was able to suppress angiogenesis [Jabr-Milane et al., 2008]. As such, PEG-modified thiolated gelatin nanoparticles are a viable platform for the delivery of therapeutic DNA to tumor mass. In addition, a system was developed for oral gene delivery. The nanoparticles-in-microsphere oral system (NiMOS) consists of type B gelatin nanoparticles encapsulated in Poly-ε-caprolactone (PCL) microspheres. Based on the successful transfection results with sFlt-1, type B gelatin nanoparticles were selected to encapsulate and deliver DNA, while PCL was selected to protect the nanoparticles from degradation in the stomach and deliver the particles to the intestine, where PCL is degraded by lipases. To evaluate the biodistribution of NiMOS, the researchers encapsulated 111In-radiolabeled gelatin nanoparticles in PCL microspheres, orally administered the formulation to fasted Winstar rats, harvested the tissues at different time points and compared the results to 111In-radiolabeled gelatin nanoparticles. The gelatin nanoparticles showed immediate and high accumulation in the large intestine whereas NiMOS accumulation was initially high in the stomach (after 1 h) [Jabr-Milane et al., 2008]. It then transferred predominately to the large intestine after 2 h. To explore the effect of this biodistribution profile on transfection, the formulations were loaded with reporter plasmids expressing β-galactosidase (CMV-βgal) or expressing GFP. DNA loaded NiMOS were orally administered to fasted Winstar rats at an oral dose of 100 μg plasmid DNA [Jabr-Milane et al., 2008].

Five days after administration, the rats were sacrificed and the GI tract was harvested for analysis. The results were compared to unloaded NiMOS formulations, naked plasmid and loaded gelatin nanoparticles. Transgene expression was evident in the small and large intestines with both reporter plasmids although GFP expression was more prominent with the loaded NiMOS formulation relative to the controls. Similar results were obtained in studies with Balb/c mice. Clearly, NiMOS is a promising system for targeted delivery of therapeutic DNA to the GI tract [Jabr-Milane et al., 2008].

7. Design of multi-functional nanocarrier system

An artificial gene-delivery vector, with a multi-component architecture is able to overcoming all the barriers, in which each component performs a different task in a planned fashion. The design of multi-functional nano-carrier is a multidisciplinary task that requires a profound understanding of the physico-chemical mechanisms that drive the assembly of such nano-particles. One among many prerequisites for a successful carrier system for nucleic acids is high stability in the extracellular environment. In addition, the biological processes that elicit the cellular uptake and intracellular processing accompanied by an efficient release of the cargo in the intracellular compartment of these gene delivery systems have to be well understood. A promising strategy to create such an interactive delivery system is to exploit the various biological stimuli. With greater understanding of physiological differences between normal and disease tissues and advances in material design, there is an opportunity to develop nano-carrier systems for target-specific drug and gene delivery that will respond to the local stimuli [Qiao et al., 2010; Mastrobattista et al., 2006]. At present, many examples of versatile, self-assembling nano-particles for the delivery of DNA can be found in literature and this number is continuously growing. In this section, emphasis is placed on the functional components that are needed for effective gene delivery and also the biological stimuli such as pH and redox potential for the synthesis of multi-functional intelligent delivery systems. Briefly, Table 1 indicates these functional carriers.

7.1. Bio-compatible, bio-degradable nano-carriers

The artificial virus should preferably be constructed from materials that are biocompatible and biodegradable to prevent carrier-induced toxicities and the accumulation of carrier components in the body. In general, lipids are well tolerated. Synthetic polymers, on the other hand, have shown to induce some cytotoxicity *in vitro* and *in vivo*. It is difficult to predict, however, which polymer will be cytotoxic and which not on the basis of the structure of the cationic polymer. In general, low-molecular-mass cationic polymers are less toxic than high-molecular-mass polymers. Peptides derived from L-amino acids are inherently biodegradable. However, when proteins or peptides contain large numbers of positively charged or exposed hydrophobic amino acids, they can destabilize biological membranes and thereby cause cytotoxicity [Mastrobattista et al., 2006].

Function	Examples	Reference
Bio-compatible, biodegradable nanocarrier	Synthetic polymers: Poly (D, L-lactide-coglycolide), Poly (L-lactic acid), Poly (epiloncaprolactone), Poly (alkylcyanoacrylates) Natural polymers: Gelatin, Chitosan, Hyaluronic acid	van Vlerken et al., 2007; Mastrobattista et al., 2006
Packaging nucleic acids into compact nanoparticles	Polyethyleimine (PEI), Polylysine (pLys)	Wagner, 2011; Walker et al., 2005
Long-circulation of nanocarrier	Polysaccharides, Polyacrylamide, Polyvinylalcohol, PEG [PEGylated polyplexes]	van Vlerken et al., 2007; Mastrobattista et al., 2006
Targeting molecules for the development of targeted NPs	Monoclonal antibody, Affibody, Aptamer, Oligopeptides, Growth factor, Vitamin	Wang et al., 2011; Wagner, 2011; Mastrobattista et al., 2006; Gu et al., 2007; van Vlerken et al., 2007; Peer et al., 2007; Alexis et al., 2008; Farokhzad et al., 2006; Zhang et al., 2001; Askoxylakis et al., 2005; Soudy et al., 2011; Kim et al., 2006; Ogris et al., 2003
Intracellular delivery	Escape from the endosomal compartment: Influenza HA2 peptide, melittin, T-domain of the diphtheria toxin, GALA peptide, pH-sensitive polymers: PEI Cytosolic un-packaging: Reduction-sensitive polyplexes Nuclear Import: SV40 from the large tumor antigen Simian virus 40, M9 from nuclear ribonucleoprotein	Eliyahu et al., 2005; Shim and Kwon, 2012; Vercauteren et al., 2012; Du et al., 2010; Schaffer et al., 2000; Bauhuber et al., 2009

Table 1. The use of different formulations with specific functions for designing of multi-functional nanocarrier systems

Polymeric nano-particles offer significant advantages over other nano-carrier platforms primarily since a remarkable flexibility in polymer matrices allows for tailoring of the nano-particle properties to meet the specific planed need. Other advantages of polymeric nano-particles include ease of production, ease of surface modification, encapsulation efficiency of the payload, payload protection, large area-to-volume, slow or fast polymer degradation and stimuli-responsive polymer erosion for temporal control over the release of drugs and feasibility of scale-up and manufacturing. Some examples of the most commonly used polymers for nano-carriers include the synthetic polymers such as poly (D, L-lactide-coglycolide) (PLGA), poly (L-lactic acid) (PLL), poly (epsiloncaprolactone) (PCL), poly (alkylcyanoacrylates) and natural polymers such as gelatin, chitosan and hyaluronic acid [van Vlerken et al., 2007; Mastrobattista et al., 2006].

7.2. Packaging nucleic acids into compact nano-particles

A prerequisite for every systemic nucleic-acid delivery system is stability in the blood stream prior to reaching its target cell. Therefore, the carrier must prevent the premature release of its load. Among the different delivery systems, nano-sized drug carriers are receiving considerable attention. Through precise selection of candidate therapeutics and appropriate functionalization of the nano-carrier systems, it is possible to develop fairly sophisticated multifunctional systems that can provide optimized anticancer therapy, a function that imparts particular use in intracellular delivery and sub-cellular localization of drugs. Reversible nucleic acid condensation by cationic proteins is a common natural process, e.g., in packaging of whole mammalian genomes into chromatin, or RNA into organelles. Compaction is also a key function of viral cores for protection against the degradative environment during infection. Nucleic acids as macromolecules are subjected to a variety of environmental factors such as pH or enzymes (e.g., nucleases) that can degrade or destroy them. Complexation of nucleic acids by cationic polymers or lipids is a widely used method to reduce their sizes and prevent their destruction by nucleases.

Reversibility is important; the delivered nucleic acid has to be accessible for subsequent transcription [Wagner, 2011]. Polyplexes are non-viral vectors consisting of DNA and polycations have shown potential in systemic targeted gene delivery in various animal models, but suffer from far lower gene transfer efficiency than viral vectors. To improve efficiency, researchers are trying to engineer synthetic vectors with virus-like qualities. For successful condensation of DNA into virus size particles, an excess of polycations is necessary, which results in a positive surface charge. The positive surface charge on particles has been shown to be generally advantageous for cell uptake [Walker et al., 2005]. Polyionic interactions, hydrogen bonding and hydrophobic interactions control the condensation of nucleic acids. In electrostatic complexes of plasmid DNA (pDNA) with polycations such as polylysine (pLys) or polyethylenimine (PEI), neutralization of approximately 10,000 negative phosphate charges of one pDNA molecule by approximately 100 polycation molecules results in compaction into "polyplexes" with sizes of 20 to >100 nm (depending on aggregation events). The polymer/pDNA core may be regarded as the engine of the delivery vehicle; for efficient and specific delivery, like in natural viruses, additional domains for cell entry and endosomal escape are required [Fig.1A & B; Wagner, 2011].

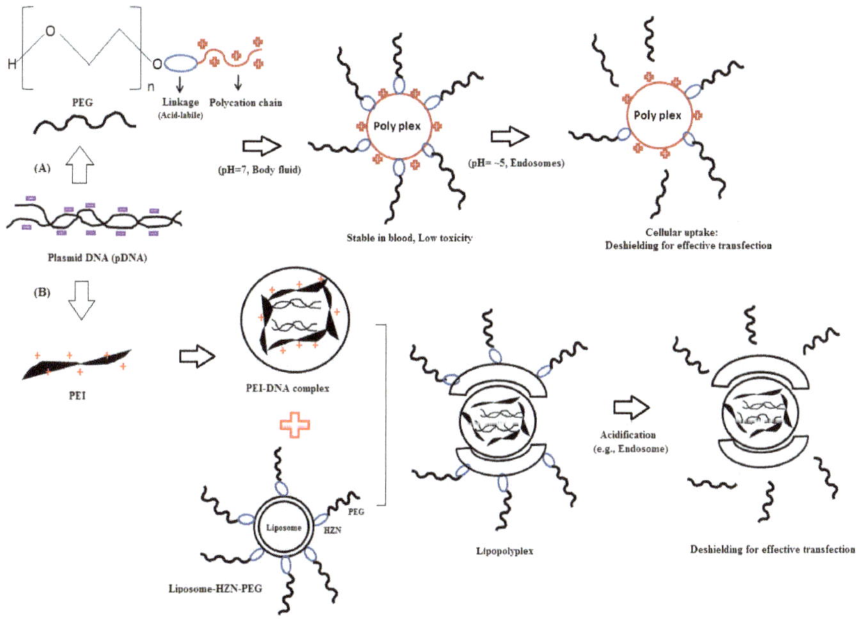

Figure 1. A) Schematic model of the pH-sensitive polyplexes: Covalent attachment of active targeting ligands e.g., peptides, proteins, aptamers and small molecules to PEG; Formation of the polycation- pDNA polyplex through charge-charge interaction; Complex shielded at physiological pH and deshielded at acidic pH. **B) pH-reversible pEGylated lipopolyplexes:** Formation of complex by mixing DNA and PEI (polyplex); Incubation of the cationic polyplexes with liposomes (liposome-Pyridylhydrazone-PEG); Shielding in extracellular compartments and deshielding in acidic medium (e.g., endosomes).

7.3. Long-circulation of nanocarrier

Both naked DNA and lipoplexes have showed rapid hepatic clearance during systemic administration. The liver elimination of lipoplexes was due to phagocytosis by Kupffer cells. Absence of any hydrophilic surface group on the particles, may lead to their interaction with plasma proteins, opsonization and removal from the circulation. The mononuclear phagocytic system (MPS) plays a key role in systemic removal of hydrophobic particles. In addition to biodegradability and biocompatibility, the non-viral carrier should be 'invisible' to the innate and acquired immune system of the patient in order to prevent unwanted immune reactions against the carrier and, consequently, rapid clearance of carriers from the blood circulation after intravenous administration. This can be achieved by adding a hydrophilic coat around the carrier. The coat can consist of a lipid bilayer or hydrophilic polymers grafted onto the surface of the carriers [Mastrobattista et al., 2006]. Among several strategies to impart particles with stealth-shielding, including surface modification with polysaccharides, polyacrylamide, and polyvinyl alcohol, surface modification with PEG and PEG co-polymers proved to be most effective, fueling its wide-spread use. PEG has a general structure of $HO–(CH_2CH_2O)_n–CH_2CH_2–OH$, including a polyether backbone that is chemically inert, with terminal hydroxyl groups that can be activated for conjugation to different types of polymers and drugs. PEG offers the advantage that it is non-toxic and non-immunogenic, leading to approval by the United States Food and Drug Administration (FDA) for internal use in humans and inclusion in the list of inactive ingredients for oral and parenteral applications [Fig. 1 A & B; van Vlerken et al., 2007]. The protective (stealth) action of PEG is mainly due to the formation of a dense, hydrophilic cloud of long flexible chains on the surface of the colloidal particle that reduces the hydrophobic interactions with the RES. The chemically anchored PEG chains can undergo spatial conformations, thus preventing the opsonization of particles by the macrophages of the RES, which leads to preferential accumulation in the liver and spleen. PEG surface modification, therefore, enhances the circulation time of molecules and colloidal particles in the blood. The mechanism of steric hindrance by the PEG modified surface has been thoroughly examined. The water molecules form a structured shell through hydrogen bonding to the ether oxygen molecules of PEG. The tightly bound water forms a hydrated film around the particle and prevents the protein interactions. In addition, PEG surface modification may also increase the hydrodynamic size of the particle decreasing its clearance, a process that is dependent on the molecular size as well as particle volume. Ultimately, this helps in greatly increasing circulation half-life of the particles [van Vlerken et al., 2007]. In cancer therapy, PEGylated polyplexes with elongated plasma circulation may take advantage of the "enhanced permeability and retention" (EPR) effect. Long-term circulating nano-particles can extravasate and passively accumulate at tumor sites due to the leakiness of tumor vessels and ineffective lymphatic efflux ("passive tumor targeting") [Wagner, 2011].

7.4. Targeting molecules for the development of targeted NPs

Appropriate packaging of nucleic acids and the use of PEG as a shield can help the complex survive within the circulation without being degraded or taken up by the mononuclear phagocyte system MPS. However, the next challenge for a PEGylated gene complex is to specifically target to cells or tissue of interest. By taking advantage of increased expression levels of receptors or antigens in diseased conditions, such as cancer, gene complexes can be targeted using specific ligands, such as antibodies, peptides, proteins, small molecules and RNA aptamer that recognize and bind to the cells of interest, resulting in high transfection efficiency [Wang et al., 2011].

Viruses are optimized for surviving in the relevant body fluids. Their surface is decorated with ligands for attachment to their target cell surface receptors. Often they use more than one receptor type for intracellular uptake into host cells. In design of synthetic nano-particles, such multivalent recognition and cell uptake mechanisms for nucleic acid delivery can be utilized [Wagner, 2011]. A simultaneous effect of the surface modification of gene carriers are that the positive surface charges are shielded, which significantly reduces the non-specific adsorption onto cell membranes. This enables targeting of the gene carriers towards specific cell types by conjugating ligands to the hydrophilic coat around the gene carrier that specifically bind internalizing cell-surface receptors. In this way, delivery of the transgene and subsequent expression can be restricted to target cells. Several different types of targeting ligands have been used for this purpose, including peptides, antibodies and vitamins. If targeting ligands are directed towards internalizing receptors, receptor binding will lead to receptor-mediated endocytosis of the targeted gene carriers, as they are small enough (< 200-300 nm). This route of uptake is to be preferred as it ensures intracellular accumulation of gene carriers in a receptor-specific way [Mastrobattista et al., 2006]. While it has been demonstrated that PEG surface modification of nano-carriers causes a greater accumulation of drug at the tumor-site by passive targeting, active targeting of the carrier can help in selection of the target cell-type within the tumor site and internalization of the nano-particles to a greater extent inside the target cells. Active targeting can be achieved by the functionalization of NPs with ligands such as proteins (mainly antibodies and their fragments), nucleic acids (aptamers), or other receptor ligands (peptides, carbohydrates and vitamins) [Gu et al., 2007]. Regardless of the targeting moiety, the principle outcome is essentially the same, mainly improved tumor cell recognition, improved tumor cell uptake, and reduced recognition at non-specific sites. PEG surface modification provides an advantage whereby the terminal groups of PEG can be functionalized to reactive groups for covalent coupling. Most commonly, PEG is functionalized to reactive carboxylic acids, amine, or sulfhydryl groups, allowing for efficient covalent attachment of the wide variety of targeting ligands by amide bonding or disulfide bridge formation [van Vlerken et al., 2007]. In this section, we describe some classes of targeting molecules.

7.4.1. Monoclonal antibodies

Monoclonal antibodies (mAb) are the first and are still the preferred class of targeting molecules. The mAb Rituximab was approved by the FDA for treating B-cell lymphoma in 1997. Another successful therapeutic mAb is Trastuzumab (Herceptin), an anti-HER2 mAb which binds to ErbB2 receptors and was approved by the FDA for treating breast cancer in 1998. Cetuximab, which binds to epidermal growth factor receptors (EGFR), was approved for treating colorectal cancer in 2004 and head/neck cancer in 2006. Bevacizumab, a tumor angiogenesis inhibitor that binds to vascular endothelial growth factor (VEGF), was approved for treating colorectal cancer in 2004. Trastuzumab and rituximab have been conjugated to poly (lactic acid) (PLA) NPs resulting in conjugates that exhibit a six-fold increase in the rate of particle uptake compared with similar particles lacking the mAb targeting. Today, over 200 delivery systems based on antibodies or their fragments are in preclinical and clinical trials. Antibodies may be used in their native state or as fragments for targeting [Imai and Takaoka, 2006; Peer et al., 2007].

7.4.2. Affibodies as targeting ligands

In recent times, a novel class of small molecules called "affibodies," which can be considered antibody mimics, have been examined for targeting. Affibodies are a class of polypeptide ligands that are potential candidates for tissue-specific targeting of drug-encapsulated controlled release polymeric nanoparticles. Affibody molecules are relatively small proteins (6-8 kDa) that offer the advantage of being extremely stable, highly soluble, and readily expressed in bacterial systems or produced by peptide synthesis. The binding affinities of affibody molecules are considerably higher compared with the corresponding antibodies. The binding pocket of an affibody is composed of 13 amino acids, which can be randomized to bind a variety of targets. In contrast to monoclonal antibody, affibody has following advantages as a targeting ligand. First, the small size of affibody (MW: 6 kDa) guarantees its tissue/cell penetration ability. Second, its functional end groups for chemical conjugation are distanced from its binding site. Moreover, affibody has a robust structure, and can be easily synthesized in a large-scale manner. All of these advantages make the affibody a valuable ligand for targeted drug delivery [Alexis et al., 2008; Manjappa et al., 2011]. Recently, anti-HER2 affibody was also employed as a targeting ligand for nano-scaled drug delivery systems. Alexis et al. conjugated the anti-HER2 affibody to poly-(D, L-lactic acid)-poly (ethylene glycol)-maleimide (PLA-PEG-Mal) copolymer for targeted delivery to cells that over-express the HER-2 antigen [Alexis et al., 2008].

7.4.3. Aptamer targeting molecules

A novel class of molecules, referred to as nucleic acid ligands (aptamers), has been developed to generate targeting agents. Aptamers are short single-stranded DNA or RNA oligonucleotides or modified DNA or RNA oligonucleotides that fold by intramolecular interaction into unique conformations with ligand-binding characteristics. Like antibodies, aptamers can be prepared to bind target antigens with high specificity and affinity. The use of aptamers as targeting molecules has several potential advantages over antibodies. Aptamers with high affinity for a target can be prepared through *in vitro* selection; a process called systemic evolution of ligands by exponential enrichment (SELEX) [Chai et al., 2011]. Conjugating aptamers to nanoparticles has shown to result in more efficient targeted therapeutics or selective diagnostics than non-targeted NPs. Farokhzad et al have developed NP-aptamer (NP-Apt) conjugates that target the prostate specific membrane antigen (PSMA), a transmembrane protein that is up-regulated in a variety of cancers, using the A10 aptamer [Farokhzad et al., 2004]. This formulation has been further evaluated *in vivo* in a tumor model of LNCaP prostate cancer cells, which express PSMA antigens, and has been shown to regress tumor size effectively following a single intra-tumor injection over a 109-day study [Farokhzad et al., 2006].

7.4.4. Oligopeptide-based targeting molecules

Recently, a number of tumor homing peptides have been reported that specifically target cancer cells and show promising results for tumor targeted drug delivery. Peptides, being smaller than other targeting ligands, have excellent tissue penetration properties and can be easily conjugated to drugs and oligonucleotides by chemical synthesis. Peptides are nearly invisible to the immune system and are not taken up in the reticuloendothelial system like antibodies and so are expected to cause minimal or no side effects to bone marrow, liver, and spleen [Gu et al., 2007]. For example, Cilengitide® is a cyclic arginine-glycine-aspartic acid (RGD) peptide that binds to the cell adhesion integrin $\alpha_v\beta_3$ on endothelial cells results in increased intracellular drug delivery in different murine tumor models and is currently in phase II clinical trials for the treatment of non-small cell lung cancer and pancreatic cancer.

Despite the success mentioned, RGD-targeted therapy still encounters many challenges. First challenge is the limitation associated with the non-specific adhesive nature of the RGD-integrin targeting system. Integrins are extracellular receptors that are not only expressed on cancer cells but also on nearly all epithelial cells and are therefore not cancer specific. Recent development of phage display screening methods has successfully isolated peptide ligands with high specificity and affinity to cell-surface hormone receptors (LHRH receptors, somatostatin receptors) and tumor vasculature antigens [Gu et al., 2007]. One of those is a dodecapeptide identified through phage display by Zhang *et al*, referred to as peptide p160. Peptide p160 displays high affinity for the human breast cancer cell lines MDA-MB-435 and MCF-7 *in vitro* with very little affinity for primary endothelial HUVEC cells [Zhang et al., 2001]. Furthermore, *in vivo* bio-distribution experiments in tumor-bearing mice, p160 showed a higher uptake in tumors than in organs such as heart, liver, lung and kidney. Relative to the RGD-4C peptide, p160 showed high accumulation in tumor versus normal organs [Askoxylakis et al., 2005; Soudy et al., 2011; Zhang et al., 2001]. Despite the potential of peptide p160 as a potent tumor homing peptide, its applicability would be largely hindered by its instability toward proteases. To overcome this, peptides have to be chemically modified so that their blood clearance is minimized in comparison with their rate of uptake at the target sites. The most common strategies used to increase peptide proteolytic stability include introduction of D- or un-natural amino acids and peptide cyclization. In a recent study, Soudy *et al* have developed analogues of cancer targeting peptide p160 to improve proteolytic stability and maintain specific affinity for breast cancer cells. These analogues are potentially safe with minimal cellular toxicity and are efficient targeting moieties for specific drug delivery to breast cancer cells [Soudy et al., 2011].

7.4.5. Growth factor or vitamin-based targeting molecules

Growth factor or vitamin interactions with cancer cells represent a commonly used targeting strategy, as cancer cells over-express the receptors for nutrition to maintain their fast-growing metabolism. Epidermal growth factor (EGF) has been shown to block and reduce tumor expression of the EGF receptor, which is over-expressed in a variety of tumor cells such as breast and tongue cancer [Peer et al., 2007].

One of the most extensively studied small molecule targeting moieties for drug delivery is folic acid (folate). The high-affinity vitamin is a commonly used ligand for cancer targeting because folate receptors (FRs) are frequently over-expressed in a range of tumor cells. It has been used as a targeting moiety combined with a wide array of drug delivery vehicles including liposomes, protein toxins, polymeric NPs, linear polymers, and dendrimers to deliver drugs selectively into cancer cells using FR-mediated endocytosis [Gu et al., 2007]. The folic acid-PEGylated PEI polyplex was evaluated as a gene carrier, and successfully delivered siRNA and pDNA to tumour cells [Kim et al., 2006].

Transferrin (Tf), an iron-binding glycoprotein interacts with Tf receptors (TfRs), which are overexpressed on a variety of tumor cells (including pancreatic, colon, lung, and bladder cancer) owing to increased metabolic rates. Direct coupling of these targeting agents to nanocarriers has improved intracellular delivery and therapeutic outcome in animal models. Tf-linked PEG-PEI was developed for tumor-selective gene delivery. The surface charge of the complexes was shielded by either PEG or a higher density of linked Tf to block undesired non-specific interactions with blood components, followed by selective targeting to tumor cells. This approach resulted in a 100-fold higher gene expression in tumor cells compared with other tissues [Ogris et al., 2003].

One challenge with targeting receptors whose expression correlates with metabolic rate, such as folate and Tf, is that these receptors are also expressed in fast growing healthy cells such as fibroblasts, epithelial and endothelial cells. Therefore, NP delivery system needs to be further refined and tuned to increase tumor selectivity [Gu et al., 2007; Peer et al., 2007].

7.5. Intracellular delivery

Non-viral vectors have to overcome multiple intracellular barriers subsequently after cellular uptake usually via endocytosis. After cellular internalization, a critical intracellular obstacle to non-viral gene delivery is degradation in the endosome/lysosome where nucleic acids are easily degraded by a mildly acidic pH and acid activated enzymes. The ability of non-viral vectors to release the nucleic acids in their intracellular targets, while surviving through low pH and digestive processes and avoiding unwanted premature decomplexation, is a key efficiency-determining requirement. The most widely believed theory in designing non-viral vectors for efficient endosomal escape is employing the "proton sponge effect" [Eliyahu et al., 2005]. Importantly, intracellular targets, where the nucleic acids are released from the vector, determine the overall gene delivery efficiency because the action sites are different for nucleic acid types. For example, plasmid DNA must be localized in the nucleus, where gene expression is initiated by transcription. However, nuclear entry is one of the major obstacles to non-viral gene delivery although nuclear translocation of plasmid DNA is crucial to achieve desired transfection efficiency. Moreover, the nuclear translocation mechanism of plasmid DNA in the cytoplasm has not yet been fully elucidated. Passive diffusion of macromolecules (e.g., plasmid DNA) in the cytoplasm is restricted by a complex network of microtubules, proteins, and various sub-cellular organelles. One explanation is the nuclear localization of plasmid DNA during cellular mitosis when the nuclear envelope disassembles. For non-dividing cells, the transport of polyplexes into the nucleus occurs only via an active transport mechanism through a nuclear pore complex that prevents molecules larger than 40 kDa from passively diffusing into the nucleus. In contrast to plasmid DNA delivery, it is obvious that transnuclear localization of siRNA should be prevented to achieve efficient RNA interference (RNAi) since siRNA acts in the cytosol, where it targets mRNA with matching sequences [Shim and Kwon, 2012]. As nano-medicines often require delivery of their therapeutic payload to specific sub-cellular locations, knowledge about intracellular trafficking might prove useful for the control of the intracellular processing of nano-particles and lead to optimization of their design [Vercauteren et al., 2012].

7.5.1. Escape from the endosomal compartment

Following internalization of peptide-DNA condensates by endocytosis, the polyplex must be able to escape the endosome so that the DNA can be delivered to the nucleus for gene expression. After endocytosis, entrapment of the vector within the acidified vesicles of the endosomal/

lysosomal system is a critical barrier to non-viral gene delivery systems. Unfortunately, the environment of the lysosomal interior is harmful for nucleic acid (NA) integrity, unless the carrier offers sufficient protection against the degradation by the acid hydrolases [Vercauteren et al., 2012]. Viruses and some pathogenic bacteria have pH-sensitive surface proteins that change conformation in mildly acidic environments such as in endosomes, and exhibit membrane-disruptive (fusogenic or endosomolytic) properties. Synthetic fusogenic peptides that mimic the sequences of these natural proteins have been confirmed to increase cytoplasmic gene delivery [Du et al., 2010]. Since escape from the endosomes is essential for efficient NA therapy, much attention has been paid to this issue, resulting in a variety of endosomolytic carriers. For example, cationic and pH-responsive lipids can be added to phospholipid carriers to assist in releasing the NAs into the cytoplasm by destabilizing the endosomal lipid bilayer in the acidic environment of the endolysosomes. Another approach is based on the coupling of fusogenic peptides to the carriers, which undergo conformational changes after their exposure to the decreasing endosomal pH values, exposing hydrophobic faces of the fusion peptide which destabilizes the endosomal membrane. Examples of these endosome-disruptive peptides are the influenza HA2 peptide, melittin, the T-domain of the diphtheria toxin or the GALA peptide [Vercauteren et al., 2012]. In an effort to translate the proton sponge activity to gene delivery peptides, histidine has been added to peptide sequences. The imidazole group of histidine has a pKa of ~ 6.0, therefore allowing it to become protonated in the acidic environment of the endosome. At physiological pH the histidines will remain neutrally charged, thereby imparting selective membrane disruption in the acidic endosome. In the past two decades, synthetic pH-sensitive polymers as endosomolytic agents have attracted great interest due to their low or non immunogenicity, which is a concern of using fusogenic proteins or peptides. Polymers such as PEI contain several secondary amines that are easily protonated in the acidic environment of the endosome. As protons are pumped in, PEI absorbs the protons leading to endosomal swelling and membrane disruption. In general, these smart polymers have both hydrophobic parts and weakly acidic groups, which afford them pH-dependent endosomolytic properties. At physiological pH, the polymers have little endosomolytic activity but undergo a conformational change at endosomal pH and show membrane-disruptive properties. This provides the polymers with reduced toxicity to the other biomembranes at neutral pH, but with the ability to facilitate endosomal escape [Fig. 1A; Du et al., 2010].

7.5.2. Cytosolic un-packaging

The final step of the gene delivery process, un-packaging of the polyplex, can limit the efficiency of gene delivery and expression. For *in vivo* polyplex gene delivery, the polycation condenses the DNA to protect it and facilitate its entry and passage through target cells. However, once inside the nucleus, in order to be processed by RNA transcription complexes, the DNA may first need to dissociate from the polycation. Strong binding of the polycations to the nucleic acids may limit the intracellular un-packing of the polyplexes which is necessary for an efficient transfection. Although some viruses have evolved highly specific and intensive mechanisms for uncoating within the cell, a synthetic polycation may not release DNA with similar high efficiency [Schaffer et al., 2000]. One of the solutions to these problems is to use degradable polycations. Although the degradable polycations whose degradation is based on the hydrolysis of an ester or amide bond have been widely used as gene carriers with decreased cytotoxicities, it is difficult to control the degradation occurring in the cytoplasm where free siRNA should be released to take action. Since the reduction potential in the cytoplasm is much higher (100 fold) than in the extracellular environments, a promising strategy to create an interactive delivery system is to exploit the redox gradient between the extra- and intra-cellular compartments, reduction-sensitive polyplexes are considered to be superior degradable candidates, especially for siRNA delivery [Bauhuber et al., 2009; Du et al., 2010].

7.5.3. Nuclear import

The nuclear envelope that separates the cell's genetic material from the surrounding cytoplasm represents a physical barrier for nuclear import of macromolecules such as pDNA. The nuclear envelope contains openings in the form of nuclear pore complexes, which allow free diffusion of molecules up to 50 kDa, corresponding to a hydrodynamic diameter of approximately 10 nm. There are several lines of evidence showing that nuclear import is a rate-limiting step for transfection of pDNA. Nuclear import of pDNA may be more challenging for transfection of non-dividing cells. Indeed, non-dividing cells showed a 90% lower expression level as compared to actively dividing cells. Strategies for nuclear import of genes have been developed following further elucidation of the endogenous nuclear import machinery [Wang et al., 2011]. In nature, large molecules with sizes up to 30 nm in diameter that require trans-nuclear transport contain nuclear localization signals (NLS) that are recognized by nuclear transport receptors like importins or transportins, and the whole complex is thereafter actively transported through NPCs [Vercauteren et al., 2012]. The nuclear localization sequence is a major player that shuttles protein–plasmid complexes through the nuclear pore. NLS-mediated active nuclear translocation involves a process starting from its interaction with cytoplasmic importins to binding of the NLS to the nuclear pore complex and the passage through the pore. Identification of the NLSs, such as SV40 from the larger tumor antigen Simian virus 40 and M9 from nuclear ribonucleoprotein, enabled design of non-viral gene vectors with nuclear targeting properties [Wang et al., 2011].

8. Designing switchable nanosystems for medical application

To enhance therapeutic efficacy while minimizing side effects, a large number of nanomaterial based platforms have been developed that allow simple delivery of genes. Based on important earlier work in the field of liposomal gene delivery and inorganic nanomaterials, the last decade has brought a broad array of new and improved nanoscale carrier platforms such as biodegradable and non-degradable polymers, dendrimers, carbon nanotubes, metallic and organic nanoparticles, quantum dots, nanogels or peptidic nanoparticles. Ideally, gene vectors should be capable of self-assembly with nucleic acids and accommodate with any type of nucleic acid or their combination. They should also target cells of interest, escape from endosomes and/or transport into nuclei. A viable gene vector for systemic delivery needs to minimize toxicity and phagocytosis and avoid non-specific interactions and self-aggregation. For potential gene delivery applications, ideal gene carriers need to combine both the targeting property and the stimulus responsiveness to enhance the bioavailability of the gene as well as to reduce the side effects. Therefore, designing stimulus-responsive nanoparticles for programmed gene delivery, which release the gene on arrival at the targeted site, is highly desired. Stimulus-responsive nanoparticles produce physical or chemical changes when subjected to external signals, including variations of macromolecular structures, solubility, surface properties, swelling and dissociation [Lehner et al., 2012]. Stimulus-responsive nanoparticles can be classified based on the type of stimulus as internally and externally controllable materials. Internal stimuli (e.g. activation by pH, redox potential, enzymes) might be controlled by a molecular mechanism highly specific for a disease and therefore improve on targeting properties. However, absolutely disease-specific internal molecular triggers are difficult to find for certain diseases. External stimuli like light, ultrasound, electromagnetic fields or ionizing radiation have the advantage of being focusable on certain body areas. This may be a significant advantage where a target cell is strongly involved in pathogenesis at one location (e.g., cancer stem cells in a cancer tissue), but of vital importance in other locations (e.g., stem cells in the bone marrow). A key challenge in externally controlled nanomaterials is tissue penetration and avoidance of undesired tissue damage in the radiation path from radiation source to target tissue. The ease of temporal control in external stimuli may represent a particular advantage for certain applications [Lehner et al., 2012]. Herein, we focus on the use of internal and biological stimuli that can be used to incorporate switch functionality into such nanocarriers and describe the clinical experience with various nanosize carrier systems as a basis for the design of new, improved, functional and "intelligent" nanosystems for gene delivery.

8.1. pH differences for stimuli-responsive delivery

The main property that is the basis of utilization of pH responsive polymers in gene delivery is the significant change in pH value within the cellular compartments. There are numerous pH gradients in physiological and pathological processes [Du et al., 2010]. The pH profile of pathological tissues, such as inflammation, infection and cancer, is significantly different from that of the normal tissue. The pH at systemic sites of infections, primary tumors, and metastasized tumors is lower than the pH of normal tissue. The pH, surface charge and density of low density lipoprotein receptors are the factors that show notable differences among the normal and tumor tissues. All these properties are known to influence the drugs' physicochemical properties and are exploited for enhanced delivery to the target site. The extracellular pH values of solid tumor are in general slightly lower than in blood or other normal tissues. Since tumors proliferate very rapidly, the vasculature of tumor is often insufficient to supply enough nutritional and oxygen needs for the expanding population of tumor cells. This results in difference in metabolic environment between the various solid tumors and the surrounding normal tissue. The insufficient oxygen in tumor leads to hypoxia and causes production of lactic acid and hydrolysis of ATP in an energy-deficient environment contributes to an acidic microenvironment, which has been found in many tumors. Most of the solid tumors have lower extracellular pH (6.5) than the surrounding tissues (pH= 7.5). The pH is compartmentalized in tumor tissue into an intracellular component (pHi), which is similar in tumor and normal tissues and an extracellular component (pHe), which is relatively acidic in tumors

[Ganta et al., 2008]. This behavior can be utilized for the preparation of stimuli responsive drug or gene-delivery systems, which can exploit the biochemical properties at the contaminated site for targeted delivery. Cellular components such as the cytoplasm, endosomes, lysosomes, endoplasmic reticulum, golgi bodies, mitochondria and nuclei are known to maintain their own characteristic pH values. It is well known that the lower pH values are found in endosomes (5.5-6.0) and lysosomes (4.5-5.5). On the basis of these discoveries, various pH/acid-sensitive polymers have been developed as carriers for pDNA, ODN or siRNA delivery [Du et al., 2010; Ganta et al., 2008].

8.1.1. Low pH-sensitive reversible shielding/masking

This part focuses on the design and synthesis of polymeric carriers that can condense a large dose of therapeutic nucleic acids into particles that can sense the differences in environmental pH. The pH-modulated or self-regulated polymers are designed to use these pH differences by incorporating appropriate structural or functional features into the basic scaffold of the polymers to improve the efficacy of gene delivery. In general, polycations (PCs), such as PEI or dendrimers (polyplexes) or with cationic lipids (lipoplexes) with positively charged surfaces are preferred for gene delivery in cell culture [Du et al., 2010]. Although, these positively charged particles are favorable for gene transfer efficiency *in vitro*, they are problematic for systemic gene targeting. Upon systemic application of positively charged cationic lipid based formulations (CL), polycations and lipopolyplexes may result in significant toxicity and/or poor efficiency due to plasma protein binding, interaction with blood cells or activation of the complement system and therefore has limited their application for *in vivo* uses via systemic administration [Du et al., 2010; Walker et al., 2005]. In general, the toxicity of cationic polymers increases with molecular weight, branched polymer morphology, and cationic charge density. A common approach for masking the surface charge of polyplexes is to coat particles with a hydrophilic polymer such as polyethylene glycol (PEG). Shielding the cationic surface by PEGylation and tailoring cationic density and polymer morphology have been popularly exploited to reduce the cytotoxicity [Shim and Kwon, 2012]. PEGylation of polyplexes prevents their aggregation, lowers toxicity, increases circulation time and improves systemic targeted gene transfer. Unfortunately, at the same time as shielding improves the properties of polyplexes for systemic application it appears to reduce its cell transfection activity due to two important barriers such as reduced cellular uptake and inadequate release of the transported gene at the target cells. The cellular uptake has been enhanced by attaching targeting ligands to the polyplexes, however, the transfection efficiency of the targeted PEG vectors often still does not reach the level of the uncoated gene vectors. This suggests that the stable shield may also hinder intracellular gene transfer steps following endosomal uptake. Therefore, it is clear that to develop an optimal nonviral system for systemic application it must have a more dynamic character [Du et al., 2010] Its surface charge must be neutralized during circulation but after reaching its target cell, the cationic surface charge should be re-exposed for efficient gene transfer. In order to solve these conflicting issues, pH-sensitive reversible shielding or masking strategies have been developed through pH-sensitive PEGylation of lipid- or polymer-based carriers as the PEG shield intended to be removable in intracellular endosomes or in the slightly acidic extracellular microenvironment of tumors. Lipoplexes and polyplexes containing a pH cleavable PEG shield were found to be less effective in gene transfer than the corresponding stably shielded particles. There is a strategy to overcome this challenge. The neutralizing shield is attached to the DNA polyplex core via an acid-labile linkage forming a shielded particle for systemic circulation. Chemical linkages that may display pH-dependent hydrolytic degradation, once internalized into endosomal and lysosomal compartments include acetal-ketal linkage, vinyl ether, orthoesters, and hydrazones. Under the acidic environment of the endosomal compartment, these linkages undergo acid-induced hydrolysis and thereby trigger deshielding of the polyplex core. Therefore, the acid-labile bioreversible shielding polymer exerts a significant impact on the outcome of transfection efficiency [Du et al., 2010].

Walker and colleagues reported reversible shielding of polyplexes with pH-triggered deshielding properties, enabled by conjugating PEG to the polycations poly-L-lysine (PLL) and PEI via a pH-sensitive hydrazone bond (PC-HZN-PEG) of acyl hydrazides or 2-pyridyl hydrazines. The reversibility of the hydrazone bond within conjugates was determined at physiological and endosomal acidic pH, identifying suitable linker systems for endosomal deshielding. The polyplexes with the acid-sensitive linkages showed much higher plasmid gene delivery efficiencies (1-2 orders of magnitude) than those with stable linkages, both *in vitro* and *in vivo* [Walker et al., 2005].

Sawant *et al.* demonstrated that the use of a lowered pH-degradable PEG-Hz-PE produced particles (polyethylene glycol-phosphatidylethanolamine conjugates) with transfection activity sensitive to changes in pH, which has a promise for site-specific transfection of tumor cells *in vivo*. In this study, the encapsulation of PEI-PE/DNA complexes into pH-sensitive micelle-like PEG-Hz-PE coat increased the stability of DNA in complete medium and increased transfection efficiency by being responsive to changes in pH. *In vivo*, the PEG2000-Hz-PE is expected to shield the PEI-PE/DNA complex in the systemic circulation and expose the complex only at the tumor sites where the pH is slightly acidic and can facilitate the removal of the PEG coat [Sawant et al., 2012].

Murthy *et al.* synthesized 'encrypted' polymeric carrier that consisted of hydrophobic, membrane disruptive methacrylate polymers onto which hydrophilic PEG chains have been grafted through acid-degradable acetal linkages; a *p*-aminobenzaldehyde acetal linkage demonstrated a suitable hydrolysis profile at endosomal pH [Murthy et al., 2003].

In 2007, Knorr *et al.* synthesized a new PEGylation reagent containing *p*-piperazinobenzaldehyde acetal linkage and a maleimide moiety which can be coupled to thiol-functionalized compounds. For reversible shielding of polyplexes, PEG-acetal-maleimide (MAL) was conjugated to PEI. At 37°C, the PEG-acetal-PEI conjugate were found to be shielded and stable. In contrast, at endosomal pH, the particles were deshielded and aggregated within 0.5 h. The reversibly shielded (PEG-acetal-PEI) polyplexes were found to have approximately 10-fold enhanced gene transfer efficiency than stable shielded polyplexes when tested on the two different cell lines, Renca-EGFR cells and K562 cells [Knorr et al., 2007].

Recently, Sethuraman *et al.* have developed pH-Responsive Sulfonamide/PEI nanoparticles that effectively target the acidic extracellular matrix of tumors, which shows a sharp pH profile, was able to shield positively charged complexes at physiological pH of 7.4. The pH sensitive polymer was able to detach from the complex when the pH environment decreased to pH= 6.6. The polymeric nanoparticle formed through electrostatic attraction is designed in such a way that the final particle is neutral. The polyplexes formed by PEI and pDNA were coated electrostatically with an ultra pH-sensitive diblock copolymer, poly (methacryloyl sulfadimethoxine)-b-PEG. The central idea of this design is that when the particles experience a decrease in pH as they extravasate into tumor tissue due to enhanced permeability and retention effect, the sulfonamide groups would lose their charge and get detached from the carrier complex. Most of the carriers developed so far do not have the high sensitivity that is required to respond to such small differences in pH between tumors and normal tissues. This is because the carboxylic acid based polymers show transitions in about one pH unit which is very broad, and that transition is much below the physiological and tumor pH range, whereas the poly(methacryloyl sulfadimethoxine) (PSD)-*block*-PEG PSD*b*-PEG polymer shows transition within 0.2 pH units between the physiological and tumor pH. These sulfonamide polymers are able to distinguish the small difference in pH between normal and tumor tissues and hence has remarkable potential in drug targeting to tumor areas [Sethuraman et al., 2008].

8.1.2. pH-dependent endosomolytic polymers

Following internalization of lipoplexes or polyplexes via the endocytic pathway, endosomal entrapment and subsequent lysosomal degradation are a major blockage that limits the efficiency of gene delivery. After cellular uptake of the gene carriers, the carrier should escape from the endosomal compartment in order to reach the cytosol and then, the nucleus. This requires dissociation of the internalized carrier from the receptors that triggered the internalization process. In addition, the membranes of the endosomes should be destabilized to allow translocation of the carriers into the cytosol [Mastrobattista et al., 2006]. Identification of endosomolytic or fusogenic components and their integration into non-viral gene delivery systems are major strategies being exploited to facilitate endosomal escape.

In the case of polyplexes, PEI and polyamidoamine (PAMAM) are two representative cationic polymers with a high efficiency of gene transfer due in part to their capability to facilitate endosomal escape. A "proton sponge effect" provides a sound explanation for the intrinsic endosomolytic activity. Upon PEI-based or PAMAM-based polyplex entry into acidic endosomes, the polymer behaves as a sponge that absorbs protons as a result of protonation of the polymer-containing amine groups (primary, secondary and tertiary). Accumulation of protons subsequently drives an influx of counter chloride ion into endosomes, leading to increased osmotic pressure and subsequent flow of water into the endosomal interior and eventually swells and ruptures endosomal membrane [Eliyahu et al., 2005].

PEIs are available in a wide range of molecular weights (MW) from 423 Da to 800 kDa and with different branching degree (from linear to branched). Generally, high MW, branched PEIs have high transfection efficiency but also high toxicity due to high cationic charge. By contrast, low MW PEIs are less toxic but less efficient as gene delivery agents. Many efforts have been directed towards creating PEI derivatives combining higher transfection efficacy and good biocompatibility. One approach to reduce the cytotoxicity, biodegradable polyethylenimine with imine linkages as acid-labile moieties were synthesized and investigated for pDNA delivery. The half-life of the acid-labile PEI was 1.1 h at pH=4.5 and 118 h at pH=7.4, suggesting that the acid-labile PEI may be rapidly degraded into non-toxic low molecular weight PEI in acidic endosome. Acid-labile PEIs showed close transfection efficiency to PEI 25KDa, but much less toxicity due to the degradation of acid-labile linkage. Therefore, the acid-labile PEIs may be useful for the development of a non-toxic polymeric gene carrier [Kim et al., 2005].

The cationic lipids have been shown to destabilize the endosomal membrane. Addition of dioleoyl phosphatidylethanolamine (DOPE) or cholesteryl hemisuccinate (CHEMS) to non-viral vectors affected the pH-sensitivity of the formulations. The mechanism behind the phenomenon, is that electrical interaction between cationic lipids and anion endosomal membranes results in the formation of ion-pairs that promote the formation of the inverted hexagonal (HII) phase and disrupt endosomal membrane. Many preparations of lipoplexes contain DOPE as a helper lipid for fusogenic functionality. The ability of DOPE to destabilize endosomal membranes is based on its propensity to acquire an inverted hexagonal phase (HII). DOPE has a small cross-section head group and a large hydrocarbon area that favors a non-bilayer structure with a cone shape that facilitates the destabilization of endosomal membranes and gene transfection. The pH-responsive component, CHEMS, being negatively charged at neutral pH stabilizes the bilayer structure, however, at acidic pH it becomes protonated and loses its stabilization property [Ma et al., 2007; Wu and Zhao, 2007].

Another approach to reduce the cytotoxicity of PEI is modification with hydrophobic moieties, such as lipids. Since lipids are the main component of cell membrane, modification with hydrophobic moieties may result in additional hydrophobic interaction between polyplexes and cell membranes, which in turn would facilitate the delivery of a payload into cells. Various hydrophobic modifications have been tried, including modification with cholesterol, myristate, dodecyl iodide, hexadecyl iodide, palmitic acid, oleic acid, stearic acid, and phosphatidylcholine. In a recent study, Sawant *et al.* developed the synthesis and characterization of a PEI-DOPE conjugate, which was explored for gene delivery *in vitro*. The modification with DOPE strongly increased the transfection efficiency of low molecular weight PEI-1.8 kDa without any negative effects on its low cytotoxicity. The PEI-PE conjugate was synthesized by reacting a phospholipid with low molecular weight PEI (PEI-1.8). It was assumed that a PEI-PE conjugate would condense DNA due to the electrostatic interaction between polycationic PEI moieties, while the lipid moieties would help to increase cell interaction of the complexes and facilitate their incorporation into lipid-based micellar systems via hydrophobic interactions [Sawant et al., 2012].

In order to take the advantages of both polycationic polymers and liposomes, Nie *et al.* have constructed programmed lipopolyplexes, featuring well compacted DNA by PEI and liposome complexing. Liposomes contain the helper lipid DOPE and a pH-cleavable PEG-hydrazone-cholesterol conjugate for shielding. Lipopolyplexes composed of DNA condensed with PEI, phospholipids including dioleoyl phosphatidyl ethanolamine (DOPE) and pH-labile ω-2-pyridyldithio polyethylene glycol α-succinimidylester (OPSS)-PEG-HZN-Chol and yielded particles of 160 nm size and a zeta potential of +7 mV. Pyridylhydrazone-based Chol-PEG was included in the liposomes for shielding in extracellular compartments and dynamic deshielding in acidic conditions such as in endosomes. In addition, this cholesterol-PEG derivative contained also a pyridyldithio moiety to provide the possibility of coupling thiol-functionalized compounds, such as receptor ligands [Fig. 1B.; Nie et al., 2011].

The endosome-escape potential of poly-histidine increases their use for delivery of nucleic acids. The imidazole ring within histidine is a major component. Under the action of an acidic endosomal interior, the weak basic nature of the imidazole ring with pKa around 6 allows its protonation and acquires cationic charges which trigger the destabilization of endosomal membranes. Accumulation of histidine residues within endosomes could elicit a proton sponge effect and destroy endosomes as a result of their increased osmolarity. Both chemistry conjugation and genetic engineering have produced a series of histidine-rich polymers and peptides as well as lipids with imidazole, imidazolinium or imidazolium polar heads. These histidylated carriers have been used to deliver nucleic acids including pDNA, mRNA or siRNA duplex *in vitro* and *in vivo* with increased transfection efficiency [Midoux et al., 2007; Martin and Rice, 2007].

The histidine-rich peptide H5WYG is a derivative of the N-terminal sequence of the HA-2 subunit of the *influenza virus* hemagglutinin in which five of the amino acids have been replaced with histidine residues. H5WYG is able to selectively destabilize membranes at a slightly acidic pH as the histidine residues are protonated. An anionic derivative of this peptide, E5WYG, in which the histidines are replaced by glutamic acid residues, is completely ineffective at membrane permeabilization at a pH= 6.8, while H5WYG can disrupt 50% of cells at pH= 6.8 and 97% of cells at pH= 6.2 within 15 minutes. H5WYG was also able to retain its activity in the presence of serum, making it possible for use *in vivo*. The most well-known non-viral DNA condensing agent is poly-L-lysine. However, PLL only exhibits modest transfection when used alone and requires the addition of an endosomolytic agent such as chloroquine or a fusogenic peptide to allow for release into the cytoplasm. To increase the transfection efficiency of polylysine without the addition of membrane-disrupting agents, a histidine-substituted polylysine can be constructed that is able to become cationic at endosomal pH [Martin and Rice, 2007].

In an attempt to facilitate endosome escape, many strategies have been developed to mimic the viral mechanism for endosome destabilization. Viruses have acquired efficient solutions for escaping from the maturating acidifying endosomes. For example, glycoproteins of enveloped viruses contain hidden fusion peptides which are exposed after endocytosis, to trigger fusion of the viral with the endosomal membrane [Wagner, 2011]. It is well-established that the influenza virus utilizes the pH-sensitive membrane-destabilizing Hemagglutinin protein (HA2) displayed on the viral coat to disrupt the endosomal membrane and enter the cytoplasm. Hemagglutinin and other fusion proteins are characterized by their unique ability to switch from an ionized and hydrophilic conformation at physiologic pH to a hydrophobic and membrane-active one in response to acidic endosomal pH gradients, which destabilizes the endosomal membrane leading to leakage of endosomal contents into the cytoplasm [Lin et al., 2010]. At neutral pH, the HA2 subunit adapts a non-helical conformation due to charge repulsion arising from ionization of glutamic and aspartic acid residues. Within the interior of the acidic endosomal compartment, however, the HA2 subunit transitions into a stable helical secondary structure due to the protonation of glutamic and aspartic acids. The hydrophobic and hydrophilic faces of the helical conformation favor endosomal membrane destabilization.

Endocytosed non-enveloped viruses such as *rhinovirus* or *adenovirus* expose lytic domains which directly disrupt the endosomal membrane, either (in case of *rhinovirus*) generating a pore large enough for crossing of the viral RNA strand into the cytoplasm or (in case of *adenovirus*) disrupting the whole endosome. Such lytic domains have been utilized in artificial settings as synthetic peptides for endosomal escape of polyplexes [Wagner, 2011].

Synthetic peptides mimicking a virus's fusogenic peptides have also been designed for delivery of nucleic acids. The amphipathic peptide, GALA, was synthesized with 30 amino acid residues with a repeated amino acid sequence (e.g., glutamic acid-alanine-leucine-alanine) that demonstrated pH sensitive fusogenic properties. A GALA peptide with a formulation based on DNA/cationic liposome/ Transferrin (Tf) complexes induced enhanced gene transfection. It is assumed that Tf-triggered internalization of the complexes by receptor-mediated endocytosis and the GALA peptide promoted endosomal destabilization and release of the genetic material into the cytoplasm [Park et al., 2010].

Modification of multifunctional envelope-type nano-devices (MENDs) with GALA peptide facilitating endosomal escape, leads to the enhanced transfection efficiency of pDNA and siRNA duplex *in vitro* and *in vivo*. To mimic envelope-type virus-like delivery systems, Sasaki *et al.* developed an artificial nanocarrier system termed as a MEND, which consists of a condensed DNA nanoparticle and lipid envelope which is further equipped with Tf, Cholesterol-GALA (Chol-GALA), or PEG-GALA to achieve target specificity and controlled intracellular trafficking, especially endosomal escape. As GALA can show fusogenic activity only at acidic pH, the direct fusion of MEND with the plasma membrane is feasible only after internalization. The Tf-MEND introduced with Chol-GALA or PEG-GALA showed a ten-fold higher transfection than that displayed by Tf-MEND. However, the simultaneous introduction of Chol-GALA and PEG-GALA enhanced the transfection efficiency more than 100-fold as compared to Tf-MEND mediated transfection. Chol-GALA and PEG-GALA operated synergistically to destabilize the envelope and endosomal membranes, respectively. Chol-GALA interacted with the envelope membrane whereas PEG-GALA penetrated into the endosomal membrane, which could destabilize the membranes and induce fusion [Sasaki et al., 2008].

A cationic counterpart of GALA is the peptide KALA which is formed by substitution of the alanine of GALA with lysine and a decrease in content of glutamic acid. KALA was the first designed peptide that could bind DNA, destabilize membranes, and mediate significant gene delivery. KALA undergoes a pH-dependent amphipathic α-helix to random coil conformational change, when the environmental pH decreased from 7.5 to 5.0. KALA can deliver both ODN and pDNA into cells [Park et al., 2010].

Several groups have focused their efforts on the development of synthetic, polymeric carriers that mimic the endosomolytic properties of fusogenic proteins and enhance the cytoplasmic delivery of therapeutic macromolecules. Recently, the ability of natural phospholipids to self-assemble into organized membrane-enclosed structures has been mimicked by amphiphilic co-polymers. The combination of a hydrophobic monomer and an ionizable co-monomer that has a more hydrophilic nature is one of the interesting strategies that have been adopted frequently for pH-responsive gene delivery. A change in pH and subsequent adjustment in the net charge causes the phase transformation depending on the hydrophobic and hydrophilic balance of the copolymer. These synthetic amphiphiles form assemblies that are remarkably similar to biological analogues, such as vesicles. Polymeric amphiphiles have much higher molecular weights than phospholipids and can self-assemble into more entangled membranes, imparting improved mechanical properties to the final structure [Park et al., 2010]. Polymer vesicles or polymersomes can combine several different polymeric compositions provided that they have the correct hydrophile/hydrophobe ratio. Particularly interesting for biomedical applications, are those copolymers that combine hydrophobic blocks with the non-antigenic properties of either PEG or biomimetic poly (2-(methacryloyloxy) ethyl phosphorylcholine) (PMPC). Indeed, the macromolecular nature of such polymersomes offers several advantages as compared to low-molecular-mass amphiphilic systems such as liposomes. PEG or PMPC polymersomes can be decorated by denser and higher molecular mass hydrophilic polymeric corona, with consequent longer circulation times than more traditional delivery systems such as stealth liposomes and other nanoparticles. Typical examples are the copolymers of methyl methacrylate (MMA) with methacrylic acid (MAc) or dimethylaminoethyl methacrylate (DMAEMA). The MMA is the hydrophobic section while MAc is the hydrophilic part of the chains. MAc is more hydrophilic at high pH when the carboxylic groups (COOH) are deprotonated, but becomes more hydrophobic when the carboxylic groups are protonated. The phase change occurs around the pKa value of the carboxylic groups, which is around 4.5-5.5. The copolymers of MMA with DMAEMA, which are hydrophilic at low pH, when the amino groups are protonated, but more hydrophobic when the amino groups are deprotonated. The key feature of these polymers is their ability to directly enhance the intracellular delivery of DNA, by destabilizing biological membranes in response to pH changes within the vesicular compartment [Park et al., 2010].

These copolymers are characterized by their unique ability to "sense" the changes in environment pH where they undergo a change from a hydrophilic, stealth-like conformation at physiologic pH to a hydrophobic and membrane-destabilizing one in response to acidic endosomal pH gradients [Lin et al., 2010]. Poly(ethylacrylic acid) (PEAA) is the first reported polymer to display a pH-dependent disruption of synthetic lipid vesicles at acidic pH= 6.3 or lower. The family of poly (alkyl acrylic acid) like poly (methyl acrylic acid) (PMAA), poly (ethyl acrylic acid) (PEAA), poly (propyl acrylic acid) (PPAA), and poly (butyl acrylic acid) (PBAA) were provided with pH-dependent, membrane destabilizing activities. These polymers are hydrophilic and stealth-like at physiological pH, but become membrane-destabilizing after uptake into the endosomal compartment where they enhance the release of therapeutic cargo into the cytoplasm [Lin et al., 2010].

Diblock copolymers PMPC-PDPA as biomimetic polymersomes were used for gene delivery made of pH-sensitive poly (2-(methacryloyloxy) ethyl-phosphorylcholine)-co-poly (2-(diisopropylamino) ethyl-methacrylate) (PMPC-PDPA) diblock copolymers. The high biocompatibility features are ascribed to PMPC residue whereas the PDPA block imparts pH responsiveness. These diblock copolymers exist as stable vesicles at physiological pH but these vesicles rapidly dissociate at around pH= 5-6 to form unimers. The phase transition of vesicles to unimers takes place because of protonation of the tertiary amine groups of PDPA chains, which transforms hydrophobic PDPA chains into a hydrophilic entity from physiological pH to mild acidic conditions. pH-responsive PMPC-PDPA vesicles release their contents upon exposure to the low pH (5.5) media in endosomes or lysosomes [Lomas et al., 2007].

Comb-like diblock copolymers with a robust membrane-destabilizing activity in response to a mildly acidic pH in the endosome were also developed. Acid-cleavable hydrazone linker has also been frequently utilized to achieve the facilitated release of nucleic acids from polyplexes. The first pH-sensitive block was the copolymer of ethyl acrylic acid (EAA) and hydrophobic methacrylate, and the second block was the copolymer of hexyl methacrylate (HMA) and trimethyl aminoethyl methacrylate (TMAEMA) grafted with N-acryloxy succinimide or β-benzyl L-aspartate N-carboxy-anhydride via acid-cleavable hydrazone linkages. These comb-like polymers exhibited a high concentration-dependent hemolytic activity in acidic solutions and degraded into smaller fragments via acid-hydrolysis of hydrazone linkages, resulting in minimized toxicity and facilitated elimination by renal excretion *in vivo*. These polymers formed siRNA complexing polyplexes that were stable even in the presence of serum and nucleases, and efficiently silenced GAPDH expression in MCF-7 breast cancer cells *in vitro* [Lin et al., 2010].

8.1.3. Low pH-sensitive siRNA/ODN–polymer conjugates

Small interfering RNA (siRNA)-based therapies have great potential for the treatment of diseases such as cancer, but an effective delivery strategy for siRNA is unclear. Benoit *et al.* developed a ternary pH responsive endosomolythic complex for the delivery of siRNA in order to sensitize drug-resistant ovarian cancer cells to doxorubicin. The electrostatic complexes were self-assembled by cationic micelles used as a nucleating core, siRNA and a pH-responsive endosomolytic polymer. Cationic micelles were formed from diblock copolymers of dimethylaminoethyl methacrylate (pDMAEMA) and butyl methacrylate (pDbB). The hydrophobic butyl core mediated micelle formation while the positively charged pDMAEMA corona enabled siRNA condensation. To enhance cytosolic delivery through endosomal release, a pH-responsive copolymer of poly (styrene-*alt*-maleic anhydride) (pSMA) was electrostatically complexed with the positively charged siRNA/micelle to form a ternary complex. Complexes exhibited size (30-105 nm) and charge (slightly positive) properties and mediated uptake in > 70% of ovarian cancer cells after 1 h of incubation [Benoit et al., 2010]. The optimized formulation of the resulting ternary nano-vector were used to deliver siRNA against polo-like kinase 1 (*plk1*), a gene up-regulated in many cancers and increased doxorubicin sensitivity in the drug-resistant ovarian cancer cells. Sensitization occurred through a p53 signaling pathway, as indicated by caspase 3/7 up-regulation following *plk1* knockdown and doxorubicin treatment, and this effect could be abrogated using a p53 inhibitor. To demonstrate the potential for dual delivery from this polymer system, micelle cores were subsequently loaded with doxorubicin and utilized in ternary complexes to achieve cell sensitization through simultaneous siRNA and drug delivery from a single carrier. These results show that knockdown of *plk1* results in sensitization of multi-drug resistant cells to doxorubicin, and this combination of gene silencing and small molecule drug delivery may prove useful to achieve potent therapeutic effects [Benoit et al., 2010].

Acid-degradable and targetable polyion complex (PIC) micelles increased the gene silencing in hepatoma cells. This multi-functional carrier was synthesized by assembling lactosylated-PEG-siRNA conjugates via acid-labile β-thiopropionate linkages into PIC micelles through the mixing with poly (L-lysine). The lactosylated-PEG-siRNA/PLL polyplexes were successfully transported into hepatoma cells in a receptor-mediated manner, releasing hundreds of active siRNA molecules into the cellular interior responding to the pH decrease in the endosomal compartment. This carrier exhibited almost 100 times enhancement in gene silencing activity and facilitating the practical utility of siRNA therapeutics [Oishi et al., 2005].

8.2. Redox-responsive nanocarriers

One of the several micro-environmental features, which have been widely exploited for improving the efficiency of nucleic acid delivery, is the redox potential gradient existing between extracellular environment and various subcellular organelles in normal as well as pathological states. The existence of a high redox potential gradient between oxidizing extracellular space and the reducing environment of subcellular organelles has been exploited mainly by incorporating a disulfide bond(s) into the structure of the delivery vectors to provide them with a capability to release the therapeutic nucleotides selectively in the subcellular reducing space. The original interest in gene delivery systems controlled by redox potential gradients was guided by the need to transiently enhance stability of the vectors during the delivery [Cheng et al., 2011; Meng et al., 2009].

The design of reduction-sensitive polymers and conjugates usually involves incorporation of disulfide linkage(s) in the main chain, at the side chain or the cross-linker in the structure of the polymers of either linear or branched structure. There are only a few examples of polyplexes where the disulfide bonds are associated with the nucleic acids [Soundara Manickam and Oupický, 2006]. Reduction-sensitive polymers and conjugates are characterized by an excellent stability in the circulation and in extracellular fluids, whereas they are prone to rapid degradation under a reductive environment present in intracellular compartments such as the cytoplasm and the cell nucleus at a time scale from minutes to hours, through thiol-disulfide exchange reactions. This quick-response chemical degradation behavior is distinct from common hydrolytically degradable polymers such as aliphatic polyesters and polycarbonates in which the ester and carbonate bonds usually exhibit gradual degradation kinetics inside body with degradation times ranging from days to weeks/or to months. This remarkable feature renders them extremely for the controlled cytoplasmic delivery of a variety of bioactive molecules including DNA, siRNA, antisense oligonucleotide (ODN), proteins, drugs, etc [Du et al., 2010].

Disulfide bonds present in the structure of polyplexes are readily reduced in the reducing intracellular environment, while largely preserved in the predominantly oxidizing extracellular space. The intracellular reduction of disulfide bonds is most likely mediated by small redox molecules like glutathione (GSH) and thioredoxin, either alone or with the help of redox enzymes. Glutathione tripeptide (g-glutamyl-cysteinyl-glycine; GSH) is the most abundant intracellular sulfhydryl present in millimolar concentrations inside the cell but only in micromolar concentrations in the blood plasma and GSH/glutathione disulfide (GSSG) is the major redox couple in animal cells [Meng et al., 2009]. Glutathione has multiple direct and indirect functions in many critical cellular processes like synthesis of proteins and DNA, amino acid transport, enzyme activity, metabolism and protection of cells. Glutathione also serves as a reductant by functioning to destroy the free radicals, hydrogen peroxide and other peroxides. It also functions as a storage form of cysteine. The intracellular glutathione concentration is an additive function of both the oxidized (GSSG) and the reduced forms (GSH) of glutathione. The glutathione redox ratio is maintained and determined by the activity of glutathione reductase, NADPH concentrations and transaldolase activity. The redox state of the GSH/GSSG couple is often used as an indicator of the overall redox environment of the cell. The large difference in reducing potential between the intracellular and extracellular milieu may be exploited for triggered intracellular delivery of a variety of bioactive molecules including DNA, siRNA, antisense oligonucleotide (ODN), proteins and low molecular weight drugs. Furthermore, of particular interest is that tumor tissues are highly reducing and hypoxic compared with normal tissues, with at least 4-fold higher concentrations of GSH in the tumor tissues over normal tissues, rendering the reducible bioconjugates valuable for tumor-specific drug and gene delivery [Meng et al., 2009]. Some examples are mentioned for the use of redox responsive nanocarrier in below:

8.2.1. The use of responsive sensitive nanocarrier for the stabilization of the carrier and decrease the cytotoxicity

A prerequisite for every systemic nucleic-acid delivery system is stability in the blood stream prior to reaching its target cell. Therefore, the carrier must prevent the premature release of its load. In order to enhance the stability of the delivery system, either the surface of the carriers was crosslinked, or the low-molecular-weight materials were sulfhydryl polymerized. Peptides containing many lysines and histidines were used for the complexation of nucleic acids, while cysteines were introduced to obtain stable and reductively degradable carriers. A series of different vehicles was built from sequences of many lysines, tryptophan, and a variable number of cysteines. All peptides obtained were able to condense DNA into particles, and exhibited increased stability after disulfide formation. The disulfide crosslinked carriers conveyed 5- to 60-fold higher gene expression as compared to their non-crosslinked analogs. The degree of gene expression was dependent on the number of incorporated cysteines, with a maximum for terminally inserted cysteines. The modification of the e-amino groups of pLL with 3-(2-aminoethyldithio) propionyl residues or their crosslinking with Dimethyl 3,3-dithiobispropionimidate (DTBP) comprises another approach utilizing reductively degradable gene carriers. These molecules were able to complex nucleotides into particles that were stable under physiological conditions but disintegrated upon treatment with GSH [Meng et al., 2009].

Read *et al.* prepared gene delivery vectors based on reducible polycations (RPCs) by oxidative polycondensation of the peptide Cys-Lys10-Cys and used to condense nucleic acids. The release of nucleic acids in these vectors relied on cleavage of the RPC in the reduced intracellular environment, eliminating the toxicity associated with high molecular weight polymers. However these polymers rely on chloroquine or cationic lipids to enhance endosomal escape and mediate transfection [Read et al., 2003].

Low molecular weight DNA condensing polypeptides were developed by substituting one to four lysine residues of Cys-Trp-Lys18 (CWK18) with cysteine groups. These polypeptides could spontaneously oxidize to form interpeptide disulfide crosslinks after binding to plasmid DNA, resulting in small stabilized DNA condensates. These reversibly cross-linked polypeptide DNA condensates were 5-60-fold more potent at mediating gene expression in HepG2 and COS-7 cells as compared to the un-crosslinked alkylated CWK18 (AlkCWK18) DNA condensates [Fig. 2 A; McKenzie et al., 2000]. In another study, in order to improve the endosomolytic properties, Histidine containing reducible polycations based on CH6K3H6C monomers (His6 RPCs) was developed, which are highly effective DNA transfection agents, provided sufficient buffering capacity and enhanced *in vitro* gene expression with rapid unpackaging following reduction in the cytoplasm without aid of chloroquine, an agent that promotes endosomal escape [Stevenson et al., 2008].

High molecular weight polypeptides containing disulfide bonds in the backbone were synthesized by an oxidative copolymerization of a histidine-rich peptide (HRP) and a nuclear localization sequence (NLS) peptide derived from the importin α-binding SV40 T antigen sequence. The synthetic approach allowed an easy synthesis of reducible copolypeptides (rCPP) with different relative contents of the HRP and NLS sequences. The rCPPs were synthesized by DMSO-mediated oxidative polycondensation. To combine two functional peptides into a single polymeric carrier, multiblock reducible copolypeptides were synthesized by randomly connecting HRP and NLS peptides via disulfide bonds into a linear polypeptide chain. Mild oxidation of the terminal Cys residues with DMSO was used. The copolypeptides show minimal cytotoxicity and transfection activity comparable to or better than control PEI polyplexes [Manickam and Oupický, 2006].

Other carriers, such as chitosan (deacetylated chitin) were also stabilized via disulfide bonds. For this purpose, the primary amino groups of low-molecular-weight chitosan were thiolated with 2-iminothiolane. These modified polymers, such as chitosanthiobutylamidines, were mixed with pDNA to form coacervates in the nanometer range [Bauhuber et al., 2009]. In a recent study, Ho *et al.* modified chitosan (CS) with extending arms consisting of disulfide spacers and arginine (Arg) residues (CS–SS–Arg) as a novel non-viral carrier for gene delivery. Cleavage of disulfide spacers by glutathione (GSH) and dithiothreitol due to thiol-disulfide exchange reactions indicates that CS–SS–Arg is likely reducible in cytoplasm. The CS–SS–Arg was allowed to condense GFP DNA to form self-organized nanoparticles with a diameter of 130 nm and zeta potential of 35 mV. The DNA was released from CS–SS–Arg/ DNA nanoparticles over time in the presence of GSH and the results suggest that the Arg-rich bioreducible CS–SS–Arg/ DNA nanoparticles are promising as a carrier for gene delivery [Ho et al., 2011].

A dilemma in non-viral nucleic acid delivery is demonstrated by considering the polymeric transfection agent PEI, which is often referred to as the gold standard for polymer-based gene carriers due to the relatively high transfection efficacy of its polyplexes. Unfortunately, efficacy and adverse reactions seem to be strongly associated with the use of PEI. A popular strategy to reduce the toxicity of polyplexes is to use low MW polycations or cationic monomers that are less cytolytic, and crosslink them with agents that can be cleaved or activated by the intracellular environment. Numerous reports describe the synthesis of carrier systems containing disulfide bonds that allow for a compaction and protection of the nucleic acid in the extracellular environment accompanied by reduced toxicity due to intracellular polymer degradation. Peng *et al.* prepared thiolated PEI (800 Da) to further oxidize into disulfide cross-linked PEI (PEI-SS), with average molecular weights of 7.1, 8.0 and 8.4 kDa depending on the degree of thiolation. Those PEI-SS had lower cytotoxicities and higher transgene expressions compared with that of the 25-kDa branched PEI (bPEI) [Peng et al., 2008].

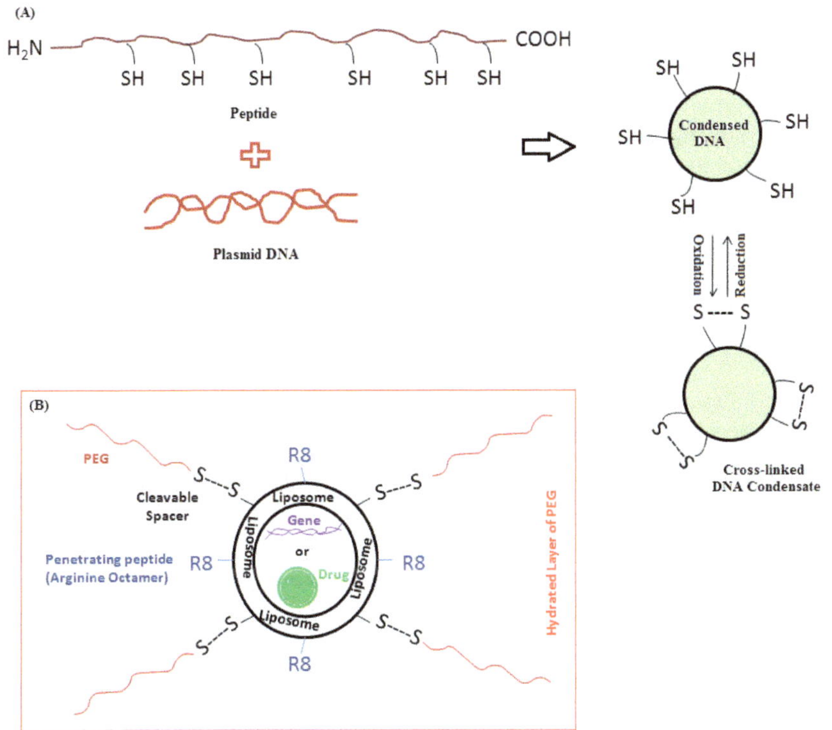

Figure 2. A) Cross-linked peptide-DNA condensates: Formation of peptide-DNA condensates through ionic binding of the peptide to the pDNA followed by interpeptide oxidation; Stabilization of the DNA condensates by reversible disulfide bonds. B) **A novel stimuli-sensitive liposome**: This carrier composes of cationic peptides (e.g., Arginine octamer) and detachable coat (e.g., PEG) for the intracellular gene or drug delivery

Kang *et al.* synthesized reducible polycations (RPC) that degrade due to changes in the intracellular reduction potential from low molecular weight (MW) bPEI 0.8 kDa via thiolation and oxidation. In this study, 2-iminothiolane was used to create thiol groups from primary amines. In this approach, a primary amine reacts with 2-iminothiolane to yield a thiol group and an amidine moiety. A procedure based on the use of 2-iminothiolane was employed in order to avoid problems associated with the use of DTBP. As a result, unlike other thiolation methods, by converting primary amines to amidine groups, the number of positive charges in the final product at a neutral pH was preserved. Moreover, the newly generated amidines contribute to the electrostatic condensation of nucleic acids. The cytotoxicity of RPC-bPEI 0.8 kDa was 8-19 times less than that of the gold standard of polymeric transfection reagents, bPEI 25 kDa. In general, the toxicity of High MW (HMW) PEI is greater than that of Low MW (LMW) PEI because HMW PEI interacts more effectively with components that are essential for cell survival such as intracellular membranes, vital proteins, and nucleic acids than its LMW counterpart. Thus, the reduced cytotoxicity of HMWRPC-bPEI 0.8 kDa may be due to the degradation of the polymer in the intracellular environment after cellular uptake [Kang et al., 2011].

In another study, Son *et al* developed a multi-functional gene carrier based on thiolated low molecular weight bPEI with functional moieties for cytoplasm-sensitive reduction, tumor targeting, and prolonged circulation in blood. The bPEI was modified with α-maleimide-ω-N-hydroxysuccinimide ester polyethylene glycol (MAL-PEG-NHS, MW: 5000) and cyclic NGR peptide for enhanced blood compatibility and tumor targeting ability. The resulting polymer (bPEI-SS-PEG-cNGR) exhibited DNA condensing capacity, a reducing property, and improved tumor targeting, suggesting that the multifunctional polymer constitutes a promising non-viral vector for cytoplasm- and tumor-specificities [Son et al., 2010].

8.2.2. Disulfides for the attachment of a shielding moiety

DOPE and N-[2-methoxypoly (ethylene glycol)-α-aminocarbonylethyl-dithiopropionate] formed a liposome that was covalently coupled to distearoylphosphatidylethanolamine (mPEG-SS-DSPE). The incorporation of the mPEG-SS-DSPE stabilized these liposomes at low pH, but the stabilizing effect was quickly reversed when the carrier was incubated with either DTT or cell-free extracts. Under these conditions, the disulfides were reduced, and thus the protecting PEG chains were cleaved, and the vehicle became degradable at low pH, releasing its load. Disulfides were used for the formation of copolymers consisting of bPEI 25 kDa and PEG of 20 or 30 kDa. The connection of PEG via DSPE led to a 125% increase in blood levels and decreased hemolysis compared to bPEI 25 kDa [Bauhuber et al., 2009].

Polyion complex (PIC) micelles are self-assembling particles with a core-shell structure formed by complexation between a pair of oppositely charged polymers having hydrophilic PEG segments. They can be utilized as gene delivery vectors with high water-solubility and colloidal stability, employing negatively charged genetic materials and cationic polymers. One approach to enhance the stability of PIC micelles is glutathione (GSH)-sensitive stabilization of PIC micelles with the core cross-linked through disulfide bonds, composed of antisense oligonucleotide and thiolated PEG-PLL block copolymer. The micelles showed sufficient colloidal stability due to the PEG shell and core cross-linking. Moreover, ODN entrapped in the micelles also displayed highly increased stability against nuclease, compared to that in the micelles without cross-linking. Release of ODN from the dissociated micelles at intracellular GSH concentration suggested the potential for intracellular ODN delivery. It is reported that PEG-peptide (PEG-SS-Cys-Trp-Lys(18): PEG-SS-CWK18) having disulfide cross-linker displayed much enhanced gene transfer efficiency compared to PEG-peptide having non-reducible cross-linker (PEG-VS-CWK18) when complexed with plasmid DNA [Kim and Kim, 2011].

8.2.3. Disulfides for the attachment of a targeting moiety

For a successful accumulation of the nucleic acid in the target cell, the delivery system requires the attachment of a specific "recognition element". However, since many targeting moieties are rather large, they hinder effective unpacking of the gene vector. Thus, inside cells, it is very important to remove them to facilitate the disassembly of the load. Here, disulfides can be quite useful, as they can be cleaved at the cell surface during cellular entry or in the cytosol [Bauhuber et al., 2009]. The frequency of sulfhydryl occurrence in Antibodies/proteins or other molecules is usually low as compared to other groups like amines or carboxylates. The use of sulfhydryl reactive chemistries thus can restrict modification to only a limited number of sites within a target molecule. N-Succinimidyl 3-(2-pyridyldithio) propionate (SPDP) is one of the most popular heterobi-functional cross-linking agents. The NHS ester end of SPDP reacts with amine groups to form an amide linkage, while the 2-pyridyldithiol group at the other end can react with sulfhydryl residues to form a disulfide linkage. The reagent is also useful in creating sulfhydryls in proteins and other molecules. Once modified with SPDP, a protein can be treated with DTT (or other disulfide reducing agents, to release the pyridine-2-thione leaving group and form the free sulfhydryl [Manjappa et al., 2011].

Iminothiolane (Traut's reagent) can react with primary amines in a ring-opening reaction that regenerates the free sulfhydryl. An example is the thiolation of antibody using Traut's reagent in the preparation of immunoliposomes. It is an excellent thiolation reagent for use in the preparation of immunotoxins. It has also been used to modify and introduce sulfhydryls into oligosaccharides from asparagines linked glycans [Manjappa et al., 2011].

8.2.4. Disulfide bonds to enhance the intracellular release of the nucleic acid

SiRNA has generated great interest as a research tool and a therapeutic agent because of its ability to efficiently silence specific genes by the mechanism of RNA interference [Vidugirienė et al., 2007]. However, siRNA cannot penetrate the cellular membrane alone and can be easily degraded by RNase; therefore, effective siRNA carriers are needed for siRNA-based therapies. In this regard, poly ion complexes (PICs) formed from nucleic acids and oppositely charged polycations have been widely studied as a promising nucleic acids carrier because of the variety of chemical designs of polycations. PICs protect nucleic acids from enzymatic degradation and show facilitated cellular uptake. Thus, PICs have demonstrated to be useful for plasmid DNA (pDNA) delivery *in vitro* and *in vivo*.

Nevertheless, there has been limited success to date in the development of PICs for siRNA delivery. In general, PICs from monomeric siRNA, which has a short structure compared to pDNA, lack stability under the physiological condition; therefore, substantial stabilization of PICs is essential to successful siRNA delivery. Meanwhile, after PICs internalize and reach the cytoplasm, they are required to efficiently release siRNA to exert its gene silencing effect. To complete such variable properties, considerable efforts have been dedicated to the design and chemical modification of polycations [Yu-Lin et al., 2011]. Takemoto *et al.* reported a new class of chemically modified siRNA, i.e., siRNA-grafted poly (aspartic acid) [PAsp (-SS-siRNA)], for PIC based siRNA delivery. PAsp (-SS-siRNA) consists of a backbone of a poly (aspartic acid) [PAsp] derivative and grafted siRNAs via a disulfide linkage. The siRNA-grafted polymer formed stable PICs due to its larger numbers and higher density of anionic charges compared with monomeric siRNA, leading to effective internalization by cultured cells. Following the endosomal escape of the PIC, the disulfide linkage of the siRNA-grafted polymer allowed efficient siRNA release from the PIC under intracellular reductive conditions. Consequently, the PIC from the siRNA-grafted polymer showed a potent gene silencing effect without cytotoxicity or immunogenicity, demonstrating a promising feature of the siRNA-grafted polymer to construct the PIC-based nanocarrier for *in vivo* siRNA delivery [Takemoto et al., 2010].

The conjugation of nucleic acids including siRNA and antisense oligodeoxynucleotide to polymer such as PEG and hyaluronic acid through a disulfide bond represents a approach to construct GSH-responsive gene delivery systems [Cheng et al., 2011]. Lee *et al.* explored the potential possibility of hyaluronic acid (HA) as a biocompatible, biodegradable, and non-cytotoxic material for delivery of siRNA. Nano-sized HA hydrogels, called HA nanogels, were prepared for target-specific intracellular delivery of siRNA to HA receptor over-expressing cancer cells. HA nanogels crosslinked with disulfide linkages were prepared by an inverse emulsion method. An aqueous phase containing thiol functionalized HA and siRNA was emulsified in an oil phase under ultrasonication, thus generating self cross-linked HA nanogels encapsulating anti-green fluorescent protein (GFP) siRNA. Release profiles of siRNA from HA nanogels were studied in response to various reductive conditions that could cleave the disulfide linkages of HA nanogels to varying extents. The HA/siRNA nanogels were readily taken up by HA receptor positive cells (HCT-116 cells) having HA-specific CD44 receptors on the surface [Lee et al., 2007]. Kam *et al.* conjugated various biological molecules, including oligonucleotides and siRNA, to phospholipid–PEG functionalized single-walled carbon nanotube (SWNT) via cleavable disulfide linkage. Due to the presence of a PEG linker, these SWNT conjugates form highly stable suspensions in aqueous solutions including physiological buffers. The SWNT carriers mediated efficient delivery and release of DNA and siRNA inside cells. Gene silencing experiments using HeLa cells displayed a two-fold higher silencing efficiency compared to lipofectamine at the same siRNA concentration. This is ascribed to a high surface area of SWNT for efficient siRNA cargo loading, high intracellular transporting ability of SWNT, and high degree of endosome/lysosome escape owing to the disulfide approach [Kam et al., 2005; Meng et al., 2009].

9. Stimuli-sensitive multi-functional nano-particulate nucleic acid delivery systems

As mentioned in the previous sections, there are some conflicting demands for overcoming different extra- and intracellular barriers met by nucleic acid-loaded nano-particles during delivery. The delivery systems, which response to only one stimulus and have less functionality, may not be efficient enough to achieve a satisfactory therapeutic effect *in vivo*. Natural gene carriers, such as viruses, have developed sophisticated mechanisms and modular biopolymer designs to overcome these barriers. The development of virus-mimicking, multi-functional gene delivery systems with features that mimic virus modular components and which transfect specific cell lines with high efficacy is considered to be a practical strategy in the future, in particular for intravenous administration. Ideal polymer-based, nucleic acid-loaded nanoparticles for potential *in vivo* applications should have several components that function at the appropriate stages during the delivery. The hierarchical nature of the synthetic carriers allows the incorporation of membrane-disrupting peptides, nucleic acid binding components, a protective coat layer, and an outer targeting ligand all in a single nanoparticle, but with functionality such that each is utilized in a specific sequence during the gene delivery process [Du et al., 2010].

The ligands on the particle surface can be used to recognize a specific cell/tissue, and facilitate cellular uptake through receptor-mediated endocytosis. A reversibly removable hydrophilic pole, such as PEG chains, provides stealth protection of the nanoparticles during their circulation in the blood as well as travelling through the ECM, and may reduce toxicity. Moieties that are responsive to different stimulus must be combined to result in an appropriate set of various trigger mechanisms at different time points. Such moieties might be cleaved in acidic environments, show good buffering capacity, be redox active or enzymatically cleavable, the pole can be removed, which might enhance the cellular uptake and/or endosomal escape. In the inner part of the nanoparticles, nucleic acids can be temporally loaded through electrostatic interaction, covalent conjugation, or physical encapsulation, which will protect the nucleic acid against enzymatic degradation. The inner part should be stable enough until delivery to the correct site (cytoplasm and/or nucleus) where it is disassembled to release the naked nucleic acid upon some kind of stimulus. In addition, it is preferred that the inner part contains endosomolytic components that help the endosomal escape. If cell penetrating peptide (CPP) is incorporated onto the surface of the inner part, cellular uptake may be further improved [Du et al., 2010]. Many experimental results emphasize that the main obstruction of CPPs is the absence of specific cellular delivery [Vivès et al., 2008]. Ideally, the design of a smart delivery system should be built in such a way that during the first phase of delivery, a non-specific cell-penetrating function is shielded by the function of cell-recognition motif which favors the concentration of the drug at the targeted cell type. Upon accumulating in the target, protecting polymer (or specific ligand) attached to the surface of the smart nanocarrier via the stimuli-sensitive bond should detach under the action of local conditions and expose the previously hidden second function (CPP) allowing for the subsequent delivery of the carrier and its cargo inside cells [Torchilin, 2008]. Such engineering of smart nanodevices has been illustrated in the work by Sawant *et al*. who developed targeted long-circulating PEGylated liposomes and PEG-phosphatidylethanolamine (PEG-PE)-based micelles possessing several functionalities. Such systems were capable of targeting a specific cell or organ by attaching the monoclonal antibody to their surface via long PEG spacer groups. Second, these liposomes and micelles were additionally modified with TATp moieties attached to the surface of the nanocarrier by using TATp-short PEG-PE derivatives. PEG-PE used for liposome surface modification or for micelle preparation was made degradable by inserting the pH-sensitive hydrazone bond between PEG and PE (PEG-Hz-PE). Under normal pH values, TATp functions on the surface of nanocarriers were "shielded" by long protecting PEG chains (pH-degradable PEG 2000-PE or PEG 5000-PE) or by long para- nitrophenyl PEG-PE (pNP-PEG-PE) moieties used to attach antibodies to the nanocarrier (non-pH degradable PEG3400-PE or PEG5000-PE). Following prolonged circulation and uptake into the tumor mass mediated by both the enhanced permeability and retention (EPR) effect and the active targeting agent on the surface of the carrier, the pH responsive bonds are cleaved in the acidic environment of the tumor, thereby releasing the high molecular weight PEG strands from the carrier and exposing the Tat-peptide for enhanced intracellular uptake and intracellular target localization, specifically located to the target tumor cells [Sawant et al., 2006; Torchilin, 2008].

Another example of a triggerable system was created by the synthesis of a liposomal carrier that was comprised of a membrane-permeable ligand and a reductively detachable PEG coating. The surface cover consisted of PEG coupled to DOPE via a thiolytically cleavable linker, while the ligand, an ariginine octamer, was immobilized onto cholesteryl hemisuccinate (CHEMS). These conjugates were mixed with dipalmitoylphosphatidylcholin (DPPC) and unmodified DOPE to form liposomes. DOPE/mPEG–DTP–DSPE liposomes were stable in plasma whereas in the presence of a reducing agent the PEG coating was effectively detached off the liposomal surface, leading to vesicle destabilization and fusion as well as complete release of the entrapped contents. Upon activation of the trigger, the arginine octamer would be exposed, causing cellular uptake of the liposome. Once in the cytosol, the remaining disulfide bonds would be cleaved, ultimately resulting in the destabilization the whole carrier [Fig. 2B; Bauhuber et al., 2009].

10. Nanoparticles mediated brain delivery systems

Nanoparticles have emerged as potential drug delivery carriers to tissues throughout the body. Yet passing the BBB is particularly difficult. The proper design of such engineered 'nanocarriers' becomes very important in transversing the impermeable membranes to facilitate drug delivery. At the same time, it is also required to retain the drug stability and ensure that early degradation of drugs from the nanocarriers does not take place. Therefore, for drugs to be successfully delivered to their target, many factors such as its size, biocompatibility, target specific affinity, avoidance of reticuloendothelial systems, stability in blood, or ability to facilitate controlled drug release need to be considered during manufacture of the NPs. As for nanocarriers to serve as good candidates for drug delivery across the BBB can be summarized as following [Bhaskar et al., 2010]: a) Particle diameter less than 100 nanometers; b) Non-toxic, biodegradable and biocompatible; c) Stable in blood (i.e., no opsonisation by proteins); d) BBB-targeted (i.e., use of cell surface, ligands, and receptor mediated endocytosis); e) No activation of neutrophils, non-inflammatory; f) No platelet aggregation; h) Avoidance of the reticuloendothelial systems; i) Prolonged circulation time; j) Scalable and cost effective with regard to manufacturing process; m) Agreeable to small molecules, peptides, proteins or nucleic acids; n) Controlled drug release or modulation of drug release profiles [Bhaskar et al., 2010].

One of the most important challenges in nano-based diagnostics and drug delivery is the functionalization of nanoparticles. At first, the combination of effective conjugation strategies is needed to develop, in a highly controlled way, specific biomolecules to the surface of nanoparticles. Some of the most prominent candidate biomolecules are cell penetrating peptides such as SynB vectors, penetratin and Tat that facilitate enhanced intracellular delivery, fluorescent dyes (rhodamine, alexa, Cy5.5), tumoral markers for brain and gene therapeutic agents for genetic therapy such as siRNA [Bhaskar et al., 2010].

Functionalization itself requires a profound knowledge of the target organ and its transport mechanisms. The BBB has several transport molecules that can potentially increase the efficiency and kinetics of nanocarriers towards brains such as, growth factors (e.g. epidermal growth factor, vascular endothelial growth factor, basic fibroblast growth factor, insulin-like growth factors (IGF-I and -II), biotin binding proteins (avidin, streptavidin, or neutravidin), insulin, albumin, leptin, lactoferrin, iron binding protein p97 (melanotransferrin), transferrin and Angiopep-2. Some agents play a pivotal role in enhancing the permeability of nanoprobes through BBB. Moreover, by altering the surface of polymeric nanoparticles on coating them with different hydrophilic surfactants, such as polysorbate 80 (Tween® 80) or other polysorbates with 20 polyoxyethylene units, biocompatible coatings of non-viral gene delivery systems, e.g. by PEG attachment for siRNA delivery show significant advantage in brain targeting [Bhaskar et al., 2010].

11. Cell penetrating peptides as efficient delivery systems

Generally, the nucleic acid delivery techniques comprise various physical and chemical methods, viral and non-viral vector systems, and uptake of naked nucleic acids [Veldhoen et al., 2008; Bolhassani et al., 2011]. All of them have certain advantages and dis-advantages and might only be appropriate if particular requirements are performed. For instance, physical and chemical methods like microinjection, electroporation or particle bombardment as well as calcium phosphate co-precipitation are highly efficient but rather harmful for the target cells and lack the potential to be applicable *in vivo*. There is general agreement that viral vector systems are the most efficient vehicles to deliver nucleic acids into cells [Veldhoen et al., 2008]. However, despite substantial efforts over the last 15 years, up to now research has failed to develop suitable and especially safe viral systems. As a result of the difficulties encountered with these viral vectors (e.g., mutagenesis and immune responses), much attention was paid to the development of safer non-viral delivery systems. Currently, liposomes and cationic polymers are used as a standard tool to transfect cells *in vitro*. These approaches are yet characterized by a significant lack of efficiency accompanied by a high level of toxicity making them mostly inadequate for *in vivo* applications [Veldhoen et al., 2008; Bolhassani et al., 2011].

Peptides acting as shuttles for a controlled cellular delivery of nucleic acids represent a new concept to bypass the problem of poor bio-availability and clinical efficacy of such macromolecules [Veldhoen et al., 2008]. The idea of using peptides as carriers goes back some 20 years when two groups discovered by chance that the HIV-1 transactivating protein Tat is taken up by mammalian cells [Frankel and Pabo, 1998; Green and Loewenstein, 1988]. Just a few years later, the Antennapedia homeodomain of *Drosophila melanogaster* was shown to act similarly [Joliot et al., 1991]. Then, it could be shown that peptides derived from Tat and Antennapedia as well as other proteins are capable of transporting macromolecular cargo molecules into cells [Fawell et al., 1994; Schwarze et al., 1999]. Based on such promising results, a rapidly expanding field focusing on the so-called cell-penetrating peptides (CPPs), also referred to as protein transduction domains (PTD) began to develop [Veldhoen et al., 2008].

Up to now numerous CPPs have been described. According to their origin, they can be grouped into three classes. The first group contains CPPs originating from naturally occurring proteins "protein derived CPPs", the second consists of chimeric CPPs composed of different protein domains and the third class includes so-called "model CPPs" which were developed according to structure-fuction relationships without any homology to natural sequences. All known CPPs are basic amino acids causing a net positive charge at physiological pH [Langel, 2002].

At present, a peptide is considered a CPP, if it shows the ability to cross a biological membrane. A cargo can be bound to the CPP covalently or non-covalently. Covalent attachment can be achieved either by expression as a fusion construct or by chemical coupling [Zatsepin et al., 2005]. In some cases, cargo and carrier bind each other non-covalently through ionic interactions. Depending on the nature of both binding partners assembly of nanoparticles may occur [Veldhoen et al., 2008].

The studies have shown that the cargo-CPP complexes are taken up by directly penetrating the cell membrane or by an endocytotic pathway. However, the precise mechanism of internalization remains elusive and strongly depends on the properties of both CPP and cargo as well as the transfection conditions and the cell lines used [Maiolo et al., 2005; De Coupade et al., 2005; El-Andaloussi et al., 2007; Bolhassani, 2011]. Recent studies indicate that the uptake mechanism of CPPs can be influenced by the attachment of cargo. For example, Richard *et al.* [Richard et al., 2003; Richard et al., 2005] reported a co-localization of Tat $^{48\text{-}59}$ with markers of clathrin-mediated endocytosis, whereas Fittipaldi *et al.* [Fittipaldi et al., 2003] found a caveolae/ lipid raft-dependent process for a Tat-GFP fusion protein and Wadia *et al.* [Wadia et al., 2004] described a macropinocytotic uptake pathway for a fusion construct of Tat peptide with Cre recombinase.

However, further information about the exact mechanism of uptake of such delivery systems is expected in the near future. Furthermore, it has been shown that even minor changes of the physical state of a CPP (e.g., exchange of certain amino acids) can alter translocation properties significantly. This particularly holds true for the attachment of large cargo molecules [Veldhoen et al., 2008]. Thus, it might not be possible to generalize results obtained with a CPP, and it might be necessary to characterize each carrier/cargo complex individually. If CPPs are proposed to be used for therapeutic purposes in the future, it is essential to focus on the attachment of functional cargos and analyze their biological effects inside the cell. Data from our lab clearly show that uptake and biological activity of a functional cargo is everything but the same. Therefore, a quantitative comparison of cargo taken up and functionally active cargo is an essential requirement in order to improve therapeutic efficacy. Indeed, only looking for efficient internalization is not sufficient [Veldhoen et al., 2008].

The successful clinical application of nucleic acid-based therapeutic strategies has been limited by the poor delivery efficiency achieved by existing vectors. The development of alternative delivery systems for improved biological activity is, therefore, obligatory. Since two decades ago that the Tat protein, and derived peptides, can translocate across biological membranes, cell-penetrating peptides have been considered one of the most promising tools to improve non-invasive cellular delivery of therapeutic molecules. Despite extensive research on the use of CPPs for this purpose, the exact mechanisms underlying their cellular uptake and that of peptide conjugates remain controversial [Trabulo et al., 2010].

There are many examples of CPP-mediated delivery of plasmid DNA into cultured cells and also *in vivo* involving the use of a non-covalent approach [Bolhassani, 2011]. While some approaches involve single component peptide vectors, the major focus has been on the association of CPPs with other non-viral gene delivery methods, such as liposomes, polyethyleneimine (PEI) or nanoparticles. In 1999, Morris and coworkers demonstrated that MPG could be used as a powerful tool for the delivery of nucleic acids. It was shown that MPG is not cytotoxic, insensitive to serum and able to efficiently deliver plasmid DNA into several different cell lines [Morris et al., 1999]. Further studies demonstrated that cell entry of the MPG/DNA particles is independent of the endosomal pathway and that the NLS of MPG is involved in both electrostatic interactions with DNA and nuclear targeting. Furthermore, it was shown that a mutation affecting the NLS of MPG prevents nuclear delivery of DNA. In an alternative study, Rittner *et al.* described the novel basic amphiphilic peptides, ppTG1 and ppTG20 (20 amino acids), and evaluated their efficiencies *in vitro* and *in vivo* as single-component gene transfer vectors. It was demonstrated that both the ppTG1 and ppTG20 peptides are able to bind nucleic acids and destabilize membranes, in a liposome leakage assay. Complexes of plasmid DNA with ppTG1 originated high levels of gene expression in cell culture experiments and, most importantly, complexes of plasmid DNA with ppTG1 or ppTG20 led to significant gene expression *in vivo* [Rittner et al., 2002]. Peptide modification has also been explored as a means to enhance gene delivery. In particular, stearic acid modification of different membrane-permeable arginine-rich peptides, such as HIV-1 Tat (48-60), HIV-1 Rev (34-50), flock house virus (FHV) coat (35-49), (RxR)4 and oligoarginines of 4-16 residues was shown to substantially increase their transfection efficiency. The mechanisms by which stearic acid modification improves plasmid DNA delivery by CPPs have been shown to involve increased efficiency of endosomal escape or enhanced cellular association, as well as higher nuclear delivery. The extensively studied Tat peptide has also been exploited for plasmid DNA delivery by different research groups, with paradoxical results [Trabulo et al., 2010, Bolhassani, 2011]. A study by Ignatovich *et al.*, demonstrated that Tat peptide is able to form complexes with plasmid DNA, which could be used for gene delivery into mammalian cells. Despite reasonably high transfection efficiency *in vitro*, low gene expression levels were detected in the liver of mice injected intravenously with DNA-Tat complexes, a fact that was attributed to inactivation of the complexes in the bloodstream due to interactions with serum albumin. Interestingly, an endocytosis-dependent mechanism was proposed for the uptake of the DNA-Tat complexes, similar to what was proposed for internalization of complexes of plasmid DNA with other polycationic carriers. A different study, by Tung *et al.*, compared the efficiency of a series of Tat peptides, containing 1–8 Tat moieties. Although, all compounds complexed with plasmid DNA, it was demonstrated that at least eight Tat peptide moieties are required in order to achieve efficient gene delivery. Sandgren *et al.* also studied the cellular uptake of complexes of plasmid DNA and the HIV-Tat derived peptide. According to this study, the Tat peptide stimulated cellular uptake of DNA in a time-, concentration- and temperature-dependent manner, while accumulating in large, acidic, cytoplasmic vesicles, followed by transfer of the cargo into the nuclear compartment and subsequent disappearance from the endolysosomal vesicles. Aiming at increasing the efficiency of the Tat peptide to deliver plasmid DNA, Lo *et al.* made several modifications to the Tat peptide, through the use of histidine and cysteine residues to enhance endosomal escape and complex stability [Trabulo et al., 2010]. Up to 7,000-fold improvement in gene transfection efficiency was observed for the Tat peptide covalently fused with 10 histidine residues (Tat-10H) over the original Tat peptide, and incorporation of two cysteine residues into this peptide resulted in an even higher efficacy (C-5H-Tat-5H-C). The association of CPPs with other non-viral delivery vectors has also been extensively investigated, aiming at exploring the possibility to combine efficient delivery, packaging and targeting moieties within the same system [Trabulo et al., 2010].

A combination of a peptide nucleic acids (PNA) with the SV40 core NLS, performed by Branden *et al.*, originated a bifunctional peptide that improved the efficacy of plasmid transfection up to 8-fold when associated with the transfection agent polyethyleneimine (PEI) [Branden et al., 1999]. Several other studies also combined PEI with CPPs. Kleemann *et al.* covalently coupled the Tat peptide to 25 kDa PEI through a heterobi-functional PEG spacer resulting in a Tat-PEG-PEI conjugate. Improved DNA reporter gene complexation and protection were observed for small (approximately 90 nm) polyplexes as well as low toxicity and significantly enhanced transfection efficiency *in vivo* [Kleemann et al., 2005]. Rudolph *et al.* demonstrated that oligomers of the Tat peptide were able to condense plasmid DNA to nanosized particles and protect DNA from nuclease degradation [Rudolph et al., 2003]. Most importantly, when DNA was pre-condensed with Tat peptides and PEI, Superfect or Lipo-fectAMINE were added to the mixture, transfection efficiency was enhanced up to 390-fold compared with the standard vectors. Similar studies by Kilk *et al.*, demonstrated that the poor transfection abilities exhibited by TP10 was significantly enhanced in the presence of PEI, increasing several fold compared to PEI alone, particularly at low PEI concentrations, therefore allowing the use of reduced PEI concentration [Kilk et al., 2005]. Using fluorescently labeled liposomes and cargos, Torchilin *et al.* demonstrated that large drug carriers, such as 200 nm liposomes, could be delivered into cells by attaching Tat peptide to the liposome surface. Next, the same group described the formation of non-covalent complexes of Tat, liposomes and DNA that were able to efficiently transfect cells both *in vitro* and *in vivo,* while being less toxic than other commonly used transfection reagents. The internalization of this system was claimed to depend on a direct cytoplasmic delivery imparted by the Tat peptide [Torchilin et al., 2001]. A study by Hyndman *et al.* showed that mixing the Tat with liposomes containing DOTAP or Lipofectin and DNA, resulted in complexes that significantly enhance transfection *in vitro* with a marked reduction in the amount of liposomes required, despite the lack of any covalent linkage of the peptide to liposomes. In this study, the use of endosomolytic agents and results from experiments performed at low temperature suggested that the endocytotic pathway was involved in the internalization of the complexes. Another report demonstrated that the increase in gene transfer of Tat-modified lipoplexes is dependent on the amount of cationic lipid in the lipoplexes and on the way, Tat was coupled to the lipoplexes. Moreover, it was shown that the cellular uptake of both Tat-modified and un-modified lipoplexes was very fast and, in contrast to previous publications, temperature-dependent [Hyndman et al., 2004]. A concept called "Programmed Packaging" was proposed by Kogure *et al.*, who developed a multi-functional envelope-type nano device (MEND), consisting of a condensed DNA core and a surrounding lipid envelope. This packaging method involves three steps: (1) DNA condensation with a polycation, (2) lipid film hydration for the electrostatic binding of the condensed DNA and (3) sonication to package the condensed DNA with lipids. MEND, having octa-arginine on the envelope for enhancing cellular uptake, showed a 1000-fold higher transfection activity than a DNA/poly-L-lysine/lipid complex prepared in similar conditions [Kogure et al., 2004]. Another study, by Khalil *et al.*, also described the high-efficiency delivery of nucleic acids to eukaryotic cells using MEND particles containing polycation-condensed nucleic acids encapsulated in an R8-DOPE lipid envelope. MEND particles were shown to be non-cytotoxic and achieved transfection efficiencies as high as *adenovirus* [Khalil et al., 2010]. In this case, the high efficiency of MEND particles was ascribed, at least in part, to R8 which was claimed to promote cellular uptake by macropinocytosis, improving intracellular trafficking towards more efficient gene expression. Along the same lines, work of the same research group demonstrated that gene expression of condensed plasmid DNA encapsulated in R8-modified nanoparticles was more than one order of magnitude higher than that of K8-modified nanoparticles, and two orders of magnitude higher than gene expression using unmodified nanoparticles. Differences in gene expression achieved with R8- and K8-modified liposomes could not be attributed to differences in cellular uptake, since both kinds of complexes were taken up primarily *via* macropinocytosis at comparable efficiencies. Moreover, it was described that modification of nanoparticles with a high density of R8 allows their escape from endocytotic vesicles *via* membrane fusion at both acidic and neutral pH, and that the guanidinium groups of arginine residues, and not only their positive charge, are important for efficient endosomal escape [Trabulo et al., 2010]. Recently, MacKay *et al.* described gene transfer using PEGylated bio-responsive nano-lipid particles (NLPs) containing plasmid DNA. In this study, the Tat peptide was attached either directly to a phospholipid (Tatp-lipid) or via a 2 kDa PEG (Tatp-PEG-lipid); incorporation of 0.3 mol% Tatp-PEG into pH-sensitive NLPs improved transfection 100,000-fold compared to NLPs. Although, Tatp-PEG-lipid could dramatically increase gene expression *in vitro*, when tested in brain and in implanted tumors, a restriction of NLP distribution to the vicinity of the infusion catheter reduced the absolute level of gene transfer [MacKay et al., 2008].

Over the last years, a research group focused on the S413-PV cell-penetrating peptide generated from the combination of 13-amino acid cell penetrating sequence derived from the Dermaseptin S4 peptide with the SV40 large T antigen nuclear localization signal [Trabulo et al., 2010]. In these studies, complexes obtained through electrostatic association of the S413-PV cell penetrating peptide with plasmid DNA are able to very efficiently mediate transfection, particularly at high peptide/DNA charge ratios (5/1 and higher). Importantly, complexes prepared with the S413-PV or reverse NLS peptides mediate transfection at significantly higher efficiencies than those containing the scrambled version of the peptide, demonstrating the importance of the cell-penetrating sequence derived from the Dermaseptin S4 peptide (amino acids 1-13) to the transfection process. Additionally, we demonstrated that ternary complexes, resulting from association of cationic liposomes to peptide/DNA complexes, are significantly more efficient in mediating transfection than the corresponding peptide/DNA or cationic liposome/DNA complexes [Trabulo et al., 2010]. In agreement with what has been described for oligonucleotides, CPPs seem to be very efficient to mediate the uptake of plasmid DNA, as well as lipoplexes and polyplexes containing DNA, surpassing the cell membrane barrier. However, the challenge of overcoming the entrapment of complexes inside endosomes has not been solved as easily as initially predicted, even taking advantage of the capacity of direct translocation to the cytoplasm of some CPPs. Nevertheless, several of the studies described above present promising strategies to overcome this limitation, such as chemical modification of the peptide backbone or coupling of CPPs to other classes of delivery vectors. Overall, accumulated evidence suggests that CPPs used in combination with other delivery systems are more likely to be effective for gene therapy purposes than CPPs alone [Trabulo et al., 2010].

12. Bioactive peptides

As antibiotic resistance increases worldwide, there is an increasing pressure to develop novel classes of antimicrobial compounds to fight infectious disease. Peptide therapeutic represents a novel class of therapeutic agents. Some of them, such as cationic antimicrobial peptides (CAMPs) and peptidoglycan recognition proteins (PGRPs), have been identified from studies of innate immune effector mechanisms, while others are completely novel compounds generated in biological systems. Currently, only selected cationic antimicrobial peptides have been licensed, and for topical applications. However, research using new approaches to identify novel antimicrobial peptide therapeutics, and new approaches to delivery and improving stability, will result in an increased range of peptide therapeutics available in the clinic for broader applications. A potentially rich source of peptide therapeutics that is being investigated by researchers is the innate immune response, the effectors of which are produced by eukaryotes to defend themselves against microbial attack [Oyston et al., 2009].

Human cancer is one of the most important causes of death in the western countries. In advanced stages of the disease, the therapeutic opportunities are still limited due to the difficulty to target specifically only cancer cells sparing healthy ones. Cancer cells have on their surface antigens that are expressed at higher levels than their normal counterparts. Often these antigens (also called tumor-associated antigens) have receptor activity and bind to specific proteins or peptides. The latter can be used for the specific delivery of anticancer drugs to cancer cells through retargeting strategies and/or for the direct modulation of cancer cell proliferation and survival interacting with cell-surface-specific receptors. These bioactive peptides can be raised against either tumor cells themselves or to the tumor microenvironment cell components (tumor vessels, tumor-associated macrophages, and fibroblasts) [Fields et al., 2009]. However, the feasibility of pharmacological application of peptides depends on absorption and bioavailability in intact forms in target tissues.

Moreover, their correct bio-distribution is sometimes hindered by biopharmaceutical obstacles, that is, protection by circulating protease-mediated degradation or specific accumulation in tumor tissues. Chemical modification of peptide backbone can increase the stability of peptides in biological fluids. Moreover, the use of delivery systems, and in particular the use of nanotechnologies, not only protects peptides from enzymatic degradation but also improves the delivery of the bioactive peptide in the target tissue. Moreover, peptide conjugation on the surface of nano-vectors can be useful for selective delivery of conventional chemotherapeutic agents in tumor tissues. The requirements for an effective and safe dermatological therapeutic or active ingredient are included as following:

1. The molecule exhibits a proven specific beneficial bioactivity that would lead to a rational demonstrable effect.
2. The bioactivity does not have a negative consequence either theoretically or experimentally due to its mechanism of action.
3. The molecule does not exhibit toxicity such as cytotoxicity, inflammation, immunogenicity, or mutagenicity.
4. The molecule is capable of reaching its desired target intact and in its active form.
5. The molecule can be formulated in such a way as to be stable, compatible with other components, and be delivered effectively to the skin [Fields et al., 2009].

Collectively, these are not easily achieved criteria. For a new technology paradigm to emerge, these criteria not only have to be met but be applicable across the wide range of product-acceptable bioactivities. Peptides have significant advantages over many other technologies in addressing these criteria primarily based upon their chemistry. Peptides consist of chains of amino acids which can be modified in many ways to increase receptor binding, increase specificity, decrease toxicity, and increase skin penetration, stability, and solubility. In this way, the field of bioactive peptides for dermatological applications has changed significantly in recent years. From modest beginnings of a single peptide capable of stimulating collagen, technological advances have created newer peptides capable of targeting most aspects of dermal health. These advances include neutralizing toxins, stimulating fibroblast scaffolding, reducing inflammation and other desirable effects [Fields et al., 2009].

13. Challenges in gene delivery for DNA vaccines

The goal of DNA vaccination is transfection of an antigen presenting cells (APC) or a bystander cell to produce antigens in an immuno-stimulatory setting. The field of genetic vaccines has so far been limited by a lack of safe and effective gene delivery systems [Nguyen et al., 2008]. We attempted to mention some barriers and solutions (e.g., viral/non-viral methods) for DNA vaccines individually.

13.1. Viral and non-viral methods for gene delivery

The main recombinant viral vectors used for gene delivery are *adenovirus, adeno-associated virus* (AAVs), *retrovirus* and *lentivirus*. The advantages of adenovirus are infection of a wide range of human cell types, ability to infect non-dividing cells and lower risk of insertional mutagenesis. However, *adenovirus* expression is short lived and *adenoviruses* can cause a severe, even lethal, inflammatory response due to prior immune exposure. AAV, which depends on *adenovirus* or another virus for replication, has also been used for gene delivery with the advantages of predictable chromosomal insertion and no known pathological consequence of infection [Nguyen et al., 2008]. The main advantage of *retroviruses*, their ability to integrate into the host genome for long-term expression, is also their main disadvantage as this integration can cause mutagenesis and potentially cancer. *Retroviruses* are also further limited by their inability to infect non-dividing cells. *Lentiviruses*, which can transfect a broad spectrum of cell types, are the most efficient method to transfect DCs *in vitro* and *in vivo*. Yang *et al.* recently reported very high levels of immune activation and therapeutic tumor rejection following immunization with a lentiviral vector engineered to target DCs by the cell surface receptor DC-SIGN [Yang et al., 2008]. In particular, Merck & Co. has advanced the use of viral DNA vaccines for HIV vaccination. While there have been some successes in using viral gene therapy and many clinical trials are currently ongoing there are currently no approved protocols. Problems with viral delivery systems include immunologic priming to the vector itself, oncogenicity due to insertional mutagenesis, difficult manufacturing and limited DNA cargo capacity [Nguyen et al., 2008]. Clinical trials have highlighted some of these safety risks as viral gene delivery has resulted in both cancer and deaths. Recently, Merck & Co. stopped its Phase III HIV *adenovirus* vaccine prompting renewed questions about the utility of viral vectors. The safety challenges and limitations of viral vectors have resulted in increased interest in non-viral approaches to gene delivery using non-viral materials. In general, the non-viral methods of DNA vaccination utilized in clinical trials, recently reviewed by Lu *et al.*, rely on physical methods. Injection of naked DNA plasmids has found limited success in humans particularly when injected intramuscularly, even though in smaller animal models naked DNA vaccination produces robust humoral and cell-mediated responses [Lu et al., 2008]. However, the rapid degradation/clearance [half-life of under 5 min if injected intravenously (IV)] of unprotected nucleic acids, poor induction of humoral immune responses in DNA vaccination in larger animals and requirement for large doses has hindered progress into clinical trials. Clinically, relevant physical methods that have been employed include electroporation, ballistics (gene gun), ultrasound and magnetofection. Encapsulation or complexation of DNA with a biomaterial can significantly enhance DNA stability, cellular uptake of DNA and final protein expression. Materials shown to possess potential for the delivery of genes include inorganic nanoparticles and surfaces that bind to or encapsulate DNA [Lu et al., 2008; Nguyen et al., 2008]. Cationic biomolecules including lipids, polysaccharides, polymers, and dendrimers can also electrostatically complex anionic DNA to facilitate transfection. Unless specifically designed to do so, DNA delivered non-virally has low potential for genomic integration [Nguyen et al., 2008]. Non-viral delivery systems for gene therapy are generally cheaper to manufacture, easily scalable from laboratory to GMP-scale production and are typically more robust for long-term storage compared to their viral counterparts. Despite achieving greater efficacy than naked DNA administration (IM, IV or otherwise), physical methods for gene delivery are often limited due to local tissue damage and insufficient gene expression. Research into non-viral gene delivery has been ongoing since the 1970s, and as understanding of the mechanisms of gene delivery has grown, the design of synthetic biomaterials has become more advanced. However, while there have been advances, non-viral methods of gene delivery generally still have lower efficacy than viruses [Nguyen et al., 2008].

13.2. Barriers to gene delivery for DNA vaccines

There are many potential blocks that must be overcome for successful DNA delivery, a process broadly defined as transfection. Plasmid DNA must first be packaged into particles. Requirements for gene delivery include protection of plasmid DNA from degradation, localization to the tissue and cell types of interest avoiding off-target distribution, minimal inactivation by interaction with serum proteins, low clearance from the blood or interstitial space and efficient transport through the extracellular matrix to the surface of target cells. Next, the DNA-containing particles must associate with cells and become internalized into them by cellular uptake processes [Nguyen et al., 2008]. Following uptake, DNA-containing particles must escape the endosomal/ phagosomal compartment into the cytoplasm and release their DNA cargo. DNA must finally translocate into the nucleus to be transcribed into mRNA and subsequently translated into protein antigen. Viruses have evolved to accomplish these steps and provide a framework for the design of synthetic delivery particles. Despite efficient uptake of particles of a variety of sizes, *in vitro* and *in vivo* transfection of DCs is still notoriously difficult to achieve. APCs are specialized not only for uptake of antigen but also rapid and efficient antigen processing. As a key role of APCs is to internalize and process pathogens for immune activation, APCs may have greater protection against foreign (viral) DNA entry into the nucleus, which may be a barrier to DNA vaccination. Whereas *in vitro* investigation of transfection efficiency in cell culture can be used to identify promising materials for transfection, there exist multiple extracellular barriers to effective DNA vaccination *in vivo*. DCs reside in the blood, in the skin (Langerhans cells), other mucosal barriers, and in lymph nodes [Nguyen et al., 2008]. macrophages (MPs) also exist in lymph nodes, as circulating precursors in the blood (monocytes) that differentiate as they enter inflamed tissue cites, and as specialized MPs lining the spleen and liver (Kupfer cells) forming the phagocytic part of the reticuloendothelial system (RES). Access to these APCs is therefore determined not only by route of injection, but also by ability of a particle to drain into lymphatic systems or activate inflammatory signals to recruit APCs. For example, Reddy *et al.* have illustrated size-based targeting of lymph-node resident DCs by accessing lymphatic vessels with 25 nm particles; lymphatic drainage and DC uptake was significantly reduced with 100 nm particles [Reddy et al., 2007]. Many cationic delivery materials, both polymeric and lipid, form vector-nucleic acid particle (VNP) complexes by electrostatic interactions with the negative charges on the phosphate groups of the DNA backbone. A net positive surface charge can facilitate transfection by interacting with the negatively charged glycoproteins at the cell membrane. However, electrostatic interactions can also rapidly lead to aggregation of these VNPs with serum proteins; as VNP-protein aggregate size increases they can be eliminated from circulation by the phagocytic MPs of the RES, deposit non-specifically in microvascular beds or crash out of solution, which may cause acute toxicity [Nguyen et al., 2008]. In addition to containing high concentrations of negatively charged proteins, plasma also has a significant ionic strength. Interactions between serum proteins, blood and interstitial fluid solutes and polycationic carrier materials can lead to competitive binding, destabilization of the VNP and subsequent premature release of the nucleic acid payload. Interaction with complement proteins, C3 and C4 in particular, can activate the innate immune responses resulting in acute inflammation and lead to severe acute toxicity or death. Mucosal surfaces and serum also contain DNase and RNase enzymes that specifically degrade nucleic acids. Condensed VNPs prevent the degradation of the nucleic acid payload by steric inhibition of these DNases/RNases. The addition of PEG and other hydrophilic polymers can be used to prevent aggregation with serum proteins and subsequent rapid clearance [Nguyen et al., 2008]. This simple functionality can sharply increase the serum half-life of a particle and prevent acute toxic events due to non-specific interactions, but also results in lower transfection efficiency and reduced cellular targeting. Toxicity at the cellular level and/or due to interactions with the immune system, liver, kidneys, or other complex organ systems can be a concern with non-viral gene delivery. For example, PEI has been shown to be an effective transfection agent but has also been reported to be toxic in animal models. Polycations such as PEI and cationic lipids such as 1, 2-dioleoyl-3-trimethylammonium-propane (DOTAP) also tend to activate complement and the reticuloendothelial system (RES) aggregate with serum proteins, and can aggregate with red blood cells as well. Some toxicity issues both *in vitro* and *in vivo* can be addressed by chemical modification of PEI [Nguyen et al., 2008]. For increased safety, biodegradable gene delivery systems have also been developed, including degradable cross-linked PEI [Kim et al., 2005], poly (ortho-esters) (POE) [Heller et al., 2000] and poly (b-amino esters) (PBAE) [Anderson et al., 2003].

13.3. Particle uptake by APCs and targeting gene delivery for DNA vaccines

Particle uptake by phagocytosis (particles > 500 nm), macropinocytosis, and receptor-mediated endocytosis are particularly important routes of entry into APCs. Delivery systems can be designed to exploit these ways. Cell-specific targeting can significantly enhance transfection efficiency and the desired therapeutic outcome. The direct conjugation of targeting moieties such as receptor ligands, peptides, sugars, aptamers and antibodies can increase cell and tissue specificity and transfection efficiency. Additionally, targeting can be based upon size-specific signals to avoid off-target affects. A variety of strategies exist for targeting APCs. First, APCs express Fc-receptors, which bind to the constant region of antibodies to facilitate uptake of antibody-coated foreign bodies. APCs also express complement receptors that help clear complement-opsonized particles [Nguyen et al., 2008]. Lectin-binding receptors, such as the mannose receptor and scavenger receptors that recognize apoptotic bodies, certain bacterial components and other non-self motifs are PRRs commonly found on APCs that can enhance particle uptake and may trigger innate immune activation. Second, unlike most other cell types, immature DCs constitutively sample their extracellular fluid environment non-specifically through macropinocytosis to maintain immune surveillance and vigilance for foreign particles, as well as to present endogenous proteins for maintenance of self-tolerance. This constant sampling may explain DC-targeting by particle size. Particle size may also influence the specific route of entry, as reviewed recently by Xiang *et al.* Particle surface characteristics also play a role in uptake, as cationic particles more readily associate with the negatively charged glycoproteins on the cell surface and promote non-specific uptake, and other surface characteristics can activate opsonization [Xiang et al., 2006]. Champion *et al.* have clarified the role of particle shape in influencing phagocytosis by MPs, as well as provided simple methods for creating materials with complex shapes and sizes to take advantage of particle physical properties. While spherical micro- and nano-particles are efficiently phagocytosed by lung alveolar MPs, phagocytosis can be inhibited by contact with odd geometries due to an inability to form the necessary actin structures. In general, size plays a more significant role with particle association with the cell surface than with internalization. These studies suggest a role for particle surface nano and micro-structure in the design of APC-targeted DNA vaccine delivery systems [Champion et al., 2007].

13.4. Biomaterials for DNA delivery: Non-polymeric biomaterials for gene delivery

Many materials have been developed for gene delivery. Early chemical methods of increasing the efficacy of gene delivery focused on co-precipitation of the DNA with salts such as calcium phosphate. More recently, inorganic materials have also been combined with polymers to form hybrid gene delivery nanoparticles. For example, textured surfaces and silica nano-particles have been shown to be effective for gene transfer *in vitro* and organically modified silica nano-particles have been shown to deliver genes *in vivo*. Gold nano-particles have also been combined with PEI for hybrid gene delivery systems. Cationic lipids have been the non-viral gene delivery vectors of choice for clinical application since Felgner first introduced their use in 1987. The cationic lipid molecule consists of a hydrophilic positively charged head group, a linker that may impart some functionality such as pH sensitivity and a hydrophobic long chain tail [Felgner et al., 1987]. A prototypical cationic lipid is DOTAP; it is the most widely used lipid for gene delivery. For *in vivo* delivery, nucleic acids are usually encapsulated into liposomes: vesicles with lipid bilayer membranes that exist as large uni-lamellar vesicles (LUVs) or multi-lamellar vesicles (MLVs). Liposomes generally consist of a single cationic lipid or a mixture of cationic lipids that facilitate nucleic acid binding and transfection, cholesterol or diolelphophatidylethanolamine (DOPE) to impart some rigidity or stability to the complex, and PEG to shield particles from aggregation, serum components, or other non-specific interactions. Lipids have been used extensively in gene therapy and are the main non-viral delivery vectors used in clinical trials. Unfortunately, some lipoplexes are toxic, interact nonspecifically with serum proteins and cells, aggregate quickly, activate the complement system, or have low *in vivo* efficacy. One promising approach that may address these problems is to increase the chemical diversity of lipid-like materials through combinatorial synthesis approaches [Nguyen et al., 2008].

14. Conclusion

Gene therapy possesses great potential for combating a variety of diseases. Initial results are promising and some technologies have advanced to clinical trials. Yet challenges remain, and despite decades of study, safe and efficient gene delivery remains a major blockage in human medicine. The current progresses of gene therapy are further focused on synthesized nano-particle technologies such as polymers (PLGA, chitosan and PEI), lipids and peptides. It is necessary to understand the effects of particle size, surface characteristics and material interactions. Research on cell penetrating peptides (CPPs) as gene/ drug delivery systems has clarified their capacity to promote the efficient internalization of therapeutic biomolecules. Despite differences in size, charge and/or structure between different bioactive molecules, it is clear that CPP-based systems appear to be very versatile and efficient delivery is achievable following proper adjustment of the carrier to the transported biomolecule. Because the development of drug, oligonucleotide or gene delivery systems is aimed at a clinical application, the design of these novel delivery vectors should consider other important issues including safety, bio-distribution, ease of manufacturing, scale-up, reproducibility and analytical and physical characterization. The advance of CPP technology depends on the development of strategies that facilitate endosomal escape and that confer cell specificity to these systems. A careful investigation of the mechanisms of internalization of CPP-cargo complexes or conjugates will greatly help the improvement of this powerful technology. However, a viable non-viral gene vector for systemic delivery depends on its capacity to bypass a series of physiological barriers and its efficiency in carrying nucleic acids to a targeted site within a cell. The concept of a multifunctional delivery system helps to solve the problems associated with various barriers. The availability of delivery devices directed towards each individual barrier, provides a basis for this direction, although the complexity in the development of multifunctional non-viral vectors is much more than a merely combination of various devices into a single system. In order to achieve the optimal gene delivery, the researchers have focused largely on the evolution of "intelligent" bio-responsive materials, as well as on the advances in formulation technologies. In this process, a number of strategies have emerged including the balances between gene packing and controlled release, and optimal control between long-circulation and intracellular trafficking that promotes safer and more efficient delivery of gene/drug in a systemic context.

Author details

Azam Bolhassani[1] and Tayebeh Saleh[2]

*Address all correspondence to: azam_bolhassani@yahoo.com

*Address all correspondence to: A_bolhasani@pasteur.ac.ir

1 Molecular Immunology and Vaccine Research Lab., Pasteur Institute of Iran, Tehran, Iran

2 Department of Nanobiotechnology, Faculty of Biological Sciences, Tarbiat Modares University, Tehran, Iran

References

[1] Abbott, A. (1992). Gene therapy: Italians first to use stem cells. Nature, , 356(6369), 465-499.

[2] Alexis, F, & Basto, P. Levy-Nissenbaum, E.; Radovic-Moreno, A.F.; Zhang, L.; Pridgen, E.; Wang, A.Z.; Marein, S.L.; Westerhof, K. & Molnar, L.K. ((2008). HER-2-targeted nanoparticle-affibody bioconjugates for cancer therapy. Chem.Med.Chem., , 3, 1839-1843.

[3] Anderson, D. G, Lynn, D. M, & Langer, R. (2003). Semi-automated synthesis and screening of a large library of degradable cationic polymers for gene delivery. Angew. Chem. Int. Ed. Engl., , 42(27), 3153-3158.

[4] Askoxylakis, V, Zitzmann, S, Mier, W, Graham, K, Krämer, S, Von Wegner, F, Fink, R. H. A, Schwab, M, Eisenhut, M, & Haberkorn, U. (2005). Preclinical evaluation of the breast cancer cell-binding peptide, p160. Clinical cancer research, , 11, 6705-6712.

[5] Bauhuber, S, Hozsa, C, Breunig, M, & Göpferich, A. (2009). Delivery of nucleic acids via disulfide-based carrier systems. Advanced Materials, , 21, 3286-3306.

[6] Benoit, D. S. W, Henry, S. M, Shubin, A. D, Hoffman, A. S, & Stayton, P. S. (2010). pH-responsive polymeric sirna carriers sensitize multidrug resistant ovarian cancer cells to doxorubicin via knockdown of polo-like kinase. Molecular pharmaceutics, , 7, 442-455.

[7] Bhaskar, S, Tian, F, Stoeger, T, Kreyling, W, Fuente, J. M, Grazú, V, Borm, P, Estrada, G, Ntziachristos, G, & Razansky, D. (2010). Multifunctional nanocarriers for diagnostics, drug delivery and targeted treatment across blood-brain barrier: perspectives on tracking and neuroimaging. Particle and Fibre Toxicology, , 7, 3.

[8] Blaese, R. M, Culver, K. W, Miller, A. D, Carter, C. S, Fleisher, T, Clerici, M, Shearer, G, Chang, L, Chiang, Y, Tolstoshev, P, Greenblatt, J. J, Rosenberg, S. A, Klein, H, Berger, M, Mullen, C. A, Ramsey, W. J, Muul, L, Morgan, R. A, & Anderson, W. F. gene therapy for ADA- SCID: initial trial results after 4 years. Science, , 270(5235), 475-480.

[9] Bolhassani, A. (2011). Potential efficacy of cell-penetrating peptides for nucleic acid and drug delivery in cancer. BBA-Reviews on Cancer, , 1816, 232-246.

[10] Bolhassani, A, Safaiyan, S, & Rafati, S. (2011). Improvement of different vaccine delivery systems for cancer therapy. Molecular Cancer, , 10(3), 1-20.

[11] Branden, L. J, Mohamed, A. J, & Smith, C. I. (1999). A peptide nucleic acid-nuclear localization signal fusion that mediates nuclear transport of DNA. Nat. Biotechnol., , 17, 784-787.

[12] Cavazzana-calvo, M, Thrasher, A, & Mavilio, F. (2004). The future of gene therapy. Nature, , 427(6977), 779-781.

[13] Cell therapy fights leukaemia. (2011). http://www.nature.com/news.

[14] Chai, C, Xie, Z, & Grotewold, E. (2011). SELEX (Systematic Evolution of Ligands by EXponential Enrichment) as a powerful tool for deciphering the protein-DNA interaction space. Methods Mol. Biol., , 754, 249-258.

[15] Champion, J. A, Katare, Y. K, & Mitragotri, S. (2007). Particle shape: a new design parameter for micro- and nanoscale drug delivery carriers. J. Control. Release, , 121(1-2), 3-9.

[16] Cheng, R, Feng, F, Meng, F, Deng, C, Feijen, J, & Zhong, Z. (2011). Glutathione-responsive nano-vehicles as a promising platform for targeted intracellular drug and gene delivery. Journal of Controlled Release. , 152(1), 2-12.

[17] De Coupade, C, Fittipaldi, A, Chagnas, V, Michel, M, Carlier, S, Tasciotti, E, Darmon, A, Ravel, D, Kearsey, J, Giacca, M, & Cailler, F. (2005). Novel human-derived cell-penetrating peptides for specific subcellular delivery of therapeutic biomolecules. Biochem. J., , 390, 407-418.

[18] DNA nanoballs boost gene therapy(2002). New Scientist, http://www.newscientist.com/article/dndna-nanoballs-boost-gene-therapy.html.

[19] Du, F. S, Wang, Y, Zhang, R, & Li, Z. C. (2010). Intelligent nucleic acid delivery systems based on stimuli-responsive polymers. Soft Matter, , 6, 835-848.

[20] El-Andaloussi, S, Johansson, H. J, Holm, T, & Langel, U. (2007). A novel cell-penetrating peptide, M918, for efficient delivery of proteins and peptide nucleic acids. Mol. Ther. , 15, 1820-1826.

[21] Eliyahu, H, Barenholz, Y, & Domb, A. J. (2005). Polymers for DNA delivery. Molecules, , 10, 34-64.

[22] Farokhzad, O. C, Jon, S, Khademhosseini, A, Tran, T. N. T, La, D. A, & Langer, R. (2004). Nanoparticle-aptamer bioconjugates. Cancer research, , 64, 7668.

[23] Farokhzad, O. C, Cheng, J, Teply, B. A, Sherifi, I, Jon, S, Kantoff, P. W, Richie, J. P, & Langer, R. (2006). Targeted nanoparticle-aptamer bioconjugates for cancer chemotherapy in vivo. Proceedings of the National Academy of Sciences, , 103, 6315-6320.

[24] Fawell, S, Seery, J, Daikh, Y, Moore, C, Chen, L. L, Pepinsky, B, & Barsoum, J. (1994). Tat-mediated delivery of heterologous proteins into cells. Proc. Natl. Acad. Sci. U.S.A., , 91, 664-668.

[25] Felgner, P. L, Gadek, T. R, Holm, M, Roman, R, Chan, H. W, Wenz, M, Northrop, J. P, Ringold, G. M, & Danielsen, M. (1987). Lipofection: a highly efficient, lipid-mediated DNA-transfection procedure. Proc. Natl. Acad. Sci. USA, , 84(21), 7413-7417.

[26] Fields, K, Falla, T. J, Rodan, K, & Bush, L. (2009). Bioactive peptides: signaling the future. Journal of Cosmetic Dermatology, , 8, 8-13.

[27] Fisher, J. (1995). Murine gene therapy corrects symptoms of sickle cell disease". Magazine of the Life Sciences.

[28] Fittipaldi, A, Ferrari, A, Zoppe, M, Arcangeli, C, Pellegrini, V, Beltram, F, & Giacca, M. (2003). Cell membrane lipid rafts mediate caveolar endocytosis of HIV-1 Tat fusion proteins. J. Biol. Chem., , 278, 34141-34149.

[29] Frankel, A. D, & Pabo, C. O. (1998). Cellular uptake of the tat protein from human immunodeficiency virus. Cell, , 55, 1189-1193.

[30] Friedmann, T, & Roblin, R. (1972). Gene therapy for human genetic disease. Science, , 175(4025), 949.

[31] Ganta, S, Devalapally, H, Shahiwala, A, & Amiji, M. (2008). A review of stimuli-responsive nanocarriers for drug and gene delivery. Journal of Controlled Release, , 126, 187-204.

[32] GaoX; Kim, K.S. & Liu, D. ((2007). Non-viral gene delivery: What we know and what is next. A.A.P.S. Journal, , 9(1), E92-E104.

[33] Gene therapy may switch off Huntington's(2003). New Scientist, http://www.news-cientist.com

[34] Gene therapy first for poor sight(2007). BBC News, http://news.bbc.co.uk

[35] Green, M, & Loewenstein, P. M. (1988). Autonomous functional domains of chemically synthesized human immunodeficiency virus Tat trans-activator protein. Cell, , 55, 1179-1188.

[36] Gu, F. X, Karnik, R, Wang, A. Z, Alexis, F, Levy-nissenbaum, E, Hong, S, Langer, R. S, & Farokhzad, O. C. (2007). Targeted nanoparticles for cancer therapy. Nano Today, , 2, 14-21.

[37] Hahn, W, Pyun, W. B, Kim, D. S, Yoo, W. S, Lee, S. D, Won, J. H, Shin, G. J, Kim, J. M, & Kim, S. (2011). Enhanced cardioprotective effects by co-expression of two isoforms of hepatocyte growth factor from naked plasmid DNA in a rat ischemic heart disease model". The Journal of Gene Medicine, , 13(10), 549-555.

[38] Heller, J, Barr, J, Ng, S. Y, Shen, H. R, Schwach-abdellaoui, K, Einmahl, S, Rothen-weinhold, A, & Gurny, R. (2000). Poly(ortho esters)- their development and some recent applications. Eur. J. Pharm. Biopharm., , 50(1), 121-128.

[39] Hyndman, L, Lemoine, J. L, Huang, L, Porteous, D. J, Boyd, A. C, & Nan, X. (2004). HIV-1 Tat protein transduction domain peptide facilitates gene transfer in combination with cationic liposomes. J. Control. Release, , 99, 435-444.

[40] Ignatovich, I. A, Dizhe, E. B, Pavlotskaya, A. V, Akifiev, B. N, Burov, S. V, Orlov, S. V, & Perevozchikov, A. P. (2003). Complexes of plasmid DNA with basic domain 47-57 of the HIV-1 Tat protein are transferred to mammalian cells by endocytosis-mediated pathways. J. Biol. Chem., , 278, 42625-42636.

[41] Imai, K, & Takaoka, A. (2006). Comparing antibody and small-molecule therapies for cancer. Nature Reviews-Cancer, , 6, 714-727.

[42] Jabr-milane, L, Van Vlerken, L, Devalapally, H, Shenoy, D, Komareddy, S, Bhavsar, M, & Amiji, M. (2008). Multi-functional nanocarriers for targeted delivery of drugs and genes. Journal of Controlled Release, , 130, 121-128.

[43] Joliot, A. H, Triller, A, Volovitch, M, Pernelle, C, & Prochiantz, A. (1991). alpha-2, 8-polysialic acid is the neuronal surface receptor of antennapedia homeobox peptide. New Biol., , 3, 1121-1134.

[44] Kaiser, J. (2009). Gene therapy halts brain disease in two boys", Science

[45] Kam, N. W. S, Liu, Z, & Dai, H. (2005). Functionalization of carbon nanotubes via cleavable disulfide bonds for efficient intracellular delivery of siRNA and potent gene silencing. Journal of the American Chemical Society, , 127, 12492-12493.

[46] Kang, H. C, Kang, H. J, & Bae, Y. H. (2011). A reducible polycationic gene vector derived from thiolated low molecular weight branched polyethyleneimine linked by 2-iminothiolane. Biomaterials, , 32, 1193-1203.

[47] Khalil, I. A, Futaki, S, Niwa, M, Baba, Y, Kaji, N, Kamiya, H, & Harashima, H. (2004). Mechanism of improved gene transfer by the N-terminal stearylation of octaarginine: enhanced cellular association by hydrophobic core formation. Gene Ther., , 11, 636-644.

[48] Kilk, K, Andaloussi, S, Jarver, P, Meikas, A, Valkna, A, Bartfai, T, Kogerman, P, Metsis, M, & Langel, U. (2005). Evaluation of transportan 10 in PEI mediated plasmid delivery assay. J. Control. Release, , 103, 511-523.

[49] Kim, Y. H, Park, J. H, Lee, M, Kim, Y. H, Park, T. G, & Kim, S. W. (2005). Polyethylenimine with acid-labile linkages as a biodegradable gene carrier. J. Control. Release, , 103(1), 209-219.

[50] Kim, S. H, Mok, H, Jeong, J. H, Kim, S. W, & Park, T. G. (2006). Comparative evaluation of target-specific GFP gene silencing efficiencies for antisense ODN, synthetic siRNA, and siRNA plasmid complexed with PEI-PEG-FOL conjugate. Bioconjugate chemistry, , 17, 241-244.

[51] Kim, Y. H, Park, J. H, Lee, M, Park, T. G, & Kim, S. W. (2005). Polyethylenimine with acid-labile linkages as a biodegradable gene carrier. Journal of Controlled Release, , 103, 209-219.

[52] Kim, T, & Kim, S. W. (2011). Bio-reducible polymers for gene delivery. Reactive and functional polymers, , 71, 344-349.

[53] Kleemann, E, Neu, M, Jekel, N, Fink, L, Schmehl, T, Gessler, T, Seeger, W, & Kissel, T. (2005). Nano-carriers for DNA delivery to the lung based upon a TAT-derived peptide covalently coupled to PEG-PEI. J. Control. Release, , 109, 299-316.

[54] Knorr, V, Allmendinger, L, Walker, G. F, Paintner, F. F, & Wagner, E. (2007). An acetal-based PEGylation reagent for pH-sensitive shielding of DNA polyplexes. Bioconjugate chemistry, , 18, 1218-1225.

[55] Kogure, K, Moriguchi, R, Sasaki, K, Ueno, M, Futaki, S, & Harashima, H. (2004). Development of a non-viral multifunctional envelope-type nano device by a novel lipid film hydration method. J. Control. Release, , 98, 317-323.

[56] Komáromy, A, Alexander, J, Rowlan, J, Garcia, M, Chiodo, V, Kaya, A, Tanaka, J, Acland, G. M, Hauswirth, W. W, & Aguirre, G. D. (2010). Gene therapy rescues cone function in congenital achromatopsia. Human Molecular Genetics, , 19(13), 2581-2593.

[57] Korthof, G. (1999). The implications of Steele's soma-to-germline feedback for human gene therapy, http://home.planet.nl

[58] Langel, U. (2002). Cell-penetrating peptides: Processes and Applications. CRC Press, Amazon.com Textbooks

[59] Lee, H, Mok, H, Lee, S, Oh, Y. K, & Park, T. G. (2007). Target-specific intracellular delivery of siRNA using degradable hyaluronic acid nanogels. Journal of Controlled Release, , 119, 245-252.

[60] Lehner, R, Wang, X, Wolf, M, & Hunziker, P. (2012). Designing switchable nanosystems for medical application. J. Control Release, , 161(2), 307-316.

[61] Levine, B. L, Humeau, L. M, & Boyer, J. MacGregor, R.R.; Rebello T.; Lu, X.; Binder, G.K.; Slepushkin, V.; Lemiale, F.; Mascola, J.R.; Bushman, F.D.; Dropulic, B.; & June, C.H. ((2006). Gene transfer in humans using a conditionally replicating lentiviral vector. Proc Natl Acad Sci U S A., , 103(46), 17372-17377.

[62] Lin, Y. L, Jiang, G, Birrell, L. K, & Sayed, M. E. H. (2010). Degradable, pH-sensitive, membrane-destabilizing, comb-like polymers for intracellular delivery of nucleic acids. Biomaterials, , 31, 7150-7166.

[63] Lo, S. L, & Wang, S. (2008). An endosomolytic Tat peptide produced by incorporation of histidine and cysteine residues as a nonviral vector for DNA transfection. Biomaterials, , 29, 2408-2414.

[64] Lomas, H, & Canton, I. MacNeil, S.; Du, J.; Armes, S.P.; Ryan, A.J.; Lewis, A.L. & Battaglia, G. ((2007). Biomimetic pH sensitive polymersomes for efficient DNA encapsulation and delivery. Advanced Materials, , 19, 4238-4243.

[65] Lu, S, Wang, S, & Grimes-serrano, J. M. (2008). Current progress of DNA vaccine studies in humans. Expert Rev. Vaccines, , 7(2), 175-191.

[66] Ma, B, Zhang, S, Jiang, H, Zhao, B, & Lv, H. (2007). Lipoplex morphologies and their influences on transfection efficiency in gene delivery. Journal of Controlled Release, , 123, 184-194.

[67] MacKayJ.A.; Li, W.; Huang, Z.; Dy, E.E.; Huynh, G.; Tihan, T.; Collins, R.; Deen, D.F. & Szoka, F.C. ((2008). HIV TAT peptide modifies the distribution of DNA nanolipoparticles following convection-enhanced delivery. Mol. Ther., , 16, 893-900.

[68] Maiolo, J. R, Ferrer, M, & Ottinger, E. A. (2005). Effects of cargo molecules on the cellular uptake of arginine-rich cell-penetrating peptides. Biochim. Biophys. Acta, , 1712, 161-172.

[69] Manickam, D. S, & Oupický, D. (2006). Multiblock reducible copolypeptides containing histidine-rich and nuclear localization sequences for gene delivery. Bioconjugate chemistry, , 17, 1395-1403.

[70] Manjappa, A. S, Chaudhari, K. R, Venkataraju, M. P, Dantuluri, P, Nanda, B, Sidda, C, & Sawant, K. K. Ramachandra Murthy, R.S. ((2011). Antibody derivatization and conjugation strategies: application in preparation of stealth immunoliposome to target chemotherapeutics to tumor. Journal of Controlled Release, , 150, 2-22.

[71] Martin, M. E, & Rice, K. G. (2007). Peptide-guided gene delivery. The AAPS journal, , 9, 18-29.

[72] Mastrobattista, E, Van Der Aa, M. A. E. M, Hennink, W. E, & Crommelin, D. J. A. (2006). Artificial viruses: a nanotechnological approach to gene delivery. Nature Reviews Drug Discovery, , 5, 115-121.

[73] Mccormick, F. (2001). Cancer gene therapy: Fringe or cutting edge? Nature, , 1, 130-141.

[74] Mckenzie, D. L, Kwok, K. Y, & Rice, K. G. (2000). A potent new class of reductively activated peptide gene delivery agents. Journal of Biological Chemistry, , 275, 9970-9977.

[75] Meng, F, Hennink, W. E, & Zhong, Z. (2009). Reduction-sensitive polymers and bioconjugates for biomedical applications. Biomaterials, , 30, 2180-2198.

[76] Midoux, P, Pichon, C, Yaouanc, J. J, & Jaffrès, P. A. (2009). Chemical vectors for gene delivery: a current review on polymers, peptides and lipids containing histidine or imidazole as nucleic acids carriers. Br. J. Pharmacol., , 157(2), 166-178.

[77] Morris, M. C, Chaloin, L, Mery, J, Heitz, F, & Divita, G. (1999). A novel potent strategy for gene delivery using a single peptide vector as a carrier. Nucleic Acids Res.,, 27, 3510-3517.

[78] Murthy, N, Campbell, J, Fausto, N, Hoffman, A. S, & Stayton, P. S. (2003). Design and synthesis of pH-responsive polymeric carriers that target uptake and enhance the intracellular delivery of oligonucleotides. Journal of Controlled Release, , 89, 365-374.

[79] Nakase, I, Kobayashi, S, & Futaki, S. (2010). Endosome-disruptive peptides for improving cytosolic delivery of bioactive macromolecules. Biopolymers, , 94, 763-770.

[80] Nguyen, D. N, Green, J. J, Chan, J. M, Langer, R, & Anderson, D. G. (2008). Polymeric materials for gene delivery and DNA vaccination. Adv. Mater., , 20, 1-21.

[81] Nie, Y, Günther, M, Gu, Z, & Wagner, E. (2011). Pyridylhydrazone-based PEGylation for pH-reversible lipopolyplex shielding. Biomaterials, , 32, 858-869.

[82] Oishi, M, Nagasaki, Y, Itaka, K, Nishiyama, N, & Kataoka, K. (2005). Lactosylated poly (ethylene glycol)-siRNA conjugate through acid-labile β-thiopropionate linkage to

construct pH-sensitive polyion complex micelles achieving enhanced gene silencing in hepatoma cells. Journal of the American Chemical Society, , 127, 1624-1625.

[83] Ogris, M, Walker, G, Blessing, T, Kircheis, R, Wolschek, M, & Wagner, E. (2003). Tumor-targeted gene therapy: strategies for the preparation of ligand-polyethylene glycol-polyethylenimine/ DNA complexes. Journal of Controlled Release, , 91, 173-181.

[84] Oyston, P. C. F, Fox, M. A, Richards, S. J, & Clark, G. C. (2009). Novel peptide therapeutics for treatment of infections. Journal of Medical Microbiology, , 58, 977-987.

[85] Park, I. K, Singha, K, Arote, R. B, Choi, Y. J, Kim, W. J, & Cho, C. S. (2010). pH-Responsive Polymers as Gene Carriers. Macromolecular rapid communications, , 31, 1122-1133.

[86] Peer, D, Karp, J. M, Hong, S, Farokhzad, O. C, Margalit, R, & Langer, R. (2007). Nanocarriers as an emerging platform for cancer therapy. Nature nanotechnology, , 2, 751-760.

[87] Peng, Q, Zhong, Z, & Zhuo, R. (2008). Disulfide cross-linked polyethylenimines (PEI) prepared via thiolation of low molecular weight PEI as highly efficient gene vectors. Bioconjugate chemistry, , 19, 499-506.

[88] Penn Medicine presents HIV gene therapy trial(2009). CROI, http://www.eurekalert.org

[89] Qiao, W, Wang, B, Wang, Y, Yang, L, Zhang, Y, & Shao, P. (2010). Cancer therapy based on nanomaterials and nanocarrier systems. Journal of Nanomaterials, , 2010, 1-9.

[90] Read, M. L, Bremner, K. H, Oupický, D, Green, N. K, Searle, P. F, & Seymour, L. W. (2003). Vectors based on reducible polycations facilitate intracellular release of nucleic acids. The journal of gene medicine, , 5, 232-245.

[91] Reddy, S. T, Van Der Vlies, A. J, Simeoni, E, Angeli, V, Randolph, G. J, Neil, O, Lee, C. P, Swartz, L. K, & Hubbell, M. A. J.A. ((2007). Exploiting lymphatic transport and complement activation in nanoparticle vaccines. Nat. Biotechnol., , 25(10), 1159-1164.

[92] Richard, J. P, Melikov, K, Vives, E, Ramos, C, Verbeure, B, Gait, M. J, Chernomordik, L. V, & Lebleu, B. (2003). Cell-penetrating peptides: A re-evaluation of the mechanism of cellular uptake. J. Biol. Chem. , 278, 585-590.

[93] Richard, J. P, Melikov, K, Brooks, H, Prevot, P, Lebleu, B, & Chernomordik, L. V. (2005). Cellular uptake of un-conjugated Tat peptide involves clathrin-dependent endocytosis and heparin sulfate receptors. J. Biol. Chem. , 280, 15300-15306.

[94] Rittner, K, Benavente, A, Bompard-sorlet, A, Heitz, F, Divita, G, Brasseur, R, & Jacobs, E. (2002). New basic membrane-destabilizing peptides for plasmid-based gene delivery in vitro and in vivo. Mol. Ther., , 5, 104-114.

[95] Roh, Y. H, Lee, J. B, Kiatwuthinon, P, Hartman, M. R, Cha, J. J, Um, S. H, Muller, D. A, & Luo, D. (2011). DNAsomes: Multifunctional DNA-Based Nanocarriers. Small, , 7(1), 74-78.

[96] Rogers, S. (1970). Gene therapy, New Sci., , 194.

[97] Rudolph, C, Plank, C, Lausier, J, Schillinger, U, Muller, R. H, & Rosenecker, J. (2003). Oligomers of the arginine-rich motif of the HIV-1 TAT protein are capable of transferring plasmid DNA into cells. J. Biol. Chem., , 278, 11411-11418.

[98] Sandgren, S, Cheng, F, & Belting, M. (2002). Nuclear targeting of macromolecular polyanions by an HIV-Tat derived peptide. Role for cell-surface proteoglycans. J. Biol. Chem., , 277, 38877-38883.

[99] Sasaki, K, Kogure, K, Chaki, S, Nakamura, Y, Moriguchi, R, Hamada, H, Danev, R, Nagayama, K, Futaki, S, & Harashima, H. (2008). An artificial virus-like nano carrier system: enhanced endosomal escape of nanoparticles via synergistic action of pH-sensitive fusogenic peptide derivatives. Analytical and bioanalytical chemistry, , 391, 2717-2727.

[100] Sawant, R. R, Sriraman, S. K, Navarro, G, Biswas, S, Dalvi, R. A, & Torchilin, V. P. (2012). Polyethyleneimine-lipid conjugate-based pH-sensitive micellar carrier for gene delivery. Biomaterials, , 33(15), 3942-3951.

[101] Scanlon, K. J. (2004). Cancer Gene Therapy: Challenges and Opportunities. Anticancer Research, , 24, 501-504.

[102] Schaffer, D. V, Fidelman, N. A, Dan, N, & Lauffenburger, D. A. (2000). Vector unpacking as a potential barrier for receptor-mediated polyplex gene delivery. Biotechnology and bioengineering, , 67, 598-606.

[103] Schwarze, S. R, Ho, A, Vocero-akbani, A, & Dowdy, S. F. (1999). In vivo protein transduction: delivery of a biologically active protein into the mouse. Science, , 285, 1569-1572.

[104] Sethuraman, V. A, Lee, M. C, & Bae, Y. H. (2008). A biodegradable pH-sensitive micelle system for targeting acidic solid tumors. Pharmaceutical Research, , 25, 657-666.

[105] Shim, M. S, & Kwon, Y. J. (2012). Stimuli-responsive polymers and nanomaterials for gene delivery and imaging applications. Advanced Drug Delivery Reviews, , 64(11), 1046-1059.

[106] Son, S, Singha, K, & Kim, W. J. (2010). Bioreducible BPEI-SS-PEG-cNGR polymer as a tumor targeted nonviral gene carrier. Biomaterials, , 31, 6344-6354.

[107] Soudy, R, Gill, A, Sprules, T, Lavasanifar, A, & Kaur, K. (2011). Proteolytically stable cancer targeting peptides with high affinity for breast cancer cells. Journal of medicinal chemistry, , 54(21), 7523-7534.

[108] Soundara ManickamD. & Oupický, D. ((2006). Polyplex gene delivery modulated by redox potential gradients. Journal of Drug Targeting, , 14, 519-526.

[109] Stevenson, M, Ramos-perez, V, Singh, S, Soliman, M, Preece, J. A, Briggs, S. S, Read, M. L, & Seymour, L. W. (2008). Delivery of siRNA mediated by histidine-containing reducible polycations. Journal of Controlled Release, , 130, 46-56.

[110] Takemoto, H, Ishii, A, Miyata, K, Nakanishi, M, Oba, M, Ishii, T, Yamasaki, Y, Nishiyama, N, & Kataoka, K. (2010). Polyion complex stability and gene silencing efficiency with a siRNA-grafted polymer delivery system. Biomaterials, , 31, 8097-8105.

[111] Torchilin, V. P, Rammohan, R, Weissig, V, & Levchenko, T. S. (2001). TAT peptide on the surface of liposomes affords their efficient intracellular delivery even at low temperature and in the presence of metabolic inhibitors. Proc. Natl. Acad. Sci. USA, , 98, 8786-8791.

[112] Torchilin, V. P. (2008). Cell penetrating peptide-modified pharmaceutical nanocarriers for intracellular drug and gene delivery. Peptide Science, , 90, 604-610.

[113] Torchilin, V. P. (2006). Multifunctional nano-carriers. Advanced Drug Delivery Reviews, , 58, 1532-1555.

[114] Trabulo, S, Cardoso, A. L, & Mano, M. Pedroso de Lima, MC. ((2010). Cell-penetrating peptides-mechanisms of cellular uptake and generation of delivery systems. Pharmaceuticals, , 3, 961-993.

[115] Tung, C. H, Mueller, S, & Weissleder, R. (2002). Novel branching membrane translocational peptide as gene delivery vector. Bioorg. Med. Chem., , 10, 3609-3614.

[116] Undercover genes slip into the brain(2003). New Scientist, http://www.newscientist.com

[117] Van Vlerken, L. E, Vyas, T. K, & Amiji, M. M. (2007). Poly (ethylene glycol)-modified nanocarriers for tumor-targeted and intracellular delivery. Pharmaceutical research, , 24, 1405-1414.

[118] Veldhoen, S, Laufer, S. D, & Restle, T. (2008). Recent developments in peptide-based nucleic acid delivery. Int. J. Mol. Sci., , 9, 1276-1320.

[119] Varkouhi, A. K, Scholte, M, Storm, G, & Haisma, H. J. (2011). Endosomal escape pathways for delivery of biologicals. Journal of Controlled Release, , 151, 220-228.

[120] Vercauteren, D, Rejman, J, Martens, T. F, Demeester, J, De Smedt, S. C, & Braeckmans, K. (2012). On the cellular processing of non-viral nanomedicines for nucleic acid delivery: Mechanisms and methods. Journal of Controlled Release, , 161(2), 566-581.

[121] Vidugiriene, J, Goueli, S, & Sužiedelis, K. (2007). RNA interference: from a research tool to a novel therapeutic agent. Acta Medica Lituanica, , 14(3), 165-169.

[122] Vivès, E, Schmidt, J, & Pèlegrin, A. (2008). Cell-penetrating and cell-targeting peptides in drug delivery. Biochimica et Biophysica Acta (BBA)-Reviews on Cancer, , 1786, 126-138.

[123] Wadia, J. S, Stan, R. V, & Dowdy, S. F. (2004). Transducible Tat-HA fusogenic peptide enhances escape of Tat-fusion proteins after lipid raft macropinocytosis. Nat. Med., , 10, 310-315.

[124] Wagner, E. (2011). Polymers for siRNA delivery: Inspired by viruses to be targeted, dynamic and precise. Accounts of Chemical Research, , 45(7), 1005-1013.

[125] Walker, G. F, Fella, C, Pelisek, J, Fahrmeir, J, Boeckle, S, Ogris, M, & Wagner, E. (2005). Toward synthetic viruses: endosomal pH-triggered deshielding of targeted polyplexes greatly enhances gene transfer in vitro and in vivo. Molecular Therapy, , 11, 418-425.

[126] Wiethoff, C. M, & Middaugh, C. R. (2003). Barriers to nonviral gene delivery. Journal of pharmaceutical sciences, , 92, 203-217.

[127] Wu, J, Zhao, X, & Lee, R. J. (2007). Lipid- based nanoparticulate drug delivery systems. Nano- particulate Drug Delivery Systems. , 89-98.

[128] Xiang, S. D, Scholzen, A, Minigo, G, David, C, Apostolopoulos, V, Mottram, P. L, & Plebanski, M. (2006). Pathogen recognition and development of particulate vaccines: does size matter? Methods, , 40(1), 1-9.

[129] Yang, L, Yang, H, Rideout, K, Cho, T, Joo, K. I, Ziegler, L, Elliot, A, Walls, A, Yu, D, Baltimore, D, & Wang, P. (2008). Engineered lentivector targeting of dendritic cells for in vivo immunization. Nat. Biotechnol., , 26(3), 326-334.

[130] Yang, Z. J, Zhang, Y. R, Chen, B, Zhang, S. L, Jia, E. Z, Wang, L. S, Zhu, T. B, Li, C. J, Wang, H, Huang, J, Cao, K. J, Ma, W. Z, Wu, B, Wang, L. S, Wu, C. T, Wang, H, Huang, J, Cao, K. J, Ma, W. Z, Wu, B, Wang, L. S, & Wu, C. T. (2009). Phase I clinical trial on intracoronary administration of Ad-hHGF treating severe coronary artery disease. Molecular Biology Reports, , 36(6), 1323-1329.

[131] Yu-lin, Y, Wen-teng, C, & Yuan-wei, S. (2011). Gene therapy using RNAi. Gene Therapy- Developments and Future Perspectives, Intech Open Access

[132] Zatsepin, T. S, Turner, J. J, Oretskaya, T. S, & Gait, M. J. (2005). Conjugates of oligonucleotides and analogues with cell penetrating peptides as gene silencing agents. Curr. Pharm. Des., , 11, 3639-3654.

[133] Zhang, J, Spring, H, & Schwab, M. (2001). Neuroblastoma tumor cell-binding peptides identified through random peptide phage display. Cancer letters, , 171, 153-164.

[134] Zhu, L, & Torchilin, V. R. (2012). Stimulus-responsive nano-preparations for tumor targeting. Integr. Biol.

Chapter 14

Cancer Gene Therapy with Small Oligonucleotides

Onur Sakiragaoglu, David Good and Ming Q. Wei

Additional information is available at the end of the chapter

1. Introduction

Although enormous advances have been made in medical research, cancer still remains as one of the leading causes of death. The effects of cancer impacts on many lives and patients' families. Also, this insidious disease represents a huge financial and socioeconomic burden to both the family and health care systems.

Cancer is a multigenetic, multicellular and multisystemic disease. Recently, the International Agency for Research on Cancer (IARC) announced that 7.6 million deaths were due to cancer and that there is on average 12.7 million new cases per year worldwide [1]. Current trends indicate that 63% of cancer deaths are from developing countries [2], [3].

Current conventional treatment options include surgery, chemotherapy and radiotherapy which can be used independently or sometimes, in combination. However, many of these treatment options are restricted to early stage tumours and even after surgery, there is still a high possibility of the tumour recurrence in these patients. In addition to the conventional treatments of cancer, there are also a number of relatively new therapies that include targeted cancer therapy, biological or immunotherapy and gene therapy. In contrast to conventional methods, these newly developed treatments can be more effective and have fewer side effects.

2. Solid tumour and its microenvironment

Cancer has two major forms: haemological cancers which are cancers arising from abnormal blood or bone marrow cells and solid tumours, which are tumours that grow into a solid mass. Traditionally, a solid mass were thought to be all rapidly dividing cells and all therapeutics were designed to stop or reverse cellular proliferation. More recent studies have determined finer details of the nature of solid tumours and their microenvironment in order to identify more specific targets for therapeutics and potential avenues for new cancer gene therapy. Hanahan and Weinberg [4] identified six hallmarks common to cancer:

Sustaining proliferative signaling: Within normal tissues, there is a carefully controlled production and release of growth-promoting signals. Cancer cells deregulate these signals and use them to their own advantage and may produce growth factor ligands for their own receptors. In addition to this autocrine proliferative stimulation, cancer cells may send signals to stimulate normal cells, within the tumour microenvironment or surrounding tissue, to supply the cancer cells with various growth factors [5], [6].

Evading growth suppressors: Cancer cells must evade the actions of tumour suppressor genes, which limit cell growth and proliferation. The two prototypical tumour suppressors encode the retinoblastoma-associated protein (RB) and tumour protein p53 (TP53) which govern the decision of cells to proliferate or to activate senescence (biological aging).

Resisting cell death: Programmed cell death by apoptosis plays an important role in cells as a natural barrier to cancer development. The structure of the apoptotic machinery and how cancer cells can avoid these mechanisms has been widely studied since beginning of last decade. Tumour cells evolve many strategies to limit or evade apoptosis. The most common one is the loss of TP53 tumour suppressor function [7].

Enabling replicative immortality: Cancer cells must have unlimited replicative potential in order to generate macroscopic tumours. Multiple studies suggest that telomeres, which are repetitive sequences at the ends of chromosomes, are centrally involved in the seemingly unlimited proliferation [8], [9].

Inducing angiogenesis: Like normal cells, tumour cells require the uptake of nutrients and oxygen as well as discharge carbon dioxide and metabolic waste. Since tumour cells grow faster than normal vasculature, tumour cells keep demanding the growth of the surrounding vasculature. The induction of angiogenesis addresses some needs in this vicious cycle, facilitating sustained expansion of neoplastic growth [10].

Activating invasion and metastasis: Metastasis is responsible for as much as 90% of cancer-associated mortality. In order for a primary tumour to metastasize it must achieve the following steps: *1) Intravasation*: At first, a cancer cell locally invades tissues in close proximity and thereby enters the microvasculature of the circulatory and lymphatic systems. *2) Extravasation:* In the microvasculature, a tumour cell maintains itself and begins its movement through the bloodstream to microvessels of distant tissues where it leaves the bloodstream. *3) Colonization:* The migrated tumour cell survives within the microenvironment of its new location and uses the local tissue for cell proliferation and a secondary macroscopic tumour formation [11].

More recent studies showed that, once a solid tumour reaches approximately 2 mm, it contains hypoxic regions as a result of the failure of angiogenesis to keep pace with abnormal tumourous tissue growth. Studies have shown that hypoxia can inhibit tumour cell differentiation and promote maintenance of cancer stem cells. Hypoxia also blocks the differentiation of mesenchymal stem/progenitor cells, which is a potential source of tumour-associated stromal cells [12]. There are also the extracellular matrix in solid tumours which is composed of complex secretions of proteins and proteoglycans produced by both neoplastic and normal stromal cells. This network continuously regulates signaling between tumour and normal stromal cells [13]. Traditionally, this microenvironment limits or prevents the effectiveness of many traditional as well as new therapies. Clearly, researchers need to develop new therapeutic strategies if we wish to successfully cure this disease. One such approach may be cancer gene therapy; however, research needs to also look at effective delivery of these agents in order to overcome the barriers set by these tumours and their microenvironment.

3. Targeted cancer therapy

Targeted cancer therapeutics are chemical agents or monoclonal antibodies that specifically inhibit the growth and spread of cancer by interfering with cell proliferation. These strategies interfere with cancer cell division and spread in different ways. Many of these therapies focus on proteins that are involved in cell signaling pathways, which form a complex communication system that governs basic cellular functions and activities. By blocking signaling pathways that make cancer cells grow and divide uncontrollably, targeted cancer therapies may induce cancer cell death through a process known as apoptosis, thus helping to stop cancer progression [18], [19].

Targeted monoclonal antibodies may also be able to modulate immune responses, which raise the possibility that these treatment strategies can be combined with other therapeutic approaches to improve clinical outcomes [20]. Many targeted therapies against tumours affect pathways that are also crucial for immune development and function. This suggests the possibility that targeted therapies may help to optimize anti-tumour immune responses from immunotherapies. Similarly, immunotherapies may serve to consolidate impressive clinical responses from targeted therapies into long-lasting clinical remissions [21]. Immunotherapy on the other hand, endeavors to stimulate a host immune response that effectuates long-lived tumour destruction.

3.1. Biological therapy

Biological therapy (immunotherapy or biotherapy,) is a method that uses a biological agent or the body's immune system, either directly or indirectly, to fight against cancer whereas traditional therapies target the tumour itself. For this reason, biological therapy can be used to lessen the side effects caused by other cancer treatments. For instance, dendritic cell-activated cytokine-induced killer cells, used after chemotherapy in patients with advanced non-small cell lung cancer, improve immune response associated with up-regulation of cytokines that are involved in the anti-tumour activity [22].

Using sipuleucel T and ipilimumab in phase III clinical trials the principle that immunotherapy can also extend cancer patient survival has been validated [23]. Sipuleucel T, which has recently been approved by the US Food and Drug Administration (FDA) for use in metastatic prostate cancer, aims to stimulate T cells that are specific for prostatic acid phosphatase (PAP), a protein that is overexpressed in prostate carcinoma cells [24]. Although the precise basis of action for sipuleucel T remains under study, treatment with this drug increases survival by an average of 4 months with minimal toxicity.

Ipilimumab, an antibody, bolsters T cell responses and potentiates tumour destruction by blocking an important inhibitory signal for activated T cells. Ipilimumab, which has recently been approved by the FDA for use in patients with advanced melanoma, enhances overall survival compared with standard care and, most notably, achieves durable benefits (more than 2.5 years) for 15–20% of treated patients [26], [27].

Agents that target interleukins have also been used in cancer therapy. Blocking IL-6 signaling is a potential therapeutic strategy for cancer characterized by pathological IL-6 overproduction [27]. Researchers have demonstrated that the recombinant immunotoxin IL6 (T23)-PE38KDEL kills IL6R-overexpressing cancer cells, and causes significant tumour regression [28]. Other studies have shown that using viral and non-viral vectors to overexpress IL-24 in human cancer cells results in inhibition of tumour growth both *in vitro* and *in vivo* [29]. Targeted therapies and cancer immunotherapies have begun to enter clinical practice recently and when they were used together they may become promising treatments; however, these combinations have not been well studied.

4. Gene therapy

Gene therapy is a relatively new method compared to other conventional treatments. It involves a therapeutic gene that is selectively delivered to a specific cell or tissue using a vector or delivery vehicle. The first successful treatment of a human disease using gene therapy techniques (as an *ex vivo* gene replacement therapy) was for the treatment of X-linked severe combined immunodeficiency (X-SCID). The replacement of the wild type gene in the bone marrow stem cells was stably expressed and conferred selective growth advantage over the defective T cells. Following treatment, eight patients were cured of this disease but unfortunately 2 patients developed abnormal white blood cell growth due to the oncogenesis ability of the retroviral vector used for gene delivery [30].

Viral vectors are the most widely used vector system for gene therapy. Within Europe and the United States, gene therapy protocols are mostly used for cancer. Cancer gene therapy research has focused mainly on melanoma, prostate cancer, ovarian cancer and leukemia [31]. Some of these protocols for cancer gene therapy include the thymidine kinase gene and the genes for immunomodulatory cytokines such as IL-2 or granulocyte-macrophage colony-stimulating factor (GM-CSF) and have been met with varying success [32]. Early clinical trials of gene therapy used *ex vivo* delivery of therapeutic genes to patients with monogenetic diseases. Such therapeutic genes, ie.: cytokine genes and viral thymidine kinase genes were transduced into autologous cells, normal cells or/and cancer cells. However, delivery of these therapeutic genes had limited efficacy due to their inability to achieve a pharmacological dose of the gene at the target tissue. *In vivo* gene therapy protocols have used mostly viral vectors for gene delivery. A large barrier for systemic gene therapy is reduced efficacy of transduction. Some of the other obstacles that affect efficacy of cancer gene therapy include: 1). identification of key target genes responsible for the disease pathology and progression; 2). identification of therapeutic genes that can inhibit disease progression; 3). optimal trans-gene expression for suppressing the target gene; and 4). delivery of therapeutic product to the target tissue at an efficacious dose [33]. Components of gene therapy for cancer can be replacement of tumour suppressor gene (p53), inhibition of oncogenes with antisense oligonucleotides, ribozymes and short inhibitory RNA, and activation of apoptosis genes [33]- [37]. However, sometimes the inhibition of the target gene and its pathway is not sufficient to inhibit the disease process because the cells have built abundant or alternative pathways to compensate [35].

The efficient transgene expression requires appropriate promoters and enhancers in order to extend the duration of transgene expression in the cell or tissue. There are two types of promoters: constitutive or inducible. The constitutive promoters can be either viral or tissue specific promoters, such as melanin for melanoma. Inducible promoters can be induced to express transgenes with hormones or small molecules. Location of enhancers is upstream of the promoters and their function is to increase transgene expression 2-100 fold if the amount of gene product is required in very high amounts in the cell. In cancer cells, the duration of transgene expression can be up to 30 days [33], [38].

5. Gene delivery

Delivery of therapeutic genes is one of the most difficult issues in gene therapy studies. All viral gene therapy strategies have significant delivery limitations and very narrow applications for cells and tissues. The best method for delivering genes will depend on the type of tissue to be targeted [36]. Commonly used vectors are retroviruses, adenoviruses, adeno-associated viruses and herpes simplex viruses. For cancer gene therapy, replication competent viruses such as the Newcastle disease virus offer a promising delivery technology for human tumour therapy [38].

In addition to viral delivery methods there are non-viral technologies that offer several advantages including less toxicity, reduced adverse immune responses and ease of producing larger quantities of vectors [39]. Chemically synthesized nanoparticles like DNA/stearyl polylysine coated lipids or DNA coated with glycine oligomers (Peptoids) offer new advances for systemic gene therapy delivery. These molecules have been shown to be effective in cancer related angiogenesis [40].

In addition, bacterium has been developed for gene delivery purposes in cancer patients. The hypoxia and solid tumour microenvironment provide a living haven for anaerobic bacteria. These so far fall into three classes. 1). Gram-positive lactic acid producing anaerobic bacteria; 2). Gram-negative intracellular, facultative anaerobes; and 3). the Gram-positive strictly anaerobic, saccharolytic/proteolytic Clostridia. Some of these modified bacterial cells, such as *Salmonella* and *Clostridium novyi* are already in phase 1 clinical studies [41].

5.1. Bacterial oncolysis

A surgeon named William B. Coley described for the first time that bacteria could be used as anticancer agents in 1890 [14]. Since then, scientists have been researching, and engineering, microorganisms such as *Clostridium, Bifidobacterium, Salmonella, Mycobacterium,* and *Bacillus* which have the ability to specifically target cancer cells and cause oncolysis. These anaerobic bacteria grow in the hypoxic core of solid tumours, where most traditional and many emerging therapeutics are unsuccessful. Due to their specificity for the tumour microenvironment, these bacteria are also promising vectors for delivering therapeutic genes to the cancer patients [15].

The hypoxic nature of solid tumours is a haven for bacterial colonization and proliferation. It has been suggested that the anaerobic nature of hypoxic-necrotic regions within tumours provide faster growth of anaerobic and facultative anaerobic bacteria. Necrotic areas may also provide purines to the further growth of bacteria [16], [17].

6. The use of small oligonucleotides for gene silencing

In 1998, Fire et al [42] discovered a mechanism, which is called RNA interference (RNAi), that moderates the activity of genes by using small single-stranded ribosomal nucleic acids.. These nucleic acids can bind to other molecules and play important roles in cells. It has been shown that small RNAs have the ability to control gene expression and other activities that were assumed to be carried out only by proteins. As a result RNAi has become a promising tool for researchers in the treatment of genetic diseases and cancer.

RNAi applications have a huge potential for use in inhibiting targets. To compare with molecular drugs, RNAi technology promises more specificity and wide range target capacity. Small RNAs that used in RNAi technology currently have been grouped into four major classes: small interfering RNAs (siRNA), short hairpin RNA (shRNA), microRNAs (miRNAs), and P-element-induced wimpy testis (PIWI) interacting RNAs (piRNA). In addition to these there are also qiRNA and other unknown small RNAs still to be discovered [43], [44].

6.1. siRNA

Synthetic siRNA was used in gene silencing firstly as an RNAi technology [45]. In the process, long dsRNA molecules were cut into 19-23 nucleotide RNAs, called siRNAs, which guide for cleaveage of complementary RNAs [46]. siRNA directly incorporates into RNA-induced silencing complex (RISC), where its guide-strand binds to and cleaves the complementary mRNA. After the cleaved mRNA is released and degraded, the RISC binds to another mRNA and starts a new cycle of cleavage [47]. siRNA can cleave its target RNA in both the cytoplasm and the nucleus [48].

Moreover, siRNAs are able to act as primers for an RNA-dependent RNA polymerase that synthesizes extra dsRNA, that results in additional siRNA, which reinforces the effect of the original siRNA [49], [50].

6.2. shRNA

Short hairpin RNA (shRNA) has been developed for long-term gene silencing [51]- [53]. shRNA is transcribed in the nucleus from short double-stranded DNA sequence with a hairpin loop. After that the shRNA transcript is processed and incorporates with RISC in the cytoplasm in a process that is the same as siRNA. However, there are some differences between siRNA and shRNA. Firstly, less than 1% of duplex siRNA remains in the cells 48 hours after introduction to the cells due to the high rate of degradation and turnover, whereas shRNA is constantly synthesized in host cells, leading to more durable gene silencing. Secondly, vector-based shRNA can only be modified by manipulating the expression strategy because it is firstly synthesized in the nucleus then transported to cytoplasm for further processes. Major component of RISC is the argonaute proteins. Within these protein family only Ago2 shows endonuclease activity to cleave shRNA in order to make it active single stranded [54].

6.3. MicroRNA

MicroRNA (miRNA) is another group of small non-coding RNAs. miRNAs are important for gene regulation and highly conserved in cells. miRNA is firstly transcribed from precursors, that are located within intergenic sequences or introns, as a primary transcript (pri-miRNA) in the nucleus. Secondly, pre-miRNA is processed by an RNase III endonuclease called Drosha and then is exported to the cytoplasm. In the cytoplasm, pre-miRNA is cleaved by Dicer, another RNase III enzyme, to make 20-23 base pair long mature miRNA that consists of both guide and passengers strands with mismatches. Mature miRNA cooperates with RISC to inhibit translation with target mRNA degradation [55].

One major difference between siRNA, shRNA, and miRNA is that both siRNA and shRNA require a complete match with the target mRNA but miRNA does not. Change in expression of a single miRNA may affect more than hundreds different genes [56]. miRNA takes part in gene regulation in different ways. Firstly miRNA binds to the 3′ UTR region of the target mRNA and repress translation [55]. Nevertheless, a number of studies have shown that miRNA can also recognize coding region or the 5′ UTR region to inhibit gene expression, although with less efficiency than at the 3′ UTR [57], [58]. Other studies have also shown that miRNA can bind to the 5′ UTR region of an mRNA and promote protein translation or can bind to DNA and induce gene expression [59], [60]. It has been stated that failure in regulation of miRNA can cause a various human diseases, including cancer [61]. Better understanding of mechanism and regulation of miRNA can contributes to develop effective RNAi therapies of cancer and other diseases.

6.4. piRNA

P-element-induced wimpy testis (PIWI) interacting RNAs (piRNAs) are small non-coding RNAs which interact PIWI proteins. These proteins are clade of argonaute proteins and are expressed predominantly in the germlines of a variety of organisms such as *Drosophila* and mammals. piRNAs help to maintain silence repetitive elements, the integrity of the genome, and the development of gametes. It has been suggested that both PIWI proteins and piRNAs are required for transposon silencing. In addition, a subset of piRNAs in *Drosophila* has been shown to function in silencing protein-coding genes [62].

piRNA–PIWI complexes are assumed to directly control transposon activity. piRNAs bound to PIWI proteins show homology-dependent target cleavage *in vitro*. Therefore, transposons are probably silenced through post-transcriptional transcript destruction [63].

piRNAs are different from siRNAs and miRNAs in several ways: 1) piRNAs consist of mostly 24–31 nucleotides whereas other non-coding small RNAs are approximately 21 nucleotides; 2) opposite to several hundred species of miRNAs, piRNAs have 50,000 cloned species; 3) many piRNAs match to the genome in clusters of 20–90 kilobases in a strand-specific manner. In some clusters, one strand is changed abruptly to another strand which suggest that these bidirectional clusters may be transcribed divergently from a central promoter, however, siRNAs and miRNAs are derived from double-stranded and short hairpin RNA precursors, respectively. 4) Some piRNAs may be involved in epigenetic regulation whereas siRNAs and miRNAs generally target mRNAs [64], [65].

7. RNAi phenomena and its use in cancer therapy

Due to their robustness and specificity, siRNA and shRNA have been extensively used to silence cancer-related gene targets. For instance, metastatic pancreatic cancer is one of the most deadly cancers. The overexpression of pancreatic duodenal homebox-1 (PDX-1) in pancreatic adenocarcinoma has been shown to act as an oncogene. A plasmid vector encoding shRNA was used to target PDX-1 expression in a pancreatic animal model. Further examination showed that the expression of PDX-1 was significantly reduced compared with that of the control group. As a result, silencing of PDX-1 expression inhibited tumour growth in malignant pancreatic cancer [66], [67].

Another example is human enhancer of zeste homolog 2 (EZH2) or p110-alpha silencing by siRNA with A systemic delivery vector in advanced prostate cancer in which tumour cells frequently metastasize to bones and regional lymph nodes. It has been shown that siRNA targeted to these proteins inhibit tumour metastasis in these cells [68]. Ryo *et al* have also shown that retrovirus-encoded shRNA was used to silence Pin1 expression in a prostate cancer model. Pin1 is a peptidyl-prolyl isomerase which catalyzes the cis/trans isomerization of peptidyl-prolyl peptide bonds [69]. It is highly overexpressed in prostate and breast cancers. Pin1 shRNA significantly inhibited tumour growth and tumour metastasis.

Angiogenesis is a charecteristic for neoplasia and tumour metastasis. The vascular endothelial growth factor (VEGF) pathway is the most important pathway in angiogenesis. siRNA has been used to selectively silence VEGF and VEGF receptors to arrest tumour growth and angiogenesis successfully. Tumour growth was markedly suppressed [70]. Moreover, the siRNA targeting VEGF receptor 2 (VEGFR2) presented a significant inhibition of tumour growth with reduced VEGFR2 expression [71]. miRNAs affect malignant process by either resulting in overexpression or downregulation of a gene product. miRNA has been used as a tumour repressor in tumours with reduced expression of tumour supressor genes or other key genes. For example, miR-26a is highly expressed in normal liver tissues but its expression is downregulated in liver tumours. Patients who have low miR-26a expression have decreased overall survival compared with patients who have high miR-26a expression [72]. Further, miR-34c, miR-145, and miR-142-5p also show tumour suppresion properties in several lung cancers. Replacement of downregulated miRNA causes discontinue the growth of lung cancer cells [73].

Due to miRNAs ability to supress tumours, miRNA gene therapy can be used for retriving miRNA gene expression and prevent tumour development. This approach is principally similar to that used for siRNA/shRNA therapeutics except that miRNAs are used to regain miRNA expression. For instance miR-34a is usually lost in human cancers especially lung cancer and prostate cancer. Using a neutral lipid emulsion (NLE), systemic delivery of synthetic miR-43a causes accumulation of miR-34a in normal lung tissues and lung tumours [74]. Furthermore, miR-34a and miR-16 are tumour suppressors of prostate cancer. miR-34a blocks metastasis of prostate cancer by repressing CD44 while miR-16 uses as target CDK1 and CDK2 genes which involves cell-cycle progression and cell proliferation [75], [76]. Another miRNA subtype miR-22 induces cellular senescence. In a breast cancer xenograft model, synthetic miR-22 induced cellular senescence and inhibited tumour growth by intratumoural delivery [77].

The effective delivery of miRNA for cancer therapy can be achieved with either plasmid or virus. Kota *et al* has shown that miR-26a, of which re-expression in liver cancer cells inhibits cyclin D2 and E2 and induces G1 arrest, was delivered into hepatocellular tumour by using adeno-associated virus where it was sucessful in inhibiting of tumour development [78].

8. Modulating key genes controlling cancer metabolism

In general, normal cells produce most of the ATP from glucose through oxidative phosphorylation [79]. On the contrary, many cancer cells produce ATP by conversion of glucose to lactate and show lower oxidative phosphorylation activity. Tumour cells keep high yields of lactic acid and produce ATP by aerobic glycolysis with or without oxygen. This phenomenon is called "Warburg effect" [80].

Accelerated glycolysis provides ATP levels to the fast proliferating tumour cells in a hypoxic environment. Along with increased glutaminolysis, it also supplies metabolic intermediates that are essential for macromolecule biosynthesis and necessary for cell growth and division

[81]. Although the conversion of pyruvate into lactate occurs in normal cells in hypoxic conditions, tumour cells produce excessive amounts of lactate even when oxygen is not a limiting factor. It has been stated that this glycolytic phenotype results from the adaptation of premalignant lesions to spasmodic hypoxia [82].

Down-regulation or completely silencing genes that are related with cancer metabolism may be the key of future methods of cancer treatment. Hexokinase II and pyruvate kinase M_2 are some of metabolic genes that have been focused on in siRNA studies. It has been shown that down-regulated hexokinase II by RNA interference resulted in increased apoptosis rate in colon cancer cells [83]. Inhibition of Pyruvate Kinase M_2, a metabolic enzyme whose expression in cancer cells results in aerobic glycolysis causes substantial tumor regression [84]. Another study have indicated that combined therapy with siRNA and cisplatin drug resulted in enhanced antitumor activity [85].

9. Silencing telomerase activity by RNAi

There are specialized, repeated structures called telomere which protect the ends of all chromosomes in eukaryotic organisms [86]. Telomeres are essential for chromosome stability. Also, it is suggested that telomeres are responsible for cellular aging since it acts as a mitotic clock [87], [88]. Telomere shortening triggers the senescence check point so-called Hayflick limit in human somatic cells [89]. Escape from this check point is the first step in cellular immortalization [90].

In most organisms the main mechanism of telomere length maintenance is carried out by telomerase, a ribonucleoprotein complex [91]. This enzyme elongates the telomeres at the 3′ end of the DNA [92]. Although the telomerase complex contains a number of components that provide telomerase activity *in vivo*, the basic components of telomerase enzyme are telomerase reverse transcriptase (TERT) and telomerase RNA [93]. Increase expression of these Proteins results in high telomerase activity and has been demonstrated in 85-90% of all human tumours [94].

Currently, attempts are underway for reducing telomerase activity which may provide a potential avenue for cancer gene therapy. Kosciolek *et al* has shown that telomerase activity in human cancer cells can be inhibited by siRNAs targeting telomerase components [95]. Human cancer cell lines were transfected with 21 nucleotide double-stranded RNA homologous to either the catalytic subunit of telomerase (hTERT) or to its template RNA (hTR). Both agents reduced telomerase activity in a variety of human cancer cell lines which included both carcinomas and sarcomas.

10. Other gene silencing approaches in cancer therapy

B cell lymphoma 2 (BCL2) is an important gene in eukaryotic cells as its expression causes uncontrolled growth by inhibiting cell death [96]. Overexpression of BCL2 protein has been reported in many types of human cancers, including leukemias, lymphomas, and carcinomas [97]. Cimmino *et al* demonstrate that miR-15a and miR-16-1 expression is inversely correlated to BCL2 expression in chronic lymphocytic leukemia (CLL) [98]. Both these miRNAs negatively regulate BCL2 at a posttranscriptional level. BCL2 repression by miR-15a and miR-16-1 induces apoptosis in a leukemic cell line model. As a result, miR-15 and miR-16 are natural BCL2 inhibitors that could be used for therapy of tumours in which BCL-2 overexpresses.

Another protein which is cyclooxygenase-2 (COX-2) enzyme has been involved in the tumourgenesis and in the progression of colorectal cancer (CRC) [99]. The use of developing RNAi-based techniques allowed researchers to better study the molecular and phenotypical loss of function of COX-2 gene by doing experiments based on a strong COX-2 silencing effects. Denkert and colleagues [100] tested the effect of an anti-COX-2 siRNA (siCOX-2) on OVCAR-3 cells derived from human ovarian carcinoma. A comparison with the COX-2 inhibitory drug NS-398 has shown that a different effect of siCOX-2 occured due to its highly specific mechanism of action. Even though COX-2 protein levels significantly reduced in both cases, NS-398 treatment induced a G0/G1 cell cycle arrest in OVCAR-3 cells but only after another factor stimulation. This effect was probably due to the action of NS-398 on other cellular targets involved in cell proliferation.

Research performed by Charames *et al* and Kobayashi *et al* demonstrated that an siRNAs can efficiently knockdown COX-2 in HT-29 human colon cancer cells and bovine Cumulus-Granulosa (CG) cells [101], [102]. Based on their results, it is clear that RNAi, compared with non-steroidal anti-inflammatory drug (NSAIDs), are more powerful and selective tools for studying *in vitro* COX-2 functioning [103]- [106].

RNAi-mediated COX-2 silencing proved to be highly effective using anti-COX-2 shRNAs (shCOX-2). In 2006, Strillaci *et al* have illustrated that an *in vitro* strategy in which COX-2 is stably knockdowned in colon cancer cells (HT- 29) [107]. There are several studies that have implicated failure of miR expression in carcinogenic mechanisms [108], [109]. miR concentrations may be increased or repressed in hepatocellular carcinoma, which suggests that these sequences may act as oncogenes or suppressors of hepatocyte transformation. Recent studies using miRNA microarrays showed that high expression of miR-21 can contribute to growth and spread of human hepatocellular cancer (HCC) by inhibiting phosphatase and tensin homolog (PTEN) tumour suppressor, whereas low levels of miR-122a which target to cyclin G1 mRNA result in increased HCC [110], [111].

One of the cancer-related genes is the multiple drug resistance (MDR1) gene which provides resistance to vinca alkaloids (vinblastine, vincristine), anthracyclins (adriamycin, daunorubicin), etoposide and paclitaxel. In order to reverse the MDR1 gene-dependent multidrug resistance (MDR), two siRNA constructs were designed to inhibit MDR1 expression by RNA interference. Some data indicate that this approach may be applicable to cancer patients to change from tumouric P-glycoprotein-dependent MDR phenotype back to a drug-sensitive one [112]. An Eppstein Barr Virus (EBV)-encoded product, latent membrane protein (LMP-1), is considered to be an oncogene playing an essential role in cell transformation and metastasis. EBV-encoded LMP-1 was inhibited by RNAi and selective inhibition of LMP-1 had anti-proliferation effect on Nasopharyngeal carcinoma (NPC) cell. RNAi could be a powerful method in further investigations of LMP-1 [113]. A recombinant adeno-associated virus type 2 vector was used to deliver shRNA targeting EBV-LMP-1 into the EBV-positive human NPC C666-1 cells. Results showed that long-term suppression of EBV-encoded LMP-1 *in vivo* is an effective way for preventing NPC metastasis [114].

One of the most important signaling pathways to control growth and proliferation of our cells is the mitogen-activated protein kinase (MAPK) pathway. Ras, which is an enzyme in this pathway, is turned to an oncogenic form in about 15% of human cancer. Suppression of tumourgenicity was done by virus-mediated RNAi to inhibit specifically the oncogenic allele of K-ras (K-rasV12) in human tumour cells [115]. Other studies have reported that the use of siRNA can further block the Ras to Map kinase cascade, at either the Raf level or through NADPH oxidase1 (Nox1)[116]- [118].

11. Conclusion

Cancer is widely recognised as one of the largest burdens to health world wide. Some main features of cancers are its ability to sustain proliferative signaling, evade growth suppressors, resist cell death, enable replicative immortality, induce angiogenesis, and activate invasion and metastasis. Until now, many methods have been developed for the treatment of cancer. Conventional treatment methods, ie.: surgery, chemotherapy and radiotherapy, are still widely used in the treatment of most cancers. However, these methods result in a high recurrence of cancer in patients. Clearly, there is an urgent need for the development of new therapies. In contrast to conventional methods, targeted gene therapy, immunotherapy, and gene therapy offer promising alternatives that are more effective and produce less side effects. Both targeted therapies and cancer immunotherapies have recently been used in clinic and these therapies can be succesful when used together, nevertheless, there are still limitations with these therapies.

Gene therapy has already begun to show great promise and is expected to be more effective in curing cancer. Targets for cancer gene therapy may include tumour suppressor genes (e.g. p53), oncogenes,and apoptosis genes. The most problematic issue for cancer gene therapy studies is the delivery of the therapheutic gene to the tumour cells. Although viral delivery methods are widely in use, there are non-viral technologies that offer several advantages that include less toxicity, reduced adverse immune responses and easier to producing large amounts of gene products. More recently, bacteria have also been used in cancer treatment. The hypoxic nature of solid tumours provides considerable conditions for growth of bacteria and bacterial colonisation. Necrotic areas can also supply purines to further facilitate growth of bacteria.

Bacterial delivery of RNA silencing tools combined with benefit of bacterial oncolysis can contribute to the treatment of cancer. Exploiting of small oligonucleic acids which are carried by spesific bacteria to cancer cells can be an effective way to cut energy supply and lysis of tumor cells.

Small oligonucleic acids can form complex secondary and tertiary structures. These nucleic acids can bind to other molecules and play an important role in cells. It has been shown that small RNAs have the ability to control gene expression and other activities that previously were assumed to be carried out only by proteins. As a result, small fragments of RNA may be tools for researchers to cure cancer. Small RNAs that are used in RNAi technology currently have been grouped into three major classes: small interfering RNAs (siRNA), microRNAs (miRNAs), and PIWI interacting RNAs (piRNA).

siRNA and shRNA have been extensively used to silence cancer-related targets. miRNA, as a tumour supressor, can be used in gene therapy for retrieving miRNA gene expression and preventing tumour development. Tumour cells keep high yields of lactic acid and produce ATP by aerobic glycolysis with or without oxygen. Accelerated glycolysis provides ATP levels to the fast proliferating tumour cells in a hypoxic environment. It is proposed that with RNA interference technologies metabolic genes in cancer cells can be silenced. Therefore tumour proliferation can be inhibited. Beside that, studies have shown that genes which are related to cancer such as Telomerase, BCL-2, COX-2 can be silenced for preventing cancer.

Author details

Onur Sakiragaoglu[1], David Good[1,2] and Ming Q. Wei[1*]

*Address all correspondence to: m.wei@griffith.edu.au

1 Division of Molecular and Gene Therapies, Griffith Health Institute and School of Medical Science, Griffith University, Gold Coast, QLD, Australia

2 School of Physiotherapy, Australian Catholic University, Banyo, QLD, Australia

References

[1] International Agency for Research on Cancer (IARC): GLOBOCAN (2008). Cancer incidence and mortality worldwide. Lyon, France: IARC. 2010.

[2] Jemal, A, Bray, F, Center, M. M, Ferlay, J, Ward, E, & Forman, D. Global cancer statistics. CA Cancer J Clin. (2011). , 61, 69-90.

[3] Ferlay, J, Shin, H. R, Bray, F, Forman, D, Mathers, C, & Parkin, D. M. Estimates of worldwide burden of cancer in 2008: GLOBOCAN 2008. Int J Cancer. (2010). , 127, 2893-2917.

[4] Hanahan, D, & Weinberg, R. The hallmarks of cancer. Cell. (2000). , 100, 57-70.

[5] Cheng, N, Chytil, A, Shyr, Y, Joly, A, & Moses, H. L. Transforming growth factor-beta signaling-deficient fibroblasts enhance hepatocyte growth factor signaling in

mammary carcinoma cells to promote scattering and invasion. Mol Cancer Res. (2008). , 6, 1521-1533.

[6] Bhowmick, N. A, Neilson, E. G, & Moses, H. L. Stromal fibroblasts in cancer initiation and progression. Nature. (2004). , 432, 332-337.

[7] Hanahan, D, & Weinberg, R. Hallmarks of cancer: the next generation. Cell. (2011). , 44, 646-674.

[8] Blasco, M. A. Telomeres and human disease: ageing, cancer and beyond. Nat Rev Genet. (2005). , 6, 611-622.

[9] Shay, J. W, & Wright, W. E. Hayflick, his limit, and cellular ageing. Nat Rev Mol Cell Biol. (2000). , 1, 72-76.

[10] Hanahan, D, & Folkman, J. Patterns and emerging mechanisms of the angiogenic switch during tumourigenesis. Cell. (1996). , 86, 353-364.

[11] Chaffer, C. L, & Weinberg, R. A. A perspective on cancer cell metastasis. Science. (2011). , 331, 1559-1564.

[12] Lin, Q, & Yun, Z. Impact of the hypoxic tumour microenvironment on the regulation of cancer stem cell characteristics. Cancer Biol Ther. (2010).

[13] Wojton, J, & Kaur, B. Impact of tumour microenvironment on oncolytic viral therapy. Cytokine Growth Factor Rev. (2010).

[14] Nauts, H. C, Swift, W. E, & Coley, B. L. The treatment of malignant tumors by bacterial toxins as developed by the late William B. Coley, M. D., Reviewed in the light of modern research. Cancer Res. (1946). , 6, 205-216.

[15] Fialho, A. M. das Gupta TK, Chakrabarty AM. Promiscuous drugs from pathogenic bacteria in the post-antibiotics era. In Patho- Biotechnology book. Landes Bioscience. (2008). , 145-62.

[16] Wei, M. Q, Mengesha, A, Good, D, & Anné, J. Bacterial targeted tumour therapy-dawn of a new era. Cancer Lett. (2007). , 259, 16-27.

[17] Al-mariri, A, Tibor, A, Lestrate, P, Mertens, P, De Bolle, X, & Letesson, J. J. Yersinia enterocolitica as a vehicle for a naked DNA vaccine encoding Brucella abortus bacterioferritin or antigen. Infect Immunol. (2002). , 39.

[18] Mok, T. S, Wu, Y. L, Thongprasert, S, Yang, C. H, Chu, D. T, Saijo, N, Sunpaweravong, P, Han, B, Margono, B, Ichinose, Y, Nishiwaki, Y, Ohe, Y, Yang, J. J, Chewaskulyong, B, Jiang, H, Duffield, E. L, Watkins, C. L, Armour, A. A, & Fukuoka, M. Gefitinib or carboplatin-paclitaxel in pulmonary adenocarcinoma. N Engl J Med. (2009). , 361, 947-57.

[19] Sandler, A, Gray, R, Perry, M. C, Brahmer, J, Schiller, J. H, Dowlati, A, Lilenbaum, R, & Johnson, D. H. Paclitaxel-carboplatin alone or with bevacizumab for non-small cell lung cancer. N Engl J Med. (2006). , 355, 2542-50.

[20] National Cancer Institute (at the National Institutes of Health) official websiteAvailable from: http://www.cancer.gov/cancertopics/treatment/types-of-treatment.

[21] Vanneman, M, & Dranoff, G. Combining immunotherapy and targeted therapies in cancer treatment. Nat Rev Cancer. (2012). , 12(4), 237-51.

[22] Li, H, Wang, C, Yu, J, Cao, S, Wei, F, Zhang, W, Han, Y, & Ren, X. B. Dendritic cell-activated cytokine-induced killer cells enhance the anti-tumour effect of chemotherapy on non-small cell lung cancer in patients after surgery. Cytotherapy. (2009). , 11(8), 1076-83.

[23] Mellman, I, Coukos, G, & Dranoff, G. Cancer immunotherapy comes of age. Nature. (2011). , 480, 480-489.

[24] Kantoff, P. W, Higano, C. S, Shore, N. D, Berger, E. R, Small, E. J, Penson, D. F, Redfern, C. H, Ferrari, A. C, Dreicer, R, Sims, R. B, Xu, Y, Frohlich, M. W, & Schellhammer, P. F. IMPACT Study Investigators. Sipuleucel T immunotherapy for castration-resistant prostate cancer. N Engl J Med. (2010). , 363, 411-422.

[25] Korman, A, Peggs, K, & Allison, J. P. Checkpoint blockade in cancer immunotherapy. Adv Immunol. (2006). , 90, 293-335.

[26] Hodi, F. S, Day, O, Mcdermott, S, Weber, D. F, Sosman, R. W, Haanen, J. A, Gonzales, J. B, Robert, R, Schadendorf, C, Hassel, D, Akerley, J. C, Van Den, W, Eertwegh, A. J, Lutzky, J, Lorigan, P, Vaubel, J. M, Linette, G. P, Hogg, D, Ottensmeier, C. H, Lebbé, C, Peschel, C, Quirt, I, Clark, J. I, Wolchok, J. D, Weber, J. S, Tian, J, Yellin, M. J, Nichol, G. M, & Hoos, A. Urba WJ. Improved survival with ipilimumab in patients with metastatic melanoma. N Engl J Med. (2010). , 363, 711-723.

[27] Robert, C, Thomas, L, Bondarenko, I, Day, O, Garbe, S, M D J. W, Lebbe, C, Baurain, C, Testori, J. F, Grob, A, Davidson, J. J, Richards, N, Maio, J, Hauschild, M, Miller, A, Jr, W. H, Gascon, P, Lotem, M, Harmankaya, K, Ibrahim, R, Francis, S, Chen, T. T, Humphrey, R, Hoos, A, & Wolchok, J. D. Ipilimumab plus dacarbazine for previously untreated metastatic melanoma. N Engl J Med. (2011). , 64, 2517-2526.

[28] Guo, Y, Xu, F, Lu, T, Duan, Z, & Zhang, Z. Interleukin-6 signaling pathway in targeted therapy for cancer. Cancer Treat Rev. (2012). , 38(7), 904-10.

[29] Guo, D. J, Han, J. S, Li, Y. S, Liu, Z. S, Lu, S. Y, & Ren, H. L. in vitro and in vivo anti-tumour effects of the recombinant immunotoxin IL6(T23)-PE38KDEL in multiple myeloma. Oncol Lett. (2012).

[30] Ramesh, R, Ioannides, C. G, Roth, J. A, & Chada, S. Adenovirus-mediated interleukin (IL) 24 immunotherapy for cancer. Methods Mol Biol. (2010). , 51, 241 70.

[31] Kohn, D. B, Sadelain, M, & Glorioso, J. C. Occurrence of leukemia following gene therapy of X-linked SCID. Nat Rev Cancer. (2003). , 3(7), 477-88.

[32] Lechanteur, C, Delvenne, P, Princern, F, Lopez, M, Fillet , G, Gielen, J, Merville M-P, & Bours V. Combined suicide and cytokine gene therapy for peritoneal carcinomatosis. Gut. (2000). , 47, 343-348

[33] Gottesman, M. Cancer gene therapy: An awkward adolescence. Cancer Gene Ther. (2003). , 10, 501-508.

[34] Scanlon, K. J. Cancer gene therapy: challenges and opportunities. Anticancer Res. (2004). A):, 501-4.

[35] Lebedeva, I, & Stein, C. A. Antisense oligonucleotides: promise reality. Ann Rev Pharmacol Toxicol. (2001). , 41, 403-419.

[36] Scanlon, K. J, Ishida, H, & Kashani-sabet, M. Reversal of the multi-drug resistant phenotype by a fos ribozyme. Proc Natl Acad Sci USA. (1994). , 91, 11123-11127.

[37] Kashani-sabet, M, & Scanlon, K. J. The Cancer Handbook, London, England: Macmillan Publisher. (2002). Chapter 91: , 1439-1449.

[38] Ohta, Y, Kijima, H, Ohkawa, T, Kashani-sabet, M, & Scanlon, K. J. Suppression of the malignant phenotype of melanoma cells by anti-oncogene ribozymes. J Invest Derm. (1996). , 106, 275-280.

[39] Kirn, D, & Scanlon, K. J. Virotherapy for cancer-current status, hurdles and future directions. Cancer Gene Ther. (2002). , 9, 959-1067.

[40] Nishikawa, M, & Huang, L. Nonviral vectors in the new Millennium: Delivery barriers in gene transfer. Human Gene Ther. (2001). , 12, 861-870.

[41] Kirchweger, G. Nanoparticles-The next big thing? Mol Ther. (2002). , 6, 301-302.

[42] Nemunaitis, J, Cunningham, C, Senzer, N, Cramm, J, & Sznol, M. Pilot trial of genetically modified, attenuated Salmonella expressing the E. coli cytosine. Cancer Gene Ther. (2003). , 10(10), 737-44.

[43] Fire, A, Xu, S, Montgomery, M. K, Kostas, S. A, Driver, S. E, & Mello, C. C. Potent and specific genetic interference by double-stranded RNA in Caenorhabditis elegans. Nature. (1998). , 391, 806-11.

[44] Farazi, T. A, Juranek, S. A, & Tuschl, T. The growing catalog of small RNAs and their association with distinct Argonaute/Piwi family members. Development. (2008). , 135(7), 1201-14.

[45] Olejniczak, M, Galka, P, & Krzyzosiak, W. J. Sequence-non-specific effects of RNA interference triggers and microRNA regulators. Nucleic Acids Res. (2010). , 38(1), 1-16.

[46] Elbashir, S. M, Harborth, J, Lendeckel, W, Yalcin, A, Weber, K, & Tuschi, T. Duplexes of nucleotide RNAs mediate RNA interference in cultured mammalian cells. Nature. (2001). , 21.

[47] Parrish, S, Fleenor, J, Xu, S, Mello, C, & Fire, A. Functional anatomy of a dsRNA trigger: differential requirement for the two trigger strands in RNA interference. Mol Cell. (2000). , 6(5), 1077-1087.

[48] Wang, Z, Rao, D. D, Senzer, N, & Nemunaitis, J. RNA Interference and Cancer Therapy. Pharm Res. (2011). , 28, 2983-2995.

[49] Robb, G. B, Brown, K. M, Khurana, J, & Rana, T. M. Specific and potent RNAi in the nucleus of human cells. Nat Struct Mol Biol. (2005). , 12, 133-7.

[50] Sijen, T, Fleenor, J, Simmer, F, Thijssen, K. L, Parrish, S, Timmons, L, Plasterk, R. H, & Fire, A. On the role of RNA amplification in dsRNA-triggered gene silencing. Cell. (2001). , 107(4), 465-476.

[51] Lipardi, C, Wei, Q, & Paterson, B. M. RNAi as random degradative PCR: siRNA primers convert mRNA into dsRNAs that are degraded to generate new siRNAs. Cell (2001). , 107, 297-307.

[52] Lee, N. S, Dohjima, T, Bauer, G, Li, H, Li, M. J, Ehsani, A, Salvaterra, P, & Rossi, J. Expression of small interfering RNAs targeted against HIV-1 rev transcripts in human cells. Nat Biotechnol. (2002). , 20, 500-5.

[53] Yu, J. Y, Deruiter, S. L, & Turner, D. L. RNA interference by expression of short-interfering RNAs and hairpin RNAs in mammalian cells. Proc Natl Acad Sci USA. (2002). , 99, 6047-52.

[54] Miyagishiand, M, & Taira, K. U. promoter-driven siRNAs with four uridine 3′ overhangs efficiently suppress targeted gene expression in mammalian cells. Nat Biotechnol. (2002). , 20, 497-500.

[55] Rao, D. D, Vorhies, J. S, Senzer, N, & Nemunaitis, J. siRNA vs. shRNA: similarities and differences. Adv Drug Deliv Rev. (2009). , 61, 746-59.

[56] Bartel, D. P. MicroRNAs: genomics, biogenesis, mechanism, and function. Cell. (2004). , 116, 281-97.

[57] John, B, Enright, A. J, Aravin, A, Tuschl, T, Sander, C, & Marks, D. S. Human MicroRNA targets. PLoS Biol. (2004). e363.

[58] Tay, Y, Zhang, J, Thomson, A. M, Lim, B, & Rigoutsos, I. MicroRNAs to Nanog, Oct4 and Sox2 coding regions modulate embryonic stem cell differentiation. Nature. (2008). , 455, 1124-8.

[59] Lytle, J. R, Yario, T. A, & Steitz, J. A. Target mRNAs are repressed as efficiently by microRNA-binding sites in the 5′ UTR as in the 3′UTR. Proc Natl Acad Sci USA. (2007). , 104, 9667-72.

[60] Orom, U. A, Nielsen, F. C, & Lund, A. H. MicroRNA-10a binds the 5′UTR of ribosomal protein mRNAs and enhances their translation. Mol Cell. (2008). , 30, 460-71.

[61] Place, R. F, Li, L. C, Pookot, D, Noonan, E. J, & Dahiya, R. MicroRNA-373 induces expression of genes with complementary promoter sequences. Proc Natl Acad Sci USA. (2008). , 105, 1608-13.

[62] Lu, M, Zhang, Q, Deng, M, Miao, J, Guo, Y, Gao, W, & Cui, Q. An analysis of human microRNA and disease associations. PLoS One. (2008). e3420.

[63] Siomi, M. C, Mannen, T, & Siomi, H. How does the royal family of Tudor rule the PIWI-interacting RNA pathway? Genes Dev. (2010). , 24(7), 636-46.

[64] Khurana, J. S, & Theurkauf, W. piRNAs, transposon silencing, and Drosophila germline development. J Cell Biol. (2010). , 191(5), 905-13.

[65] Kim, V. N. Small RNAs just got bigger: Piwi-interacting RNAs (piRNAs) in mammalian testes. Genes Dev. (2006). , 20(15), 1993-1997.

[66] Lin, H, & Yin, H. A novel epigenetic mechanism in Drosophila somatic cells mediated by Piwi and piRNAs. Cold Spring Harb Symp Quant Biol. (2008). , 73, 273-81.

[67] Liu, S. H, Patel, S, Gingras, M. C, Nemunaitis, J, Zhou, G, Chen, C, Li, M, Fisher, W, Gibbs, R, & Brunicardi, F. C. PDX-1: demonstration of oncogenic properties in pancreatic cancer. Cancer. (2011). , 117, 723-33.

[68] Liu, S, Ballian, N, Belaguli, N. S, Patel, S, Li, M, Templeton, N. S, Gingras, M. C, Gibbs, R, Fisher, W, & Brunicardi, F. C. PDX-1 acts as a potential molecular target for treatment of human pancreatic cancer. Pancreas. (2008). , 37, 210-20.

[69] Takeshita, F, Minakuchi, Y, Nagahara, S, Honma, K, Sasaki, H, Hirai, K, Teratani, T, Namatame, N, Yamamoto, Y, Hanai, K, Kato, T, Sano, A, & Ochiya, T. Efficient delivery of small interfering RNA to bone-metastatic tumors by using atelocollagen in vivo. Proc Natl Acad Sci U S A. (2005). , 102(34), 12177-82.

[70] Ryo, A, Uemura, H, Ishiguro, H, Saitoh, T, Yamaguchi, A, Perrem, K, Kubota, Y, Lu, K. P, & Aoki, L. Stable suppression of tumourigenicity by Pin1-targeted RNA interference in prostate cancer. Clin Cancer Res. (2005). , 11, 7523-31.

[71] Takei, Y, Kadomatsu, K, Yuzawa, Y, Matsuo, S, & Muramatsu, T. A small interfering RNA targeting vascular endothelial growth factor as cancer therapeutics. Cancer Res. (2004). , 64, 3365-70.

[72] Schiffelers, R. M, Ansari, A, Xu, J, Zhou, Q, Tang, Q, Storm, G, Molema, G, Lu, P. Y, Scaria, P. V, & Woodle, M. C. Cancer siRNA therapy by tumour selective delivery with ligand targeted sterically stabilized nanoparticle. Nuc Acids Res. (2004). e149.

[73] Ji, J, Shi, J, Budhu, A, Yu, Z, Forgues, M, Roessler, S, Ambs, S, Chen, Y, Meltzer, P. S, Croce, C. M, Qin, L. X, Man, K, Lo, C. M, Lee, J, Ng, I. O, Fan, J, Tang, Z. Y, Sun, H. C, & Wang, X. W. MicroRNA expression, survival, and response to interferon in liver cancer. N Engl J Med. (2009). , 361, 1437-47.

[74] Liu, X, Sempere, L. F, Galimberti, F, Freemantle, S. J, Black, C, Dragnev, K. H, Ma, Y, Fiering, S, Memoli, V, & Li, H. DiRenzo J, Korc M, Cole CN, Bak M, Kauppinen S,

Dmitrovsky E. Uncovering growth-suppressive MicroRNAs in lung cancer. Clin Cancer Res. (2009). , 15, 1177-83.

[75] Trang, P, Wiggins, J. F, Daige, C. L, Cho, C, Omotola, M, Brown, D, Weidhaas, J. B, Bader, A. G, & Slack, F. J. Systemic delivery of tumour suppressor microRNA mimics using a neutral lipid emulsion inhibits lung tumours in mice. Mol Ther. (2011). , 19, 1116-22.

[76] Liu, C, Kelnar, K, Liu, B, Chen, X, Calhoun-davis, T, Li, H, Patrawala, L, Yan, H, Jeter, C, Honorio, S, Wiggins, J. F, Bader, A. G, Fagin, R, Brown, D, & Tang, D. G. The microRNA miR-34a inhibits prostate cancer stem cells and metastasis by directly repressing CD44. Nat Med. (2011). , 17, 211-5.

[77] Takeshita, F, Patrawala, L, Osaki, M, Takahashi, R. U, Yamamoto, Y, Kosaka, N, Kawamata, M, Kelnar, K, Bader, A. G, Brown, D, & Ochiya, T. Systemic delivery of synthetic microRNA-16 inhibits the growth of metastatic prostate tumours via downregulation of multiple cell-cycle genes. Mol Ther. (2010). , 18, 181-7.

[78] Xu, D, Takeshita, F, Hino, Y, Fukunaga, S, Kudo, Y, Tamaki, A, Matsunaga, J, Takahashi, RU, Takata, T, Shimamoto, A, Ochiya, T, Tahara, H, & mi, . -22 represses cancer progression by inducing cellular senescence. J Cell Biol. 2011; 193:409-24.

[79] Kota, J, Chivukula, R. R, Donnell, O, Wentzel, K. A, Montgomery, E. A, Hwang, C. L, Chang, H. W, Vivekanandan, T. C, Torbenson, P, Clark, M, Mendell, K. R, & Mendell, J. R. JT. Therapeutic microRNA delivery suppresses tumourigenesis in a murine liver cancer model. Cell. (2009). , 137, 1005-17.

[80] Rolfe, D. F, & Brown, G. C. Cellular energy utilization and molecular origin of standard metabolic rate in mammals. Physiol Rev. (1997). , 77, 731-758.

[81] Warburg, O. Ueber den stoffwechsel der tumouren. (Constable, London, (1930).

[82] Mazurek, S, & Eigenbrodt, E. The tumour metabolome. Anticancer Res. (2003). , 23, 1149-1154.

[83] Gatenby, R. A, & Gillies, R. J. Why do cancers have high aerobic glycolysis? Nat Rev Cancer. (2004). , 4, 891-899.

[84] Peng, Q, Zhou, J, Zhou, Q, Pan, F, Zhong, D, & Liang, H. Silencing hexokinase II gene sensitizes human colon cancer cells to 5-fluorouracil. Hepatogastroenterology (2009). , 56(90), 355-60.

[85] Goldberg, M. S, & Sharp, P. A. Pyruvate kinase M2-spesific siRNA induces apoptosis and tumor regression. J Exp Med. (2012). , 209(2), 217-24.

[86] Guo, W, Zhang, Y, Chen, T, Wang, Y, Xue, J, Zhang, Y, Xiao, W, Mo, X, & Lu, Y. Efficacy of RNAi targetting of pyruvate kinase M2 combined with cisplatin in a lung cancer model. J Cancer Res Clin Oncol. (2011). , 137(1), 65-72.

[87] Blackburn, E. H, & Gall, J. G. A tandemly repeated sequence at the termini of the extrachromosomal ribosomal RNA genes in Tetrahymena. J Mol Biol. (1978). , 120(1), 33-53.

[88] Zakian, V. A. Telomeres: Beginning to understand the end. Science. (1995). , 270, 1601-1607.

[89] Harley, C. B. Telomere loss: Mitotic clock or genetic time bomb? Mutat Res. (1991). , 256, 271-282.

[90] Hayflick, L. The limited in vitro lifetime of human diploid cell strains. Exp Cell Res. (1965). , 37, 614-636.

[91] Wright, W. E, & Shay, J. W. The two-stage mechanism controlling cellular senescence and immortalization. Exp Gerontol. (1992). , 27, 383-389.

[92] Greider, C. W, & Blackburn, E. H. The telomere terminal transferase of Tetrahymena is a ribonucleoprotein enzyme with two kinds of primer specificity. Cell. (1987). , 51(6), 887-98.

[93] Shcherbakova, D. M, Zvereva, M. E, Shpanchenko, O. V, & Dontsova, O. A. Telomerase: structure and properties of the enzyme, characteristics of the yeast telomerase. Mol Biol (Mosk). (2006). , 40(4), 580-94.

[94] Nakamura, T. M, Morin, G. B, Chapman, K. B, Weinrich, S. L, Andrews, W. H, Lingner, J, Harley, C. B, & Cech, T. R. Telomerase catalytic subunit homologs from fission yeast and human. Science. (1997). , 277(5328), 955-9.

[95] Kim, N. W, Piatyszek, M. A, Prowse, K. R, Harley, C. B, West, M. D, Ho, P. L, Coviello, G. M, Wright, W. E, Weinrich, S. L, & Shay, J. W. Specific association of human telomerase activity with immortal cells and cancer. Science. (1994). , 266, 2011-2015.

[96] Kosciolek, B. A, Kalantidis, K, Tabler, M, & Rowley, P. T. Inhibition of Telomerase Activity in Human Cancer Cells by RNA Interference. Mol Can Ther. (2003). , 2, 209-216.

[97] Cory, S, & Adams, J. M. The Bcl2 family: regulators of the cellular life-or-death switch. Nat Rev Cancer. (2002). , 2, 647-656.

[98] Sanchez-beato, M, Sanchez-aguilera, A, & Piris, M. A. Cell cycle deregulation in B-cell lymphomas. Blood. (2003). , 101, 1220-1235.

[99] Cimmino, A, Calin, GA, Fabbri, M, Iorio, MV, Ferracin, M, Shimizu, M, Wojcik, SE, Aqeilan, RI, Zupo, S, Dono, M, Rassenti, L, Alder, H, Volinia, S, Liu, CG, Kipps, TJ, Negrini, M, Croce, CM, & mi, . -16 induce apoptosis by targeting BCL2. Proc Nat Acad Sci USA. 2005; 102(39):13944-9.

[100] DuBois RNAbramson SB, Crofford L, Gupta RA, Simon LS, Van De Putte LB, Lipsky PE. Cyclooxygenase in biology and disease. FASEB J. (1998). , 12(12), 1063-73.

[101] Denkert, C, Furstenberg, A, Daniel, P. T, Koch, I, Kobel, M, Weichert, W, Siegert, A, & Hauptmann, S. Induction of G0/G1 cell cycle arrest in ovarian carcinoma cells by

the antiinflammatory drug NS-398, but not by COX-2-specific RNA interference. Oncogene. (2003). , 22(54), 8653-61.

[102] Charames, G. S, & Bapat, B. Cyclooxygenase-2 knockdown by RNA interference in colon cancer. Int J Oncol. (2006). , 28(2), 543-9.

[103] Kobayashi, S, Sakatani, M, Kobayashi, S, Okuda, K, & Takahashi, M. Gene silencing of cyclooxygenase-2 mRNA by RNA interference in bovine cumulus-granulosa cells. J Reprod Dev. (2007). , 53(6), 1305-11.

[104] Bozza, P. T, Payne, J. L, Morham, S. G, Langenbach, R, Smithies, O, & Weller, P. F. Leukocyte lipid body formation and eicosanoid generation: cyclooxygenase-independent inhibition by aspirin. Proc Nat Acad Sci USA. (1996). , 93(20), 11091-6.

[105] Grilli, M, Pizzi, M, Memo, M, & Spano, P. Neuroprotection by aspirin and sodium salicylate through blockade of NFkappaB activation. Science. (1996). , 274(5291), 1383-5.

[106] Elder, D. J, Halton, D. E, Hague, A, & Paraskeva, C. Induction of apoptotic cell death in human colorectal carcinoma cell lines by a cyclooxygenase-2 (COX-2)-selective nonsteroidal anti-inflammatory drug: independence from COX-2 protein expression. Clin Cancer Res. (1997). , 3(10), 1679-83.

[107] Lim, J. T, Piazza, G. A, Han, E. K, Delohery, T. M, Li, H, Finn, T. S, Buttyan, R, Yamamoto, H, Sperl, G. J, Brendel, K, Gross, P. H, Pamukcu, R, & Weinstein, I. B. Sulindac derivatives inhibit growth and induce apoptosis in human prostate cancer cell lines. Biochem Pharmacol. (1999). , 58(7), 1097-107.

[108] Strillacci, A, Griffoni, C, Spisni, E, Manara, M. C, & Tomasi, V. RNA interference as a key to knockdown overexpressed cyclooxygenase-2 gene in tumour cells. Brit J Cancer. (2006). , 94(9), 1300-10.

[109] Calin, G. A, & Croce, C. M. MicroRNA signatures in human cancers. Nat Rev Cancer. (2006). , 6, 857-866.

[110] Esquela-kerscher, A, & Slack, F. J. Oncomirs-microRNAs with a role in cancer. Nat Rev Cancer. (2006). , 6, 259-269.

[111] Meng, F, Henson, R, Wehbe-janek, H, Ghoshal, K, Jacob, S. T, & Patel, T. MicroRNA-21 regulates expression of the PTEN tumour suppressor gene in human hepatocellular cancer. Gastroenterology. (2007). , 133, 647-658.

[112] Gramantieri, L, Ferracin, M, Fornari, F, Veronese, A, Sabbioni, S, Liu, C. G, Calin, G. A, Giovannini, C, Ferrazzi, E, Grazi, G. L, Croce, C. M, Bolondi, L, Negrini, M, & Cyclin, G. is a target of miR-122a, a microRNA frequently down-regulated in human hepatocellular carcinoma. Cancer Res. (2007). , 67, 6092-6099.

[113] Nieth, C, Priebsch, A, Stege, A, & Lage, H. Modulation of the classical multidrug resistance (MDR) phenotype by RNA interference (RNAi). FEBS Lett. (2003). , 545, 144-150.

[114] Li, G, Li, X. P, Peng, Y, Liu, X, & Li, X. H. Effective inhibition of EB virus encoded latent membrane protein-1 by siRNA in EB virus (+) nasopharyngeal carcinoma cell. Zhonghua Er Bi Yan Hou Tou Jing Wai Ke Za Zhi. (2005). , 40, 406-410.

[115] Li, X, Liu, X, Li, C. Y, Ding, Y, Chau, D, Li, G, Kung, H. F, Lin, M. C, & Peng, Y. Recombinant adeno-associated virus mediated RNA interference inhibits metastasis of nasopharyngeal cancer cells in vivo and in vitro by suppression of Epstein-Barr virus encoded LMP-1. Int J Oncol. (2006). , 29, 595-603.

[116] Brummelkamp, T. R, Bernards, R, & Agami, R. Stable suppression of tumourigenicity by virus-mediated RNA interference. Cancer Cell. (2002). , 2, 243-247.

[117] Hingorani, S. R, Jacobetz, M. A, Robertson, G. P, Herlyn, M, & Tuveson, D. A. Suppression of BRAFV599E in human melanoma abrogates transformation. Cancer Res. (2003). , 63, 5198-5202.

[118] Sumimoto, H, Miyagishi, M, Miyoshi, H, Yamagata, S, Shimizu, A, Taira, K, & Kawakami, Y. Inhibition of growth and invasive ability of melanoma by inactivation of mutated BRAF with lentivirus-mediated RNA interference. Oncogene. (2004). , 23(36), 6031-9.

[119] Mitsushita, J, Lambeth, J. D, & Kamata, T. The superoxidegenerating oxidase Nox1 is functionally required for Ras oncogene transformation. Cancer Res. (2004). , 64, 3580-3585.

Chapter 15

Poly(amino ester)s-Based Polymeric Gene Carriers in Cancer Gene Therapy

You-Kyoung Kim, Can Zhang, Chong-Su Cho,
Myung-Haing Cho and Hu-Lin Jiang

Additional information is available at the end of the chapter

1. Introduction

Gene therapy is a novel approach that broadly defined as the transfer of genetic material into a cell, tissue, or whole organ, with the goal of curing a disease or at least improving the clinical status of a patient [1]. Gene therapy refers to local or systemic administration of a nucleic acid construct that can prevent, treat and even cure diseases by changing the expression of genes that are responsible for the pathological condition [2]. As a form of molecular medicine, gene therapy hold great promises to provide new treatments for a large number of inherited and acquired diseases, such as cancer. It has also been considered as suitable substitute for conventional protein therapy, since it can overcome inherent problems associated with administration of protein drugs in terms of bioavailability, systemic toxicity and manufacturing cost [3].

There are two essential components in current gene therapy: an effective therapeutic genetic agent and the gene delivery system [4, 5]. The most extensively studied approach involves the delivery of plasmid DNA (pDNA) for expressing therapeutic transgenes. Considerable efforts have been made in plasmid design. This includes removal of extraneous CG dinucleotides, incorporation of scaffold/matrix attached region sequences to prolong expression, promoter selection for gene expression, and improving plasmid entry into the nucleus [6]. The recently emerged RNA interference (RNAi) has also become recognized as pivotal cellular regulator of genetic events and a useful tool in elucidating pathways during stages of development, pathogenesis and senescent cell regulation [7]. RNAi encompasses the range of endogenous or synthetic short double or single stranded oligonucleotides, including microRNAs (miRNAs), small interfering RNAs (siRNAs), short hairpin RNAs (shRNAs), piwi interacting RNAs (piRNAs) and antisense oligonucleotides (ASOs) [8]. The intracellular delivery of genetic agents for RNAi such as siRNA takes benefits from existing expertise in pDNA transfer, as they share common properties. However, they face distinct challenges due to apparent differences in size, stability of the formed nucleic acid complexes, the location and mechanism of action [9].

Naked genetic therapeutics is vulnerable to enzyme degradation, rapid clearance by renal filtration, poor cellular uptake due to anionic charges of the phosphate backbone, inefficiently escape from endosome into cytosol. Therefore, the development of gene vectors for effectively carrying genes into cells has made a great deal of progress in recent years [5, 10]. Vectors as gene delivery system that have been developed fall into two broad categories: viral and non-viral vectors. Vectors based upon many different viral systems, including retroviruses, lentiviruses, adenoviruses, and adeno-associated viruses (AAV) (Table 1), currently offer the best choice for efficient gene delivery [11, 12]. They are all highly efficient in specific circumstances, but the potential risks of undesired immune response and the risk of insertional mutagenesis following long term viral gene transfer and toxic side reactions have raised concerns [13-15].

Virus	Genome	Size	Advantages	Disadvantages
Retrovirus	ssRNA	7-10 kb	Long-term expression	Application is limited to replicating cells Possibility of insertional mutagenesis
Adenovirus	dsDNA	36 kb	Capable of very efficient episomal gene transfer in a wide range of cells and tissues Easy to grow in large amounts	The host response to the virus appears to limit the duration of expression and the ability to repeat dosing
AAV	ssDNA	5 kb	Structurally simple Provoke less of a host-cell response	Extremely difficult to grow in large amounts

Table 1. Viral vector delivery systems [12].

Although viral vector has the advantages in terms of gene transfer efficiency, non-viral gene therapy has the advantage over viral vector therapies with its ability to target specific cells, being less immunogenic and non-integrating into the host genome, low production cost, scalability despite most studies showing less sustained gene expression [16-18]. Non-viral vectors have been investigated even more aggressively since the death of a patient in a virus-based gene therapy trial [19] and the occurrence of leukemia following gene therapy of children with X-linked severe combined immune deficiency using a retroviral gene therapy vector [20]. Previous efforts focused primarily on cationic lipid/DNA complexes frequently composed of combinations of N-[1-(2,3-dioleyloxy)propyl]-N,N,N-trimethylammonium chloride (DOTMA) [21], dioleoyl phosphatidylethanolamine (DOPE) [22], and dimethylaminoethane-carbamoyl cholesterol (DC-Chol) [23]. These complexes stabilize incorporated DNA against physical and enzymatic damage. On the other hand, numerous agents poly(L-lysine), polyethylenimine (PEI), chitosan, dendrimers etc. have now been extensively investigated as polymer-based non-viral vector gene delivery systems [24, 25]. The success of these agents is directly correlated with their ability to overcome issues of low efficiency and inconsistent preparation that have plagued previous non-viral vector delivery systems.

Among polymeric vectors, the wildly used PEI with appropriate molecular weight can electrostatically interact with negatively charged phosphate groups of genetic agents to form particulate polyelectrolyte complexes, which exhibit superior transfection efficiency due to high buffering capacity [26]. However, high molecular weight of PEI shows high cytotoxicity, and when further decreasing the molecular weight, both cellular toxicity and transfection efficiency are decreased [27]. Polyethylene glycol (PEG) was conjugated to PEI to ameliorate its cell cytotoxicity and develop functionality which limit its clinical application [28-32]. However, free PEI is not easily biodegradable in cellular space, which may remain additional safety concerns. Therefore, it calls for the development of functional biocompatible materials with favorable gene transfer efficiency to substitute for PEI [33, 34]. Poly(amino ester)s-based polymers are a promising class of polymeric gene vector due to their biocompatibility [35-37]. Poly(amino ester)s can be synthesized by Michael addition reaction using functional amines including a primary and a secondary amine to diacrylate ester [38]. The ease in synthesis and lack of byproducts make them even more favorable gene vector candidates with biocompatibility and biodegradability properties [38-43].

Here, we are focused on recent progress of different strategies of functionalization of synthetic biocompatible poly(amino ester)s and the applications of these. The characterization of physicochemical properties, degradation kinetics, transfection efficiency and toxicity in vitro and in vivo were covered in this chapter.

2. Poly(amino ester)s-based gene therapy

Poly(amino ester)s are promising and efficient gene delivery vectors due to their high transfection efficiency and biocompatibility, which were first synthesized by Langer et al. [44-46].

2.1. Poly(amino ester)s synthesis and degradation kinetics

2.1.1. Linear poly(amino ester)s

Varieties of linear poly(amino ester)s are synthesized by Michael addition reaction of small molecular weight monomers and diacrylate monomers. The Langer group initially investigated the synthesis of poly(β-amino ester)s via the addition of N,N′-dimethylethylenediamine, piperazine, and 4,4′-trimethylenedipiperidine to 1,4-butanediol diacrylate as shown in Fig. 1(A). They reported that addition of secondary amines to diacrylate moieties results into tertiary amines which do not participate in subsequent addition reaction, that otherwise leads to polymer branching or cross linking.

One of the major merit of poly(β-amino ester)s is degradation. Due to the hydrolysis of the ester bonds in the polymer backbones, poly(β-amino ester)s can easily degraded. The degradation of poly(β-amino ester)s presents a particularly attractive basis for the development of new polymeric gene carriers for two reasons: firstly, poly(β-amino ester)s degrade into nontoxic byproducts to increase the safety of gene carrier; secondary, degradation of poly(β-amino ester)s will increases the transfection efficiency. While complexation of DNA with cationic polymers is required to compact and protect DNA during early events in the transfection process, DNA and polymer must ultimately decomplex to allow efficient transcription [44]. In view of this requirement, degradable poly(β-amino ester)s could play an important role in "vector unpackaging" events in the cells [44, 47]. As shown in Fig. 1(C), the polymers degraded more slowly at pH 5.1 than at pH 7.4, and at pH 5.1 each polymer having a half-life of approximately 7-8 h. In contrast, polymers 1 and 3 [Fig. 1(B)] were completely degraded in less than 5 h at pH 7.4. These results are consistent with the pH-degradation profiles of other amine-containing polyesters, such as poly(4-hydroxy-L-proline ester), in which pendant amine functionalities are hypothesized to act as intramolecular nucleophilic catalysts and contribute to more rapid degradation at higher pH [44]. The degradation of polymer 2 occurred more slowly at pH 7.4 than at pH 5.1 due to the incomplete solubility of polymer 2 at pH 7.4 and the resulting heterogeneous nature of the degradation mileu [44].

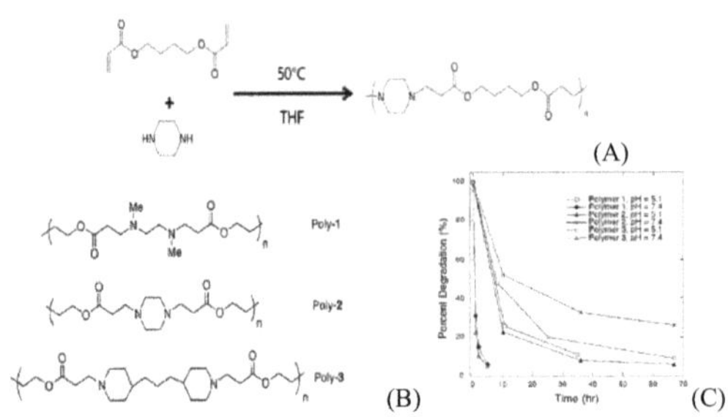

Figure 1. The synthesis of poly(β-amino ester)s from butanediol diacrylate and piperazine (A) and degradation of polymer 1-3 at 37 °C at pH 5.1 and 7.4 (B and C). [Source from Ref. [44]].

After that, the same group reported a parallel approach suitable for synthesis of hundreds to thousands of structurally unique poly(amino ester)s and application of these libraries to rapid and high throughput identification of new gene delivery agents and structure-function trends although they did not report the degradation profiles of poly(amino ester)s in this study [38]. The high throughput method indicated that synthesis of poly(β-amino ester)s are easy to controlable. The advantage of combinatorial chemistry and automated high throughput synthesis is that it has revolutionized modern drug discovery by rapid synthesis and evaluation with greater precision. As shown in Fig. 2, 140 different poly(β-amino ester)s were synthesized from the 7 diacrylate monomers and 20 amine-based monomers as a screening library. Polymerization reactions were conducted simultaneously as an array of individually labeled vials and the reactions were performed in methylene chloride at 45 °C for 5 days.

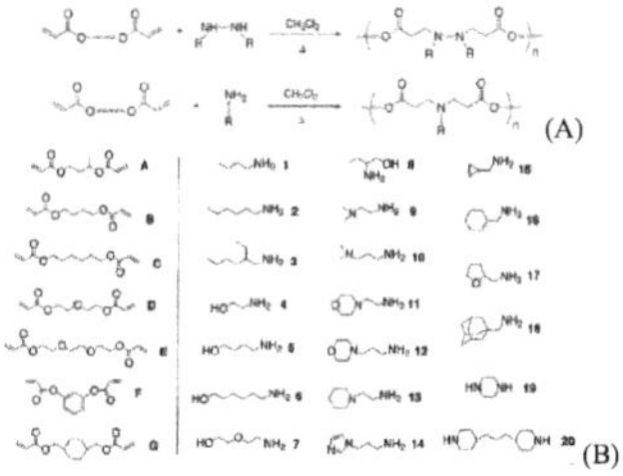

Figure 2. Synthesis of poly(β-amino ester)s. Poly(β-amino ester)s were synthesized by the conjugate addition of primary or bis(secondary amines) to diacrylates using methylene chloride solvent (A) and diacrylate (A-G 7 set) and amine (1-20) monomers chosen for the synthesis of an initial screening library (B). [Source from Ref. [38]].

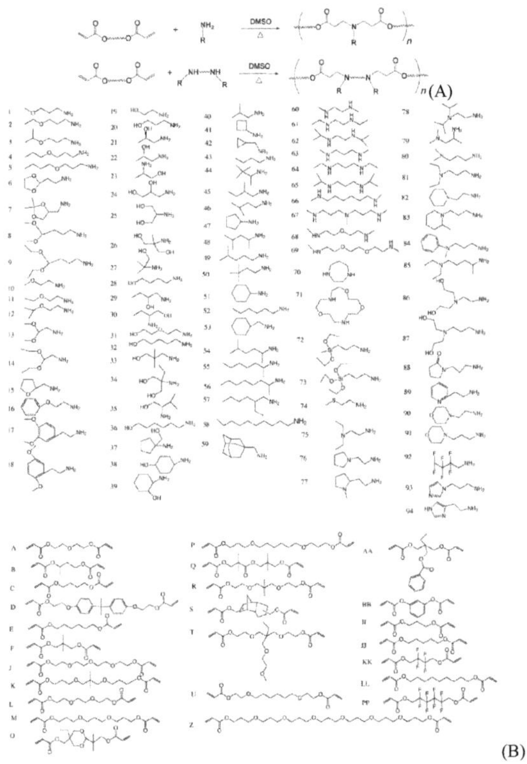

Figure 3. Synthesis of poly(β-amino ester)s. Poly(β-amino ester)s were synthesized by the conjugate addition of primary or bis(secondary amines) to diacrylates using DMSO solvent (A). Amino (numbers) and diacrylate (letters) monomers (B). [Source from Ref. [48]].

Based high throughput methods, in 2003, Anderson synthesized over 2,350 poly(β-amino ester)s as shown in Fig. 3 [48]. Polymerization reactions were performed in 1.6M DMSO at 56 °C for 5 days. Anderson et al. observed that reaction conditions such as optimum temperature and solvent play an important role during the synthesis of poly(β-amino ester)s. Even though maximizing monomer concentration in reaction is desirable to obtain high molecular weight poly(β-amino ester)s and it leads to insoluble gel formation [49].

Park et al. reported the synthesis of linear poly(amino ester)s from three different molecular weights of PEG diacrylate and low molecular weight PEI As shown in Fig. 4 [37].

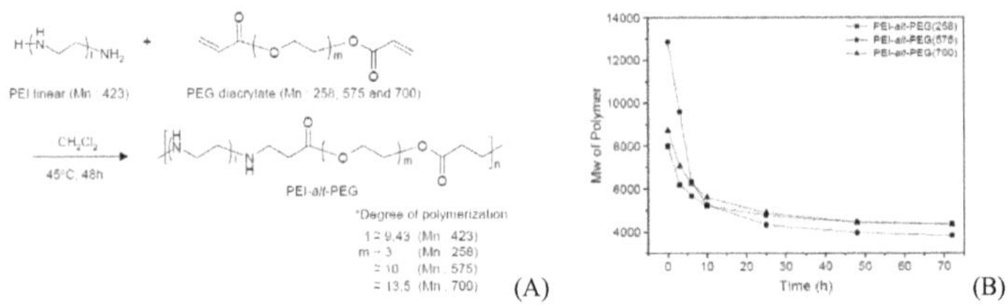

Figure 4. Proposed reaction scheme for copolymer formation (A) and degradation of copolymers (B). [Source from Ref. [37]].

It was found that molecular weights of poly(amino ester)s were maintained relatively constant at about 4kDa during the degradation aftger 72 h regardless of molecular weight of PEG diacylate. However, half life was observed depending on molecular weight of PEG diacrylate. Poly(β-amino ester)s composed of PEG diacylate (Mn: 575) showed an half life of 8 h while that of 25 h for poly(β-amino ester)s with PEG diacylate (Mn: 700). This rapid degradation in case of linear poly(β-amino ester)s is plausible as even few cleavages may reduce chain length rapidly with quick drop in molecular weight [37].

2.1.2. Branched poly(amino ester)s

Liu et al. synthesized the branched poly(amino ester)s by the polymerization of 1-(2-aminoethyl)piperazine (AEPZ) with 1,4-butanediol diacrylate (BDA), which was carried out by adding BDA dropwise to an equimolar solution of AEPZ in chloroform at 45 °C as shown in Fig. 5 [50]. After the polymerization was performed for around 72 h, a water-soluble polymer, BDA-AEPZ, was obtained by precipitating the solution into acetone containing HCl. The molecular weight of BDA-AEPZ was around 5126 with a polydispersity index of 1.52 as determined by GPC.

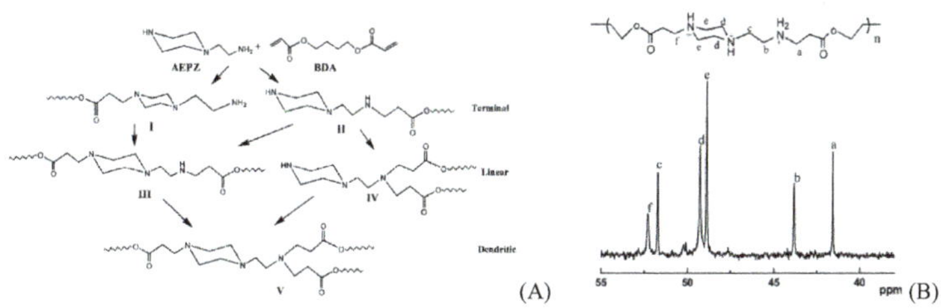

Figure 5. Possible routes of the Michael addition polymerization of trifunctional amine monomers and diacrylates (A) and the structure of poly(amino ester)s obtained and enlarged ^{13}C-NMR (INVGATE) spectrum of methylene carbons attached to the hydrochloride salts of amines in BDA-AEPZ (B). [Source from Ref. [50]].

The polymerization of AEPZ with diacylate monomers was reported but branched poly(amino ester)s with primary, secondary and tertiary amines were supposed to be formed based on unsolidified experimental conditions, suggesting that secondary amines are more reactive than primary ones in case of trifunctional amines [50]. Wu et al. also synthesized protonated hyperbranched poly(amino ester)s and characterized as gene delivery carriers as shown in Fig. 6(A) [51]. It was found that all these hyperbranched poly(amino ester)s degraded in a controlled manner within 50 days and it was speculated that this phenomenon may be due to the lesser water accessibility of the ester groups in hyperbranched sturctures [Fig. 6(B)].

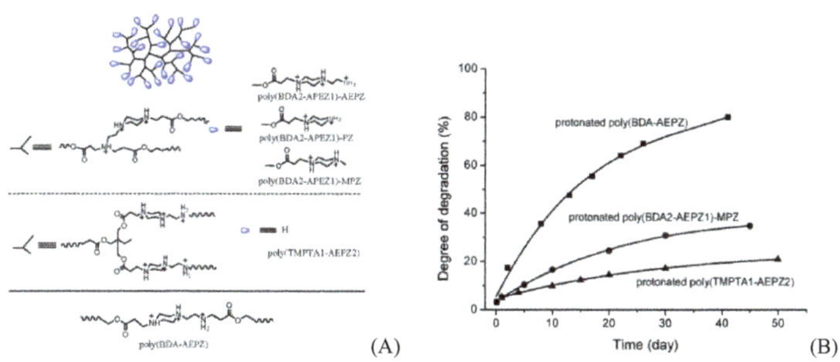

Figure 6. Structure of linear and hyperbranched poly(amino ester)s obtained via Michael addition polymerization of trifunctional amines with diacrylates and triacrylates (A) and comparison of the hydrolysis profiles of protonated hyperbranched poly(BDA2-AEPZ1)-MPZ, hyperbranched poly(TMPTA1-AEPZ2), and linear poly(BDA-AEPZ) in aqueous solutions (B). [Source from Ref. [51]].

Cho's group also reported the synthesis of branch poly(amino ester)s by Michael addition, based on hydrophobic polycaprolactone diacrylate and low molecular weight PEI [Fig. 7(A)] [40]. It was simply an indication of application of ester linkage which supports the easy degradation leaving nontoxic building blocks, thereby increased transfection efficiency and reduced cytotoxicity. The branched poly(amino ester)s showed controlled degradation with the half life of 4-4.5 days as shown in Fig. 7(B).

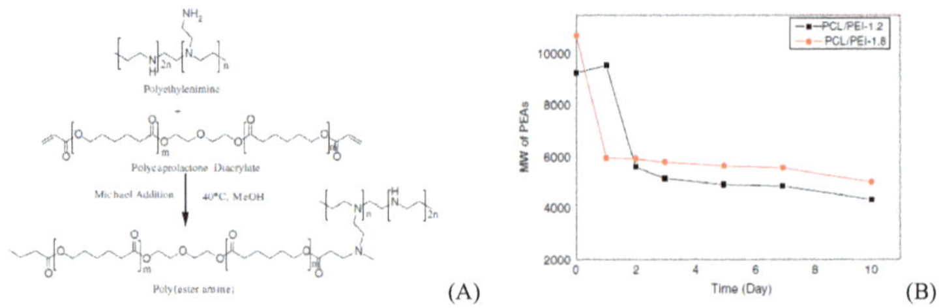

Figure 7. The synthetic scheme of PEAs by Michael addition (A) and degradation of PEAs (PCL/PEI-1.2 and PCL/PEI-1.8) (B). [Source from Ref. [40]].

Same group also reported another degradable branched poly(amino ester)s based on poloxamer diacrylate and low molecular weight PEI [52]. These hyperbranched poly(amino ester)s can be easily synthesized by Michael type addition reaction between poloxamer diacrylate and low molecular weight PEI [Fig. 8(A)] and the hyperbranched poly(amino ester)s showed slow degradation at physiological conditions which was greatly dependent on hydrophilicity of poloxamer [Fig. 8(B)].

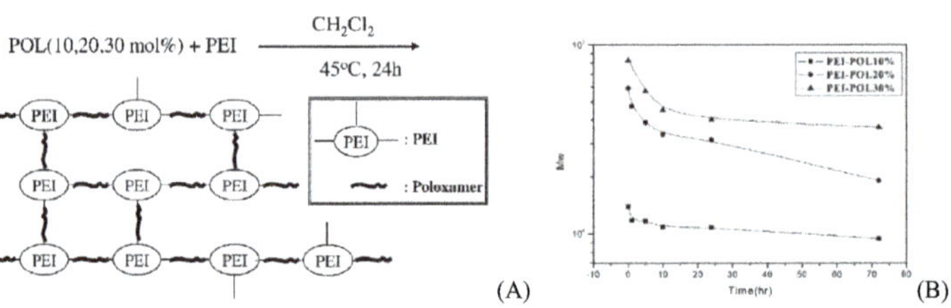

Figure 8. Synthetic scheme of PEA by Michael addition reaction (A) and degradation of PEAs (B). PEAs were dissolved in 0.1 M PBS, and incubated at 37 °C with 100 rpm. [Source from Ref. [52]].

All together, poly(amino ester)s can be easily synthesized by Michael type addition reaction and showed good degradation profiles due to the hydrolysis of the ester bonds in the polymer backbones.

2.2. Characterization of poly(amino ester)s/DNA complexes

2.2.1. DNA condensation and protection

One prerequisite of a polymeric gene carrier is DNA condensation [53]. Polycation-mediated gene delivery is based on the electrostatic interactions between the positive charged polycation and negatively charged phosphate groups of DNA [32]. As shown in Fig. 9(A), retardation of DNA migration begins at poly(β-amino ester)s/DNA ratios as low as 0.1:1 (w/w) and migration is completely retarded at poly(β-amino ester)s/DNA ratios above 5:1 (w/w) [34]. Condensation protects the DNA from degradation by nucleases, and the compact particles can be taken up by cells via natural processes such as adsorptive endocytosis, pinocytosis and phagocytosis [32]. DNA in the complexes was protected from nuclease attack whereas the naked DNA was degraded. This result suggests that intact DNA could be delivered by poly(β-amino ester)s into cells without degradation [Fig. 9(B)] [34].

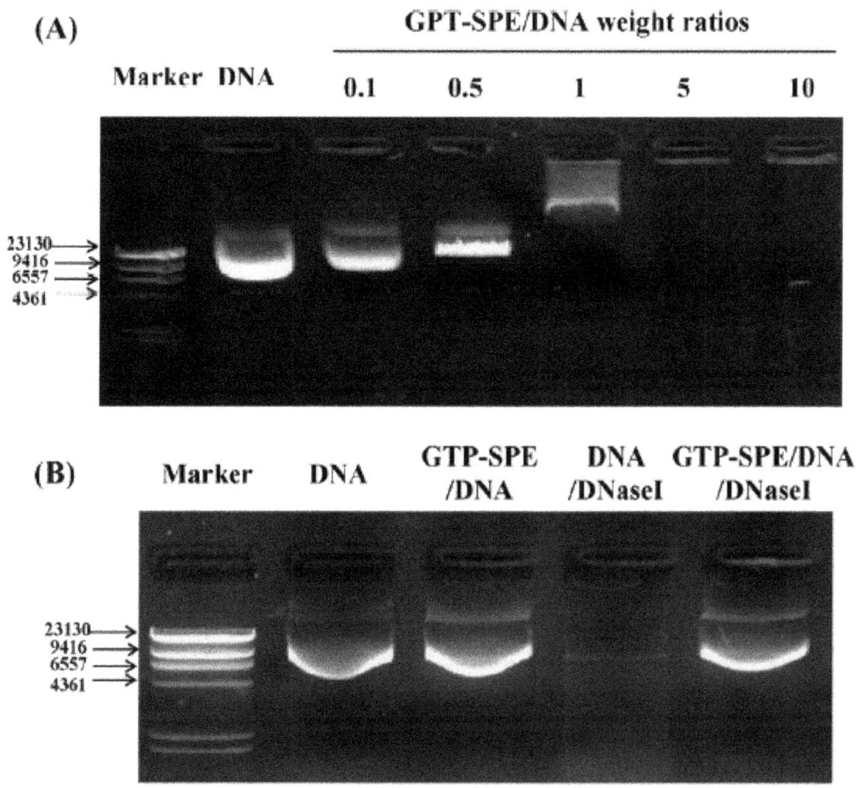

Figure 9. DNA condensation and protection study. Agarose gel electrophoresis of poly(β-amino ester)s (GPT–SPE)/DNA complexes at various weight ratios (A) and DNA protection and release assay (B). [Source from Ref. [34]].

2.2.2. Particle sizes and surface charges of poly(amino ester)s/DNA complexes

Surface properties, such as particle size and surface charge of the complex, are necessary to assure its uptake by cells [53]. In particular, the particle size of a complex is an important factor that influences the access and passage of the complex through the targeting site. Successful gene carrier depends on its ability to condense negatively charged DNA into nanosized particles with positive charges so as to enter into the cells [54]. Compact particles of small size are usually obtained only at higher N/P ratios, resulting in complexes with a strong positive net charge. For most cell types, the poly(amino ester)s/DNA complexes size requirement is on the order of 200 nm or less [55]. As shown in Fig. 10(A), poly(β-amino ester)s formed complexes with diameters in the range of 50-150 nm at DNA/polymer ratios above 1:2. A positive surface charge of polyplexes is necessary for binding to anionic cell surfaces, which consequently facilitates uptake by the cell [30, 56]. The surface charge of poly(β-amino ester)s/DNA complexes has been examined in terms of ζ-potential. The ζ-potentials for complexes were on the order of +10 to +15 mV at DNA/polymer ratios above 1:1, and the complexes did not aggregate extensively over an 18h period as shown in Fig. 10(B).

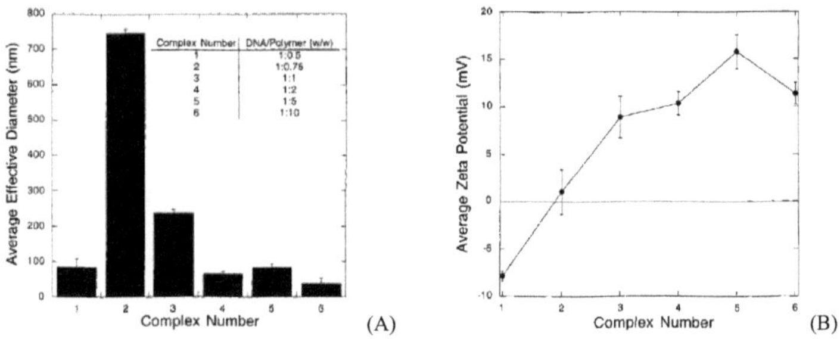

Figure 10. Average effective diameters (A) and ζ-potentials (B) of DNA/polymer complexes formed from pCMV-Luc plasmid and poly(β-amino ester)s (polymer 3) (Mn = 31000) as a function of polymer concentration. [Source from Ref. [44]].

2.3. Toxicity and transfection considerations of poly(amino ester)s/DNA complexes *in vitro*

Safe and efficient delivery of genes is critical for the successful application of gene therapy. In fact, it is the only major obstacle in the expansion of gene therapy from bench to beside. Many vectors with high transfection efficiency show high toxicity while vectors with low toxicity are poor in transfecting cells. Optimum balance between these two parameters is a key to the success in gene therapy [57-59]. As biodegradable polymers are designed to contain a combination of various functional components, it is likely that engineered systems for non-viral gene delivery, especially with the application of biodegradable ester linkage will eventually be constructed. This biodegradable linkage approach to vector development is giving way to a safety profile where low molecular weight amine contain monomers are couples with acylate linkers to yield high molecular weight poly(amino ester)s with reduced toxicity and enhanced transfection efficiency.

Jere et al. evaluated cytotoxicity of mini-library of poly(amino ester)s in 293T and HeLa cells by MTS assay [59]. In order to measure maximum possible cytotoxicity, poly(amino ester)s were administered in increasing concentrations to 293T cells as shown in Figs. 11(A) and (B). In both cell lines, poly(amino ester)s obtained from R106 to R113 exhibited very high cytotoxicity which further increased with increase in weight ratios, while poly(amino ester)s obtained from R114, R115 and R116 showed good cell viability at lower ratios but significant cytotoxicity at higher weight ratios. Excellent cell viability and uniform transfection pattern were observed with poly(amino ester)s obtained from R117 to R121. Slight cytotoxicity was observed at higher mass ratios (90:1 and 110:1) (viability above 80% in all ratios) indicating that cytotoxicity was highly sensitive to monomer ratio and varied drastically even with small change in monomer concentration. It was reported that the cytotoxicity of cationic polymers is probably caused by polymer aggregation on cell surfaces, impairing important membrane functions. Also, the cationic polymers may interfere with critical intracellular processes of cells: in particular, the primary amine was reported to disrupt PKC function through disturbance of protein kinase activity [60, 61]. On the other hands, in 293T cells, poly(amino ester)s obtained from R106 to R113 showed some transfection at lower weight ratios but it was suddenly decreased with increased weight ratios which may be because of low cell viability at these ratios [Fig. 11(C)]. Poly(amino ester)s obtained from R114 to R119 showed intermediate transfection while poly(amino ester)s obtained from R120 and R121 gave good transfection. However, in HeLa cells slightly different transfection pattern was observed as shown in Fig. 11(D)]. Poly(amino ester)s obtained from R106 to R115 failed to give significant transfection. On the other hand, poly(amino ester)s obtained from R116 to R119 showed intermediate transfection which was slowly increased from R116 to R119. Transfection was highest with poly(amino ester)s obtained from R120 and R121 and it was increased with increasing weight ratios till 90:1 after that it again decreased due to increased cytotoxicity. It was also reported that in addition to factors such as chemical structure and polymer molecular weight, either amine or acrylate terminated also plays a significant role in determining transfection efficiency of poly(amino ester)s [46]. Excess of amine monomers results into amine terminated polymer which effectively binds with cell membrane and promotes its uptake whereas acrylate terminated polymers has poor cellular entry and transfection efficiency.

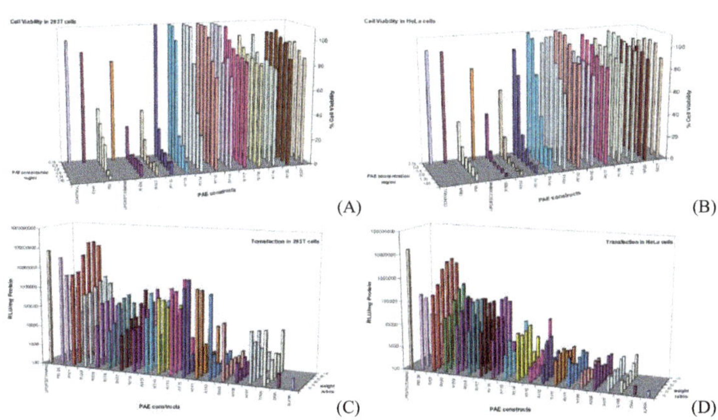

Figure 11. Cytotoxicity of PAEs at various concentrations in 293T cell line (A) and HeLa cell line (B); and transfection efficiency of PAE/DNA complexes in serum free-media at various mass ratios in 293T cells (C) and HeLa cells (D). [Source from Ref. [59]].

2.4. Toxicity and transfection considerations of poly(amino ester)s/DNA complexes *in vivo*

Intravenous administration as one of the most commonly used methods in gene therapy area even most gene therapy vectors, as well as other biomolecules and potential engineered drugs, has short elimination half-lives due to the serum proteins in the blood stream. In vivo transfection efficiency of the poly(amino ester)s was studied after intravenous administration into mice [62]. As shown in Fig. 12, the quantity of luciferase was determined in lung, liver, spleen, kidney and heart after 24 h intravenous administration of polymer/DNA complexes. Fig. 12 shows luciferase gene expression in various mouse organs after intravenous administration of the polymer/DNA complexes via the tail vein. As shown in Fig. 12, injection of polymer/DNA complexes resulted in transfection primarily in the lung which is in agreement with previous results [63, 64]. Verbaan et al. suggested two mechanisms regarding this phenomenon of predominant gene expression in the lung; firstly, because the lung is the first organ encountered by polyplexes after tail vein injection, the positively charged polyplexes may electrostatically interact with the negatively charged membranes of the endothelial cells in the lung, secondly, the physical trapping of large aggregates formed by the interaction of polyplexes with blood components like serum proteins and erythrocytes [63, 64]. Also, the poly(amino ester)s/DNA complexes showed the highest transfection activity in the lung regardless of N/P ratio. This may be caused by the positive charge of the poly(amino ester)s/DNA complexes like PEI 25K/DNA complexes. In contrast to PEI 25K/DNA complexes, the poly(amino ester)s/DNA complexes had high transfection in the liver because the liver is the main organ for gene accumulation and subsequent degradation [62]. Plank et al. reported that opsonization of the polyplexes led to a rapid clearance by the mononuclear phagocytic system (MPS) [65]. Uptake by the MPS would be in agreement with the observed liver and spleen accumulations. In addition, the presence of discontinuous or fenestrated endothelia in the vascularization of the liver and spleen may facilitate the gene accumulation in these tissues [66]. The poly(amino ester)s/DNA complexes showed higher transfection efficiency than golden standard PEI 25K/DNA ones, and the luciferase activity was increased in all organs except kidney with increase of N/P ratio indicating that poly(amino ester)s/DNA complexes function efficiently after intravenous administration.

Implantable infusion pumps have been developed as an one of therapy methods for a number of diseases, and there has been remarkable progress in endoscopic and laparoscopic surgical techniques. This progress in surgical techniques and devices could make intraperitoneal administration a conventional and feasible approach for future clinical applications [67]. Intraperitoneal gene delivery may provide a strategy for the treatment of a variety of diseases, including cancer. Zugates et al. synthesized parallel end-modification of poly(β-amino ester)s by the conjugate addition of amines to diacrylate monomers as shown in Fig. 13 [68].

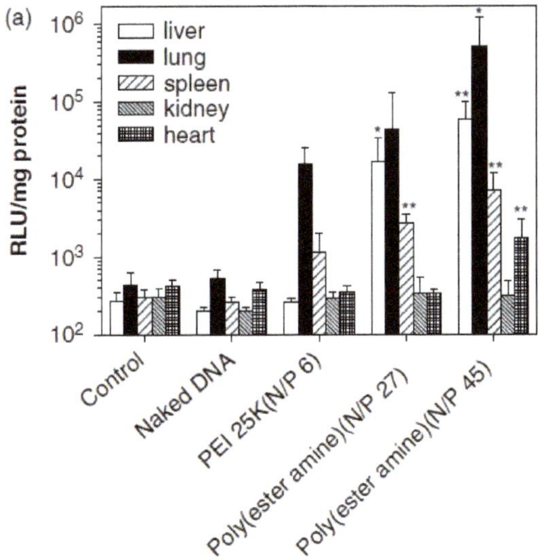

Figure 12. Tissue distribution of poly(amino ester)s/DNA (gWIZ-Luc) complexes administered by intravenous injection and inhalation at various N/P ratios. ($*p < 0.1$; $**p < 0.05$, Student's t-test, two-tailed). [Source from Ref. [62]].

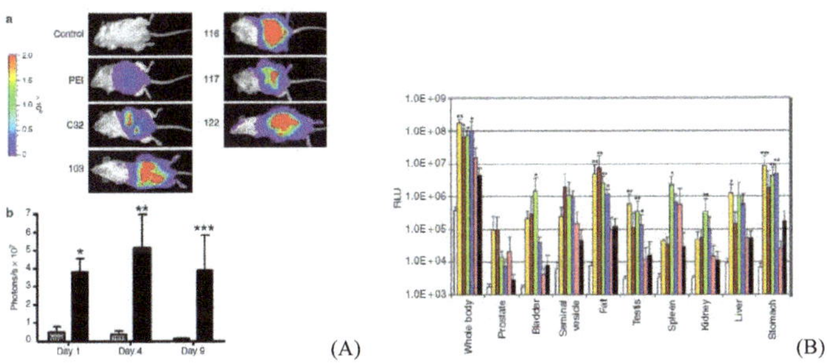

Figure 13. Intraperitoneal gene delivery in mice (A). (a) Whole-body optical images of luciferase expression in FVB/J mice 6 hours after intraperitoneal injection of polymer/DNA complexes. Images show the highest expression obtained for each polymer. The control mouse was injected with 120 μl of 50 mM NaAc buffer, pH 5.2. Pseudocolor images representing emitted bioluminescence are superimposed over grayscale images. Relative light units (RLUs)/pixel are indicated in the color scale bar on the left. (b) Quantification of whole-body luciferase expression at various times after intraperitoneal injection of C32- (hatched) and C32-117-delivered (solid) DNA. Statistically significant differences between C32 and C32-117 at a given time point are indicated. n = 4 for each treatment group. $*P < 0.05$; $**P < 0.01$; $***P < 0.001$. Organ distribution of gene expression (B). Quantification of luciferase expression in whole body and individual organs 6 hours after intraperitoneal injection of polymer/DNA complexes in FVB/J mice. Results are expressed as mean transfection levels (± SD) for a buffer control (white), C32-103 (yellow), C32-116 (red), C32-117 (green), C32-122 (blue), C32 (pink), and jet-polyethylenimine (jet-PEI) (black). n ≥ 3 for each treatment group. [Source from Ref. [68]].

High transfection levels were observed after intraperitoneal injection of polymer/DNA complexes. End-modified polymers resulted in whole-body reporter protein expression more than an order-of magnitude higher than that for jet-PEI. They also outperformed the best poly(β-amino ester)s synthesized to date, C32, with overall expression levels 4- to 12-fold higher. They found that sustained expression past 1 week both with modified C32 and with C32, but modified C32 was expressed at significantly higher levels, reflecting its enhanced delivery capabilities. This effect was most evident between the C32-116 and C32-117 polymers, where the latter displayed 5- to 65-fold higher delivery to the bladder, spleen, liver, and kidney. The only difference between these two diaminopropane end-capping reagents is the ethyl versus dimethyl branching.

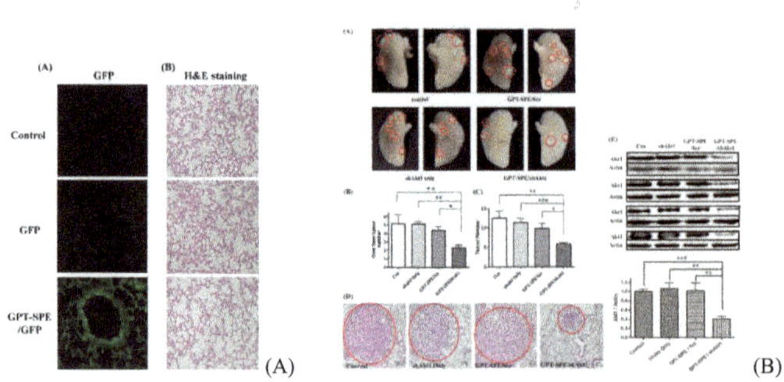

Figure 14. A) In vivo analysis after aerosol administration to lungs. Two days after exposure, mice were sacrificed and lungs were collected for the detection of GFP signal and Hematoxylin & Eosin staining. (A) Transfection efficiency study: GFP expression analysis (magnification: 200×). B) Lung histopathology study: Hematoxylin & Eosin staining (magnification: 200×, scale bar represents 50 μm). (B) Therapeutic efficiency of GPT–SPE as aerosol gene delivery carrier in lung tumor bearing K-*ras*^{LA1} mice: aerosol delivery of GPT–SPE/Akt1 shRNA significantly inhibited lung tumor numbers: (A) Lungs showing numerous visible lesions (red circle represents tumor tissues). (B) Total tumor numbers ($n = 4$, $*p < 0.05$, $**p < 0.01$). (C) Tumor size over 1 mm tumor numbers ($n = 4$, $*p < 0.05$, $**p < 0.01$, $***p < 0.001$). Aerosol delivery of GPT–SPE/Akt1 shRNA significantly suppressed lung tumor progression through the Akt signaling pathway. (D) Histopathological characteristics. Red circle indicates the incidence in the lungs (magnification: 200×, scale bar represents 50 μm). (E) Western blot analysis of Akt1 protein expression in the lungs and bands-of-interest were further analyzed by densitometer ($n = 4$, $**p < 0.01$, $***p < 0.001$).

One of the most non-invasive approaches to drug/gene delivery is via inhalation. Gene therapy to the lung can potentially be exploited for the treatment of both genetic and acquired diseases. However, any therapeutic approach for the respiratory tract must take into account the heterogeneity of the cellular targets in the lung: epithelial cells, alveolar cells, vascular cells, serous cells in the sub-mucosal glands and a number of other cell types [69]. Our group developed spermine-based biocompatible poly(β-amino ester)s as an aerosol delivery gene carrier [34]. As shown in Fig. 14 (A-A), GFP signal was dominant in the lungs with GPT–SPE/GFP complexes-exposed group compared to the control and naked GFP-exposed groups. No necrosis, degeneration, metaplasia, anaplasia in pneumocytes, atelectasis, or emphysema were detected [Fig. 14 (A-B)]. These results indicate that GPT–SPE functions safely and efficiently in aerosol delivery system. Significant anticancer effects of GPT–SPE/Akt1 shRNA complexes in the lungs through aerosol inhalation were observed in lung tumor bearing K-*ras*^{LA1} mice [Fig. 14 (B)] without toxicity [Table 2]. These result indicating that poly(β-amino ester)s (GPT-SPE) could be a safe and efficient gene carrier in aerosol-administered lung cancer gene therapy.

	Con	GPT-SPE
(A) Routine CBC		
WBC ($\times 10^3$ cells/μL)	6.71 ± 2.06	5.41 ± 0.97
RBC ($\times 10^6$ cells/μL)	9.89 ± 0.66	10.26 ± 0.55
HGB (g/dL)	13.37 ± 1.30	13.47 ± 1.54
HCT (%)	46.50 ± 3.68	48.83 ± 2.63
MCV (fL)	47.43 ± 0.51	47.60 ± 0.26
MCH (pg)	13.50 ± 0.61	13.47 ± 0.38
MCHC (g/dL)	28.73 ± 0.64	28.40 ± 0.44
CHCM (g/dL)	27.80 ± 0.66	26.70 ± 0.66
RDW (%)	16.33 ± 1.37	16.43 ± 0.40
HDW (g/dL)	1.97 ± 0.31	1.87 ± 0.04
PLT ($\times 10^3$ cells/μL)	2084.00 ± 250.32	1778.33 ± 637.72
MPV (fL)	8.70 ± 0.30	8.60 ± 0.10
(B) Platelet parameters		
PDW (%)	60.27 ± 3.98	52.46 ± 0.36
PCT (%)	1.57 ± 0.30	1.39 ± 0.55
MPC (g/dL)	18.90 ± 0.36	16.36 ± 0.70
MPM (pg)	1.39 ± 0.02	1.20 ± 0.04
Large Pit ($\times 10^3$ cells/μL)	47.43 ± 0.51	41.63 ± 0.26

CBC, complete blood count; WBC, white blood cell; RBC, red blood cell; HGB, hemoglobin; HCT, hematocrit; MCV, mean cell volume; MCH, mean corpuscular hemoglobin; MCHC, mean corpuscular hemoglobin concentration; CHCM, mean cell hemoglobin concentration; RDW, red cell distribution width; PLT, platelets; MPV, mean platelet volume; PDW, platelet distribution width; PCT, plateletcrit; MPC, mean platelet component; MPM, mean platelet mass; Large Pit, large platelets.

Table 2. Toxicological analysis. Blood samples were collected for routine examination and to assess the potential toxicity of GTP–SPE. [Source from Ref. [34]].

2.5. Targeting considerations

Targeting confers another important criterion in gene delivery. To increase specificity and safety of gene therapy further, the expression of the therapeutic gene needs to be tightly controlled within the target tissue. Targeted gene expression has been analyzed using tissue-specific promoters (breast-, prostate-, and melanoma-specific promoters) and disease-specific promoters (carcinoembryonic antigen, HER-2/neu, Myc-Max response elements, DF3/MUC). Alternatively, expression could be regulated externally with the use of radiation-induced promoters or tetracycline-responsive elements [70]. Recently, Arote et al. coupled folic acid moiety to the poly(amino ester)s backbone using PEG (MW: 5000 Da) as a linker for targeting of folate receptor, a tumor associated glycosylphosphatidylinositol anchored protein [71]. As shown in Fig. 15, folate-PEG-poly(amino ester)s (FP-PAEs) showed marked anti-tumor activity against folate receptor-positive human KB tumors in nude mice with no evidence of toxicity during and after therapy using the TAM67 gene. Anti-tumor activity with PAEs without folic acid moiety (PEGylated-PAEs, P-PAEs) proved ineffective against a xenograft mice model than that with FP-PAEs at the same dose, suggesting that FP-PAEs is a highly effective gene carrier capable of producing a therapeutic benefit in a xenograft mice model without any signs of toxicity.

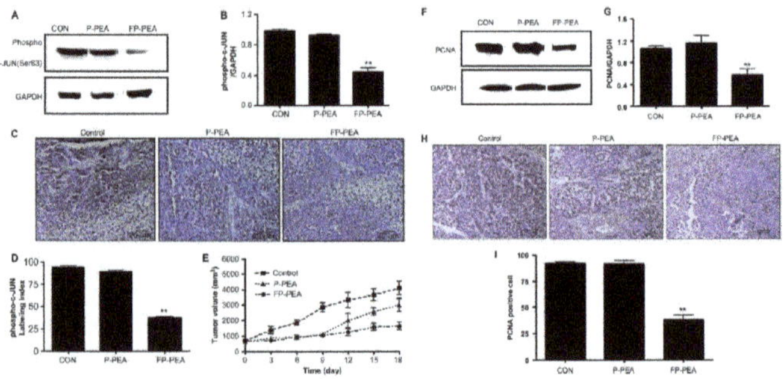

Figure 15. Effect of FP-PEAs/TAM67 complexes on tumor growth. The tumor volume in BALB/c mice bearing KB cells was recorded every 3 d. Tumor tissue homogenates were subjected to western blot analysis. Blots were probed with antibodies as indicated. (A) Expression level of phospho-c-Jun. (B) The bands-of-interest were further analyzed by densitometer. (C) Immunohistochemical analysis of phospho-c-Jun in the tumors. Dark brown color indicates the phospho-c-Jun expression (magnification, X 400; bar = 20 μm). (D) Comparison of phospho-c-Jun labeling index in tumors. phospho-c-Jun positive staining was determined by counting 10 randomly chosen fields per section, determining the percentage of DAB positive cell per 100 cells at X 400 magnification. (E) Suppression of tumor growth by FP-PEAs/TAM67 complexes (F) Expression level of PCNA. (G) The bands-of-interest were further analyzed by densitometer. (H) Immunohistochemical analysis of PCNA in the tumors. Dark brown color indicates the PCNA expression (magnification, X 400; bar = 20 μm). (I) Comparison of PCNA labeling index in tumors. PCNA positive staining was determined by counting 10 randomly chosen fields per section, determining the percentage of DAB positive cell per 100 cells at X 400 magnification. (*, $P < 0.05$; **, $P < 0.01$ compared with control; #, $P < 0.05$; ##, $p < 0.01$ compared with vector control; $n = 4$). [Source from Ref. [71]].

3. Conclusion

Gene therapy shows tremendous promise for a broad spectrum of clinical applications. Development of a safe and efficient gene delivery system is one of the main challenges to be solved before this strategy can be adopted for routine use in clinical trails. As a degradable cationic polymeric gene carrier, poly(amino ester)s comprise many desirable properties in the context of gene delivery, including condensation of DNA into nanoscale-size particles and protects DNA from endogenous nucleases and efficiently deliver DNA with low toxicity. The need for clinical application of poly(amino ester)s, more comprehensive preclinical investigations such as exact quality control (QC) of polymer, pharmacokinetics and toxicological studies should be performed.

Author details

You-Kyoung Kim[1], Can Zhang[1], Chong-Su Cho[2], Myung-Haing Cho[3] and Hu-Lin Jiang[1]

1 School of Pharmacy, China Pharmaceutical University, Nanjing,, P. R. China

2 Department of Agricultural Biotechnology, Seoul National University, Seoul,, Korea

3 College of Veterinary Medicine, Seoul National University, Seoul,, Korea

References

[1] Verma IM, Somia N. Gene therapy -- promises, problems and prospects. Nature 1997;389:239-42.

[2] Bhavsar MD, Amiji MM. Polymeric nano- and microparticle technologies for oral gene delivery. Expert Opin Drug Deliv 2007;4:197-213.

[3] Ledley FD. Pharmaceutical approach to somatic gene therapy. Pharm Res 1996;13:1595-614.

[4] Park TG, Jeong JH, Kim SW. Current status of polymeric gene delivery systems. Adv Drug Deliv Rev 2006;58:467-86.

[5] Su CH, Wu YJ, Wang HH, Yeh HI. Non-viral gene therapy targeting cardiovascular system. Am J Physiol Heart Circ Physiol 2012.

[6] Rogers ML, Rush RA. Non-viral gene therapy for neurological diseases, with an emphasis on targeted gene delivery. J Control Release 2012;157:183-9.

[7] Elbashir SM, Harborth J, Lendeckel W, Yalcin A, Weber K, Tuschl T. Duplexes of 21-nucleotide RNAs mediate RNA interference in cultured mammalian cells. Nature 2001;411:494-8.

[8] Monaghan M, Pandit A. RNA interference therapy via functionalized scaffolds. Adv Drug Deliv Rev 2011;63:197-208.

[9] Scholz C, Wagner E. Therapeutic plasmid DNA versus siRNA delivery: Common and different tasks for synthetic carriers. J Control Release 2012;161:554-65.

[10] Shen H, Sun T, Ferrari M. Nanovector delivery of siRNA for cancer therapy. Cancer Gene Ther 2012;19:367-73.

[11] Verma IM, Weitzman MD. Gene therapy: twenty-first century medicine. Annu Rev Biochem 2005;74:711-38.

[12] Smith AE. Viral vectors in gene therapy. Annu Rev Microbiol 1995;49:807-38.

[13] Wu TL, Ertl HC. Immune barriers to successful gene therapy. Trends Mol Med 2009;15:32-9.

[14] Woods NB, Bottero V, Schmidt M, von Kalle C, Verma IM. Gene therapy: therapeutic gene causing lymphoma. Nature 2006;440:1123.

[15] Parkes RJ, Hart SL. Adhesion molecules and gene transfer. Adv Drug Deliv Rev 2000;44:135-52.

[16] Perez-Martinez FC, Guerra J, Posadas I, Cena V. Barriers to non-viral vector-mediated gene delivery in the nervous system. Pharm Res 2011;28:1843-58.

[17] Kim SS, Garg H, Joshi A, Manjunath N. Strategies for targeted nonviral delivery of siRNAs in vivo. Trends Mol Med 2009;15:491-500.

[18] Lee M, Kim SW. Polyethylene glycol-conjugated copolymers for plasmid DNA delivery. Pharm Res 2005;22:1-10.

[19] Ferber D. Gene therapy. Safer and virus-free? Science 2001;294:1638-42.

[20] Kohn DB, Sadelain M, Glorioso JC. Occurrence of leukaemia following gene therapy of X-linked SCID. Nat Rev Cancer 2003;3:477-88.

[21] Felgner PL, Gadek TR, Holm M, Roman R, Chan HW, Wenz M, et al. Lipofection: a highly efficient, lipid-mediated DNA-transfection procedure. Proc Natl Acad Sci U S A 1987;84:7413-7.

[22] Farhood H, Serbina N, Huang L. The role of dioleoyl phosphatidylethanolamine in cationic liposome mediated gene transfer. Biochim Biophys Acta 1995;1235:289-95.

[23] Kao MC, Law SL, Chuang TC, Lin YS. In vitro gene transfer in mammalian cells via a new cationic liposome formulation. Oncol Rep 1998;5:625-9.

[24] Liu F, Huang L. Development of non-viral vectors for systemic gene delivery. J Control Release 2002;78:259-66.

[25] Uchida E, Mizuguchi H, Ishii-Watabe A, Hayakawa T. Comparison of the efficiency and safety of non-viral vector-mediated gene transfer into a wide range of human cells. Biol Pharm Bull 2002;25:891-7.

[26] Godbey WT, Wu KK, Mikos AG. Poly(ethylenimine) and its role in gene delivery. J Control Release 1999;60:149-60.

[27] Godbey WT, Wu KK, Mikos AG. Poly(ethylenimine)-mediated gene delivery affects endothelial cell function and viability. Biomaterials 2001;22:471-80.

[28] Jiang HL, Xu CX, Kim YK, Arote R, Jere D, Lim HT, et al. The suppression of lung tumorigenesis by aerosol-delivered folate-chitosan-graft-polyethylenimine/Akt1 shRNA complexes through the Akt signaling pathway. Biomaterials 2009;30:5844-52.

[29] Jiang HL, Kim YK, Arote R, Jere D, Quan JS, Yu JH, et al. Mannosylated chitosan-graft-polyethylenimine as a gene carrier for Raw 264.7 cell targeting. Int J Pharm 2009;375:133-9.

[30] Jiang HL, Kwon JT, Kim EM, Kim YK, Arote R, Jere D, et al. Galactosylated poly(ethylene glycol)-chitosan-graft-polyethylenimine as a gene carrier for hepatocyte-targeting. J Control Release 2008;131:150-7.

[31] Lungwitz U, Breunig M, Blunk T, Gopferich A. Polyethylenimine-based non-viral gene delivery systems. Eur J Pharm Biopharm 2005;60:247-66.

[32] Kircheis R, Wightman L, Wagner E. Design and gene delivery activity of modified polyethylenimines. Adv Drug Deliv Rev 2001;53:341-58.

[33] Arote RB, Jiang HL, Kim YK, Cho MH, Choi YJ, Cho CS. Degradable poly(amido amine)s as gene delivery carriers. Expert Opin Drug Deliv 2011;8:1237-46.

[34] Jiang HL, Hong SH, Kim YK, Islam MA, Kim HJ, Choi YJ, et al. Aerosol delivery of spermine-based poly(amino ester)s/Akt1 shRNA complexes for lung cancer gene therapy. Int J Pharm 2011;420:256-65.

[35] Akinc A, Lynn DM, Anderson DG, Langer R. Parallel synthesis and biophysical characterization of a degradable polymer library for gene delivery. J Am Chem Soc 2003;125:5316-23.

[36] Anderson DG, Peng W, Akinc A, Hossain N, Kohn A, Padera R, et al. A polymer library approach to suicide gene therapy for cancer. Proc Natl Acad Sci U S A 2004;101:16028-33.

[37] Park MR, Han KO, Han IK, Cho MH, Nah JW, Choi YJ, et al. Degradable polyethylenimine-alt-poly(ethylene glycol) copolymers as novel gene carriers. J Control Release 2005;105:367-80.

[38] Lynn DM, Anderson DG, Putnam D, Langer R. Accelerated discovery of synthetic transfection vectors: parallel synthesis and screening of a degradable polymer library. J Am Chem Soc 2001;123:8155-6.

[39] Zhong Z, Song Y, Engbersen JF, Lok MC, Hennink WE, Feijen J. A versatile family of degradable non-viral gene carriers based on hyperbranched poly(amino ester)s. J Control Release 2005;109:317-29.

[40] Arote R, Kim TH, Kim YK, Hwang SK, Jiang HL, Song HH, et al. A biodegradable poly(amino ester)s based on polycaprolactone and polyethylenimine as a gene carrier. Biomaterials 2007;28:735-44.

[41] Arote RB, Hwang SK, Yoo MK, Jere D, Jiang HL, Kim YK, et al. Biodegradable poly(amino ester)s based on glycerol dimethacrylate and polyethylenimine as a gene carrier. J Gene Med 2008;10:1223-35.

[42] Hong SH, Kim JE, Kim YK, Minai-Tehrani A, Shin JY, Kang B, et al. Suppression of lung cancer progression by biocompatible glycerol triacrylate-spermine-mediated delivery of shAkt1. Int J Nanomedicine 2012;7:2293-306.

[43] Yin Q, Shen J, Chen L, Zhang Z, Gu W, Li Y. Overcoming multidrug resistance by co-delivery of Mdr-1 and survivin-targeting RNA with reduction-responsible cationic poly(beta-amino esters). Biomaterials 2012;33:6495-506.

[44] Lynn DM, Langer R. Degradable Poly(β-amino esters): Synthesis, Characterization, and Self-Assembly with Plasmid DNA. J Am Chem Soc 2000;122:10761-8.

[45] Zugates GT, Anderson DG, Little SR, Lawhorn IE, Langer R. Synthesis of poly(beta-amino ester)s with thiol-reactive side chains for DNA delivery. J Am Chem Soc 2006;128:12726-34.

[46] Akinc A, Anderson DG, Lynn DM, Langer R. Synthesis of poly(beta-amino ester)s optimized for highly effective gene delivery. Bioconjug Chem 2003;14:979-88.

[47] Luo D, Saltzman WM. Synthetic DNA delivery systems. Nat Biotechnol 2000;18:33-7.

[48] Anderson DG, Lynn DM, Langer R. Semi-automated synthesis and screening of a large library of degradable cationic polymers for gene delivery. Angew Chem Int Ed Engl 2003;42:3153-8.

[49] Anderson DG, Akinc A, Hossain N, Langer R. Structure/property studies of polymeric gene delivery using a library of poly(beta-amino esters). Mol Ther 2005;11:426-34.

[50] Liu Y, Wu D, Ma Y, Tang G, Wang S, He C, et al. Novel poly(amino ester)s obtained from Michael addition polymerizations of trifunctional amine monomers with diacrylates: safe and efficient DNA carriers. Chem Commun (Camb) 2003:2630-1.

[51] Wu D, Liu Y, Jiang X, He C, Goh SH, Leong KW. Hyperbranched poly(amino ester)s with different terminal amine groups for DNA delivery. Biomacromolecules 2006;7:1879-83.

[52] Kim TH, Cook SE, Arote RB, Cho MH, Nah JW, Choi YJ, et al. A degradable hyperbranched poly(amino ester)s based on poloxamer diacrylate and polyethylenimine as a gene carrier. Macromol Biosci 2007;7:611-9.

[53] Jiang HL, Kim YK, Arote R, Nah JW, Cho MH, Choi YJ, et al. Chitosan-graft-polyethylenimine as a gene carrier. J Control Release 2007;117:273-80.

[54] Arote RB, Lee ES, Jiang HL, Kim YK, Choi YJ, Cho MH, et al. Efficient gene delivery with osmotically active and hyperbranched poly(amino ester)s. Bioconjug Chem 2009;20:2231-41.

[55] Wagner E, Ogris M, Zauner W. Polylysine-based transfection systems utilizing receptor-mediated delivery. Adv Drug Deliv Rev 1998;30:97-113.

[56] Kunath K, von Harpe A, Fischer D, Petersen H, Bickel U, Voigt K, et al. Low-molecular-weight polyethylenimine as a non-viral vector for DNA delivery: comparison of

physicochemical properties, transfection efficiency and in vivo distribution with high-molecular-weight polyethylenimine. J Control Release 2003;89:113-25.

[57] Cristiano RJ. Viral and non-viral vectors for cancer gene therapy. Anticancer Res 1998;18:3241-5.

[58] Jere D, Jiang HL, Arote R, Kim YK, Choi YJ, Cho MH, et al. Degradable polyethylenimines as DNA and small interfering RNA carriers. Expert Opin Drug Deliv 2009;6:827-34.

[59] Jere D, Yoo MK, Arote R, Kim TH, Cho MH, Nah JW, et al. Poly (amino ester) composed of poly (ethylene glycol) and aminosilane prepared by combinatorial chemistry as a gene carrier. Pharm Res 2008;25:875-85.

[60] Wong K, Sun G, Zhang X, Dai H, Liu Y, He C, et al. PEI-g-chitosan, a novel gene delivery system with transfection efficiency comparable to polyethylenimine in vitro and after liver administration in vivo. Bioconjug Chem 2006;17:152-8.

[61] Jiang HL, Kwon JT, Kim YK, Kim EM, Arote R, Jeong HJ, et al. Galactosylated chitosan-graft-polyethylenimine as a gene carrier for hepatocyte targeting. Gene Ther 2007;14:1389-98.

[62] Park MR, Kim HW, Hwang CS, Han KO, Choi YJ, Song SC, et al. Highly efficient gene transfer with degradable poly(amino ester)s based on poly(ethylene glycol) diacrylate and polyethylenimine in vitro and in vivo. J Gene Med 2008;10:198-207.

[63] Verbaan F, van Dam I, Takakura Y, Hashida M, Hennink W, Storm G, et al. Intravenous fate of poly(2-(dimethylamino)ethyl methacrylate)-based polyplexes. Eur J Pharm Sci 2003;20:419-27.

[64] Ferrari S, Moro E, Pettenazzo A, Behr JP, Zacchello F, Scarpa M. ExGen 500 is an efficient vector for gene delivery to lung epithelial cells in vitro and in vivo. Gene Ther 1997;4:1100-6.

[65] Plank C, Mechtler K, Szoka FC, Jr., Wagner E. Activation of the complement system by synthetic DNA complexes: a potential barrier for intravenous gene delivery. Hum Gene Ther 1996;7:1437-46.

[66] de Wolf HK, Luten J, Snel CJ, Oussoren C, Hennink WE, Storm G. In vivo tumor transfection mediated by polyplexes based on biodegradable poly(DMAEA)-phosphazene. J Control Release 2005;109:275-87.

[67] Santana A, Hyslop S, Antunes E, Mariano M, Bakhle YS, de Nucci G. Inflammatory responses induced by poly-L-arginine in rat lungs in vivo. Agents Actions 1993;39:104-10.

[68] Zugates GT, Peng W, Zumbuehl A, Jhunjhunwala S, Huang YH, Langer R, et al. Rapid optimization of gene delivery by parallel end-modification of poly(beta-amino ester)s. Mol Ther 2007;15:1306-12.

[69] Lemkine GF, Demeneix BA. Polyethylenimines for in vivo gene delivery. Curr Opin Mol Ther 2001;3:178-82.

[70] Dachs GU, Dougherty GJ, Stratford IJ, Chaplin DJ. Targeting gene therapy to cancer: a review. Oncol Res 1997;9:313-25.

[71] Arote RB, Hwang SK, Lim HT, Kim TH, Jere D, Jiang HL, et al. The therapeutic efficiency of FP-PEA/TAM67 gene complexes via folate receptor-mediated endocytosis in a xenograft mice model. Biomaterials 2010;31:2435-45.

Permissions

The contributors of this book come from diverse backgrounds, making this book a truly international effort. This book will bring forth new frontiers with its revolutionizing research information and detailed analysis of the nascent developments around the world.

We would like to thank Dr. Ming Wei and Dr. David Good, for lending their expertise to make the book truly unique. They have played a crucial role in the development of this book. Without their invaluable contribution this book wouldn't have been possible. They have made vital efforts to compile up to date information on the varied aspects of this subject to make this book a valuable addition to the collection of many professionals and students.

This book was conceptualized with the vision of imparting up-to-date information and advanced data in this field. To ensure the same, a matchless editorial board was set up. Every individual on the board went through rigorous rounds of assessment to prove their worth. After which they invested a large part of their time researching and compiling the most relevant data for our readers. Conferences and sessions were held from time to time between the editorial board and the contributing authors to present the data in the most comprehensible form. The editorial team has worked tirelessly to provide valuable and valid information to help people across the globe.

Every chapter published in this book has been scrutinized by our experts. Their significance has been extensively debated. The topics covered herein carry significant findings which will fuel the growth of the discipline. They may even be implemented as practical applications or may be referred to as a beginning point for another development. Chapters in this book were first published by InTech; hereby published with permission under the Creative Commons Attribution License or equivalent.

The editorial board has been involved in producing this book since its inception. They have spent rigorous hours researching and exploring the diverse topics which have resulted in the successful publishing of this book. They have passed on their knowledge of decades through this book. To expedite this challenging task, the publisher supported the team at every step. A small team of assistant editors was also appointed to further simplify the editing procedure and attain best results for the readers.

Our editorial team has been hand-picked from every corner of the world. Their multi-ethnicity adds dynamic inputs to the discussions which result in innovative outcomes. These outcomes are then further discussed with the researchers and contributors who give their valuable feedback and opinion regarding the same. The feedback is then collaborated with the researches and they are edited in a comprehensive manner to aid the understanding of the subject.

Apart from the editorial board, the designing team has also invested a significant amount of their time in understanding the subject and creating the most relevant covers. They scrutinized every image to scout for the most suitable representation of the subject and create an appropriate cover for the book.

The publishing team has been involved in this book since its early stages. They were actively engaged in every process, be it collecting the data, connecting with the contributors or procuring relevant information. The team has been an ardent support to the editorial, designing and production team. Their endless efforts to recruit the best for this project, has resulted in the accomplishment of this book. They are a veteran in the field of academics and their pool of knowledge is as vast as their experience in printing. Their expertise and guidance has proved useful at every step. Their uncompromising quality standards have made this book an exceptional effort. Their encouragement from time to time has been an inspiration for everyone.

The publisher and the editorial board hope that this book will prove to be a valuable piece of knowledge for researchers, students, practitioners and scholars across the globe.

List of Contributors

Shintaro Fumoto and Koyo Nishida
Graduate School of Biomedical Sciences, Nagasaki University, Japan

Shigeru Kawakami
Graduate School of Pharmaceutical Sciences, Kyoto University, Japan

Mitsuru Hashida
Graduate School of Pharmaceutical Sciences, Kyoto University, Japan
Institute for Integrated Cell-Material Sciences (iCeMS), Kyoto University, Japan

Tranum Kaur
Department of Biophysics, Punjab University, Chandigarh, India

Roderick Slavcev
School of Pharmacy, University of Waterloo, Kitchener, Ontario, Canada

Lynn F. Gottfried and David A. Dean
Department of Pediatrics, University of Rochester Medical Center, Rochester, NY, USA

J. Teissié
CNRS; IPBS (Institut de Pharmacologie et de Biologie Structurale), Toulouse, France
Université de Toulouse, Toulouse, France

Qiana L. Matthews, Linlin Gu, Alexandre Krendelchtchikov and Zan C. Li
Department of Medicine, Division of Infectious Diseases, The University of Alabama, Birmingham, AL, USA

Matthias Renner
Department of Medical Biotechnology, Paul-Ehrlich-Institut, Langen, Germany

Juraj Hlavaty
Christian-Doppler Laboratory for Innovative Immunotherapy, University of Veterinary Medicine, Vienna, Austria
Institute of Virology, Department of Pathobiology, University of Veterinary Medicine, Vienna, Austria

Toshihiro Nakajima, Toshimitsu Itai, Hiroshi Wada and Toshie Yamauchi
GenomIdea, Inc., Midorigaoka, Ikeda, Osaka, Japan

Yasufumi Kaneda
Division of Gene Therapy Science, Department of Molecular Therapeutics, Graduate School of Medicine, Osaka University, Yamada-oka, Suita, Osaka, Japan

Eiji Kiyohara
Division of Gene Therapy Science, Department of Molecular Therapeutics, Graduate School of Medicine, Osaka University, Yamada-oka, Suita, Osaka, Japan
Department of Dermatology, Graduate School of Medicine, Osaka University, Yamadaoka, Suita, Osaka, Japan

Koichi Miyake and Takashi Shimada
Department of Biochemistry and Molecular Biology, Division of Gene Therapy Research Center for Advanced Medical Technology, Nippon Medical School, Japan

Yosuke Morodomi
Department of Thoracic Oncology, National Kyushu Cancer Center, Japan

Makoto Inoue and Mamoru Hasegawa
DNAVEC Corporation, Japan

Tatsuro Okamoto and Yoshihiko Maehara
Department of Surgery and Science, Graduate School of Medicine, Kyushu University, Japan

Yoshikazu Yonemitsu
R&D Laboratory for Innovative Biotherapeutics, Graduate School of Pharmaceutical Sciences, Kyushu University, Japan

Yadollah Omidi and Jaleh Barar
Ovarian Cancer Research Center, Perelman School of Medicine, University of Pennsylvania, Philadelphia, PA, USA
Research Center for Pharmaceutical Nanotechnology, Faculty of Pharmacy, Tabriz University of Medical Sciences, Tabriz, Iran

George Coukos
Ovarian Cancer Research Center, Perelman School of Medicine, University of Pennsylvania, Philadelphia, PA, USA
Ludwig Center for Cancer Research, University of Lausanne, Lausanne, Switzerland

Mohamed Amessou
Department of Pathology, Wayne State University School of Medicine, Detroit, Michigan, USA

Mustapha Kandouz
Department of Pathology, Wayne State University School of Medicine, Detroit, Michigan, USA
Karmanos Cancer Institute, Wayne State University, Detroit, MI, USA

Ghazala Khan
Division of Science, University of Bedfordshire, Park Square, Luton, UK

Suzanne E. Brooks
Cancer Sciences Division (MP824), Southampton University Hospitals, University of Southampton, Southampton, UK

Frances Denniss
Department of Haematological Medicine, King's College London School of Medicine, The Rayne Institute, London, UK

Dagmar Sigurdardottir
Department of Immunology, Institute for Cell Biology, University of Tübingen, Tübingen, Germany

Barbara-ann Guinn
Division of Science, University of Bedfordshire, Park Square, Luton, UK
Cancer Sciences Division (MP824), Southampton University Hospitals, University of Southampton, Southampton, UK
Department of Haematological Medicine, King's College London School of Medicine, The Rayne Institute, London, UK

Azam Bolhassani
Molecular Immunology and Vaccine Research Lab., Pasteur Institute of Iran, Tehran, Iran

Tayebeh Saleh
Department of Nanobiotechnology, Faculty of Biological Sciences, Tarbiat Modares University, Tehran, Iran

Onur Sakiragaoglu and Ming Q. Wei
Division of Molecular and Gene Therapies, Griffith Health Institute and School of Medical Science, Griffith University, Gold Coast, QLD, Australia

David Good
Division of Molecular and Gene Therapies, Griffith Health Institute and School of Medical Science, Griffith University, Gold Coast, QLD, Australia
School of Physiotherapy, Australian Catholic University, Banyo, QLD, Australia

You-Kyoung Kim, Can Zhang and Hu-Lin Jiang
School of Pharmacy, China Pharmaceutical University, Nanjing, P. R. China

Chong-Su Cho
Department of Agricultural Biotechnology, Seoul National University, Seoul, Korea

Myung-Haing Cho
College of Veterinary Medicine, Seoul National University, Seoul, Korea

www.ingramcontent.com/pod-product-compliance
Ingram Content Group UK Ltd.
Pitfield, Milton Keynes, MK11 3LW, UK
UKHW022206051026
15624UKWH00001B/19

9 781632 420992